Renal Physiology

PEOPLE AND IDEAS

Renal Physiology

PEOPLE AND IDEAS

Edited by Carl W. Gottschalk,
Robert W. Berliner, and
Gerhard H. Giebisch

American Physiological Society
BETHESDA, MARYLAND

Library of Congress Catalog Card Number: 87-18665
International Standard Book Number: 0-683-03671-8
Printed in the United States of America by
Waverly Press, Inc., Baltimore, Maryland 21202
Distributed for the American Physiological Society by
The Williams & Wilkins Company, Baltimore, Maryland 21202

Preface

THIS book is the second in a series on the history of people and ideas published by the American Physiological Society in conjunction with its centennial. The first, *Circulation of the Blood: Men and Ideas*, appeared in 1982 and was a reissue of a book first published in 1964 by Oxford University Press. Other books on the development of our understanding of endocrine function and on membrane transport processes are in preparation.

Each chapter in this series is written by a scientist who has contributed importantly to contemporary developments in the area and is broadly knowledgeable in the field. The insider's view, while not without its own bias, provides a special insight that ought to be part of the historical record of the discipline.

We anticipate that the perspective of each author will be especially meaningful to other scientists. We all carry with us our own historical record based on personal experience as to how our area of science has evolved. This written record is a documentation of some of the successes and failures that are part of the landscape of experimental science. A scientific society has a unique opportunity to provide this view, which might otherwise not be preserved.

Because physiology has played such an important role in the development of modern medicine, the documentation of its advances has interest for a broader audience. The history of people and ideas in physiology is part of the development of modern medicine and modern biology and is presented to further our understanding of the process of scientific discovery. All who benefit from modern medicine (and who has not?) owe some debt to those whose lives and ideas are chronicled here.

PAUL C. JOHNSON

Table of Contents

I

Evolution of Renal Physiology From Earliest Times to William Bowman

LEON G. FINE

EARLIEST TIMES

CENTURIES of apparently fruitless debate over the nature of body fluids preceded the first glimmerings of a constructive interest in the function of the kidneys. Little of substance in this regard was retrieved by the Greeks from the earlier sophisticated Minoan culture, and it was contact with the civilizations of the Euphrates and the Nile that first stirred the inquisitiveness of the early Greeks to probe the structure and function of the human body. Egyptian papyri, however, illustrate a very incomplete knowledge of anatomy. Although animal anatomy, especially that of the liver, was known to the Mesopotamians, who used this organ for divination, no such dignity was accorded the kidneys, which were relegated to an inglorious position in the interests of prescientific humankind. It was the gradual refinement of thought on the origin and nature of body fluids by early Greek writers that inevitably brought the role of the kidneys into focus, and it is through this door that the understanding of the evolution of renal physiology must be approached.

The Greeks (500–50 B.C.)

It seems that Empedocles of Agrigento (b. 490 B.C.) must be accorded the distinction of being the first to teach that the heart is at the center of the vascular system and that the blood, which was regarded as the seat of "innate heat" and the container of the "pneuma" or life spirit, is discharged from this organ to the rest of the body (32). The Empedoclean doctrine asserted that the essence of all things can be resolved into four elements: air, fire, water, and earth; it exerted considerable influence on the Ionians (29), whose own Anaximenes (b. 545 B.C.) had earlier expounded, "*As our soul, being air, sustains us so pneuma and air pervade the whole world*" (32). Although persistent interest in the pneumatic doctrine is evident in the writings of Diogenes of Apollonia (fifth century B.C.) (34), alternative theories were emerging. Heracleitus of Ephesus (ca. 540–480 B.C.), who was probably responsible for the treatise "On Regimen" in the Hippocratic collection of writings, proposed that all life is a balance of fire and water, the properties of which determine all physical and mental functions (32).

Hippocrates of Cos (b. 460 B.C.) is represented by a body of literature much of which may have arisen from the pens of his contemporaries (13). The impact of these collected writings on future generations was enormous, undoubtedly because they represented the first exposition of the primacy of accurate observation in medical practice. Although this approach was applied to disease states, there is no evidence that systematic dissection of animals was customarily practiced at the time. The doctrine of the four humors described in "On the Nature of Man" by Polybus (ca. 390 B.C.), the son-in-law of Hippocrates, captivated the minds of philosophers and physicians for centuries (32). This doctrine held that blood, phlegm (pituita), black bile (melancholia), and yellow bile (choler) constitute the living body and respectively correspond to the four elements, fire, water, earth, and air, that constitute nonliving matter [Fig. 1; (31)].

It was not long before an eclectic approach arose that incorporated the views of both Empedocles and Polybus. Such a view is evident in the writings of Diocles of Carystus (fourth century B.C.) (16). The great philosophers Socrates (ca. 470–399 B.C.) and Plato (ca. 428–348 B.C.) made no contribution to the physiological thinking of the time, and the field floundered until the advent of the great philosopher-scientist Aristotle.

Aristotle (384–322 B.C.), the son of a physician, was unsurpassed as a systematizer of scientific knowledge. In his *Historia animalium* he described the anatomy of the kidneys and pointed out the fact

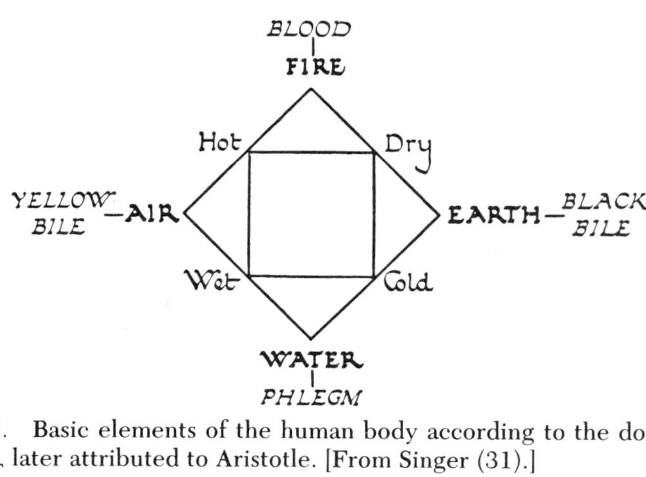

Figure 1. Basic elements of the human body according to the doctrine of Polybus, later attributed to Aristotle. [From Singer (31).]

that in all animals the right kidney is higher than the left (2). Because this is clearly opposite to that in humans, a fact not noted by Aristotle, one can only assume that he had little knowledge of the human kidney. Aristotle described the cavity in the middle of the kidney (i.e., the renal pelvis) (Fig. 2) but did not comment on the obvious difference between the multipapillate human kidney and the unipapillate structure of many other species. He studied the kidneys of the turtle, ox, and bison and erroneously concluded that kidneys are absent in birds and fishes. He gave no insight into the function of kidneys, and although he adhered to the doctrine of humors, his curiosity about the nature of urine and its relationship to the fluids of the body was apparently not aroused.

The Alexandrians (300–250 B.C.)

After the loss of Athenian liberty and the breakup of the Alexandrian empire (following the death of Alexander in 323 B.C.), Alex-

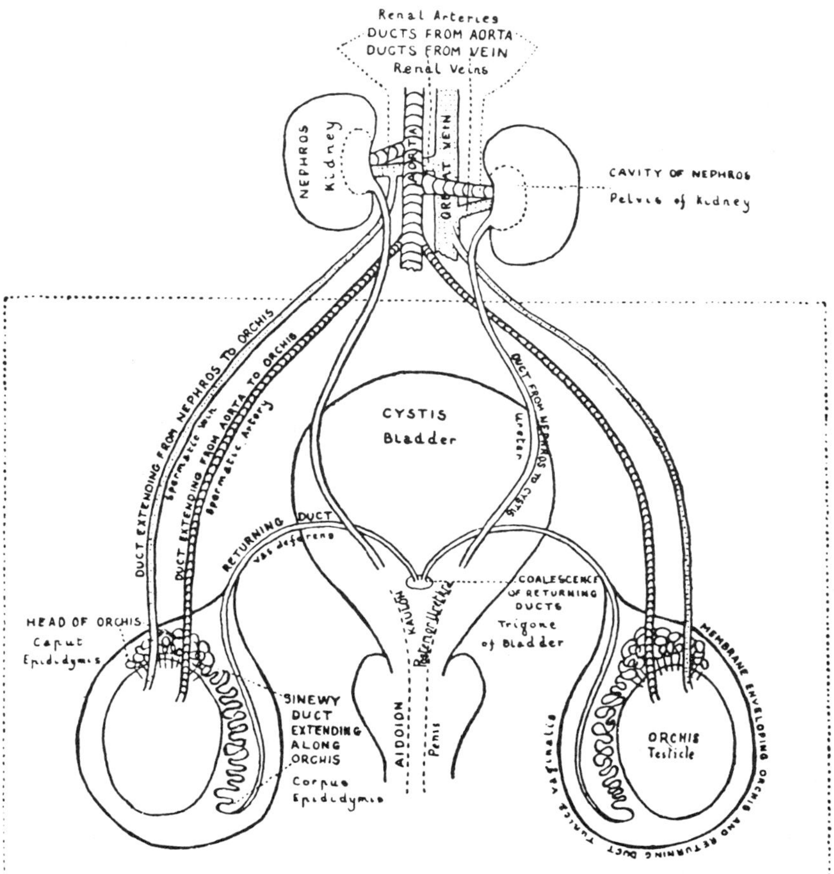

Figure 2. Aristotelian concept of the kidneys, showing the right higher than the left, each possessing a cavity. [From Singer (32).]

andria became the center of the scientific world. The establishment of a library and museum and the origin of anatomy as a scientific discipline allowed this center to hold sway for centuries. The two figureheads of the anatomical movement were Herophilus of Chalcedon (ca. 335–280 B.C.) and Erasistratus of Ceos (ca. 290 B.C.). The former, according to Galen, was the first to dissect both human and animal bodies in public, but it was the latter who must be considered the "Father of Physiology." It was only because Galen took such delight in ridiculing the ideas of Erasistratus that they (if accurately represented) were documented for posterity. Of great interest are the views of Erasistratus on the function of the kidney, which can be distilled from Galen's *On the Natural Faculties* (11).

Erasistratus knew (according to Galen) that urine is secreted in the kidneys but failed to adequately explain why or how it occurs other than to state that urine is "attracted" into the kidneys. The commonly held idea was that the upper part of the kidney received blood and that the watery residue, being heavy, percolated down through the kidneys and was discharged from the lower part through the ureter. It was also believed that the kidneys received blood not from the aorta but from the vena cava, so that the great unresolved dilemma was: If the watery fluid falls downward in the vena cava, how does it enter the kidneys, which lie on either side but not below it?

Galen

Galen (A.D. 131–201) of Pergamum in Mysia (Asia Minor) was one of the most brilliant physiologists of all time and can lay justifiable claim to being the first experimental renal physiologist. He made observations on fluid balance and on the origin of urine that were innovative and completely revolutionary.

Galen's system of physiology is illustrated in Figure 3. He was a pneumatist and believed that the pneuma or spirit was inhaled through the trachea into the lungs and thence passed through a "vein-like artery" (i.e., the pulmonary vein) to the left ventricle where it was admixed with blood. The blood, in turn, was derived from the nutrients absorbed from the intestine (chyle), which were processed by the liver. He believed that the liver converted chyle into venous blood, which was endowed with a living substance (natural spirit) and ebbed and flowed in the venous system. Impurities in blood that reached the right side of the heart were removed by the artery-like vein (pulmonary artery) that extended into the lungs, which expired them. Once cleansed, this blood left the right ventricle and reentered the general circulation. A small portion permeated the interventricular septum and entered the left ventricle, drop by drop, where it encountered the inhaled pneuma, a "vital spirit" (as opposed to the "natural spirit" from the intestines) that was distributed throughout internal blood.

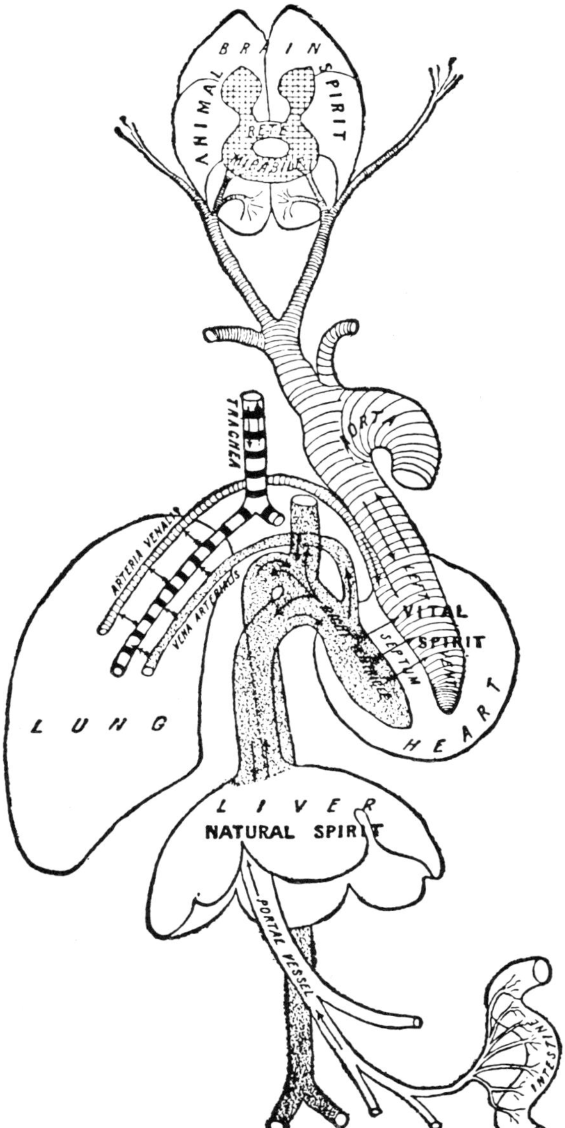

Figure 3. Physiological system of Galen. [From Singer (31).]

It is evident from this system that Galen considered the lungs, rather than the kidneys, the principal "purification system" of the body. Nevertheless in Book I of *On the Natural Faculties* considerable effort is spent explaining the origin of urine (11). Galen firmly believed that every organ in the body has the innate capacity to attract substances of its own special quality and that the kidneys are no exception to this rule. He pointed out that every butcher is aware of the fact that the kidneys are connected to the bladder by the ureters. He further pointed out that people who suffer from dysuria or retention of urine experience pain in the loins, which points to a connection between bladder and kidneys. This simple fact, says Galen, clearly refutes the "ingenuity" of Asclepiades (first century B.C.), who believed that the bladder is a sponge or a piece of wool that absorbs vapors formed from ingested fluid and converts it into fluid. Galen was incredulous that the "*Compact and impervious nature of the bladder*" with "*two strong coats*" was not apparent to seemingly observant people: "*Why do vapors not pass through the peritoneum and the diaphragm by this analogy and fill the whole abdominal cavity and thorax with water?*" "*How does one explain the fact,*" he asked "*that when the bladder is filled with water or tied at its neck and squeezed all round, it does not let anything out but retains its contents? Does this not refute the idea of inlets via the ureters?*" In order to answer this question, Galen experimented on a living animal, perhaps the first well-devised renal physiology experiment described. In Book I, chapter 13, of *On the Natural Faculties* (11) he wrote:

Now the method of demonstration is as follows. One has to divide the peritoneum in front of the ureters, then secure these with ligatures, and next, having bandaged up the animal, let him go (for he will not continue to urinate). After this one loosens the external bandages and shows the bladder empty and the ureters quite full and distended—in fact almost on the point of rupturing; on removing the ligature from them, one then plainly sees the bladder becoming filled with urine.

When this has been made quite clear, then, before the animal urinates, one has to tie a ligature round his penis and then to squeeze the bladder all over; still nothing goes back through the ureters to the kidneys. Here, then, it becomes obvious that not only in a dead animal, but in one which is still living, the ureters are prevented from receiving back the urine from the bladder. These observations having been made, one now loosens the ligature from the animal's penis and allows him to urinate, then again ligatures one of the ureters and leaves the other to discharge into the bladder. Allowing, then, some time to elapse, one now demonstrates that the ureter which was ligatured is obviously full and distended on the side next to the kidneys, while the other one—that from which the ligature had been taken—is itself flaccid, but has filled the bladder with urine. Then, again, one must divide the full ureter, and demonstrate how the urine spurts out of it, like blood in the operation of venesection; and after this one cuts through the other also, and both being thus divided, one bandages up the animal externally. Then when enough time seems to have elapsed, one takes off the bandages; the bladder will now be found empty, and the whole region between the intestines and the peritoneum full of urine, as if the animal were suffering from dropsy. Now, if anyone will but test this for himself on an animal, I think he will strongly condemn the rashness of Asclepiades, and if he also learns the reason why nothing regurgitates from the bladder into the ureters, I think he will be persuaded by this also of the forethought and art shown by Nature in relation to animals.

In Galen's opinion this simple experiment conclusively proved that it is the kidneys, not the bladder, that form urine.

To the question "*How is the urine formed in the kidneys and how is it propelled to the bladder?*" Galen responded with only two alternatives to the first part: either the kidneys "attract" urine or the veins exert a propulsive action. He pointed out that if the latter alternative were true, not only urine but also the whole of the blood would be squeezed into the kidneys. Because this does not occur, he concluded that the kidneys exert their own attraction on urine. Furthermore:

If the kidneys are like sieves and readily let the thinner serous portion [i.e., urine] *through and keep out the thicker portion, then the whole of the blood contained in the vena cava must go to them just as the whole of the urine is thrown into the filters. Further, the example of milk being made into cheese will show clearly what I mean. For this too, although it is all thrown into the wicker strainers, does not all percolate through; such part of it as is too fine in proportions to the width of the meshes passes downwards and this is called whey; the remaining thick portion, which is destined to become cheese, cannot get down since the pores of the strainers will not admit it. Thus it is that, if the blood-serum has similarly to percolate through the kidneys the whole of the blood must come to them and not merely one part of it.*

Galen also found it improbable that the kidneys act as filters because the blood would have to fall into them from the vena cava. Because the kidneys are positioned on either side of the vena cava, this cannot be the case and "*they obviously exert traction; for this is the only remaining alternative.*"

Galen provided yet another argument against the sieve hypothesis: if the thin, serous part of blood passed through the kidney as through a sieve, the thick sanguineous portion remaining in the veins would obstruct the blood flowing in from behind, which would therefore have first to run back into the vena cava to empty the veins going to the kidneys and by so doing (i.e., reversing flow) would prevent a second quantity of impurified blood from entering the kidneys. Because there is no obvious power to cause this to-and-fro motion of the blood in the renal veins (the arteries are not mentioned), this possibility is highly unlikely.

Next Galen turned his attention to the nature of the "attractive force" of the kidneys. He astutely observed that it cannot be due to the "*tendency of matter to fill a vacuum for if this were so, nobody would have ever died of retention of urine since no more can flow into a vacuum than has run out.*"

In addressing the argument that urine is simply the residual matter from the nutrition of the kidneys, Galen demonstrated his innate grasp of the concept of fluid balance:

The amount of urine passed every day shows clearly that it is the whole of the fluid drunk which becomes urine, except that which comes away with the dejections or passes off as sweat or insensible perspiration. This is most easily recognized in winter in those who are doing no work but are carousing, especially if the urine be thin and diffusible; these people rapidly pass almost the same quantity as they drink

Galen considered it impossible that organs as small as the kidneys could contain four whole "congii" (~12 quarts, the amount of urine passed if a very large amount of fluid were drunk). It is thus unlikely that the kidneys produce urine as a consequence of their own nutrition but that "*what one drinks goes to the kidneys.*"

The foregoing illustrates just how far ahead of his time Galen was and how independent was his thinking in relation to the existing dogma, upon which he rarely loses an opportunity to heap repetitive scorn. Not content, however, with deducing the mechanisms of urine formation described above, he turned his attention to another philosophical question in *De usu partium* (*On the Usefulness of the Parts of the Body*) (12) and asked: Why does the kidney have the structure that it does? The question is overambitious, as his answers reveal; nevertheless Galen's logic is interesting to contemplate.

After concluding that the watery component of blood is necessary for the distribution of nutrients, Galen reasoned that when the work of the thin fluids is completed they should be eliminated from the body and that the kidneys are the hollow instruments whereby this is achieved. Because the arteries to the kidneys are almost as large as the veins and because he had previously shown that they contain blood and not air (as claimed by Erasistratus), Galen concluded that the kidneys "*relieve the blood of its watery portion.*" This was an important departure from the prevailing notion that urine was the residue from the nutrition of the kidneys. Without the knowledge that the direction of blood flow is different in the renal artery and the renal vein, he could only conclude that the kidneys purify the blood carried by both vessels. This was the first time that the concept of separation of fluid from the blood was proposed as the principal excretory function of the kidneys.

Galen's logic is fascinating: Because the kidneys attract the serous portion of the blood, he felt it unreasonable that the two organs should be exactly opposite each other since each would exert a pull in the opposite direction; thus one kidney is placed higher (more caudally) than the other. The right kidney is higher than the left because blood coming from the liver via the hepatic veins is on the right and "*it is easier for every body with an attractive faculty to exert it in a straight line.*" (Because in humans the left kidney is higher than the right, Galen must have been describing the condition in some primate species in which the opposite is the case.)

How are the kidneys able to achieve this separation of fluid without loss of blood into the ureter? Here Galen finds the answer in the texture of the renal substance. He argues that the spleen is porous and loose textured and thus allows blood to percolate through the organ; the kidneys, in contrast, are dense, and it is this property that imparts to them the ability to retard the escape of blood.

As bizarre as many of Galen's arguments may seem today, his absolute insistence on providing an explanation for every phenomenon, no matter how trivial, set the stage for serious contemplation of all biological events and provided the first suggestion that the phenomena of nature could be investigated with simple logic.

From Galen to the Middle Ages (A.D. 200–1500)

During the centuries that followed the seminal observations of Galen, nothing substantive was contributed to the knowledge of the structure and function of the kidney. The rise of Mohammedanism gave expression to the minds of the great Moslem physicians ar-Rāzī (or Rhazes) (865–932) and Ibn Sīnā (or Avicenna) (980–1037), whose anatomical and herbal texts were translated into Latin and were enormously popular in the Middle Ages. Jewish physicians including Isaac Judaeus (855–955) and Moses Maimonides (1135–1204) likewise added to the compendium of drugs and formulations for the treatment of a variety of ailments. An eleventh-century Persian manuscript by Ismail of Jurjani gave complete directions for the examination of urine (13).

The remains of classical learning were preserved in monasteries during the period that Christianity replaced the paganism of the Roman Empire (ca. A.D. 400–1200), but no attempt was made to advance theoretical knowledge. A decline occurred in all that seemed to be promising up to the time of Galen. Superstitions, formulas, incantations, and illogical rules governed the practice of medicine.

A notable exception to this decay was the center of learning that arose in Salerno around the year 1000. The advent of Constantine brought crude Latin translations of the Arabic scholars to this center in southern Italy, and the works of Galen, including the lore of the pulse and of urine, received fresh attention; medicine flourished as an independent science until the decline of Salerno (ca. 1200).

A glimmer of light appeared amidst the stagnation of centuries with the advent of the early universities in the thirteenth century. Medical faculties arose (e.g., that of Bologna in 1156) and teaching focused on the theoretical rather than the clinical aspects of medicine. It was here that public dissection was practiced. Initially the examination of the human body was for purposes of gathering evidence for legal processes, but with time postmortem examination evolved into the study of anatomy (13).

Among the early surgeons of Bologna was William of Saliceto (1210–1280). His best-known contribution was a description of dropsy (edema) associated with sclerosis of the kidneys (19) that appeared in his *Liber Magistri Guglielmi placentini de Saliceto in scientia medicinali* of 1490. The medical and surgical traditions of Bologna were transplanted to the University at Montpellier in southern France by Henri de Mondeville (1270–1320), and from the pen of his fellow student Mondino de Luzzi (ca. 1270–1326) arose the first practical manual of anatomy (Fig. 4), which discusses the application of anatomical and physiological principles to medicine (23). The importance of this work was highlighted after the invention of printing: it passed through no fewer than thirty-nine separate editions and translations.

Concomitant with the gradual evolution of anatomy, crude at-

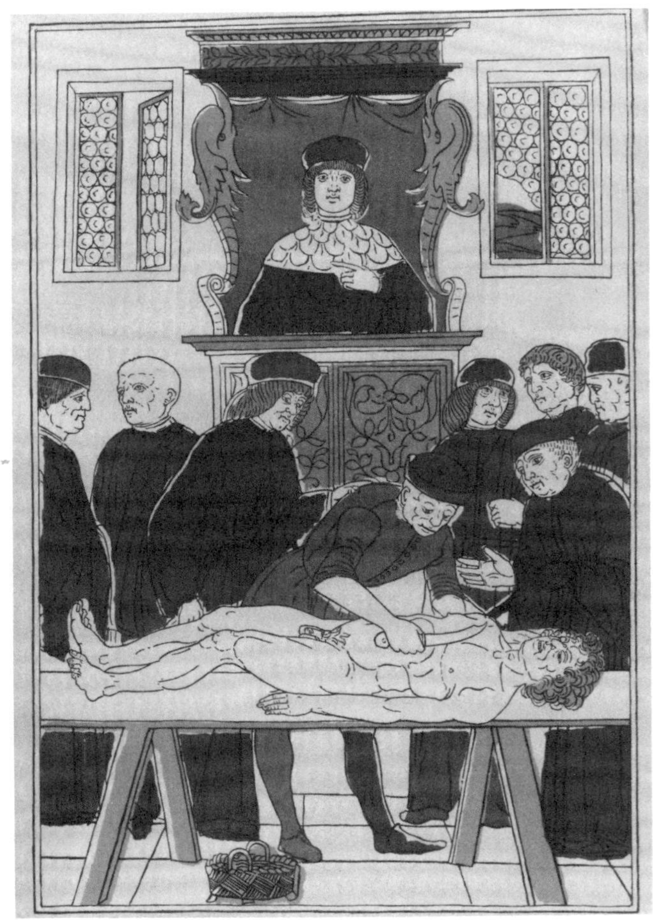

Figure 4. Anatomical dissection by Mondino de Luzzi. [From Ketham (17).]

tempts evolved to utilize urine as a means of understanding alterations in bodily function. The practice of uroscopy (water casting) became a favorite theme of the illustrators of the time, and the urinal became the emblem of medical practice in the Middle Ages. In Ketham's *Fasciculus medicinae* (17) of 1493, for instance, there is an illustration (Fig. 5) of two pages presenting urine in tulip-shaped glass containers for inspection by doctors in gowns and skull caps. In the same volume is an illustration (Fig. 6) of a circle of urine glasses that "*sets forth the colors of the urine and the verdicts derived from them.*" Similar circles of urine glasses have been traced by Sudhoff to early fifteenth-century manuscripts (17), and entire texts on urine and its use in diagnosis appeared during the latter part of the fifteenth century (27).

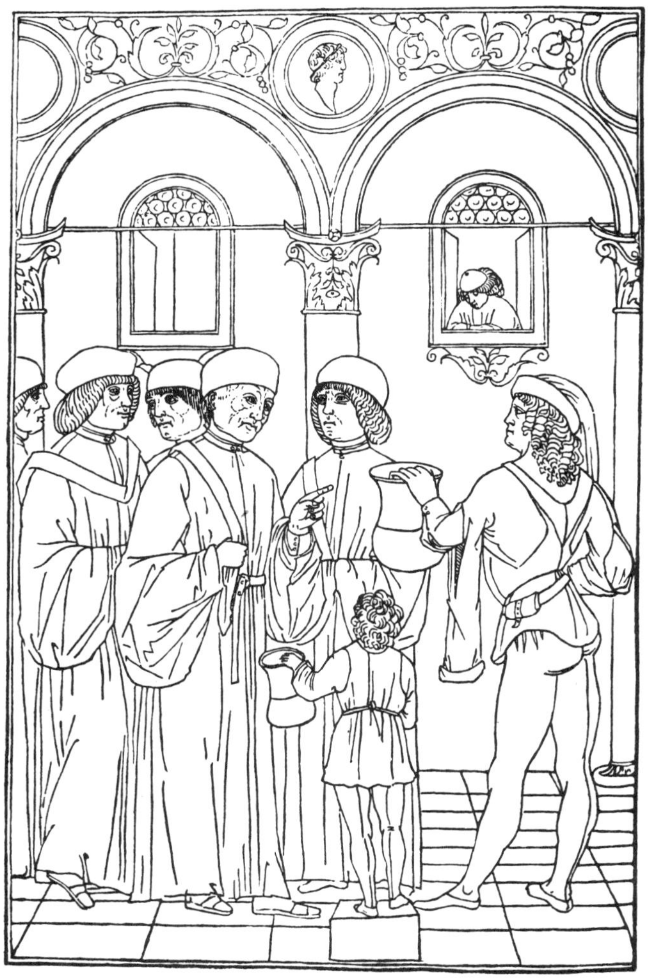

Figure 5. Uroscopy: examination of urine for diagnosis and prognosis. [From Ketham (17).]

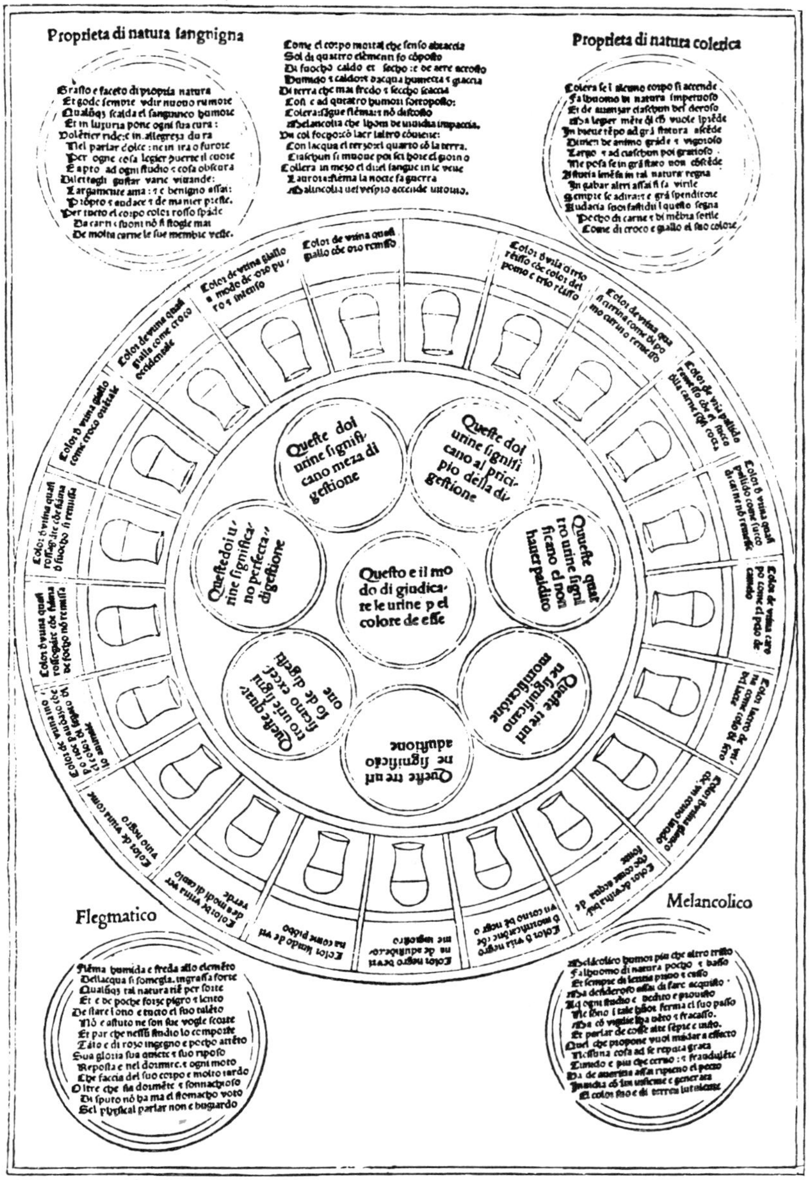

Figure 6. Circle of urine glasses indicating the diagnostic principles derived from different colors and sediments. [From Ketham (17).]

Da Vinci and Vesalius

Leonardo da Vinci (1452–1519), in his role as anatomist, suffered the same fate as Eustachio fifty years later. The disappearance of his work for a long period deprived him of the recognition he deserved as a depictor of human anatomy. There is little question that the aesthetic qualities of da Vinci's anatomical works exceed those of all who preceded him and probably those of most of his successors. His depiction of human kidneys in their correct position in the abdomen was the most accurate in existence (Fig. 7). Nevertheless his attempt to represent the Galenical system in humans appears to be drawn

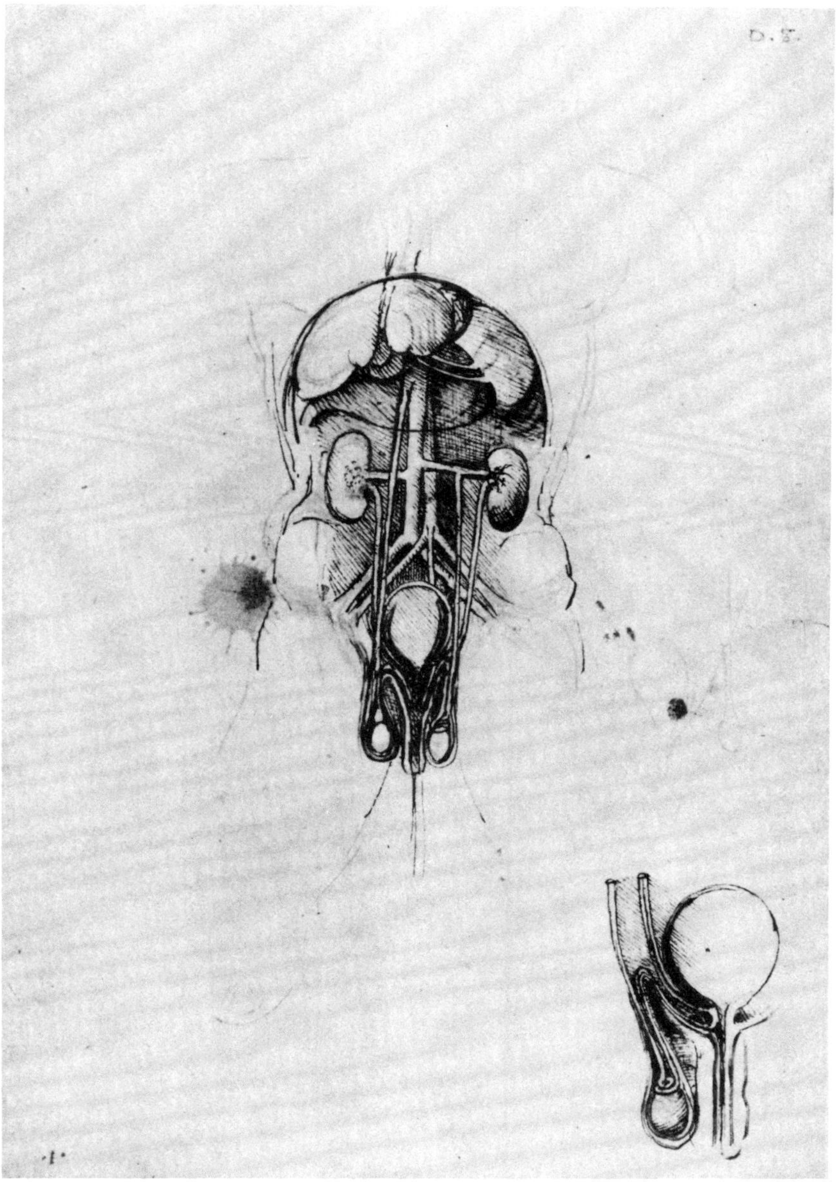

Figure 7. Leonardo da Vinci's depiction of the anatomy of the human kidneys showing the right renal artery emerging from the aorta caudally to the left. [From O'Malley and Saunders (26).]

from dissections in animals. For instance, the heart shows ventricles with moderator bands (as in oxen) and the vena cava opens into the right ventricle. His depiction of the kidney is cursory. Written on the illustration of a single left kidney are the words, "*cut it through the middle and depict how the passages for the urine are closed and how they distil it*" [i.e., the urine] (Fig. 8). According to O'Malley and Saunders (26), da Vinci thought that the papillae of the kidney

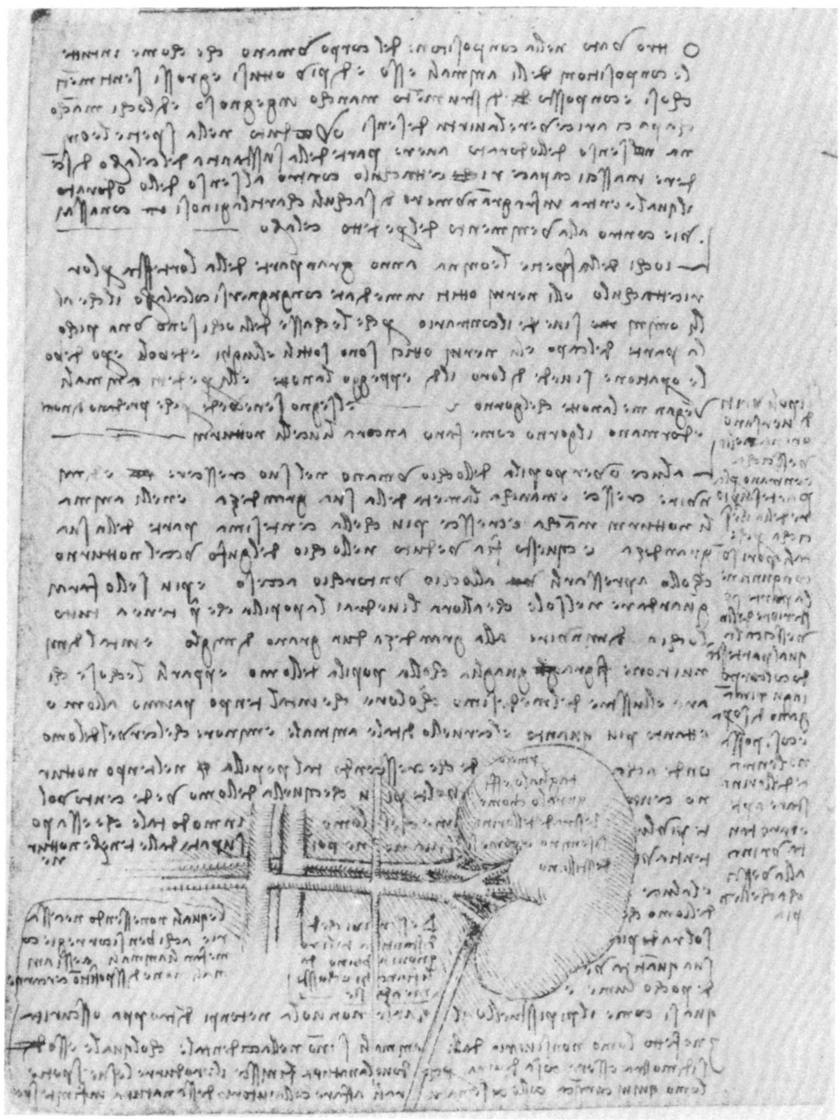

Figure 8. Leonardo da Vinci's depiction of the kidney. Only the writings overlying the kidney refer to this organ. [From O'Malley and Saunders (26).]

resembled minute alembics for the distillation of urine, a view proposed by Gabriel Zerbi (d. 1506).

The publication of *De humani corporis fabrica libri septem* by Andreas Vesalius (1514–1564) stands out as one of the first major contributions to the knowledge of the human body that was based on careful observation rather than on inflexible dogma (33). Despite the magnitude of his overall contribution, Vesalius depicted the kidneys incorrectly (Fig. 9). According to the dogma of Galen, the right is shown higher than the left. Illustrations of transected kidneys show the pelvicalyceal system to be that of the unipapillate dog kidney despite the fact that they were represented as human. Vesalius shows the "sieve theory" of Galen in two figures that depict the kidney being divided by a sieve (Fig. 9). Blood was supposed to enter the upper chamber, and urine was supposed to filter into the lower chamber that leads into the ureter. By comparing this conceptual kidney with a real bisected kidney, Vesalius essentially eliminated the long-held belief in urine straining that had remained extant since Galen.

Eustachio

The first description of the microscopic tubular structures within the renal parenchyma is generally attributed to Bellini (10), who in 1662 published his anatomical treatise on the kidney, *Exercitatio*

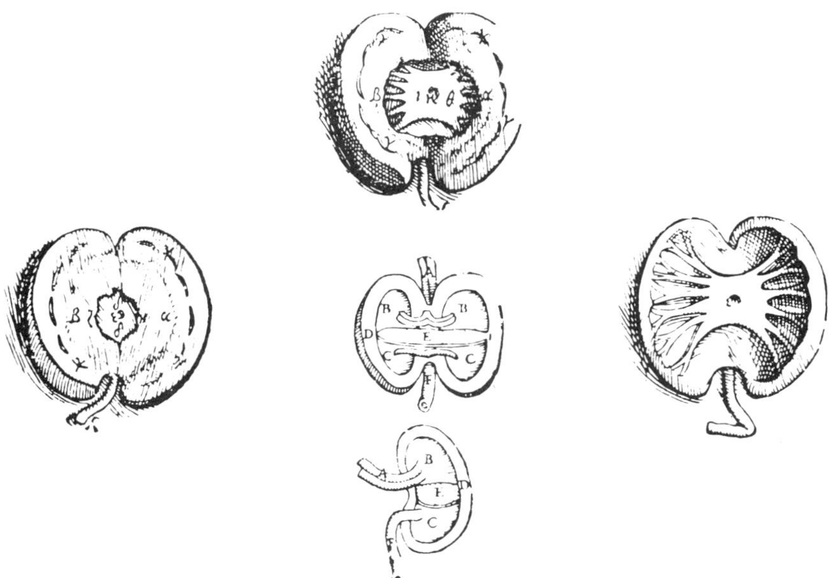

Figure 9. Vesalius's depiction of the kidney. *Top, right,* and *left* figures depict bisected dog kidneys. *Center* and *bottom* figures depict the false doctrine of Galen regarding the straining of urine. [From Vesalius (33).]

anatomica de structura et usu renum (3). However, lying forgotten in the papal archives was a splendid anatomical work written by Bartolommeo Eustachio (1520–1574), which contained information about the kidney that preceded the observations of Bellini by nearly a century and that surpassed the quality of his illustrations by a wide margin.

Eustachio's first anatomical treatise, *Opuscula anatomica* (7), was published in 1564. Of greatest interest is the fifth plate in this volume, in which a human kidney is bisected sagittally to reveal the renal pyramids with their papillae opening into the pelvicalyceal system. Also shown is a kidney in which the renal parenchyma is absent, revealing the anatomical relationships of the arteries, veins, and pelvicalyceal system within the kidney. The accuracy of these illustrations is remarkable (Fig. 10) and includes a correct depiction of the arcuate vessels forming arches at the corticomedullary junction and the interlobar vessels that supply the anatomically distinct "lobes" of the kidney. He was also the first to describe the suprarenal glands (Fig. 11).

After Eustachio's death in 1574, his assistant inherited his anatomical plates (forty-seven, including the original seven on the kidney) and these ultimately found their way to the Vatican library where they lay in complete anonymity for a century and a half. In 1714 the physician to Pope Clement XI, Giovanni Maria Lancisi (1654–1720), discovered the plates and added his own descriptions to all except the first eight, for which Eustachio's commentary was available (13). He published a text entitled *Tabulae anatomicae* (18), containing the forty-seven plates prepared during Eustachio's lifetime (19), which brought the work of Eustachio to the attention of the world. There is little doubt that if the plates had appeared one hundred and fifty years earlier, Eustachio would have ranked with Vesalius as founder of modern anatomy.

The work of Eustachio received further glory at the hands of Bernhard Siegfried Albinus (1697–1770), the finest anatomist of his day. His atlas entitled *Explicatio tabularum anatomicarum* (1) was published in 1744 and contained new copper engravings by the Dutch artist Jan Wandelaar (6). Of all the editions containing Eustachio's illustrations of the kidney, only the original *Opuscula anatomica* of 1564 contains a detailed description of the kidney. A recent survey of this work, containing the translation below, has shown that Eustachio, not Bellini, was the first to observe the structure of the renal tubules (9).

Eustachio described the renal vessels in chapter 43 of the *Opuscula anatomica* (7) as follows:

After these things have been accurately observed the membrane of the kidney [the insertion of the capsule in the hilar region] *is pulled back and forth so as to expose the branches of the vessels, no less dextrously than felicitously. Indeed these branches are spread out like*

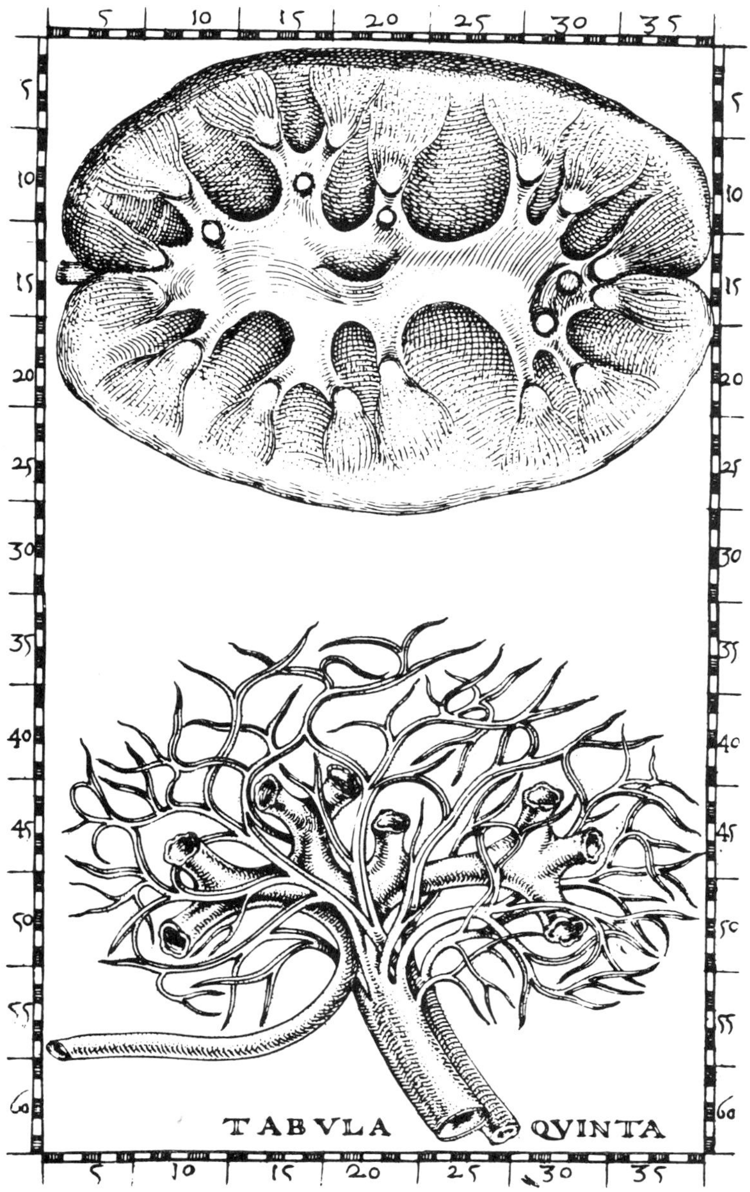

Figure 10. Eustachio's dissection of the human kidney. *Top*, the pelvicalyceal system; *bottom*, vascular anatomy. [From Lancisi (18).]

the digits of the goose [foot] *and are supported from above and in between by the same type of membrane. They reach the depth of the kidney supported and surrounded by soft, uneven flesh. However, in order that you may see the distribution and the pattern of the* [blood] *vessels, care of another kind must be employed. First the substance of the curved part of the kidney* [cortex] *must be incised in different*

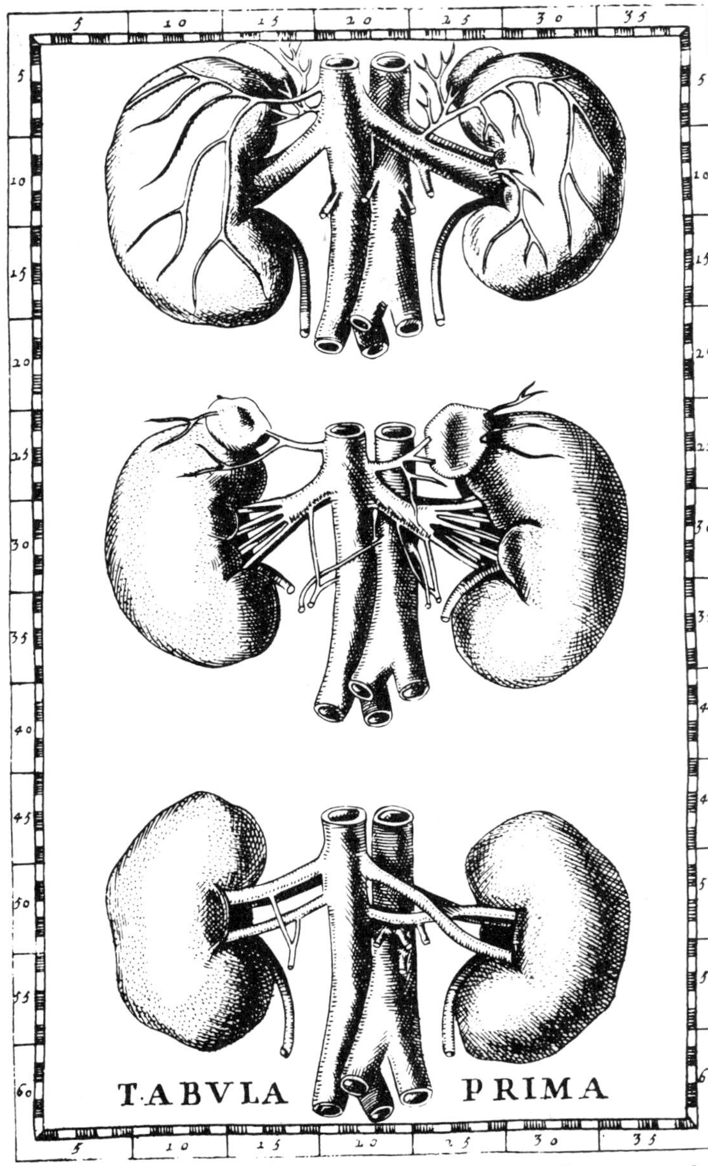

Figure 11. Eustachio's depiction of the kidneys and suprarenal glands. [From Lancisi (18).]

planes, both transverse and oblique. By compressing with the fingers you will immediately see that drops of blood trickle out [indicating that the blood vessels extend to the outermost cortex]. *Carefully scrape the substance* [of the kidney] *with the dull side of the scalpel* [and] . . . *the finer branches of the vessels will become visible. Then with the scalpel inserted into the draining vessels you will be able to observe their wondrous and elegant arrangement. Also you will see that those same branches do not terminate in the renal sinus but end not far from the outer boundary of the edge of their humped parts* [corticomedullary function] *on account of their fineness.*

In chapter 37 Eustachio described his definitive observations on the structure of the renal parenchyma:

Although the kidneys appear to have been designated as bodies with vertical lines extending from their centers to their circumferences, lines of this type are nowhere more distinct than in those segments which we have indicated, and represent small glandules resembling the nipples of the breast [papillae] [Fig. 10]. *Although many think that they are fibers of the kidney, some think that they are branches of the blood vessels which are as fine as hairs. For my part, I think that there are certain furrows and small canals* [tubules] *in the substance of the kidney which are carved out for flowing liquids and fluids. It is through these* [tubules] *that the urine is filtered into the renal cavity* [pelvis].

For if one wished to contemplate the ingenuity of nature in many of its facets it should not be so amazing to anyone that the furrows or small canals, which are distinct within the substance of the kidney, should filter [distill] *the urine.*

Eustachio had clearly described the renal collecting tubules that later came to be known as the ducts of Bellini or collecting ducts. He was unable to understand the process of urine formation but was somewhat dissatisfied with Galen's failure to emphasize the attractive function of the bladder. Eustachio, however, marvelled at how "*the urine penetrates from the ureters into the bladder by some wondrous artifice of nature; whether, as Galen believed, when the covers* [valves] *of both vessels* [ureters] *are opened, an exit may be provided for the urine, or whether, as we have demonstrated (and a fact that Galen himself sometimes acknowledged) an exit may open through a complicated route, but the return may be closed.*"

Bellini

Lorenzo Bellini (1643–1704) was an Italian anatomist who made a substantial contribution to the knowledge of the anatomy and physiology of the kidney by demonstrating that the substance of the kidney is composed of anatomical subunits, i.e., renal tubules. Although Eustachio had made this observation earlier, Bellini was apparently unaware of it when he made his observations. Bellini, a pupil of Borelli (1608–1679), published his classic text *Exercitatio anatomica de structura et usu renum* (3) in 1662 when he was nineteen years old.

Bellini first attacked the prevailing concept that the kidneys are made of a hard, solid, fleshy substance. He demonstrated that this substance was an aggregate of vessels:

Having cut through any part of the kidney, certain fibers or filaments extending from the outer surface to the hollow pelvis are quite plainly visible. [See Fig 12.] *In order that you may see them more clearly you may separate a particular slender portion with your fingers . . . and then it will appear more distinctly that these fibers are continuous from the outermost surface even to the hollow of the pelvis.*

When these filaments (tubules) were compressed, Bellini observed water welling up everywhere. With the bravado of the true investigator, he showed that "*if you are not afraid to present this to your tongue you will discover a certain saltiness and, in some, the taste of*

Fig. IX

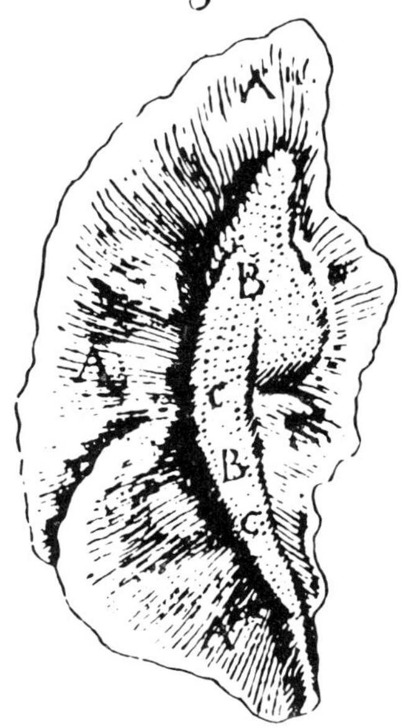

Fig. X

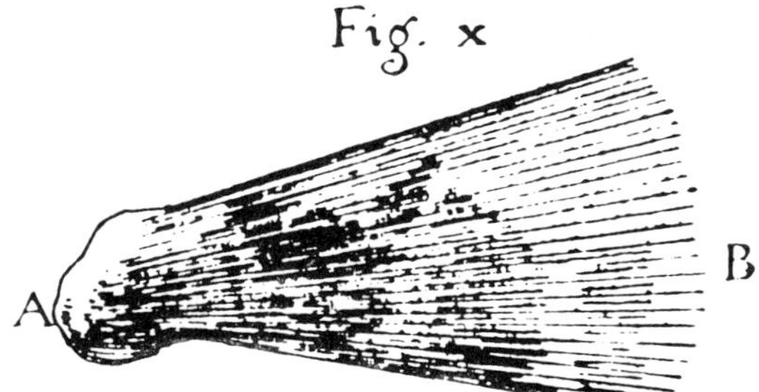

Figure 12. Bellini's depiction of collecting tubules. *Top*, the opening of the collecting tubules at the tip of the papilla; *bottom*, an isolated papilla with collecting ducts converging at the tip. (Note the "verruca" at the tip of the papilla.) [From Bellini (3).]

urine." He observed that the same "juice" arises from a kidney that had been sectioned. With the use of a magnifying lens, he observed that when tubules are compressed "*the urine is very clearly seen welling out as if pushing forth from so many little water pipes. . . . From these things one can confidently infer that the substance of the kidney . . . is nothing else than . . . a mass of canalicular and capillary spaces through which urine flows into the pelvis.*"

Bellini made further observations that demonstrated his ability as a microanatomist. He observed that when liquids were injected into the renal artery they exuded onto the surface of the kidney that had been stripped of its capsule. He reasoned that the minute arterial branches must open into "*a little space which, although it could not be perceived by sense yet reason persuades, and the glass clearly confirms, that it occurs.*" This being the case, he reasoned that arterial blood comes into contact with two classes of vessels, the veins and the "renal vessels" or tubules. Serum separated from blood enters the tubules, whereas blood, having been separated from its serous humor, enters the veins. Thus the "*secretion* [of the urine] *occurs neither by attraction nor by familiarity but by sympathy and is accomplished solely by the configuration of the vessels producing it.*"

The foregoing requires that the credit for the suggestion that urine is separated from blood by a distinct arrangement of anatomical structures goes to Bellini. All this he achieved without the aid of a microscope. His work was known to Malpighi and undoubtedly provided an important stimulus for further investigation.

It is clear that Bellini's "mechanical" explanation came remarkably close to the process of glomerular filtration; the only component he had failed to observe was the glomerulus, which effects the straining off of protein-free fluid from the blood.

Malpighi

Only four years after Bellini's description of the kidney, Marcello Malpighi (1628–1694) published his classic essay on the kidney, "De viscerum structura," in *Opera omnia* (1666) (20). This work was a landmark in understanding renal function because of its great detail and clarity and was unsurpassed until Bowman's paper of 1842 nearly two centuries later. So precisely were the kidneys described by Malpighi that he apparently did not feel the need to use illustrations. This is indeed surprising in light of the magnificent plates that accompany his embryological and botanical works. His work on the kidney (the edition of 1669) was translated into English in 1925 (14).

Malpighi first described the lobular appearance of the external surface of the kidney and correctly concluded that this is the vestige of the lobular structure of the fetal kidney. The interior of the kidney is also clearly divided into many-sided pyramids, each with a discrete blood supply. He then dramatically described the "*very small round bodies, like a coil of small worms*" on the surface of the kidney. The glomeruli (which appropriately were subsequently called Malpighian corpuscles) were seen to be attached to the tortuous vessels (i.e., tubules) that, "*after short, sharp convolutions close to the outer surface, run in a straight course toward the pelvis.*" He failed to notice the hairpin loops in the medulla of the kidney.

In examining the substance of the renal cortex, Malpighi noted that it consists of innumerable little canals that he identified as excretory vessels. He was able to trace these urinary vessels (i.e., the straight portion of the terminal nephron that Bellini had observed) to the outermost surface of the kidney, noting correctly that the terminal segments (which we now regard as the "origin" of the nephron) were reflected inward to find their ultimate ends beneath the surface.

Malpighi described the "glands" of the kidney (i.e., the glomeruli), "*attached like apples to the blood vessels, the latter swollen with the black liquid* [which he injected] *and stretched out into the form of a beautiful tree.*" He was frustrated at not being able to perceive the precise structure of these glands and, in fact, did not appreciate that they contained a capillary tuft. Rather he considered them to be surrounded by the terminal buds of the blood vessels, thus being stained the same color as the vessels when a dye was perfused into the renal artery. Dye injected into the veins similarly arrived at the glands, albeit less predictably.

Having concluded that both arteries and veins are in direct connection with the glomeruli, Malpighi addressed the more difficult question of whether the urinary vessels (i.e., tubules) were similarly connected. He acknowledged that he had never been able to observe liquids perfused through the renal arteries penetrating into the tubules. He even attempted to highlight the connection (the existence of which, he was convinced, must be present) by ligating the ureter and renal veins of a live dog to produce a kidney swollen by the blood driven into it. Despite the fact that a connection between glands and urinary vessels was suggested, it was "*not such as satisfied the senses in all particulars.*" Malpighi was sufficiently sophisticated as an investigator to realize that the negative findings were a consequence of the limitations of his techniques and continued to believe in the connection between glomeruli and tubules, using as his analogy the invariable connection between all glands and their excretory ducts.

Malpighi was able to ascertain that all urinary vessels terminate at the tips of the papillae, but he firmly denied the existence of the "verruca" at these locations, as was depicted in the illustration of Bellini (Fig. 12).

The final chapter of "De renibus" is devoted to a consideration of the function of the kidney. Malpighi assumed that the glands were responsible for separating urine from blood; however, the precise mechanism by which this was achieved eluded him. He clearly stated that the excreting bodies probably have little pores through which small particles (salty or sulfurous) can pass but not those of large size or different shape. All particles of use to the organism are retained, whereas those of no use are eliminated. He supported this contention by observing that when blood is thinned urine may become bloody; when it grows thicker bleeding subsides. Not content with playing the role of anatomist and physiologist, Malpighi relied on his expertise as a physician to draw pathophysiological conclusions. He felt that most diseases of the kidney spring from diseases of the blood entering the kidneys. He cited gout as an example of a systemic disorder in which the kidneys are affected.

Having established to his satisfaction that the glands were the source of the fluid component of the urine, Malpighi turned his attention to the urinary vessels. Drawing on his extensive knowledge of comparative anatomy and physiology, he noted that in birds urine is "*coarser and more compact*" than in humans and that this property leads to "*the formation of hairs within the narrow tubules as the urine becomes solidified.*" He did not deduce that this propensity to form a solid material was due to removal of water by the tubules, but he did surmise that removal or addition of certain substances by the tubules allows the salts and liquids to more easily adopt the form of hairs.

Malpighi's contribution to the understanding of renal function cannot be overestimated. His work on the kidney followed Bellini's by only four years, yet his insight and the detailed nature of his observations appear to belong to a different scientific era. Physiological thought, however, had not reached the level of sophistication that could have exploited Malpighi's anatomical observations to further elaborate the fundamentals of renal function. Concepts such as glomerular filtration and tubular reabsorption required another two hundred and fifty years to become established.

Ruysch, Bertin, Schumlansky, and Müller

As so often happens in the evolution of science, subsequent observations seemed to confuse rather than to refine and advance the observations of Malpighi. Frederik Ruysch (1638–1731) had been taught to inject blood vessels by the anatomist Jan Swammerdam. When he injected diffusible dyes into the renal artery, Ruysch observed that the dyes passed from the glomerular tufts into the tubules. He erroneously concluded that the tubules were in continuity with the renal microvessels (28) and proposed that the kidney possessed exhalant arteries with open mouths that opened directly into the excretory canals (tubules). Despite this mistake Ruysch must be credited with producing the first illustration that clearly demonstrated that the convoluted tubules constitute the bulk of the renal cortex (Fig. 13). These figures were subsequently reproduced in

Manget's compilation of anatomical works by famous anatomists, the *Theatrum anatomicum* (22).

In 1774 the French anatomist Exupère Joseph Bertin (1712–1781) wrote a memoir on the kidney in which he stated that urine is formed both by glands and by blood vessels (4). He considered that the glands described by Malpighi were the terminations of the tubules, which were smaller than the secretory glands that he considered to be present in the kidney. He erred on certain points, such as his concept of secreting glands, but he was the first to notice that the cortical substance extended into the interior of the kidney. These extensions of the cortex subsequently became known as the columns of Bertin, which separate the pyramids of the kidney. He was also astute enough to conclude that, because the number of orifices that open into the papilla is significantly smaller than the number of tubules, several tubules must unite before reaching the papilla.

The first person to refute Ruysch's contention that tubules are continuations of arterioles was Antoin Ferrein (1693–1769), professor of anatomy and surgery in Paris. By filling the renal arteries with colored fluid, he failed to alter the whiteness of the tubules, but he missed the mark by stating that the tubules do not end in the glands of Malpighi (8). He did, however, confirm Bertin's contention by direct observation that tubules unite as they converge towards the papilla.

The obscure Russian physician Alexander Schumlansky finally confirmed Malpighi's contention that glomeruli and tubules communicate (30). His depiction (Fig. 14) was inaccurate only in the

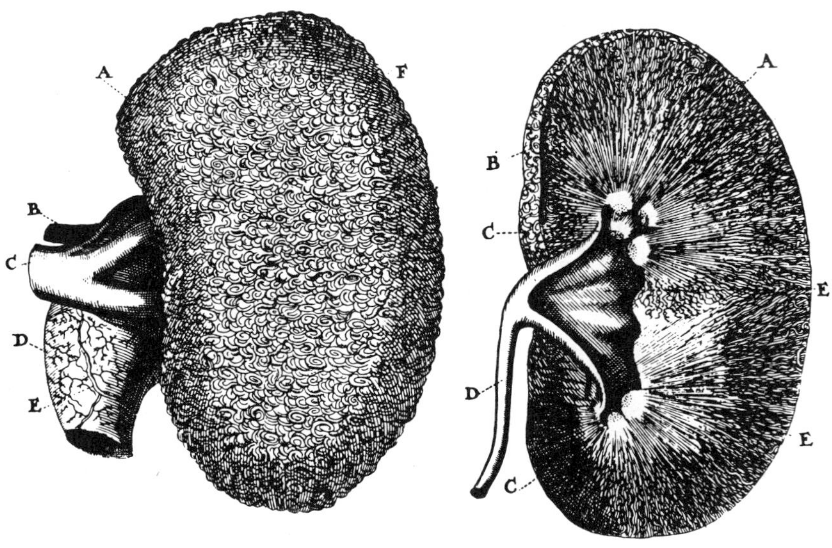

Figure 13. Ruysch's depiction of convoluted tubules in the kidney cortex. [From Manget (22).]

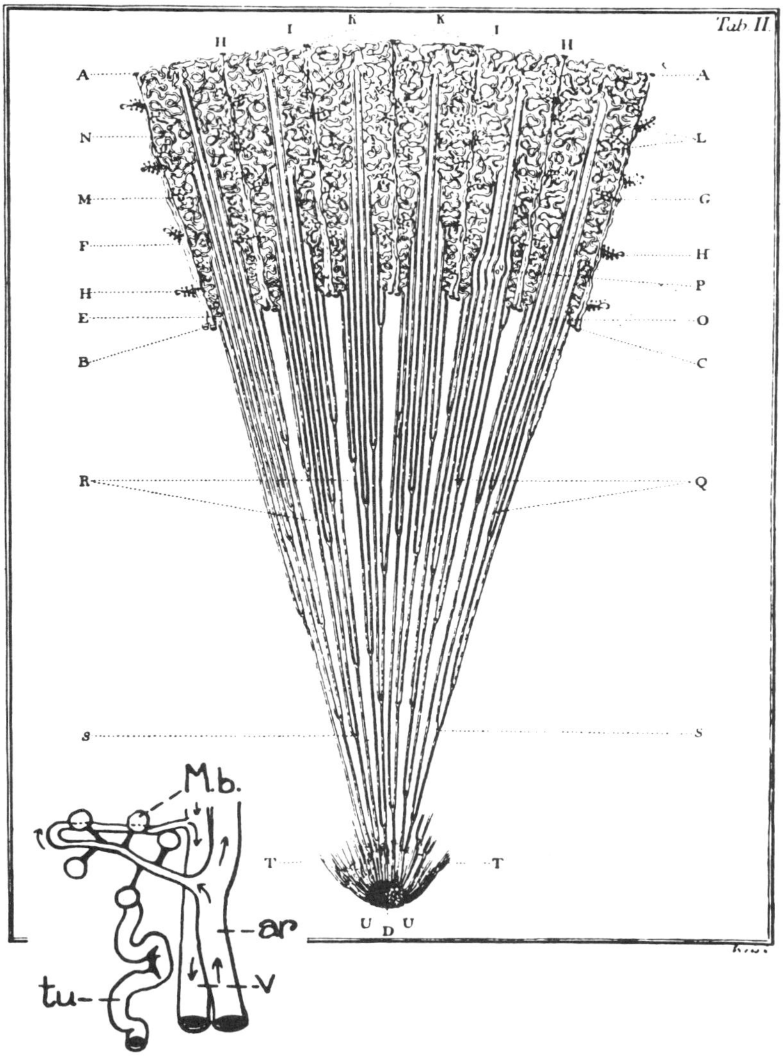

Figure 14. Schumlansky's diagram of six renal lobules depicting the connection of the tubules conveying towards the papilla. *Inset*, Maluf's drawing of glomerular connections to the tubules. (Glomeruli are shown much smaller than their actual size.) [From Maluf (21).]

inappropriately small size of glomeruli, which was later more clearly illustrated by Maluf (21).

That glomeruli definitely do not communicate with the tubules was propounded emphatically, but quite erroneously, by Johannes Peter Müller (1801–1858). Müller, who was one of the eminent members of the Berlin School of modern scientific medicine, authored the *Handbuch der Physiologie des Menschen fur Vorlesungen* (25), which was issued in several parts between 1833 and 1840 and became the standard textbook of physiology on the continent, in Britain, and in the United States. In the *Handbuch* Müller states:

Among the tubuli uriniferi of the cortical substance lie the acini of Malpighi, bodies larger than the urinary canals and visible even with the naked eye. Schumlansky has drawn them much too small. They ... consist wholly of convoluted blood vessels ... and are simply receptacles for blood and not, as Schumlansky supposed, the beginning of the tubule uriniferi. The convoluted tubule uriniferi themselves are the seat of the secretion of the urine.

Müller expanded on these views in his book *De glandularum secernentium structura* (24) and emphasized, "*That the urinary ducts terminate in the Malpighian bodies is most certainly a false assertion.*"

Bowman

William Bowman (Fig. 15), stimulated (and presumably irritated) by the apparent finality of Müller's conclusions, was prompted to investigate the matter further. Bowman, who had joined the medical department of King's College in 1837, was appointed junior demonstrator in anatomy and curator of the museum at that institution. At the age of 25, he was elected a fellow of the Royal Society. A year later he published his classic paper "On the Structure and Use of the Malpighian Bodies of the Kidney, with Observations on the Circulation Through that Gland" (5). This work became the most definitive contribution to the microscopic anatomy of the kidney since Malpighi and was accurate in all of its details.

Why was Bowman able to elucidate the structure of the glomerulus

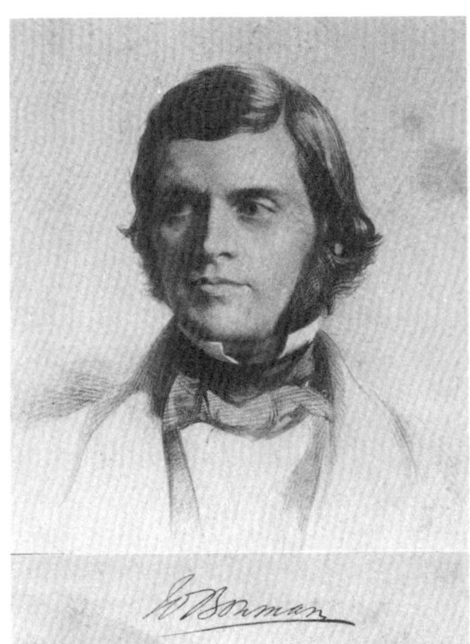

Figure 15. William Bowman (1816–1892). [Original engraving given to C. W. Gottschalk by Joseph T. Wearn.]

with greater success than his predecessors? The answer, notwithstanding Bowman's investigational prowess, was to some extent determined by the technical progress that had been made by others and by the fact that his initial observations were obviously at variance with the conclusions reached by Müller. First, Bowman's optical equipment was far superior to that available to Malpighi; second, a method of vascular injection had been employed by Doyere of Paris, in which the combination of lead acetate and potassium dichromate resulted in the precipitation of lead dichromate, which allowed small blood vessels to be outlined with clarity; and finally, the use of thin microscopic slices allowed the continuity of anatomical structures to be determined with certainty (21).

Bowman's investigations included a wide variety of species, including parrots and boa constrictors! He noted:

The Malpighian bodies I saw to be a rounded mass of minute vessels invested by a cyst or capsule of precisely similar appearance to the basement membrane of the tubes. Seeing these similar tissues in such close proximity, it was not easy to resist the conviction that the capsule was the basement membrane of the tubes expanded over the vessels.

However, Bowman was unable to gain an unequivocal view of this continuity. It was here that the method of vascular injection allowed the critical observation to be made, for "*the injected material had in many instances burst through the tuft and, being extravasated into the capsule, had passed off along the tube.*" He was now able to construct the anatomy of the nephron with great clarity, and the single plate in his paper (5), containing seventeen separate figures, illustrates more effectively than many lines of text how precisely he appreciated the structure of the nephron. The afferent and efferent arterioles, respectively supplying and emerging from the glomerulus (the "*portal system of the kidney*" as Bowman termed it), and the peritubular capillary plexuses are shown with clarity and precision. His graphic depiction of the human nephron (Fig. 16) is a medical classic. The only lapses were his failure to appreciate that the glomerular capillaries are lined externally by epithelial cells that are in continuity with those of the capsule and his oversight of the hairpin looping of the tubules in the medulla, subsequently discovered by Friedrich Henle in 1862 (15).

Did Bowman's revealing anatomical insights lead him to an appreciation of the function of the glomerulus? His own words could not be more explicit:

It would indeed be difficult to conceive a disposition of parts more calculated to favour the escape of water from the blood than that of the Malpighian body. A large artery breaks up in a very direct manner into a number of minute branches each of which suddenly opens into an assemblage of vessels of far greater aggregate capacity than itself and from which there is but one narrow exit. Hence must arise a very

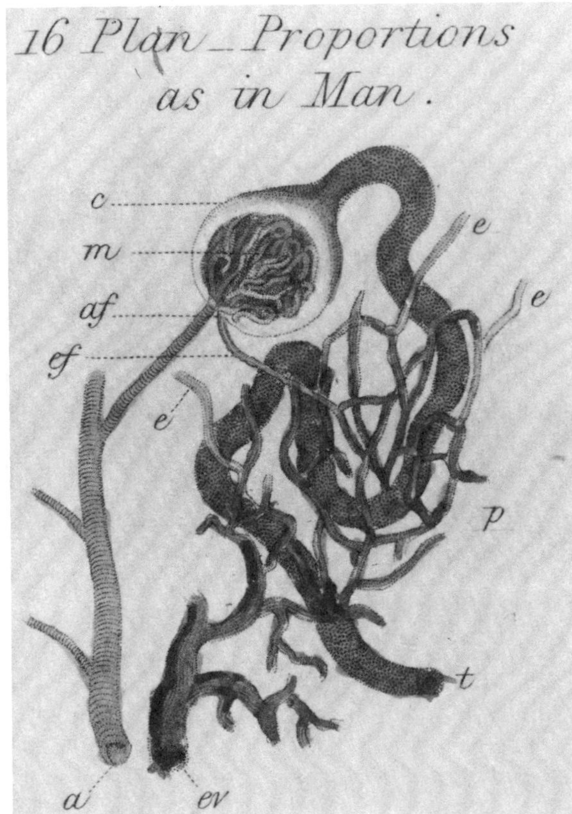

Figure 16. Bowman's depiction of the proportions of the human nephron. [From Bowman (5).]

abrupt retardation in the velocity of the current of blood. The vessels in which this delay occurs are uncovered by any structure. They lie bare in a cell from which there is but one outlet, the orifice of the tube. . . . Why is so wondrous an apparatus placed at the extremity of each uriniferous tube if not to furnish water to aid in the separation and solution of the urinous products from the epithelium of the tube. . . . The secretion is brought from the tubules of the gland in a fluid state and only becomes solid by the reabsorption of its aqueous portion after it has traversed the tortuous canals where it was formed.

Although Bowman did not articulate the concept of filtration in physicochemical terms, his clear understanding of the existence of two separate processes now recognized as glomerular filtration and tubular reabsorption and his precise description of the anatomy of the nephron became the basis for all future studies on the physiology of the kidney.

BIBLIOGRAPHY

1. ALBINUS, B. S. *Explicatio tabularum anatomicarum Barth. Eustachii.* Leiden: Johannum Arnoldum Langerak, Johannum Hermannum Verbeck, 1744.
2. ARISTOTLE. *Historia animalium,* translated by A. L. Peck. Cambridge, MA: Harvard Univ. Press, 1965. (Loeb Classical Library, vol. 437.)
3. BELLINI, L. *Exercitatio anatomica de structura et usu renum.* Florentiae: Ex typografia sub signo Stellae, 1662.
4. BERTIN, M. Memoire pour servir de l'histoire des reins. *Hist. Acad. R. Sci. Mem. Math. Phys.* 77, 1744.
5. BOWMAN, W. On the structure and use of the Malpighian bodies of the kidney with observations on the circulation through that gland. *Phil. Trans. R. Soc. Lond.* (Part 1): 57, 1842.
6. CHOULANT, L. *History and Bibliography of Anatomic Illustration,* translated by M. Frank. New York: Hafner, 1962.
7. EUSTACHIO, B. *Opuscula anatomica.* Venice: Vincent Luchinus exudebat. 1564.
8. FERREIN. Sur la structure de viscères nommés glandulus et particulierment sur celle des reins et du fore. *Hist. Acad. R. Sci. Mem. Math. Phys.* 489, 1749.
9. FINE, L. G. Eustachi's discovery of the renal tubule. *Am. J. Nephrol.* 6: 47–50, 1986.
10. FULTON, J. F. *Selected Readings in the History of Physiology.* Springfield, IL: Thomas, 1966, p. 350.
11. GALEN. *On the Natural Faculties,* translated by A. J. Brock. Cambridge, MA: Harvard Univ. Press, 1916. (Loeb Classical Library, vol. 71.)
12. GALEN. *On the Usefulness of the Parts of the Body,* translated by M. Talmadge. Ithaca, NY: Cornell Univ. Press, 1968, vol. 1. (Translated from *De usu partium.*)
13. GARRISON, F. H. *An Introduction to the History of Medicine.* Philadelphia, PA: Saunders, 1929.
14. HAYMAN, J. M., JR. Malpighi's "Concerning the structure of the kidneys." *Ann. Med. Hist.* 7: 242–263, 1925.
15. HENLE, J. Zur Anatomie der Niere. *Abh. Ges. Wiss. Göttingen, Math. Physik. K1.* 10: 223, 1862.
16. JAEGER, W. W. *Diokles von Karyostos. Die Griechische Medizin und die Schule des Aristoteles.* Berlin: de Gruyter, 1938.
17. KETHAM, J. DE. *Fasciculo di Medicina,* edited by K. Sudhoff. Florence, Italy: Lier, 1925. (Momenta Medica Ser.)
18. LANCISI, G. M. *Tabulae anatomicae Bartolomaei Eustachii.* Rome: Ex officina typografia Francisci Gonzagae, 1714.
19. MAJOR, R. H. Kidney diseases. In: *Classic Descriptions of Disease.* Springfield, IL: Thomas, 1978, p. 527.
20. MALPIGHI, M. De viscerum structura. In: *Opera omnia.* (1666) London: Scott, 1686, p. 87–100.
21. MALUF, N. S. R. The centenary of Bowman's exposition of the renal unit (1842–1942). *Ann. Med. Hist.* 4: 427, 1942. (ser. 6.)
22. MANGET, J. J. *Theatrum anatomicum.* Geneva: Cramer and Perachon, 1717.
23. MONDINO DE' LUZZI. *Anathomia.* Pavia: Antonius de Carchano, 1487.
24. MÜLLER, J. De glandularum secernentium structura penitiori earumque

prima formatione in homine atque animalibus. Leipzig: Leopoldi Vossii, 1830.
25. Müller, J. *Handbuch der Physiologie des Menschen für Vorlesungen.* Coblenz: J. Holscher, 1834, vol. 1.
26. O'Malley, C. D., and J. B. de C. M. Saunders. *Leonardo da Vinci on the Human Body.* New York: Schuman, 1952.
27. Pinder, U. *Epiphanie medicorum.* Nuremburg: Friedrich Peypus, 1506.
28. Ruysch, F. Thesaurus magnus et regius qui est decimus thesaurorum anatomicorum. In: *Opera omnia anatomico-medico-chirurgica.* Amsterdam: Janssonio-Waesbergios, 1729, vol. II.
29. Sarton, G. *Introduction to the History of Science. From Homer to Omar Khayam.* Baltimore, MD: Williams & Wilkins, 1927, vol. 1.
30. Schumlansky, A. *Disseratio inauguralis anatomica de structura renum.* Argentorati: Lorenzii & Schuleri, 1782.
31. Singer, C. *A Short History of Medicine.* New York: Oxford Univ. Press, 1928.
32. Singer, C. The Greeks to 50 BC. In: *A Short History of Anatomy and Physiology From the Greeks to Harvey.* New York: Dover, 1957.
33. Vesalius, A. De renibus. In: *De humani corporis fabrica libri septem.* Basileae: Ex officina Johannis Oporini, 1543, p. 514–517.
34. Wiberg, J. The medical science of ancient Greece. The doctrine of the heart. *Janus* 41: 225, 1937.

II

Renal Blood Flow and Dynamics of Glomerular Filtration: Evolution of a Concept from Carl Ludwig to the Present Day

KLAUS THURAU, JOHN M. DAVIS, AND DIETER A. HÄBERLE

RENAL HEMODYNAMICS

Der schöpferische Geist des Menschen
ist damit ausgezeichnet . . .
"etwas zu denken das niemand zuvor gedacht hat
wenn er etwas sieht was jeder sieht."

Man's creative intellect is distinguished
by the ability . . .
"to think something which no-one ever thought before
whilst seeing something which everybody sees."

Arthur Schopenhauer
(1788–1860)

PHYSIOLOGISTS today gain knowledge by the application of two principles introduced into physiology in the early part of the last century. First, they employ a hypothetico-deductive method in that their scientific endeavour begins with a "working hypothesis," the correctness of which is then established by systematic experimental examination of its logical consequences. This "new" method stands in stark contrast to the inductive method advocated by Francis Bacon (1561–1626) and John Stuart Mill (1806–1873), a conflict of which the scientists of the period were well aware, as an essay by Justus von Liebig in 1863 shows.[1] As a rule this experimental examination generates observations that require further hypotheses for their explanation, and so the process results in the gradual development of concepts that in truth are systems of more or less well substantiated hypotheses reflecting the imagination of individual researchers. Second, physiologists employ physicochemical methods to carry out experiments, a procedure that originated in a temporary constellation of certain philosophical systems at the beginning of the nineteenth century (see next section).

Both of these principles are particularly relevant to the theme of this chapter because the creation of our modern concepts of renal blood flow and the dynamics of glomerular filtration by Carl Ludwig (Fig. 1) in 1842 is intimately related to the introduction of this new scientific method into physiology and because the development of the concept in the following century and a half is an excellent example of scientific evolution by progressive interaction between observations and the ideas and imagination of outstanding people.

Accordingly, and given our intention to restrict our considerations to ideas that have become generally accepted components of our modern view of renal function, we first address Carl Ludwig's scientific thought and his theory of urine formation. In the second part of this chapter, we attempt to show how the subsequent scientific disputes developing out of Ludwig's concepts led eventually to observations that occasioned the Belgian pathologist Norbert Goormaghtigh to propose a control mechanism, located in the juxtaglomerular apparatus, that functionally relates renal blood flow and glomerular filtration to tubular reabsorption. Finally, we show how years later this idea was experimentally confirmed and developed.

Carl Ludwig's Concept

Ludwig's Mechanistic Paradigm

We accept today as self-evident that physiological functions are the expression of universal, meaningfully ordered, physicochemical processes that, for that very reason, can be analyzed and understood by recourse to the theoretical and experimental methods of physics and chemistry. This approach, which in retrospect was so successful,

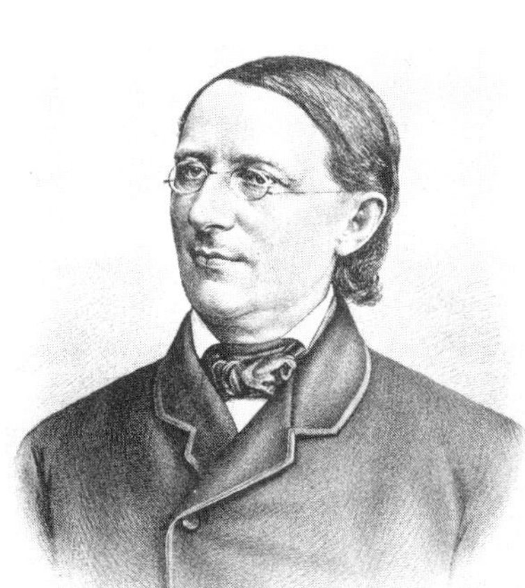

Figure 1. Carl Friedrich Wilhelm Ludwig (1816–1895).

was in fact the real and revolutionary innovation in Ludwig's 1842 hypothesis (34) that saw urine formation as the result of a simple biophysical process of ultrafiltration in the glomeruli and was an unprecedented departure from the then-current views.

Physiology at that time was a system of natural philosophy based on vitalism, divine revelation, and other metaphysical notions. Physical methods, although in use in physiological investigation since the time of Stephen Hales (1677–1761) and raised to new heights by workers like François Magendie (1783–1855) and Johannes Müller (1801–1858), were still questioned as being sufficient or appropriate means of gaining insight into the processes of life. In order to realize his scientific ideas, Ludwig thus had to challenge the traditional philosophies by the adoption of this new weltanschauung. In this he was not alone. Joined by three other scientific "revolutionaries" Emil du Bois-Reymond, Hermann von Helmholz, and Ernst Wilhelm von Brücke and supported by the newly emerging esteem in which physics was held and the writings of scientific naturalists like Karl Vogt, Jakob Moleschott, and Ludwig Büchner, these researchers regarded the living organism as a kind of machine in which physicochemical processes were responsible for all the phenomena of life, and which, for that very reason, could be investigated solely by physicochemical methods.

Characteristic of this new approach are the following words of Carl Ludwig, taken from the introduction to his *Lehrbuch der Physiologie des Menschen* (*Textbook of Human Physiology*), which he published as a young professor in Zürich in 1852:

In accordance with this experience, it is concluded that all the phenomena of the animal body are the consequence of simple attractions and repulsions (between a limited number of chemical atoms) such as can be observed when these elementary components collide.[2] *This conclusion will be irrefutable, when it is proven, with mathematical precision, that the above mentioned elementary conditions are so ordered, with respect to direction, time and mass, in the animal body that all the accomplishments of the living or dead organism must, of necessity, follow from their interactions.*[3]

In the chapter "Sitz der Seele" ("Seat of the Soul") he wrote:

According to the one group of hypotheses, a special substrate, the soul, is responsible for the intellectual functions. This substrate, like the luminiferous ether, pervades the finite cerebral mass. The adherents of the numerous gradations of realistic philosophic systems are agreed, insofar as they can decide on a view at all, that the manifestations of the soul result from a certain sum of conditions present in brain and blood, since with the creation, development and passing of the brain and with alterations in the composition of the blood, intellect, feeling and will appear, disappear or change. He who accepts conclusions drawn from analogy as valid, and who, by virtue of his knowl-

edge is able to compare thoroughly the manifestations of the soul with other natural phenomena will be, if forced to choose, in no doubt with which of the two views he concurs.[4]

It is nonetheless characteristic of the scientific integrity of the new approach that Ludwig continued, "*He who demands irrefutable proof for one or the other of the philosophies will have to admit that such is not yet available.*"[5]

Ludwig's Concept of Renal Function

Given Ludwig's materialist-mechanist view of life and the circumstance of his initial employment at the Marburg Anatomical Institute at which his first tasks, under the direction of Hermann Nasse, were concerned with the structure of renal vasculature, it is probably not surprising that he was the first (albeit more intuitively than experimentally) to understand correctly the mechanism of filtrate formation and its reabsorption and at the same time to have the appropriate strength of character to present these considerations in such a way that they very rapidly assumed a central position in contemporary scientific discussion.

Dynamics of Glomerular Filtration

Ludwig based his concepts of renal function on the following observations, gained from the literature and from his own experiments during the period from his appointment at Marburg in 1841 to the publication of his Habilitation dissertation[6] (34) in 1842 and his two-volume text book (35, 36) in 1852 and 1856.

1. Blood is a protein-containing solution; in addition, "*proteins have a substantial chemical affinity for water and many aqueous solutions (and to some extent also for fats).*"[7] In the context of these discoveries, Ludwig carried out a variety of model experiments on the reabsorption of concentrated and diluted urine by blood through semipermeable membranes. He found that the fluid components of blood "*penetrate the intact vascular walls. This process, termed secretion, is opposed by a further process, reabsorption.*"[8] He thought this secretion through "thierische Häute" (animal membranes) occurred through minute openings and that the passage of fluid through these openings did not lead to any change in the fluid's composition. However, this did not hold for protein-containing solutions, since the rate of filtration of such solutions through animal membranes diminished with time, presumably because (as he put it) the pores gradually clog up. Furthermore the rate of filtration rose with increasing blood pressure. Using sheep intestine as a model membrane, he studied both these phenomena with defibrinized serum at various hydrostatic pressures.

2. From his dye-injection experiments with the anatomist Bünger in Marburg, Ludwig was well aware of the structure of the renal

vascular system, in particular the two capillary beds, the glomerular and the peritubular, in series (Fig. 2A).

3. By this time the laws of hydraulics applied to symmetrically branched tubes were well known. Using these laws Ludwig performed experiments on models, and from the analysis of these experiments he was able to predict the hydrostatic pressure and flow profiles in the vascular bed of the kidney (Fig. 2B).

4. The chemical composition of urine and blood was sufficiently well known to lead to the recognition of the fact that urine is not a product of the kidney's own chemical activity but rather the principal components of urine are already present in blood. Conversely, it was

A

B

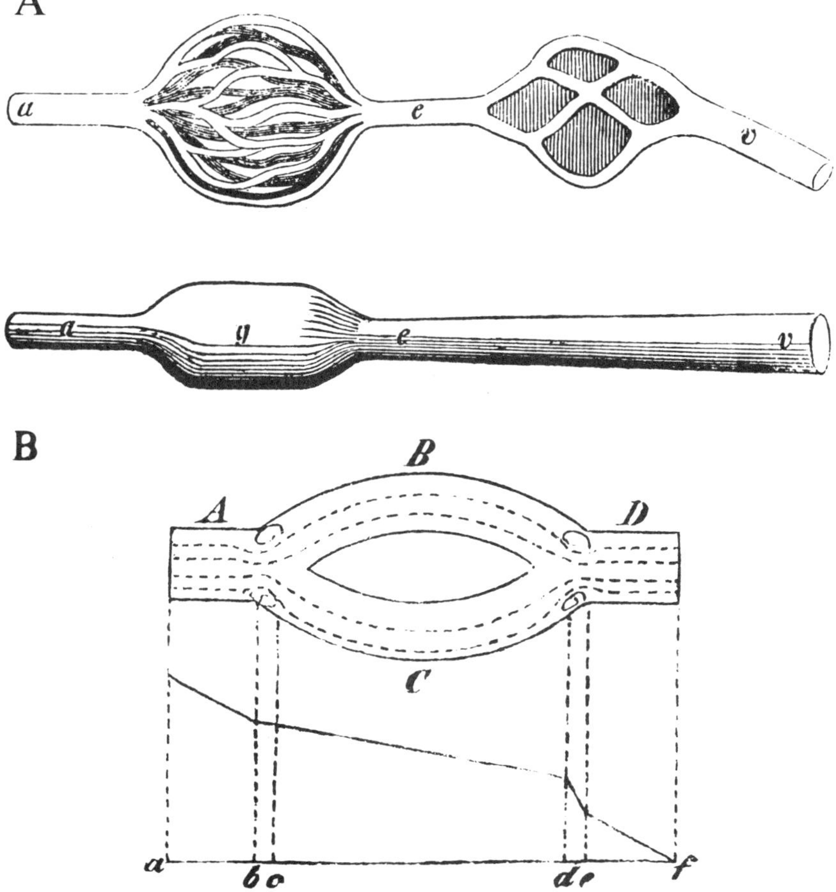

Figure 2. *A: top,* Ludwig's representations of renal microvasculature including capillary beds of glomerulus (*left*), and peritubular network (*right*). *Bottom,* representation of relative total cross-sectional areas of different vascular segments. a, Afferent arteriole; e, efferent arteriole; g, glomerulus; v, venule. *B:* representation of pressure profile across capillary bed.

also apparent that substances such as urea are excreted at far higher concentrations than at those present in blood. It followed then that, if these substances entered urine solely by glomerular filtration as Ludwig proposed, a substantial fraction of filtered solvent had to have been reabsorbed through the tubular walls back into the blood.

5. Finally and probably of more fundamental importance than these facts, Ludwig strictly applied the principle of seriously considering only such theory as could be experimentally investigated with the methods of physics and chemistry, and he assessed the correctness of such theory according to its physicomechanistic plausibility (see Ludwig's Mechanistic Paradigm, p. 32). This principle enabled him to reject other theories on the origin of urine, for example, the vitalist view or the view put forward by Johannes Müller in his textbook (1835) that regarded the kidney as a gland and ascribed the responsibility for urine formation to the renal nerves.

Ludwig's strict application of his mechanistic philosophy had doubtlessly been further consolidated during his period as an Assistant in Bunsen's laboratory at Marburg. Considering this and the anatomical structure of the glomerulus, it is in no way surprising that even at this early stage he was able to speculate that the process of glomerular filtration might be regulated by the contraction of the muscular walls of the afferent or efferent arterioles, with the consequent slowing of blood flow. He regarded the filtration part of his hypothesis as the most plausible and firmly based. The different compositions of blood and urine suggested to him, at least for a time, that only reabsorptive and diffusive processes occurred in the renal tubules, that is, reabsorption of the fluid filtered in the glomerulus and diffusive transport of the other urinary components.

Reabsorption of the Filtrate

Ludwig's efforts to interpret urine as an ultrafiltrate of blood were based, as described in the previous section, on the structure of the renal glomerulus and the relevant laws of hydrodynamics and ultrafiltration as well as on parallels observed in blood and urine composition. However, the credibility of the hypothesis required that Ludwig also explain the differences in blood and urine composition. This he did simply, based on differing epithelial permeabilities and "endosmosis." Ironically it was probably the strict application of his principle of attempting to account for life processes purely in terms of physics and chemistry or, conversely, the fear of lending support to the vitalist view of life (should this principle not be applied with the utmost consequence) that led him in his early writings to such a simplified, and in the final analysis, wrong view of tubular reabsorptive mechanisms. This approach was already clear in his Habilitation dissertation (34) in which he wrote about the vitalist theory of urine secretion by the glomeruli and tubules:

Another notion, accepted up till now, proposes that the kidneys themselves are furnished with the ability to attract urea, which, in its passage into the tubules draws with it water and solutes, with the exception of albumin and fats. This theory, begotten of naturalistic philosophy or some even more miserable doctrine, has found adherents solely for the reason that it has never been investigated. Not to speak of the fact that the absence of albumin from the urine cannot be explained by such an attraction unless the proteins and fats be rejected in toto, since otherwise the dissolved albumin etc. would be transported similarly to the dissolved salt. It is ridiculous to maintain that a body be attracted by another body and, at the same time, be repelled by it, without there being a further process for separating them, and that is supposedly what happens in the kidney![9]

In any case Ludwig modified his view of the reabsorptive process, together with his view of the basic mechanism of ultrafiltration across animal membranes, in parallel with the general development of science. In his earlier writings, in the period from the preparation of his Habilitation dissertation (34) to the publication of volume 2 of the first edition of his textbook (36) in 1856, he was forced to disregard the possibility of a mechanistically explainable transport process in the epithelial cells, if for no other reason than the impossibility of the experimental verification of such a concept. However, by the time the second edition of volume 2 was published in 1861, he was clearly contemplating such a process as a possible explanation for the reabsorption of NaCl. In the context of a consideration of how the rapidly diffusible urea accumulates in urine, whereas the relatively poorly diffusible NaCl disappears back into the bloodstream, he wrote, "*Thus, all other conditions being held constant, it remains to assume that either some special component of the tubular wall reduces the rate of diffusion* [of urea], *or that the NaCl is reabsorbed back into the bloodstream by some force, analogous to chemical force.*"[10] Here was a major change in a substantial part of Ludwig's hypothesis.

What led Ludwig to this volte-face? In 1842 Julius Robert Mayer, a young physician from Heilbronn, had published a brief essay in *Liebig's Annals* entitled "Bemerkungen über die Kräfte in der unbelebten Natur" ("Observations on the forces in inanimate nature") in which the fundamental law of conservation of energy was expressed for the first time. At about the same time (1843), similar findings had been published by the English physicist James P. Joule. Conceptually, it was then not such a great step from this to the view that cells may be able to transform force (as energy was then termed) in a physicochemical sense from one form into another. In addition, in 1858 Rudolf Virchow, a student of Johannes Müller, had published his "Zellularpathologie" in which the phenomenon "illness" was ascribed to derangements of normal cellular processes. By the end of that decade, the concept that cells could by themselves accomplish selective transport processes was thus fully consistent with contemporary scientific thought and in no way represented a retrograde grasp at vitalistic principles.

As far as can be ascertained, Ludwig's 1861 version of his views on reabsorption was his final written opinion on that theme. Indeed, in the remaining thirty-four years of his life, there were only five additional publications from his laboratory concerning the kidney. Beginning in the 1870s, Ludwig's filtration theory was the subject of vigorous and concerted attacks by Rudolf Heidenhain (1834–1897), Professor of Physiology in Breslau since 1859. Heidenhain absolutely rejected Ludwig's biophysical filtration theory in favor of secretory phenomena, not only in renal glomeruli but also with respect to the formation of lymph, a subject that occupied Ludwig's attention for practically all of his scientific career. Although reportedly deeply aggrieved and greatly distressed by Heidenhain's acerbic attacks (61), Ludwig apparently made no attempt to defend his view of renal function in general or of glomerular filtration in particular. There are a number of possible reasons for this: apart from the fact that he had turned his attention to the experimental investigation of other aspects of physiology, the phenomenon of endosmosis, which had played a central role in the original theory of the reabsorption of the filtrate, had been largely explained by the work of Traube, Pfeffer, and others; indeed the osmolarity of biological fluids was by this time able to be measured by freezing-point depression. It must have become obvious to Ludwig that his theory was never going to be able to account for the excretion of osmotically concentrated or dilute urine, and apart from measurements of renal hemodynamics and physicochemical analyses of blood and urine, Ludwig had no other investigative techniques at his command. Ludwig was not the last worker to be stumped by the problem of the osmotic concentration of urine: indeed the question was not settled until Kuhn and Wirz in Basel solved the riddle of the medullary countercurrent system seventy years later.

Nevertheless there is evidence (albeit circumstantial) that Ludwig never discarded his view that reabsorption of the glomerular filtrate by active involvement of the renal tubular epithelium was an essential component of urine formation. In 1906 his former Assistant Rudolf Metzner wrote:

Ludwig's hypothetical assumption that the glomerular filtrate is concentrated by water reabsorption during its passage through the renal tubules is strongly supported by recent studies. Simple diffusion, however, plays only the most minor of roles, one must assume an active process in the epithelia of the loop of Henle, convoluted tubules and probably also the collecting ducts, especially since this water removal is coupled to a selective reabsorption which in turn is partly dependent on the requirements of the organism, implying that both functions are, to a certain extent, independent of each other. Uric acid, phosphoric acid and exogenous substances are excreted by a genuine secretion into the tubules . . . The kidney is capable of synthesising exogenous substances from their components (hippuric acid synthesis).[11]

To summarize:

There is no crass disagreement between Ludwig's and Bowman-Heidenhain's theories. Ludwig never denied a secretory activity of the renal epithelia in the excretion of uric acid etc., Heidenhain did not absolutely reject the existence of reabsorption. Heidenhain's objections against the existance of glomerular filtration have been shown, however, to be invalid.[12]

This remarkably farsighted and conciliatory article of Metzner's deserves special comment. Metzner was born in Leipzig in 1858 and, following his graduation there as a medical practitioner in 1889, he came to Ludwig's institute as an Assistant. After his period with Ludwig and a sojourn in Freiburg where he achieved his Habilitation in 1893, he was appointed to the Chair of Physiology in Basel in 1895, where he remained for the rest of his career. He retired from the university in 1924 and died in Riehen (near Basel) in 1935. In 1906 and 1907 he contributed a number of chapters to Nagel's *Handbuch der Physiologie des Menschen*, including the chapter on urine formation and excretion from which the previous two quotations are taken. Because Metzner was not primarily active in this area [his main interests were muscle and sensory physiology and histology (11)] it is reasonable to assume that the views expressed in that chapter reflect the general tenor, if not the detail, of the views on renal function existing in the Leipzig institute in the final phase of Ludwig's activity. However, the article has an interest beyond the direct link to Ludwig. Metzner thoroughly and critically reviewed a large volume of experimental evidence that he treated with all consequence—accepting those arguments that could not validly be rejected—and came to the conclusion that urine formation could best be explained by a three-component process: ultrafiltration of a large volume of fluid at the glomerulus; reabsorption of most of the filtrate and solutes, actively mediated by the tubular epithelium; and secretion of certain urinary components, also actively mediated by the tubular epithelium. Thus Metzner had proposed a theory of urine formation more complete and considerably closer to our current concept than Cushny's "modern theory" published in the famous monograph some ten years later (7). Cushny, for example, still rejected secretion, and it wasn't until the second edition of that monograph in 1926 that he conceded that something of that nature had to occur. By this time, of course, Cushny had had access to the early pioneering studies of Wearn and Richards on filtration (71) and of Marshall and Vickers (38) on secretion. It must be added here that, for reasons unknown to us, Metzner's important contribution went all but unnoticed.[13] He received none of the credit that he undoubtedly deserved; this was subsequently accorded to others.

Development of Concepts After Carl Ludwig

Quantification of Glomerular Filtration Rate

By the 1860s Ludwig had developed an incomplete though, insofar as it had been formulated, correct concept of renal function. However, the next generation of researchers were unable, for the time being, to do much with it because the means for its experimental verification were still limited to measurements of blood pressure, renal blood and urine flow, and blood and urine composition. (Against this background, Richards's endeavors to develop micromethods for the direct investigation of nephron function cannot be too highly regarded. The outstanding contributions of Richards and his colleagues are the subject of the chapter by Windhager in this volume.)

The most acceptable component of Ludwig's theory of urine formation remained that of glomerular ultrafiltration, particularly in view of Starling's substantiation in the 1890s (64, 65). Because knowledge of its magnitude was clearly of decisive importance in the dispute over whether urine formation is a process of filtration and selective reabsorption or of secretion, it is not surprising that researchers began to look for ways to quantify the filtration rate by means of various urinary parameters.

Attempts to Measure Glomerular Filtration Rate by Blocking Reabsorption

By the turn of the century, many substances capable of increasing urine flow (and altering urine composition) were known to renal physiologists. These include the poisons sublimate ($HgCl_2$) and phlorizin and the poorly reabsorbable salts and sugars (osmotic diuretics). Two groups of experiments of this type are of historical interest.

In 1902 Galeotti (13) observed a massive increase in urine flow and the approach of urine composition toward that of plasma water in dogs chronically treated with sublimate. Because subsequent histological examination revealed essentially normal glomeruli but severely damaged tubules, he concluded that the composition and, in particular, the volume of excreted urine corresponded to that of the glomerular ultrafiltrate. This quite clever conceptual approach had to fail, as we know today, because of the considerable fall in glomerular filtration rate (GFR) under those conditions.

A second attempt along similar lines began from the following observations: in rising concentrations sulfates and phosphates (compared with NaCl) stimulate lymph flow as a consequence of their osmotic activity and thus their ability to draw water from tissues (32). In addition these poorly absorbable salts diminish water absorption from the intestine (8). These observations led other workers to examine the effect of these substances on urine flow (6, 18, 25), and it was Cushny (6) and Meyer and Halsey (see ref. 44) in particular who recognized the analogy between the diuretic effect and the diarrhea-promoting effect of these substances. Unfortunately these experiments, too, did not lead to the desired goal of quantifying GFR because it was not possible to achieve sufficiently high concentrations of the salts in plasma. However, this approach was not entirely fruitless because it led directly to the idea that the excretion rate of such substances might yield information on GFR.

Attempts to Measure GFR From the Excretion Rate of a Marker: Clearance Principle

On 9 July 1870, Adolf Fick, a former student and subsequently a close and lifelong friend of Carl Ludwig, read a paper to the Physikalisch-Medizinische Gesellschaft in Würzburg in which he described his principle for determining cardiac output (10). As far as can be established, Heidenhain was the first to apply this principle to the kidney. In 1883, in his article on urine formation in Hermann's *Handbuch der Physiologie* (24), he calculated the filtration rate required to account for the observed daily urea excretion (35 g) on the assumption that, as implied by Ludwig's theory, urea entered urine solely by filtration.[14] These considerations, the fact that urinary chromogens are highly concentrated during antidiuresis and poorly concentrated during diuresis, and the existence of such "osmotic diuretics" as the sulfates led Cushny to the idea that there may be substances that are filtered but not reabsorbed and thus are always present in urine. Cushny (7) rather confusingly and imprecisely termed them "no-threshold" substances, but it was realized that the excretion rate of such substances might be used to estimate GFR. The problem, how to find a nonreabsorbable marker for GFR without a reference substance that by definition had to be nonreabsorbable, must have been irritating. A partial solution was achieved with the realization that nonreabsorbed substances might be expected to have high urine-to-plasma (U/P) concentration ratios. Mayrs, working in Cushny's department in Edinburgh, eliminated urea from consideration by showing that it had a lower U/P ratio than sulfate, phosphate, or creatinine (39), a finding also very difficult to reconcile with Cushny's views on reabsorption. Although Mayrs clearly appreciated the criteria for a GFR marker (40), he unfortunately selected sulfate, which (unknown to him) did not meet these criteria.

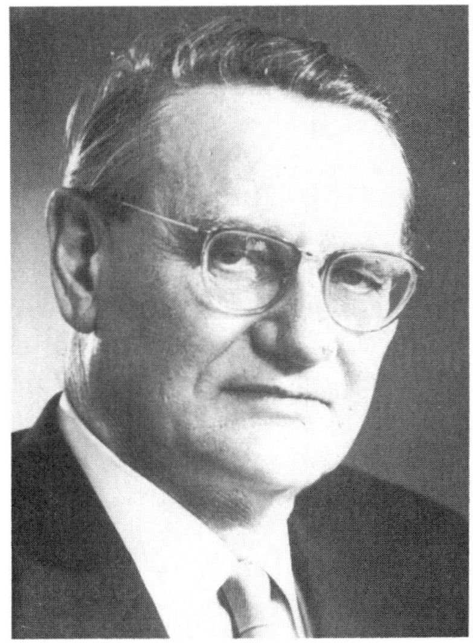

Figure 3. Poul Brandt Rehberg (1895–1985).

A turning point came in 1926 as a result of the investigations of the young Danish physiologist Poul Brandt Rehberg (Fig. 3). Born on the island of Fyn (Funen), Denmark, he graduated MSc from the University of Copenhagen in 1921 and was appointed to an Assistantship in August Krogh's zoophysiological laboratory at that University. In 1926 two papers appeared in *The Biochemical Journal* in which he published the results of the studies undertaken for his doctorate (50, 51). In these papers, remarkable for their perspicuity at a time when it must have been difficult to achieve any genuine overview of renal function, Rehberg analyzed the current hypotheses and, basically accepting Cushny's "modern theory," concluded that to be suitable GFR markers, genuine no-threshold substances must all be excreted with similar U/P ratios if their plasma concentrations were drastically raised by exogenous administration. In experiments on himself, he found that only creatinine had the required high U/P ratio and proposed creatinine clearance as a measure of GFR, which he calculated to be 100–150 ml/min. Thus it was Rehberg who was the first to become aware of the probable high rate of filtration and, consequently, reabsorption in the human kidney. Using this as a reference value, Rehberg then showed that some of Cushny's no-threshold substances were indeed reabsorbed, and thus in terms of quantifying GFR, the concept of threshold/no-threshold substances, as Cushny had conceived it, was as impracticable as the earlier approaches.

The search for the ideal marker was finally resolved in 1934 by a series of inspired experiments in two American laboratories. The problem of threshold/no-threshold substances was circumvented by examining substances foreign to the body and physiologically inert. In Philadelphia Richards et al. (56) had arrived at inulin, which was known to Richards from his student days with the bacteriologist Philip Hiss at Columbia. Of high molecular weight (~5,000) and thus poorly diffusible in biological membranes, inulin is not metabolized in the body. Using the micropuncture techniques systematically developed by him and his colleagues, Richards subsequently delivered the evidence that inulin fulfilled the criteria of a GFR marker (55). In Homer W. Smith's Laboratory in New York, James A. Shannon (62) arrived at the same conclusion after working through a series of unmetabolized sugars. With the advent of inulin, an unequivocal and exact method was available to measure GFR, and thus the road was open to investigate the dynamics of the process of glomerular filtration. Notwithstanding this, Rehberg's introduction of creatinine clearance as an index of GFR remains a landmark, and the continued use of creatinine clearance today, particularly in clinical medicine and research, bears testimony to this man's contribution.

Dynamics of Glomerular Filtration: Pressures and Resistances

As described in Dynamics of Glomerular Filtration, p. 34, in the course of his model investigations into glomerular filtration, Carl Ludwig had also carried out studies into the dynamics of the process. He had clearly recognized that renal blood flow and glomerular filtration had to be related to each other because the afferent and efferent arteriolar flow resistances play central roles in both phenomena. He had even speculated that regulation of these resistances could render GFR and renal blood flow independent of change in systemic arterial pressure (36).

Glomerular Capillary Pressure

In the context of his views on the formation of urine, Ludwig and his students, particularly Goll (14) and Hermann (26), had carried out studies on the dependency of urine production on arterial and venous blood pressure and on renal blood flow and ureter pressure. These experiments were of limited heuristic value partly because of the incompleteness of the concept, as far as reabsorption was concerned, and partly because experiments with Ludwig's *Stromuhr* (flowmeter) were vulnerable to criticism because of the necessary transection of the renal vessels and hence the renal nerves. Claude Bernard had assumed that renal nerves regulated both renal blood flow and tubular activity, as in the salivary glands. Thus it is probably understandable that researchers turned primarily to experiments in which glomerular capillary pressure could be measured, but not the relationship between renal blood flow and glomerular capillary pressure, which doubtlessly would have led sooner to the understanding of the glomerular filtration process. Two experimental approaches were adopted: *1*) what was the maximum spontaneously achieved ureter pressure at which urine production just stopped[15] and *2*) what was the minimum arterial blood pressure at which urine production, and thus filtration, just continued[16]? Even before the turn of the century, both experimental approaches yielded values of glomerular capillary pressure remarkably close to modern direct measurements.

Based on these experiments, the glomerular capillary pressure in canine kidneys was initially estimated to be ~80 mmHg, an estimate subsequently adjusted to two-thirds of the mean aortic pressure. However, despite these sophisticated and extensive experiments, the approach was not altogether satisfactory because of the extreme experimental conditions and the unavoidable interference with the parameter under investigation. It was thus obvious that a further method had to be sought, with which glomerular capillary pressure could be estimated under undisturbed filtration conditions. This was achieved in the 1950s in an ingenious indirect approach by John Pappenheimer and colleagues (49), who used the molecular-sieving theory. Based on investigations in muscle capillaries and assuming, as Ludwig had postulated, that filtration occurred through pores, Pappenheimer calculated from the clearance relationships of myoglobin, egg albumin, creatinine, and hemoglobin that these hypothetical pores had a radius of 35–40 Å. Applying Poiseuille's law and assuming a value for the filtration-barrier thickness, a filtration coefficient was calculated. From this value and knowing (or assuming) GFR, filtration fraction, and plasma protein concentration, a hydrostatic pressure gradient of 20 mmHg can be calculated to be necessary to overcome the resistance to flow through the filtration barrier. Taking the mean glomerular capillary oncotic pressure and the presence in Bowman's capsule into account, a glomerular capillary pressure of about 60–80 mmHg can be finally calculated. Direct measurement of this parameter remains a problem today. Although the first direct measurements were made by Richard's colleagues Hayman (23) and White (72) in the 1920s in amphibia, it was not until about forty years later that similar measurements could be made in mammals; Brenner and co-workers (3) then successfully employed the servonulling apparatus of Wiederhielm et al. (73) in a mutant strain of rat (the Munich-Wistar rat) with glomeruli frequently accessible from the renal surface. Although measurements with this technique in dogs (access to glomeruli was gained surgically) yielded values of 56–61 mmHg, which is consistent with the estimates of Pappenheimer, it appears that considerable variability exists among strains and species, and in those animals in which no direct measurements have been made, the issue must still be regarded as open.

Pre- and Postglomerular Flow Resistance

Given a value for glomerular capillary pressure, the pressure profile along the renal vascular bed can be estimated, and assuming blood flow values, resistance to flow in the various vascular segments can be quantified. Indeed it was Ludwig who carried out the first attempts in this field by measuring renal venous blood flow with his *Stromuhr*. However, he failed to pursue these experiments, presumably for the reasons mentioned in the previous section. Until the turn of the century, many different means other than the *Stromuhr* had been tried. Ludwig had already carried out the first experiments with the isolated perfused kidney—for colloid in his perfusion solution he had used gum arabic! Defibrinated blood or blood to which an extract of leeches (heparin!) had been added was used. To maintain oxygenation, the isolated pulmonary circuit was used. In 1883 Cohnheim (another former Ludwig colleague) and Roy (5) introduced the oncometer, a form of plethysmograph, to gain an index of renal blood flow, and of course, blood flow had been measured directly by intermittent collection of the renal venous effluent or by measuring the linear velocity through a vessel of known cross-sectional area. In essence these procedures all delivered similar information: that renal blood flow was extremely high; estimates for humans ranged from 300 to 2,000 liters/day. Clarity was finally achieved with the invention of the *Thermostromuhr* (1927–1929) by the physiologist Hermann Rein (52), then in Freiburg and subsequently in Göttingen. With this instrument an accurate, continuous record of absolute mean flow in an unopened blood vessel was obtained for the first time. Due to the highly favorable frequency response of the instrument, rapid regulatory adjustments of blood flow could be readily resolved and thus the way was open for a thorough investigation of the relationships between arterial pressure, renal blood flow, and GFR. Given that the original intellectual impulse was Ludwig's, it is beyond the scope of this chapter to trace in detail the subsequent development in this area. Suffice it to say that the "missing" parameter, the directly measured glomerular capillary pressure, meant that the calculations of arteriolar resistances remained rather speculative. Subsequent to the introduction of the servonulling device (see the previous section), the literature has expanded explosively, and the matter continues to be one of intense scientific interest. For a more detailed summary of this literature, the reader is referred to the excellent review of Arendshorst and Gottschalk (1).

Autoregulation

The concept of renal autoregulation developed gradually over sixty years or more. Although Ludwig had to be content with pure speculation on the regulation of the afferent and efferent arteriolar resistances, Cohnheim and Roy's oncometer (5) had provided the first concrete evidence well before the turn of the century. These experiments showed that renal volume remained initially constant with increasing blood pressure. Even Metzner (44) remarked on the independence of renal vascular tone from systemic vascular tone.

In 1911 Burton-Opitz and Lucas (4) apparently made the first direct observation of the constancy of renal blood flow when arterial blood pressure was raised by stimulation of the splanchnic nerves. Similar observations were made thirteen years later in Dublin by O'Connor (46), who in addition raised blood pressure by catecholamine injection. Although O'Connor's findings are not easy to interpret, he was sufficiently prescient to repeat his initial findings in animals in which the kidneys were denervated and the adrenals ligated. He was thus certain that the pressure independency he had observed was an intrarenal mechanism. In a series of publications of Rein and colleagues in the 1930s (22, 48, 53, 54), in which the constancy of renal blood flow despite pressure changes in the presence or absence of the renal nerves was confirmed, Rein left no doubt that he considered this to be an autonomous (i.e., intrarenal) mechanism.

At about the same time (the early 1930s) Medes and co-workers (41, 42) used Rein's *Thermostromuhr* simultaneously with Rehberg's creatinine clearance and showed that GFR and renal blood flow generally move parallel to each other and that the "autonomous blood flow regulation" renders not only blood flow but also GFR independent of systemic blood pressure variations. This finding was confirmed in 1947 by Forster and Maes (12) in denervated kidneys in animals with demedullated adrenals.

Until this time there had been no reason to seriously consider, insofar as the issue had ever arisen, that renal blood flow was anything other than uniformly distributed throughout the renal parenchyma. The first inklings that this might not be the case came as a consequence of studies of the function of the renal medulla (see the next section).

Intrarenal Regulatory Mechanisms

Tubuloglomerular Feedback Mechanism

The above findings of autoregulatory phenomena (see the previous section), made possible by the introduction of the *Thermostromuhr* and creatinine clearance, required substantial supplementation of Ludwig's concept for their explanation. It fell to the Belgian pathologist Norbert Goormaghtigh (Fig. 4) to recognize the critical relationships, or at least to foresee them, because the definitive experiments were not to be made for another thirty years or more.

Norbert Goormaghtigh, whose name is as intimately associated with the juxtaglomerular apparatus (JGA) as with the University of

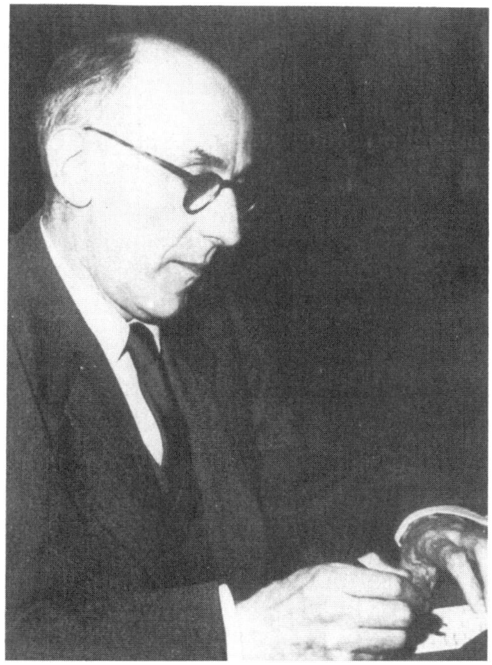

Figure 4. Norbert Goormaghtigh (1890–1960).

Ghent, was born in Ostende, Belgium. A brilliant student, at age twenty-three he qualified as a medical practitioner in 1913 and immediately turned to research in two areas that remained lifelong interests: carcinogenesis and the adrenal gland. After World War I, he returned to Ghent and was awarded his doctorate for a thesis entitled "La cortex surrénale humaine dans les plaies de l'abdomen et aux périodes intéressantes de la vie sexuelle." His appointment to the Chair of Morbid Anatomy at Ghent saw him, as one obituary in 1969 put it, as the inheritor of an excellent library and several good quality microscopes but no laboratory, no refrigeration, no modern autopsy room, and no animal house. However, the record of his publications shows little evidence of these shortcomings. His interests in the physiology and pathology of the endocrine system slowly gained the upper hand, as studies on the adrenals, the reproductive system, insulin, and arterial hypertension show. This last theme recurred consistently throughout Goormaghtigh's entire scientific career and, with the renal-adrenal-hypothalamic "axis," was undoubtedly the background against which he viewed his findings in the JGA. The two productive decades of the 1920s and 1930s came to an abrupt halt with the start of World War II. Despite conditions in occupied Belgium and considerable anxiety for the personal safety of his family, he continued to work and publish as best he could.

After the war he felt himself called upon to accept a number of administrative posts, culminating in the Rectorship of the University of Ghent during 1949–1950, at the price of continued interruption to his research and disturbance to his health. He died in Laethem-Saint-Martin, near Ghent, Belgium, in 1960 in his seventieth year.

The idea that a vascular bed might react to an increase in perfusion pressure by increasing its flow resistance was not new. In 1902 W. M. Bayliss (2), at University College, London, had ascribed this reaction (albeit without unequivocal evidence) to intrinsic properties of smooth muscle cells. What was surprising in the case of the kidney was the extent of this reaction. In subsequent years the role of vascular nerves was examined in this context; it was finally suggested that this phenomenon in mammalian kidneys may be explained by the process of glomerular recruitment, which was thought to occur in the amphibian kidney! Goormaghtigh was intrigued by earlier findings of the anatomist Karl Peter (49a). In his celebrated study on renal anatomy published in 1909, Peter had noted that the ascending limb of the loop of Henle invariably made contact with the vascular pole of its parent glomerulus. In 1925 the Amsterdam anatomist J. H. C. Ruyter (57) described large, granulated "epithelioid" cells in the walls of the afferent arteriole just prior to its entry into the glomerulus, and suggested (albeit very hesitantly) that this structure may in some way regulate blood flow. Strangely, as he remarked, he was able to find these cells only in mice and rats, that is, in no other species. Two years later, in a very brief communication (with no illustrations), Oberling (45) also reported a distinct group of cells at the same site, this time in the human kidney. Recognizing the potential importance of the structure, Goormaghtigh (15) reinvestigated the juxtaglomerular region in cats and humans and confirmed the presence of large, granular cells in the wall of the afferent arteriole that he termed *afibrillar* cells; this generated some confusion because Ruyter (57) had particularly remarked on the presence of myofibrils, the number of which was inversely related to the degree of granulation and from which he correctly inferred the origin of the granular cell. Goormaghtigh also described a second population of small cells, lacis cells, in the angle between the afferent and efferent arterioles; these cells had not previously been described and now bear his name. In addition he described the rich innervation of the structure.

These observations led him to a number of speculations on the function of this complex. He considered the granular cells as some form of sensory receptor, the "metabolism" of which was regulated by blood chemistry or blood pressure and which in turn, through a nervous reflex, regulated arteriolar tone. The mechanism thus regulated blood flow to the glomerulus, protecting it, as he put it, from toxic substances in the blood and particularly from raised blood pressure. In the concept of the metabolic influence of granular cells on nerve endings, an endocrine, or more accurately paracrine, element can already be recognized.

In 1933 Zimmermann (75) described the characteristic form of tubular cells in that portion of the thick ascending limb of the loop of Henle that makes contact with the vascular pole of the glomerulus; he coined for them the name *macula densa.* Goormaghtigh (16) incorporated this tubular element into his hypothesis in 1937, regarding it as a further component of the JGA. With regard to its role, he wrote:

Since the cells of these plaques [i.e., macula densa] *are in no way related to the capillaries, their function is different from the other elements of the nephron. Taking into account our interpretation of the function of the tissue complex at the vascular pole in the kidney, this structure . . . might communicate the events in the corresponding tubular segment to the intraglomerular circulation. In this context, this group of epithelial cells may be regarded as a sensory plaque, placed downstream from the most important functional segment of the nephron, thus resulting in the possibility of an automatic regulation of the glomerular circulation, controlled either by the "emptiness" or "fullness" of the intercalated segment or by the physico-chemical composition of the passing urine.*[17]

In a series of experiments in the following years, Goormaghtigh noted hypertrophy and hyperplasia of granular cells under a variety of conditions, including chronic administration of vitamin D_2, eclampsia, essential hypertension, acute or chronic experimental hypertension, and in renal ischemia induced by partial renal artery occlusion by unilateral application of a Goldblatt clip. Goormaghtigh had been well acquainted with endocrine cells and processes from his earlier work, and these observations led him to amend his hypothesis (17) in 1939 in that he explicitly conceived of the granular cells as being endocrine cells containing a hypertensive principle that he thought was probably renin, which had been discovered at the turn of the century by the well-known Finnish physiologist and former Ludwig student, Robert Tigerstedt. Thus by 1939 Goormaghtigh had completed, as far as a morphologist was able, his concept of the functional role of the JGA. This concept is all the more remarkable because it was built on conclusions reached solely by intellectual analysis of structural relationships. The fact that Goormaghtigh promoted this concept with all consequence for years thereafter, despite other interests and duties and the fact that as a pathologist he had practically no opportunity for its direct experimental verification, suggest that he was well aware that the JGA was an important connecting link between tubular and glomerular function and between salt and water balance and blood pressure regulation.

During the next twenty-five years, the physiological implications of Goormaghtigh's ideas, although not forgotten, were not systematically followed up. Two causes, apart from the obvious interruption and consequences occasioned by the outbreak of World War II, lay at the root of this delay. First, the famous "Goldblatt experiment," in which this juxtaglomerular structure and the intrarenal renin-angiotensin system were stimulated and systemic blood pressure was elevated, led to pathophysiological considerations being uppermost in the minds of many researchers, and the question of the renal physiological role was somewhat submerged by the clinical relevance of these findings. Second, there was no adequate methodological access to this structure in which vascular and tubular elements were united and present, as it were, in every nephron.

In the early 1960s, however, changing circumstances led to the renascence of Goormaghtigh's ideas. In those years two phenomena were the center of attention in many laboratories, namely, the autoregulation of renal blood flow and GFR and the balance between filtration rate and tubular volume reabsorption. In addition the spread and development of micropuncture in the late 1950s had given physiologists a powerful tool with which to approach these problems at the individual-nephron level. In light of mounting information on volume reabsorption and its dependency on tubular cell metabolism, autoregulation appeared more as an integrated part of a tubuloglomerular balance than as an isolated phenomenon. Thus in these years two hypotheses attempting to account for the intrarenal mechanisms of autoregulation of renal blood flow and GFR were put forward, one by Thurau (67) at the Second International Congress of Nephrology (1963) in Prague and the other by Guyton (20). The hypotheses had one feature in common; namely, they both incorporated a negative-feedback loop at the JGA so that a rise in renal perfusion pressure, followed initially by a rise in GFR and tubular flow rate, led subsequently to a change in the physicochemical characteristics of the tubular fluid in the macula densa segment. This change was, as Goormaghtigh had suggested, detected by the macula densa, transduced in some manner within the JGA complex, and finally resulted in a decrease of GFR, thus reestablishing the filtration rate existing prior to the increase in blood pressure. The two hypotheses conflicted, however, on a number of substantial points such as the nature of the detected signal and the nature of the vasoactive response. On the basis of a computer model, Guyton suggested that the signal was a fall in tubular fluid osmolarity. Thurau, on the other hand, proposed that an increased intratubular flow rate, resulting from the rise in GFR, was translated by the reabsorptive characteristics of the thick ascending limb into an elevated NaCl concentration at the macula densa; this then served as the signal for the local activation of the renin-angiotensin system in the JGA and subsequent afferent arteriolar vasoconstriction. The idea of a flow-dependent NaCl-concentration signal at the macula densa was at that time by no means unrealistic because micropuncture studies had just revealed the early distal NaCl concentration to be quite low, which suggested that the thick ascending limb reabsorbed more salt than water. The actively lowered NaCl concentration immediately offered itself as the flow-dependent signal for a tubuloglomerular feedback. Although Guyton's idea was not subjected to experimental examination until some years later, Thurau soon delivered the first evidence for his hypothesis by means of a simple experiment. He hypothesized that if a rise in the NaCl concentration in tubular fluid at the macula densa were to lead to a drastic fall in filtration, this should be reflected in a simultaneous reduction in proximal tubular diameter. The first experiment took place on 28 February 1964 during a stay in Carl Gottschalk's laboratory in Chapel Hill and clearly showed that retrograde injection of 150 mM NaCl from an early distal puncture site to the macula densa led, within seconds, to a reduction of proximal tubular diameter. Isotonic mannitol solution injected in the same fashion had no effect.

In a series of sophisticated studies begun in 1965 (see ref. 59), Jürgen Schnermann and colleagues in Thurau's laboratory subsequently succeeded in giving this concept a solid and convincing experimental foundation. Thus the concept of a tubuloglomerular feedback regulation of GFR emerged, a mechanism adjusting GFR (in effect) to the reabsorptive capacity of the nephron. Constancy of GFR with increasing blood pressure thus appeared to be a consequence of a constant reabsorptive capacity of the tubular epithelium. Despite the mass of evidence accumulated in the intervening twenty years, it is probably not an exaggeration to say that much of it is unavoidably circumstantial or inferential due to the inaccessability of the JGA to direct investigation. Also, final solutions to aspects that are still unclear—the precise nature of the tubular signal and its detection by the macula densa, the detailed nature of transduction within the JGA, and the mediation of the vasoactive response—will most likely have to wait for new methodological or theoretical impulses.

Regional Distribution of Renal Blood Flow

As noted previously there had been no serious reason to doubt the homogeneity of intrarenal blood flow distribution until the 1940s. However, this situation changed substantially in the following two decades. In 1942 and again in 1951, the Swiss physical chemist Werner Kuhn and colleagues (21, 30) proposed that the structures of the renal medulla constitute a countercurrent system that could account for the osmotic concentration of urine. The possibilities of this proposal were immediately recognised by the young physiologist Heinrich Wirz, then recently returned to Basel from a stay in Homer

Smith's New York laboratory. Together with Kuhn and Hargitay (a student), Wirz (74) presented the first experimental evidence for this mechanism in 1951. Although championed vigorously by Wirz for the remainder of that decade, general acceptance of the idea was slow to come. One exception was the response of the group of young workers in the Göttingen laboratory of Kurt Kramer, who from the middle 1950s on amassed much evidence in support of this hypothesis. It was Kramer (Fig. 5), a circulatory physiologist of note and a former student of Hermann Rein (and practically the latter's successor to the Chair of Physiology at Göttingen), who recognized the special demands that such a mechanism must make on its blood circulation in supplying the metabolic needs of the tissue, carrying away excess solute and water, and yet not washing out the osmotic gradient. He thus hypothesized that medullary circulation must be qualitatively and quantitatively different from that in the renal cortex. Certainly this idea was justified by the unique vascular anatomy of the medulla, with its long, hair pin–looped vasa recta running parallel to the loops of Henle and with its entire blood flow derived exclusively from the efferent arterioles of the small population of juxtamedullary glomeruli. The idea that cortical and medullary circulations were functionally different was not new to Kramer. Some years earlier he had devoted a major study (28) to the experimental examination of the proposal of Trueta et al. (69) (then warmly debated) that medullary circulation acted as a shunt for renal circulation under certain circumstances. Although this concept proved incorrect, it certainly served to stimulate awareness of the unique nature of medullary circulation. In a series of studies over a period

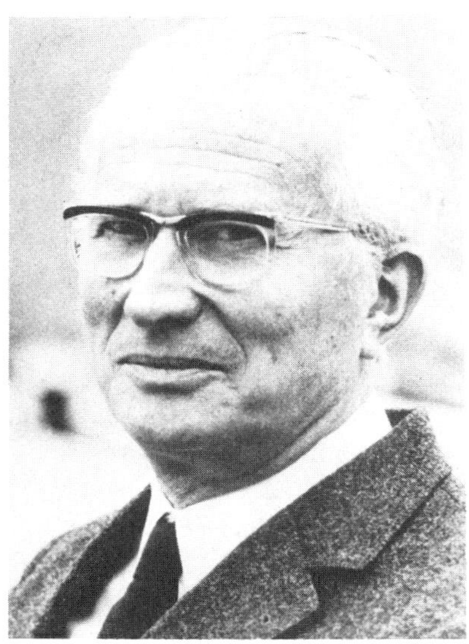

Figure 5. Kurt Kramer (1906–1985).

of years, Kramer and his associates (9, 29, 43, 68) employed an ingenious instrument, the origins of which lay in the noninvasive photoelectric oximeter that Kramer had developed in the 1930s. Now, with the assistance of his subsequently long-serving technician Heinz Brechtelsbauer, this device was modified to record dye-dilution curves of Evans blue or indocyanine green at various depths of the cortex and medulla, from which the various circulatory parameters could be calculated. They noted a much-prolonged mean transit time for blood flowing through the medulla, compared with that in the cortex, and quantified, for the first time, the relatively low medullary blood flow. Similar conclusions were reached in Washington at much the same time by Lawrence Lilienfeld et al. (31), who used the accumulation of radiolabeled albumin as an index of medullary blood flow. These findings not only demonstrated the heterogeneity of intrarenal blood flow distribution but also established a new, important functional role for renal blood flow that is distinctly different from that conceived by Ludwig. In subsequent years much interest has been devoted to the possibility that alterations in intrarenal blood flow distribution might be physiologically important. However, as Ofstad and Aukland (47) recently noted, the methods available to date are not yet adequate to confirm the existence of such a phenomenon, let alone to decide its physiological significance.

Epilogue

This brief survey, which was intended to be a treatment of the knowledge and ideas of the most influential researchers in the field of renal blood flow and the dynamics of glomerular filtration, has become, *peu á peu*, more of a history of the development of this topic. Perhaps this was inherently unavoidable; two reasons may be offered. First, notwithstanding our proposition that our present-day concepts of this subject correspond largely to those of Ludwig and Goormaghtigh, even those workers did not develop their hypotheses in vacuo. Both drew heavily on the pre- and coexisting ideas and observations of other scientists; indeed as has been shown, through continual contact, communication, and exchange with their scientific contemporaries, they continued to develop and amend their theories throughout their entire careers, as is characteristic of genuine scientists. Moreover these hypotheses would never have achieved the validity they enjoy today had it not been for the numerous other workers who devised methods and instruments allowing these hypotheses to be examined in all detail: methods and instruments to which Ludwig and Goormaghtigh never had access. Thus our present-day concepts of renal blood flow and glomerular filtration dynamics are not only those of Carl Ludwig and Norbert Goormaghtigh but are also the product of a historical development. Second, despite the many new areas of physiological research, the hypotheses of Ludwig and Goormaghtigh remain the subject of intense scientific interest because they still contain purely descriptive and speculative elements. Such problems we mention only briefly. We accept today that the glomerular filtration rate is mainly regulated by variation of pre- and postglomerular flow resistances. How and to what extent the two resistances cooperate in this regulation is still a subject of scientific discussion. Only when techniques become available that allow the continuous and simultaneous recording of glomerular capillary pressure, glomerular plasma flow, and filtration rate in the same nephron, without the interruption of the tubulo-glomerular feedback control loop, will it be possible to settle this question. A further question of considerable interest is the variability of the resistance against which filtration takes place, that is, the virtual K_f. In recent years it has been shown that this parameter is influenced by various hormone systems and that it appears to be a function of the glomerular plasma flow itself. Although much has been learned about the structural organization of the glomerular filtering membrane, the mechanisms underlying these phenomena are totally unclear. Ludwig, for instance, discussed the possibility of interactions between the ultrafiltrate and the ultrafilter; these interactions take the form of solute polarization, alterations at the pore openings, and solute-filter interaction within the pores themselves. Furthermore, on the basis of his model experiments, he envisaged a nonlinear relationship between pressure and filtration rate. Interestingly, recent results of the Australian anatomist Graeme Ryan prompted speculative explanations very much in the spirit of Ludwig's ideas (58). Fixing superficial glomeruli in situ, that is, with blood flow and filtration persisting up to the instant of fixation, Ryan was able to show that albumin does not penetrate the filtering membrane at all, but is held up at the endothelial fenestrae. This contrasts with earlier observations in kidneys fixed after nephrectomy (i.e., with no blood flow or filtration), which showed molecules the size of albumin and even larger penetrating the filter and held back only by the slit diaphragm. Thus, as predicted by Ludwig, the functional characteristics of the filtration barrier depend on glomerular blood flow and filtration.

With respect to the intrarenal mechanisms controlling blood flow and filtration rate, the uncertainties are even greater. Although it appears certain that the enzyme renin and the local production of vasoactive angiotensin II at the JGA are involved in the regulation process, exactly how they are involved and what the other components of the regulatory mechanism(s) are remain to be established. Given the structural complexity of the JGA, it will not be surprising if the regulatory mechanism turns out to be rather complex. The JGA "classically" consists of three cell types: the macula densa cells, the circumjacent lacis or Goormaghtigh cells, and the renin-containing (granular) myoepithelial cells in the arteriolar wall. In addition two further cell types may well be intimately involved with JGA function: the peripolar cells, apparently in free communication with Bowman's space, and the mesangial cells. Our knowledge of the functional characteristics of these five cell types is, at best, exiguous and fragmentary. The macula densa cells appear to have much lower levels of Na^+-K^+-ATPase than do other cell types. The Goormaghtigh, mesangial, and granular cells all have intracellular myofibrils. These three cell types appear to be extensively linked by gap junctions and thus represent a functional syncytium. The functional significance of these findings is unknown. Although there is good evidence that these structures function together as a paracrine system strongly influencing GFR and blood flow, there is newer evidence that this function may itself be modulated by products from endothelial cells and by sympathetic nerve activity. In addition there is also evidence of unknown, intracellular effects of renin.

The extent of our ignorance and the complexity of the biochemical and biophysical processes in this system is, in a certain sense, comparable to the circumstances under which Ludwig proposed his revolutionary hypothesis of urine formation, although, of course, it is not for a moment suggested that the overall scientific moment of the two situations is in the least comparable. Nevertheless, before a scientist of our time would attempt to publish such an innovative and daring hypothesis, he or she would most likely (given the more empirical and pragmatic approach to science today) first seek much more information and data and second devote time to the development of techniques that would enable him or her to make the necessary observations. Moreover the available technical potential and the willingness and availability of colleagues to join in the investigation of the problem are certainly most important criteria for the success of such a plan. In other words the process has gained a substantial component of scientific management, or as Peter Medawar (41a) put it, the practicability of the project is decisive. The ability to assess this correctly is certainly one of the most important requirements of the modern scientist.

We are deeply indebted to our teacher Kurt Kramer (1906–1985), to whom this chapter is dedicated.

NOTES

1 *Über Francis Bacon von Verulam und seine Methode der Naturforschung* (Munich 1863).

2 Ludwig defines the elementary components of which all living organisms are composed as atoms, electricity, and the luminiferous ether with which he also equates warmth.

3 "*Dieser Erfahrung entsprechend zieht man den Schluss, dass alle vom thierischen Körper ausgehenden Erscheinungen eine Folge der einfachen Anziehungen und Abstossungen* (einer begrenzten Anzahl chemischer Atome)

sein möchten, welche an jenen elementaren Wesen bei einem Zusammentreffen derselben beobachtet werden. Diese Folgerung wird unumstösslich, wenn es gelingt mit mathematischer Schärfe nachzuweisen, es seien die erwähnten elementaren Bedingungen nach Richtung, Zeit und Masse im thierischen Körper derartig geordnet, dass aus ihren Gegenwirkungen mit Nothwendigkeit alle Leistungen des lebenden und todten Organismus herfliessen" (ref. 35, p. 2).

[4] *"Nach der einen Gruppe der Hypothesen, liegt den geistigen Funktionen eine besondere Substanz, die Seele, zu Grunde, welche dem Lichtäther ähnlich, zwischen den wägbaren Massen der Hirnsubstanz schwebt. . . . Die Anhänger der zahllosen Abstufungen realistischer Weltanschauung haben sich, insofern sie sich überhaupt zur Bildung einer Vorstellung entschliessen konnten, darüber geeinigt, dass die Seelenerscheinungen resultieren aus einer gewissen Summe im Hirn und Blut enthaltener Bedingungen, weil mit dem Entstehen, der Entwicklung und dem Vergehen des Hirns und mit dem Wechsel in der Blutzusammensetzung Verstand, Empfindung und Wille kommen, schwinden oder sich ändern. Wer den Schluss aus Analogien gelten lässt uind durch seine Kenntnisse befähigt ist zu gründlichen Vergleichungen der Seelenerscheinungen mit den übrigen Naturereignissen, wird, wenn er wählen muss, nicht zweifelhaft sein, welcher von beiden Meinungen er zustimmen soll"* (ref. 35, p. 452).

[5] *"Wer aber einen unumstösslichen Beweis für eine der beiden Anschauungen verlangt, wird eingestehen, dass er noch nicht geliefert sei"* (ref. 35, p. 452).

[6] The principle prerequisite for appointment to the permanent staff of a German university as a lecturer ("Privat-Dozent") was the preparation, submission, and publication of a substantial dissertation, which was subject to adjudication by scientific peers.

[7] *"Eiweissstoffe haben zum Wasser und zu vielen wässerigen Lösungen (und zum Theil auch zu Fetten) eine grosse Adhäsionsverwandtschaft"* (ref. 35, p. 45).

[8] *"durchbrechen auch die unverletzte Gefässwand. Diesem Vorgang, den mal als Absonderung (secretio) bezeichnet, steht ein anderer, die Aufsaugung (resorptio) entgegen"* (ref. 36, p. 141).

[9] *"Alia opinio quae adhuc probatur, docet, renes ipsos attractione ad uream esse instructos, hancque in transitu aquam et substantias seri aqua solutas, excepto albumine et sapone secum ferre. Haec sententia, profecta ex philosophia illa naturali aut doctrina etiam miseriori, ea sola de causa sectatores invenit, guod nunguam examini est subjecta. Ut omittamus tali attractione, nisi corpore proteini et sapones omnio repelluntur, quia alioquin albumen solutum etc. pariter ac salia soluta traductum iri, absentiam albuminis in urina explicari non posse; ridiculum est, statuere, corpus corpore attrahi ut statim reddatur, quin alio processu affinitatis separetur, id quod in renibus fit"* (ref. 34, p. 15).

[10] *"Somit bleibt unter Aufrechterhaltung der anderen Bedingungen entweder nur übrig, eine besondere Struktur in der Kanälchenwandung anzunehmen, die die Diffusionsgeschwindigkeit herabsetzt, oder zu unterstellen, daß das NaCl unter Umständen durch eine der chemischen analoge Kraft in das Blut zurückgenommen werde."* (ref. 37, p. 428).

[11] *"Die hypothetische Annahme Ludwigs, das Glomerulusfiltrat werde auf seinem Wege durch die Harnkanälchen durch Wasserresorption konzentriert,*

hat durch die neueren Untersuchungen eine starke Stütze erhalten. Eine einfache Diffusion ist dabei allerdings nur zum geringsten Teile im Spiele, es muß dafür eine aktive Tätigkeit der Epithelien in den Henleschen Schleifen, in den Tub. contort. und wohl auch in den Sammelröhren in Anspruch genommen werden, zumal da mit dieser Wasserentziehung eine auswählende Rückresorption gelöster Bestandteile verbunden ist, wobei zum Teil das Bedürfnis des Organismus entscheidet; daraus ergibt sich aber, daß beide Funktionen bis zu einem gewissen Grade unabhängig voneinander verlaufen können. Harnsäure, Phosphorsäure und blutfremde Stoffe werden in den Harnkanälchen. . . . . durch echte Sekretion abgeschieden Die Niere . . . Lat die Fähigkeit, blutfremde Stoffe aus ihren Komponenten aufzubauen (Hippursäuresynthese)" (ref. 44, p. 291–292).

[12] *"Ein schroffer Gegensatz zwischen Ludwigscher und Bowman-Heidenhainscher Theorie besteht nicht; Ludwig hat nie die sekretorische Tätigkeit der Nierenepithelien in bezug auf Abscheidung der Harnsäure usw. geleugnet, Heidenhain sich ebenfalls nicht durchaus ablehnend gegen das Bestehen einer Rückresorption verhalten. Die Einwände Heindenhains gegen das Bestehen eioner Glomerulusfiltration haben sich allerdings nicht als stichhaltig erwiesen"* (ref. 44, p. 292).

[13] The article, cited in passing by Cushny (7) and Marshall and Vickers (38), was the subject of a short study by Kenney (27). As far as can be ascertained, the article has not been cited elsewhere.

[14] He calculated a GFR of 70 liters/day, which in view of his estimate of renal blood flow of 123 liters/day would have meant an impossible increase in hematocrit and which he thus rejected as being ridiculous. This was a substantial component of his argument against filtration.

[15] The first measurement of this pressure was 7–10 mmHg, reported by Loebell (33), a student of Ludwig's. Hermann (26), similarly a student of Ludwig's, later measured values of ~40 mmHg. Heidenhain (24) reported a maximum of 63 mmHg at an arterial blood pressure of 100–105 mmHg, a value consistent with that of Starling (64), who found a value 32 mmHg below aortic pressure.

[16] Measurements of Goll (14), Ustimowitsch (70), and von Schröder (60), all students of Ludwig, showed that urine production just continued at an aortic pressure of 40 mmHg; Grützner (19) measured ~30 mmHg. Because, according to Wundt (cited in ref. 66), these values had to be reduced by 20% to account for the pressure drop across the preglomerular resistance, one arrives at pressures of 24–32 mmHg, values closely resembling those of the plasma oncotic pressure measured by Starling (63).

[17] *"Puisque les cellules de ces plaques . . . n'ont aucun rapport avec les capillaires, leur fonction est distincte des autres éléments du tube. Compte tenu de notre interprétation de la fonction du complexe tissulaire du pôle vasculaire du rein, le dispositif anatomique . . . permet éventuellement á la circulation intra-glomérulaire d'être renseignée sur ce qui se passe dans le tube correspondant. Dans cette éventualité le groupe de cellules épithéliales envisagé ici aura la valeur d'une plaque sensorielle placée en aval des segments fonctionnels les plus importants du nephron: d'où la possibilité d'un réglage automatique de la circulation glomérulaire commandé soit par l'état de vacuité ou de plénitude du segment intercalaire soit par l'état physico-chimique de l'urine qui y passe"* (16).

BIBLIOGRAPHY

1. Arendshorst, W. J., and C. W. Gottschalk. Glomerular ultrafiltration dynamics: historical perspective. *Am. J. Physiol.* 248 (*Renal Fluid Electrolyte Physiol.* 17): F163–F174, 1985.
2. Bayliss, W. M. On the local reactions of the arterial wall to changes of internal pressure. *J. Physiol. Lond.* 28: 220–231, 1902.
3. Brenner, B. M., J. L. Troy, and T. M. Daugharty. The dynamics of glomerular ultrafiltration in the rat. *J. Clin. Invest.* 50: 1776–1780, 1971.
4. Burton-Opitz, R., and D. Lucas. The blood supply of the kidney. V. The influence of the vagus nerve upon the vascularity of the left organ. *J. Exp. Med.* 13: 308–313, 1911.
5. Cohnheim, J., and C. S. Roy. Untersuchungen über die Cirkulation in den Nieren. *Virchows Arch. Pathol. Anat. Physiol. Klin. Med.* 92: 424–448, 1883.
6. Cushny, A. R. On diuresis and the permeability of the renal cells. *J. Physiol. Lond.* 27: 429–450, 1902.
7. Cushny, A. R. *The Secretion of the Urine*, 2nd ed. London: Longmans, Green, 1926.
8. Cushny, A. R., and G. B. Wallace. Über Darmresorption und die salinischen Abfuhrmittel. *Pfluegers Arch. Gesamte Physiol. Menschen Tiere* 77: 202–209, 1899.
9. Deetjen, P., H. Brechtelsbauer, and K. Kramer. Hämodynamik des Nierenmarks. III. Mitteilung. Farbstoffpassagezeiten in äussere Markzone und V. Renalis. Die Durchblutungsverteilung in der Niere. *Pfluegers Arch. Gesamte Physiol. Menschen Tiere* 297: 281–293, 1964.
10. Fick, A. Über die Messung des Blutquantums in den Herzventrikoln. In: *Verhandlungen der Physitalisch-Medizinischen Gesellschaft in Würzburg*. Würzburg, Germany: Stahel, 1872. (Neve Folge. Bana II, Sitzung am 9 Juli, 1870.)
11. Fischer, I. *Biographisches Lexikon hervorragender Ärzte (1880–1930)*, 3rd ed. Munich, FRG: Urban & Schwarzenberg, 1962, vol. 2, p. 1031.
12. Forster, R. P., and J. P. Maes. Effect of experimental neurogenic hypertension on renal blood flow and glomerular filtration rates in intact denervated kidneys of unanaesthetised rabbits with adrenal glands demedullated. *Am. J. Physiol.* 150: 534–540, 1947.
13. Galeotti, G. Über die Arbeit, welche die Nieren leisten, um den osmotischen Druck des Blutes auszugleichen. In: *Archiv für Physiologie*, edited by E. Du Bois-Reymond. Leipzig, Germany: Veit, 1902, p. 200–242.
14. Goll, F. Über den Einfluss des Blutdrucks auf die Harnabsonderung. *Z. Rat. Med. N.F.* 4: 78–100, 1854.
15. Goormaghtigh, N. Les segments neuro-myo-artériels juxtaglomérulaires du rein. *Arch. Biol.* 43: 575–591, 1932.
16. Goormaghtigh, N. L'appareil neuro-myo-artériel juxtaglomérulaire du rein; les réactions en pathologie et ses rapports avec le tube urinifère. *C. R. Séances Soc. Biol. Fil.* 124: 293–296, 1937.
17. Goormaghtigh, N. Une glande endocrine dans la paroi des artérioles rénales. *Brux. Med.* 19: 1541–1549, 1939.
18. Gottlieb, R., and R. Magnus. Über die Beziehungen der Nierenzirkulation zur Diurese. *Arch. Exp. Pathol. Pharmakol.* 45: 223–258, 1901.

19. Grützner, P. Beiträge zur Physiologie der Harnsekretion. *Pfluegers Arch. Gesamte Physiol. Menschen Tiere* 11: 370–386, 1875.
20. Guyton, A. C. Theory for autoregulation of glomerular filtration rate and blood flow in each nephron by the juxtaglomerular apparatus (Abstract). *Physiologist* 6: 194, 1963.
21. Hargitay, B., and W. Kuhn. Das Multiplikationsprinzip als Grundlage der Harnkonzentrierung in der Niere. *Z. Elektrochem. Angew. Phys. Chem.* 55: 539–558, 1951.
22. Hartmann, H., S. L. Ørskov, and H. Rein. Die Gefässreaktion der Niere im Verlaufe allgemeiner Kreislaufregulationsvorgänge. *Pfluegers Arch. Gesamte Physiol. Menschen Tiere* 238: 239–250, 1937.
23. Hayman, J. M. Estimations of afferent arteriole and glomerular capillary pressures in the frog kidney. *Am. J. Physiol.* 79: 389–409, 1927.
24. Heidenhain, R. Die Absonderung der festen Harnbestandtheile. In: *Handbuch der Physiologie*, edited by L. Hermann. Leipzig, Germany: Vogel, 1883, vol. 5, pt. 1, p. 279–373.
25. Heidenhain, R. Versuche und Fragen zur Lehre von der Lymphbildung. *Pfluegers Arch. Gesamte Physiol. Menschen Tiere* 49: 209–301, 1891.
26. Hermann, M. Über den Einfluss des Blutdruckes auf die Sekretion des Harns. *Sitzungsber. Akad. Wiss. Wien Math. Naturwiss. Cl. Abt. 2* 45: 317–351, 1862.
27. Kenney, R. A. *The Metzner Theory of Urine Formation.* The Hague: Junk, 1957.
28. Kramer, K. Zur Vasomotorik des intrarenalen Kreislaufs. *Sitzungsber. Ges. Befoerd. gesamten Naturwiss. Marburg* 75: 26–45, 1952.
29. Kramer, K., K. Thurau, and P. Deetjen. Hämodynamik des Nierenmarks. I. Mitteilung. Capilläre Passagezeit, Blutvolumen, Durchblutung, Gewebshämatocrit und O_2-Verbrauch des Nierenmarks in situ. *Pfluegers Arch. Gesamte Physiol. Menschen Tiere* 270: 251–269, 1960.
30. Kuhn, W., and K. Ryffel. Herstellung konzentrierter Lösungen aus verdünnten durch blosse Membranwirkung. *Hoppe-Seyler's Z. Physiol. Chem.* 276: 145–178, 1942.
31. Lilienfeld, L. S., H. C. Maganzini, and M. H. Bauer. Bloodflow in the renal medulla. *Circ. Res.* 9: 614–617, 1961.
32. Limbeck, R. von. Zur Lehre von der Wirkung der Salze. Über die diuretische Wirkung der Salze. *Arch. Exp. Pathol. Pharmakol.* 25: 69–86, 1889.
33. Loebell, C. E. *De conditionibus quibus secretiones in glandulus perificiuntur.* Marburg, Germany: Elwert 1849 (Inaugural Dissertation).
34. Ludwig, C. *De viribus physicis secretionem urinae adjuvantibus.* Marburg, Germany: Elwert, 1842.
35. Ludwig, C. *Lehrbuch der Physiologie des Menschen.* Heidelberg, Germany: Winter, 1852, vol. 1.
36. Ludwig, C. *Lehrbuch der Physiologie des Menschen.* Leipzig, Germany: Winter, 1856, vol. 2.
37. Ludwig, C. *Lehrbuch der Physiologie des Menschen*, 2nd ed. Leipzig, Germany: Winter, 1861, vol. 2.
38. Marshall, E. K., and J. L. Vickers. The mechanism of the elimination of phenolsulphonephthalein by the kidney—a proof of secretion by the convoluted tubules. *Bull. Johns Hopkins Hosp.* 34: 1–7, 1923.
39. Mayrs, E. B. The relative excretion of urea and some other constituents of the urine. *J. Physiol. Lond.* 56: 58–68, 1922.

40. Mayrs, E. B., and J. M. Watt. Renal bloodflow and glomerular filtration. *J. Physiol. Lond.* 56: 120–124, 1922.
41. Medes, G., and C. J. Bellis. The effect of altering renal blood pressure on glomerular filtration. *Am. J. Physiol.* 107: 227–229, 1934.
41a. Medawar, P. B. *The Art of the Soluble.* London: Methuen, 1967.
42. Medes, G., and J. F. Herrick. Blood flow to the kidney and creatinine clearance. *Proc. Soc. Exp. Biol. Med.* 31: 116–119, 1933.

43. Meier, M., H. Brechtelsbauer, and K. Kramer. Hämodynamik des Nierenmarks. IV. Mitteilung. Farbstoffverdünnungskurven in verschiedenen Abschnitten des Nierenmarks. *Pfluegers Arch. Gesamte Physiol. Menschen Tiere* 279: 294–304, 1964.
44. Metzner, R. Die Absonderung und Herausbeförderung des Harnes. In: *Handbuch der Physiologie des Menschen*, edited by W. Nagel. Braunschweig, Germany: Vieweg, 1906, vol. 2, pt. 1, p. 207–335.
45. Oberling, C. L'existence d'une housse neuro-musculaire au niveau des artères glomérulaires de l'homme. *C. R. Acad. Sci. Paris* 184: 1200–1202, 1927.
46. O'Connor, J. M. On glomerular control of the kidney bloodflow. *J. Physiol. Lond.* 59: 200–212, 1924.
47. Ofstad, J., and K. Aukland. Renal circulation. In: *The Kidney. Physiology and Pathophysiology*, edited by D. W. Seldin and G. Giebisch. New York: Raven, 1985, vol. 1, p. 471–496.
48. Opitz, E., and D. H. Smyth. Nierendurchblutung bei Reizung des Carotis-Sinus. *Pfluegers Arch.* 238: 633–637, 1937.
49. Pappenheimer, J. R., E. M. Renkin, and L. M. Borrero. Filtration, diffusion and molecular sieving through peripheral capillary membranes. A contribution to the pore theory of capillary permeability. *Am. J. Physiol.* 167: 13–46, 1951.
49a. Peter, A. Untersuchungen über Bau und Entwicklung der Niere. Jena, Germany: Fischer, 1909.
50. Rehberg, P. B. Studies on kidney function. I. The rate of filtration and reabsorption in the human kidney. *Biochem. J.* 20: 447–460, 1926.
51. Rehberg, P. B. Studies on kidney function. II. The excretion of urea and chloride analysed according to a modified filtration reabsorption theory. *Biochem. J.* 20: 461–480, 1926.
52. Rein, H. Die Thermostromuhr. Ein Verfahren zur fortlaufenden Messung der mittleren absoluten Durchflussmengen in uneröffneten Gefässen in situ. Z. *Biol.* 87: 394–418, 1927.
53. Rein, H. Vasomotorische Regulationen. *Ergeb. Physiol.* 31: 28–72, 1931.
54. Rein, H., and R. Rössler. Die Abhängigkeit der vasomotorischen Blutdruckregulation bei akuten Blutverlusten von den thermoregulatorischen Blutverschiebungen im Gesamtkreislaufe. Z. *Biol.* 89: 237–248, 1929.
55. Richards, A. N., P. A. Bott, and B. B. Westfall. Experiments concerning the possibility that inulin is secreted by the renal tubules. *Am. J. Physiol.* 123: 281–298, 1938.
56. Richards, A. N., B. B. Westfall, and P. A. Bott. Renal excretion of inulin, creatinine and xylose in normal dogs. *Proc. Soc. Exp. Biol. Med.* 32: 73–75, 1934.
57. Ruyter, J. H. C. Über einen merkwürdigen Abschnitt der vasa afferentia in der Mäuseniere. *Z. Zellforsch. Mikrosk. Anat.* 2: 242–248, 1925.

58. Ryan, G. B., and M. J. Karnovsky. Distribution of endogenous albumin in the rat glomerulus: role of haemodynamic factors in glomerular barrier function. *Kidney Int.* 9: 36–45, 1976.
59. Schnermann, J., and J. P. Briggs. Function of the juxtaglomerular apparatus: local control of glomerular hemodynamics. In: *The Kidney: Physiology and Pathophysiology*, edited by D. W. Seldin and G. Giebisch. New York: Raven, 1985, vol. 1, p. 669–697.
60. Schröder, W. von. Über die Wirkung des Coffeins als Diureticum. *Arch. Exp. Pathol. Pharmakol.* 22: 39–61, 1887.
61. Schröer, H. *Carl Ludwig. Begründer der messenden Experimentalphysiologie.* Stuttgart, FRG: Wissenschaftliche Verlagsgesellschaft, 1967.
62. Shannon, J. A. The excretion of inulin by the dog. *Am. J. Physiol.* 117: 405–413, 1935.
63. Starling, E. H. On the absorption of fluids from the connective tissue spaces. *J. Physiol. Lond.* 19: 312–326, 1896.
64. Starling, E. H. The mechanisms of the secretion of urine. In: *Textbook of Physiology*, edited by E. A. Schaefer. Edinburgh, UK: Pentland, 1898, vol. 1, p. 639–661.
65. Starling, E. H. The glomerular functions of the kidney. *J. Physiol. Lond.* 24: 317–330, 1899.
66. Tammann, G. Die Thätigkeit der Niere im Lichte der Theorie des osmotischen Drucks. *Z. Phys. Chem.* 20: 180–197, 1896.
67. Thurau, K. Fundamentals of renal circulation. In: *Proc. 2nd Int. Cong. Nephrol., Prague.* Amsterdam: Excerpta Med., 1963, p. 51–61.
68. Thurau, K., P. Deetjen, and K. Kramer. Hämodynamik des Nierenmarks. II. Mitteilung. Wechselbeziehung zwischen vasculärem und tubulärem Gegenstromsystem bei arteriellen Drucksteigerungen, Wasserdiurese und osmotischer Diurese. *Pfluegers Arch. Gesamte Physiol. Menschen Tiere* 270: 270–285, 1960.
69. Trueta, J., A. E. Barclay, P. M. Daniel, K. J. Franklin, and M. M. L. Pritchard. *Studies of the Renal Circulation.* Springfield, IL: Thomas, 1947.
70. Ustimowitsch, C. Experimentelle Beiträge zur Theorie der Harnabsonderung. *Ber. Verh. Königlich-Sächischen Gesselseh. Wiss. Leipzig Math.-Phys. Cl.* 22: 430–470, 1870.
71. Wearn, J. T., and A. N. Richards. Observations on the composition of glomerular urine with particular reference to the problem of reabsorption in the renal tubules. *Am. J. Physiol.* 71: 209–227, 1924.
72. White, H. L. Observations on the nature of glomerular activity. *Am. J. Physiol.* 90: 689–703, 1929.
73. Wiederhielm, C. A., J. W. Woodbury, S. Kirk, and R. F. Rushmer. Pulsatile pressures in the microcirculation of frog's mesentery. *Am. J. Physiol.* 207: 173–176, 1964.
74. Wirz, H., B. Hargitay, and W. Kuhn. Lokalisation des Konzentrierungsprozesses in der Niere durch direkte Kryoskopie. *Helv. Physiol. Pharmacol. Acta* 9: 196–207, 1951.
75. Zimmermann, K. W. Über den Bau des Glomerulus der Säugerniere. *Z. Mikrosk. Anat. Forsch. Leipz.* 32: 176–278, 1933.

III

Clearance Concept in Renal Physiology

STANLEY E. BRADLEY

CLEARANCE CONCEPT

IN 1928 Donald D. Van Slyke (see Fig. 2) and associates (25) introduced the word "clearance" to indicate the urinary output of urea per minute relative to its concentration in blood, defining it as the volume of blood completely "cleared" of urea per minute when urine flow exceeds 2 ml/min. Fifteen years later Homer W. Smith [see Fig. 6; (42)] wrote: "*In my opinion this word has been more useful to renal physiology than all the equations ever written. In recent years,*" he added, "*it has broken loose from the excretion of urea and, taking conceptual wings, has become a generalized notion applicable to all aspects of renal excretion.*" Smith's admittedly somewhat startling assertion has found its justification in major contributions to our understanding of kidney function that can be ascribed in part to attention focused by an apt and useful term on a potentially effective new methodology and on the body of concepts from which it has emerged. The fundamental concept itself can be traced, in fact, as far back as July 1870 to a meeting of the Physikalisch-Medizinische Gesellschaft in Würzburg at which Professor Adolf Fick (see Fig. 4) presented a very short paper outlining a method of measuring cardiac output in dogs (14a). Fick's method depended on much the same mathematical formulation introduced by Van Slyke, but it was used for measuring carbon dioxide clearance by the lungs and, in doing so, for evaluating total blood flow (or cardiac output) through the lungs. In this seemingly ambiguous statement, that clearance measures simultaneously an excretion of a solute and a volume of fluid flow, lies a source of some confusion in the understanding and application of the clearance principle.

Van Slyke was interested in his own formulation chiefly as an appropriate approach to the measurement of a solute (urea) excreted by the kidneys. Smith and other physiologists, in contrast, found it a suitable tool for the estimation of glomerular filtration rate (GFR) and renal blood flow. In the course of physiological studies, the successful use of clearance techniques for measurement of flows, however, also made it possible to obtain meaningful information on the mechanism and quantitative aspects of renal conservation and elimination of solutes. It may be said that Van Slyke and Smith stood at the convergence of two different lines of conceptual thought that led to the introduction of clearance methods: one was determined by an urgent need to understand renal disease and was dominated therefore by clinicians; the other was designed to improve the understanding of normal renal function and was dominated therefore by physiologists.

Clinical Approach to Clearance Conceptualization

Since urea retention has been recognized for many years as a cardinal sign of renal functional insufficiency, it is not surprising that clinicians tended to focus a major effort on understanding, controlling, and forecasting the course of renal disease in terms of this phenomenon. Urea was discovered as long ago as 1773 by H. M. de Rouelle (1718–1779) in Paris and was characterized there in 1784 by A. F. de Fourcroy (1755–1809), who named it "urée." The analytical determination of urea remained so unreliable, however, and required such tedious and time-consuming manipulation for extraction and gravimetric measurement that physicians found little immediate use for it. By 1836 R. Bright (1789–1858) at Guy's Hospital in London was familiar with the rise in blood urea in patients with chronic renal disease; he described one instance (case 6) among 100 patients with "albuminous urine" in whom blood urea reached a value of 1,500 mg% in association with an equivalent reduction in urinary urea content. He mentioned by name several other London physicians who had made similar observations. By this time the work of Friedrick Wöhler (1800–1882) and Justus von Liebig (1803–1873) [two brilliant students of J. J. Berzelius (1779–1848), Professor of Medicine and Pharmacy in Stockholm] had already resulted in epoch-making contributions to knowledge of urea. Wöhler, working in Berlin in 1828, was the first to succeed in synthesizing urea and, by doing so, lifting the curtain on the modern era of organic synthesis. His close and lifelong friend, von Liebig, Ordinarius (full professor) in Chemistry at the University of Giessen and later at Munich, won worldwide recognition for the development of an improved (but still impractical) method of urea determination and, more importantly, for his studies of nitrogen metabolism that placed urea in a modern biochemical perspective.

Despite these advances clinical acceptance was slow in coming until the studies of Léon Ambard (Fig. 1) and his associates in Paris and later in liberated Strasbourg, where he was named Professor of Experimental Medicine at the new French University in 1919. Am-

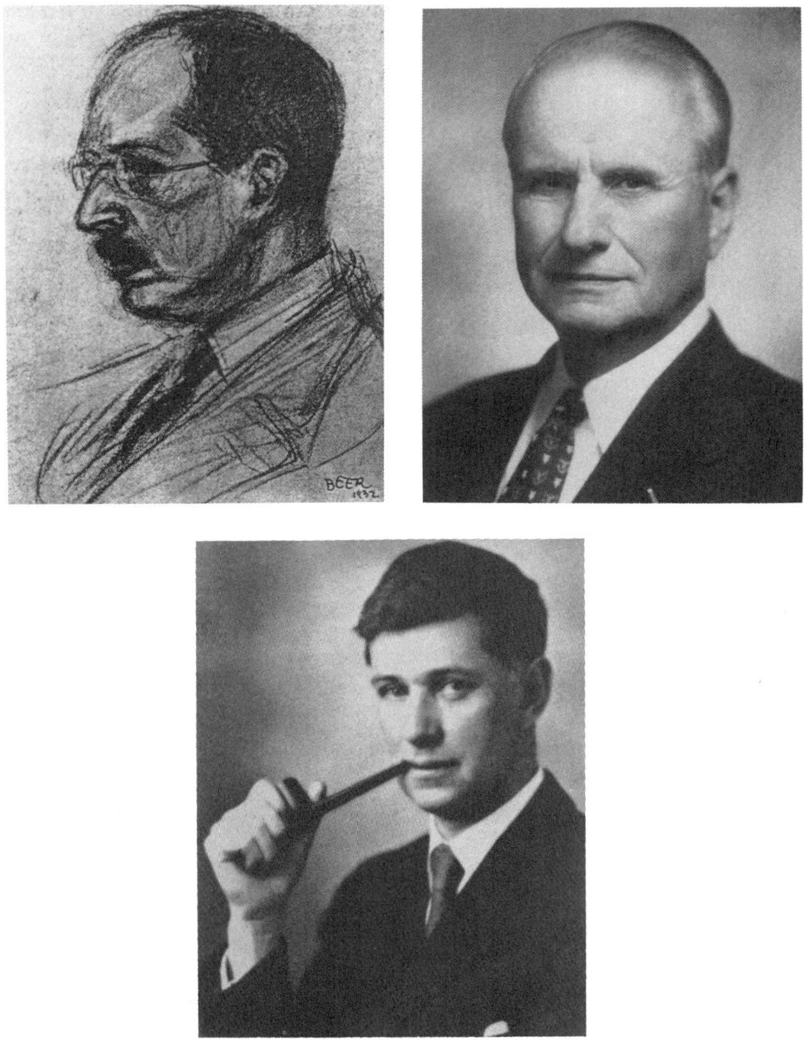

Figure 1. Pioneers of the clinical approach to the clearance concept in renal physiology: Léon Ambard (1876–1962) (*top, left*); Franklin C. McLean (1888–1968) (*top, right*); Thomas Addis (1881–1949) (*bottom*). [From Beer (6) and McLean (24).]

bard received his medical degree from the University of Paris in 1905, and after hospital training he became head of the laboratory of the Clinique des Maladies des Voies Urinaires at the Hôpital Necker, still today a major center of nephrology. There he embarked upon studies of the relationship between urea concentrations in blood and urine under varied conditions of urea and water loading; these studies yielded new approaches to the problems of renal functional change and diagnosis of renal diseases. His overriding objective was to find a predictable and constant interrelation between blood and urine levels and urine flow in normal animals in order to arrive at a reliable diagnostic index that would change only as a result of renal function impairment. It must have seemed to Ambard that the elaboration of additional controversial theory in this domain offered a much less satisfactory approach than did recourse to direct experimentation. Over the course of more than a decade, Ambard and his associates published a series of papers that inspired many other investigators—particularly in American laboratories, among them those of Van Slyke in New York, of Thomas Addis in San Francisco, and of E. K. Marshall, Jr. in Baltimore—to examine urinary urea excretion. In these publications Ambard presented experimental evidence that led him to define what he called the "laws of urea excretion" that could be summarized as a mathematical expression for the relationship between blood (B) and urine (U) concentrations of urea and urine flow (V) (3, 4). The resulting value came to be known as "Ambard's coefficient" or "constant" and may be written simply, omitting empirical constants and correction for body weight, as

$$\text{Ambard's coefficient} = B^2/(UV\sqrt{V}) \qquad (1)$$

Ambard's conclusion that this ratio between the square of the blood level and urinary excretion of urea is relatively constant in the absence of renal disease was confirmed by many workers, and his coefficient was widely used for years thereafter, especially in Europe, as a clinical test of renal functional efficiency. Nevertheless, Ambard's data were sharply criticized because they depended on an old unreliable and nonspecific sodium hypobromide method of urea analysis in which nitrogen is released from alcohol-extracted material by hyperbromide treatment of nitrogen-containing compounds and is measured gasometrically. Confirmatory work in 1914 by Franklin C. McLean [Fig. 1 (23)] in Van Slyke's laboratory proved particularly supportive because he used, at first, a new and more reliable colorimetric method of measuring urea that had been developed in Boston by Folin and Denis (12) and then somewhat later, an even better method introduced by Marshall (18) based on the use of specific soybean urease. McLean had joined the Van Slyke group after leaving his post as Professor of Pharmacology at the University of Oregon where he had initiated studies of the Ambard coefficient. He brought to his work an interest in mathematical manipulation that stimulated him to modify Ambard's equation, inverting it to obtain what he called an "index of urea excretion." The inversion was made primarily to emphasize more accurately the direct relationship between the index and urinary urea output, on one hand, and the inverse relationship between index and blood level, on the other. His formulation was

$$\text{McLean's index} = (UV\sqrt{V})/B^2 \qquad (2)$$

It may be noted that this reformulation (i.e., the inversion) prefigures the ultimate clearance equation and in doing so indicates Ambard's view that urinary and blood concentrations are of prime importance in determining urea excretion. Since maintenance of a putatively constant coefficient (or index) requires use of B^2 and $\sqrt{V}$, as in Ambard's experiments, these factors were not eliminated.

CLEARANCE CONCEPT

Although Ambard's and McLean's findings (as well as those of other workers) clearly showed that the blood level is directly related in some manner to urea output, its relative importance remained uncertain. Marshall, in the Department of Physiological Chemistry at the Johns Hopkins University, reported with D. M. Davis in 1914 (20) that urea excretion is directly proportional to the blood level and not to its square as long as urine flow is high. A similar finding was reported by Thomas Addis (Fig. 1) and C. K. Watanabe (2) at Stanford University in 1916; using Ambard's formulation they also found that urinary concentration seemed to vary inversely with urine flow under these circumstances. In gathering these data with their own from studies of themselves and of dogs, Austin, Stillman, and Van Slyke (5) found that these conclusions hold when urine flow is higher than 2.5 liters/day (a value they designated the so-called "augmentation limit") but fail to do so at lower flows. The data for which they used McLean's inverted Ambard equation indicated that urea excretion below the augmentation limit increases "*approximately . . . in proportion to the square root of the rate of volume output of urine per unit of body weight.*" In a second paper published seven years later (1928), these observations were reassessed and restated much more simply, eliminating the square of the blood concentration and the square root of the urine concentration: "*Expressed in other words,*" Moeller, McIntosh, and Van Slyke (25) pointed out, "*with abundant urine the urea excretion per minute equals the urea contained in a constant volume of blood. This volume of blood in a normal adult is about 75 cc.*" These new insights, clearly influenced by McLean's revision of the Ambard equation, which endowed it with the dimensions of volume flow per unit time, led Van Slyke and his group to conclude that the hypothetical constant volume of blood is that "*which one minute's excretion suffices to clear of urea when the urine volume is large enough to permit maximal urea output,* [which] *we for convenience term the maximal blood urea clearance.*" They presented it as

$$C_m = UV/B \qquad (3)$$

where C_m is maximal blood urea clearance. In a paper published in November of the same year, Addis (1) discussed application of the same simplified formulation (the "excretion ratio") as a measure of functional renal mass in Bright's disease; in a footnote he observed that his colleague G. B. Barnett had pointed out that "*the ratio was the volume of blood freed of urea.*" The birth of the term "clearance" and its association with a fluid volume was confused, however, by its use to express a movement of solute and by retaining the square root of V at lower flows in "standard clearance" (C_s)

$$C_s = (U\sqrt{V})/B \qquad (4)$$

Donald Dexter Van Slyke (Fig. 2) deserves special mention in this account, not only because he was successful in finding a word of power about which a variety of ideas, new and old, crystallized as a base for a new renal physiology, but also because he contributed so importantly to knowledge of many areas essential to an understanding of the role of the kidney. His genius in conceiving and devising new methods (particularly in gasometric technology) clarified and opened up new approaches that he successfully exploited in unraveling puzzles of enzyme kinetics, acid-base balance, renal amino acid and ammonia excretion, gas and electrolyte equilibria in the blood, and nitrogen metabolism. In his moving obituary tribute to Van Slyke in 1972, A. B. Hastings (15) wrote only a few words about Van Slyke's work on clearance for lack of space in which to describe the overwhelming intellectual legacy Van Slyke left behind. Van Slyke was a New Yorker, born and bred. He grew up in upstate New York, the son of L. L. Van Slyke, who served as Chief Agricultural Chemist in the State Agricultural Experiment Station for fifty years. The younger Van Slyke received a doctorate in organic chemistry from

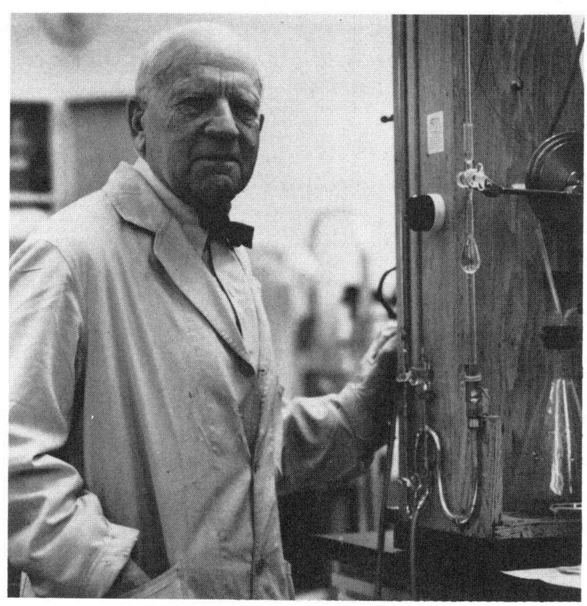

Figure 2. Donald Dexter Van Slyke (1883–1971) at Brookhaven National Laboratory standing in front of a Van Slyke gasometer not long before his death at age eighty-eight.

the University of Michigan in 1909 and shortly thereafter joined P. H. Levene as an assistant at the Rockefeller Institute. In 1914 he was named Chemist of the newly founded Rockefeller Institute Hospital where he devoted his life to full-time investigation. He retired in 1949 to embark upon a new career as Assistant Director of Biology and Medicine at the Brookhaven National Laboratory, which had just opened its doors and where he worked until his death in 1971. Van Slyke was a stocky, laconic, pleasant, frank, and open man with a gift for friendship and effortless kindness that made his penetrating criticisms all the more welcomed and appreciated. It is not surprising therefore that Van Slyke set in motion the next stage of clearance conceptualization by a characteristic act of courtesy and kindness.

In 1928, shortly after the publication of Van Slyke's definitive description of the "maximal" and "standard" urea clearances, William Goldring (1898–1981) (see Fig. 6 *top*) an instructor in the Department of Medicine at New York University College of Medicine (as it was called at that time), traveled uptown to look for Addis, who was at the Rockefeller Institute Hospital working in collaboration with Van Slyke. Goldring wanted to discuss with Addis his own work on a method Addis had introduced for the quantification of urinary excretion of "formed elements." As it happened, however, Goldring failed to find Addis but was welcomed by Van Slyke himself. In the words of Herbert Chasis (see Fig. 6 *top*; (8)], a medical student working at that time at Bellevue Hospital with Goldring, who was later his close associate:

Goldring, while waiting for Addis, visited with Van Slyke about renal function testing. Van Slyke suggested that the urea clearance might be helpful in studying changes in renal function in patients with acute febrile disease. Goldring took his suggestion back with him to Bellevue and studied patients with pneumonia and erysipelas during their acute febrile stage and during convalescence.

Failing to find a consistent pattern of change in his data, Goldring sought the help of Homer W. Smith, the recently appointed Professor and Chairman of the Department of Physiology in the medical school. Smith, a physiologist interested chiefly in comparative physiology of the kidney with special reference to its evolution and role in regulating the composition and volume of body fluids, mulled over the data without finding a rational explanation for the changes observed. He emerged with the conviction that understanding the renal excretion of any solute would require knowledge of the amount of the solute moving from the blood into the glomerular filtrate for subsequent processing by the tubules during movement from the glomerulus to the urine. With this idea in mind, Smith set out to find a suitable substance, the clearance of which would depend solely on glomerular filtration without subsequent reabsorption or secretion by the tubules. In doing so, his action was determined by current theory of the mechanisms of urine formation (glomerular filtration–tubular reabsorption) and by his realization that the clearance formulation could be best employed to measure movement of a definable fluid volume rather than of a solute. The validity of both filtration and tubular reabsorption as factors in urine formation rested on a century of work and contention in physiological laboratories throughout the world, principally in Europe. This endeavor had been directed not to the evaluation of the excretion or retention of solutes such as urea, so important to clinicians, but to understanding the fluid movements involved in renal function, in particular, transrenal water flow from blood to urine. This physiological approach was successful in refining the fundamental basis of the clearance concept that was to make it a useful instrument for investigation of glomerulotubular function.

Physiological Approach

From Bowman and Ludwig to Fick

Of necessity any advance in the comprehension of renal functional mechanisms requires an accurate and detailed knowledge of the microanatomy of the kidney, knowledge that was lacking at the beginning of the nineteenth century. Lorenzo Bellini (1643–1704) had described the tubules of the kidney in 1662; Marcello Malpighi (1628–1694), the glomeruli and their connection with the arteries in 1666; and Frederick Ruysch (1638–1731), the glomerular capillaries in 1729 (46); however, it was not until 1842 that descriptions consonant with present-day knowledge appeared. These we owe to the work of two young men of the same age: William Bowman (1816–1892), a demonstrator in anatomy at King's College in London, and Carl Friedrich Ludwig (1816–1895), prosector in anatomy at the University of Marburg in Germany.

Both published almost simultaneously (1842) the results of microdissection and vascular injection studies of the kidneys of a wide variety of mammals: Bowman in *Philosophical Transactions of the Royal Society of London* and Ludwig in an Habilitationsschrift. Each clearly presented the relationship between the glomerular capillary tufts and the tubules and the disposition of vessels and nephrons within the kidney. Each man realized the suitability of the glomerulus as an apparatus for the separation of water and solute from the blood, but Ludwig, with more sophistication, dealt with glomerulotubular function hypothetically in terms of intravascular pressures and endosmosis.

Bowman was to become an outstandingly successful and pioneering contributor to the anatomy and physiology of the eye and to ocular surgery, while Ludwig continued to grow as a medical scientist and became the foremost physiologist of his day in Germany (on a par with Claude Bernard in France). He produced a generation of disciples who carried his teachings throughout the world to dominate medicine in Europe and America. Figure 3, which shows the Ludwig School's "Stammbaum" as given by Rothschuh (35), lists a most impressive constellation of famous men in physiology. The Ludwig theory of urine formation as a consequence of glomerular filtration and differential endosmotic tubular reabsorption was important for the clearance formulation not because it contained an adumbration of the clearance concept but because it stimulated intense controversy and calculations designed to test its validity, which led directly to the use of clearance techniques in renal physiology. Moreover we owe the first description of the clearance equation to Ludwig's early friend and student, Adolf Fick (Fig. 4), who brought forward in 1870 the first clearly and accurately stated proposal for its use, not in study of the kidney, however, but for measurement of cardiac output.

Fick came from an unusually gifted family in Kassel (13). His oldest brother was Professor of Anatomy at Marburg where Carl Ludwig worked from 1841 to 1849 before going to Zurich as Professor of Anatomy and Physiology. Fick's initial predilection for mathematical studies brought him, also, to Marburg where it may be supposed that his brother's influence led him to change his course to medicine and where he became acquainted with Ludwig. After taking his degree at Marburg and completing his training there, young Fick followed Ludwig to Zurich in 1852 to take up a position as prosector. He remained there for sixteen years before accepting an invitation to take the Chair in Physiology at the University of Würzburg where he remained for the rest of his life. In Zurich he was quickly recognized as an outstanding investigator after his definitive exploration and clarification of the principles governing the diffusion of a solute in fluids (Fick's law), which he developed mathematically from Fourier's theory of heat. Although he was primarily interested in the physiology of muscle, Fick was a general physiologist, adept and knowledgable in many areas, as evidenced by his textbooks, among them the *Compendium der Physiologie des Menschen* (11), which went through four editions between 1860 and 1891. Although Fick presented a report describing his principle before the Würzburg Physikalisch-Medizinische Gesellschaft in July 1870, only a brief synopsis of his talk, presumably written by the Secretary, was published in its proceedings (32). A fuller description is given by Fick himself, however, in the third edition (1882) of his *Compendium*. Curiously enough, reference to the new idea does not seem to appear in the second edition (1874), although experimental data are included there to illustrate quantitatively the uptake of oxygen and release of carbon dioxide by blood perfusing the lungs. The account given in the third edition follows a discussion of pul-

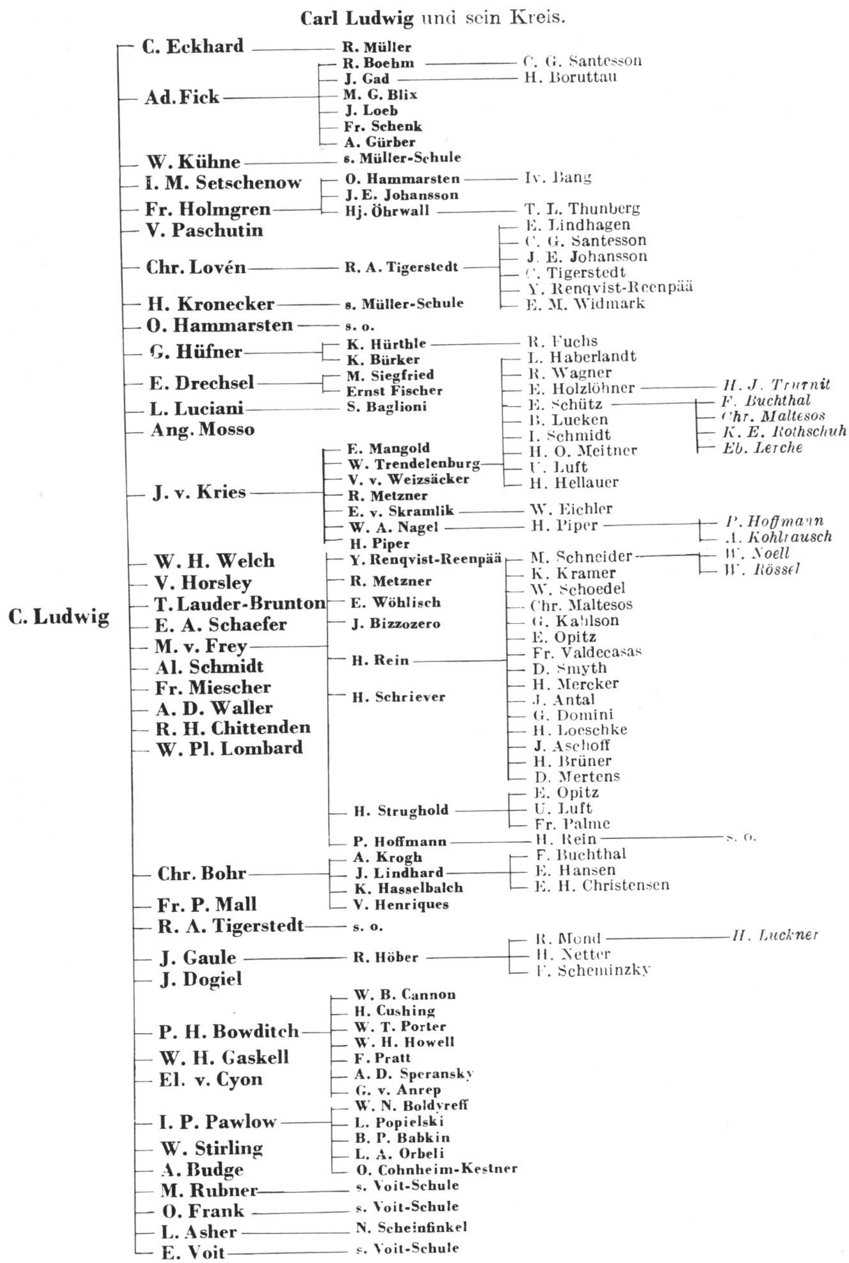

Figure 3. The Ludwig School. This intellectual pedigree presents the names of the most important trainees who worked closely with Carl Ludwig (1816–1895) in Leipzig. The list of German students is reasonably complete; of those coming from abroad, less so. Their students, in turn, were difficult to trace in many instances. [From Rothschuh (35).]

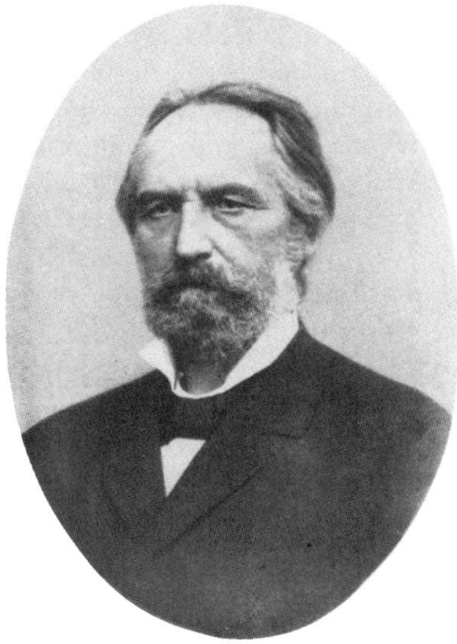

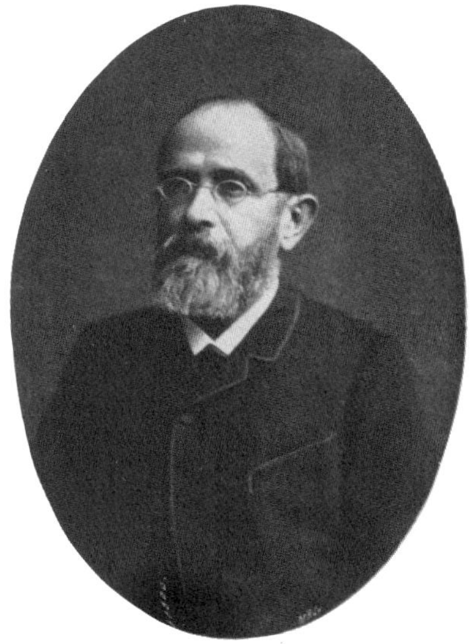

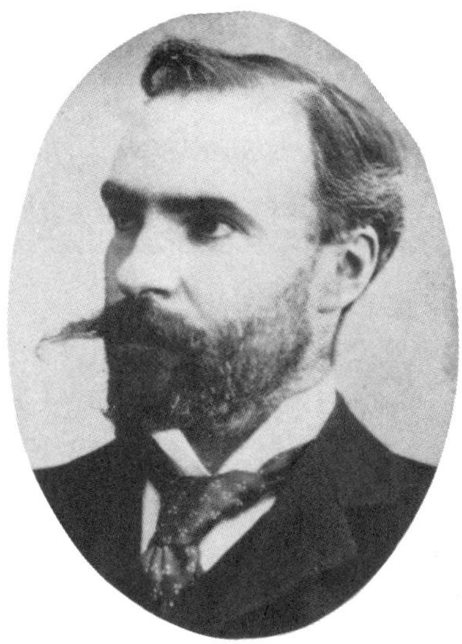

Figure 4. Pioneers of the physiological approach to the clearance concept in renal physiology. *Top left*, Adolf Fick (1829–1901); *right*, Rudolf P. H. Heidenhain (1834–1897); and *bottom*, Arthur R. Cushny (1866–1926) during his years at Michigan. [From Rothschuh (34), Grützner (14), and Vaughan (51).]

monary carbon dioxide excretion under conditions of varied respiratory rate and depth. The following excerpt is taken from it:

The value of the minute output of carbon dioxide makes it possible to estimate the magnitude of total blood flow in normal adult persons. If we assume an output of 270 milliliters of carbon dioxide (measured at 0°C and 760 mm Hg pressure) as seen with quiet breathing at 12 respirations per minute we may ask: how many milliliters of blood must flow through the lungs each minute to account for the change from the venous to the arterial state on giving up 270 milliliters of carbon dioxide? In order to calculate this, one must know how much carbon dioxide is given up by each 100 milliliters of venous blood to become arterial. In man, it is admittedly not yet known how much the (mixed) venous carbon dioxide content exceeds the arterial. In numerous studies of blood gases in dogs we know that, on the average, every 100 milliliters of venous blood gives up 4.4 milliliters carbon dioxide in the change from the venous to the arterial state (measured at 0°C and 1 M. Hg pressure or 5.8 milliliters measured at 0°C and 760 mm Hg). If we make the admittedly somewhat arbitrary assumption that venous and arterial blood in man do not differ materially from that in the dog, then so many times 100 milliliters of blood must flow through the lungs as 5.8 is contained in 270 in order to give up just 270 in one minute. If one carries out the computation indicated it is evident that, in round numbers, 4600 milliliters of blood pass through the lungs in each minute or 76 milliliters per second, therefore also across some total cross-section of the vasculature, as for example, the cross-section of the aorta. If one assumes further that the heart contracts 70 times each minute then a ventricle will eject 4600/70 or 66 milliliters of blood with each systole.

It can be seen that Fick's computation here employs an expression resembling that described above for urea clearance

$$\begin{aligned} CO_2 \text{ clearance} &= CO_2 \text{ output (ml/min)}/[(A - V)CO_2] \\ &= \text{cardiac output} \end{aligned} \tag{5}$$

where $(A - V)CO_2$ is the peripheral arterial–central venous concentration difference for CO_2 (ml/ml). Here, also, the clearance expression yields unquestionably a value for fluid flow (not solute movement) per unit time, a volume that is by no means "hypothetical." Fick did not attempt to use his discovery in studies of other organs. This application seems first to have been made in 1883 by Rudolf P. H. Heidenhain (Fig. 4) in the Department of Physiology at the University of Breslau (now Wroclaw in Poland) for the estimation of glomerular filtration rate.

Heidenhain's Contribution

Heidenhain, son of a Prussian medical family (his father and five brothers were physicians), was born in Marienwerder, began his studies in the natural sciences at the University of Königsberg in East Prussia (now Kaliningrad in the Soviet Union) and then studied medicine in Halle where the teaching of A. W. Volkmann (1800–1877), Professor of Anatomy and Physiology, awakened an enthusiasm for physiological research. In his teaching Volkmann stressed physical principles and studies of physiological optics and hemodynamics, an emphasis in harmony with the growing critical spirit of the time, which rejected the vitalism that had informed all thought of biological activity and function up to this period. Heidenhain completed his medical education at the University of Berlin (1854) and embarked upon graduate work there with Emil du Bois-Reymond (1818–1896).

The Berlin laboratory of anatomy and physiology had been directed by Johannes Müller for more than twenty years and had reached a peak of exciting productivity. Müller was widely recognized as an original thinker of great genius who had gathered together unusually outstanding students, as Rothschuh's Stammbaum (33) for him strikingly shows (Fig. 5). In his own intellectual development, Müller was remarkably ambivalent, dedicated on one hand to unbiased and penetrating experimental investigation and on the other to a spiritual view of life that made it difficult for him "*to be convinced of the strict validity of physical laws in the organism,*" as his associate of many years, du Bois-Reymond, observed. Thus young Heidenhain found himself in a most stimulating atmosphere, one in which tension between the older vitalistic view and the newer physicochemical approach was evident but not restrictive. Du Bois-Reymond, who was to take over direction of the Institute after Müller's early death in 1858, was in fact one of the leaders of the growing movement to abandon vitalistic beliefs; he sought to prove the cogency of his position through the success of his contributions to knowledge of nerve and muscle physiology. Undoubtedly, however, Heidenhain was influenced both by Müller and by du Bois-Reymond.

In 1856 Heidenhain returned to Volkmann in Halle; one year later he was promoted to Privatdozent after acceptance of his Habilitationsschrift, which dealt with the determination of blood volume. Shortly after his marriage to Volkmann's daughter in 1858, Heidenhain was called at the age of twenty-five to take the Chair in Physiology as successor to K. B. Reichert at the University of Breslau where he remained until his death in 1897. Heidenhain is described as a short, lively man whose strength of character was evident at once on his move to Breslau in the manner in which he won respect in dealing graciously with a student strike against him, whom they called the "green foreign professor" (14). He continued to be successfully productive in studies of muscular activity, in development of the Heidenhain-Pavlov pouch with his student Pavlov, and most extensively in explorations of the function of glandular tissues: liver, pancreas, salivary glands, and gastric mucosa.

From his studies of urinary excretion of the dye indigo carmine, he came to the conclusion that urine formation depends solely on active tubular (and glomerular) secretion. When he reviewed "Excretory Processes" for Hermann's massive *Handbuch der Physiologie*

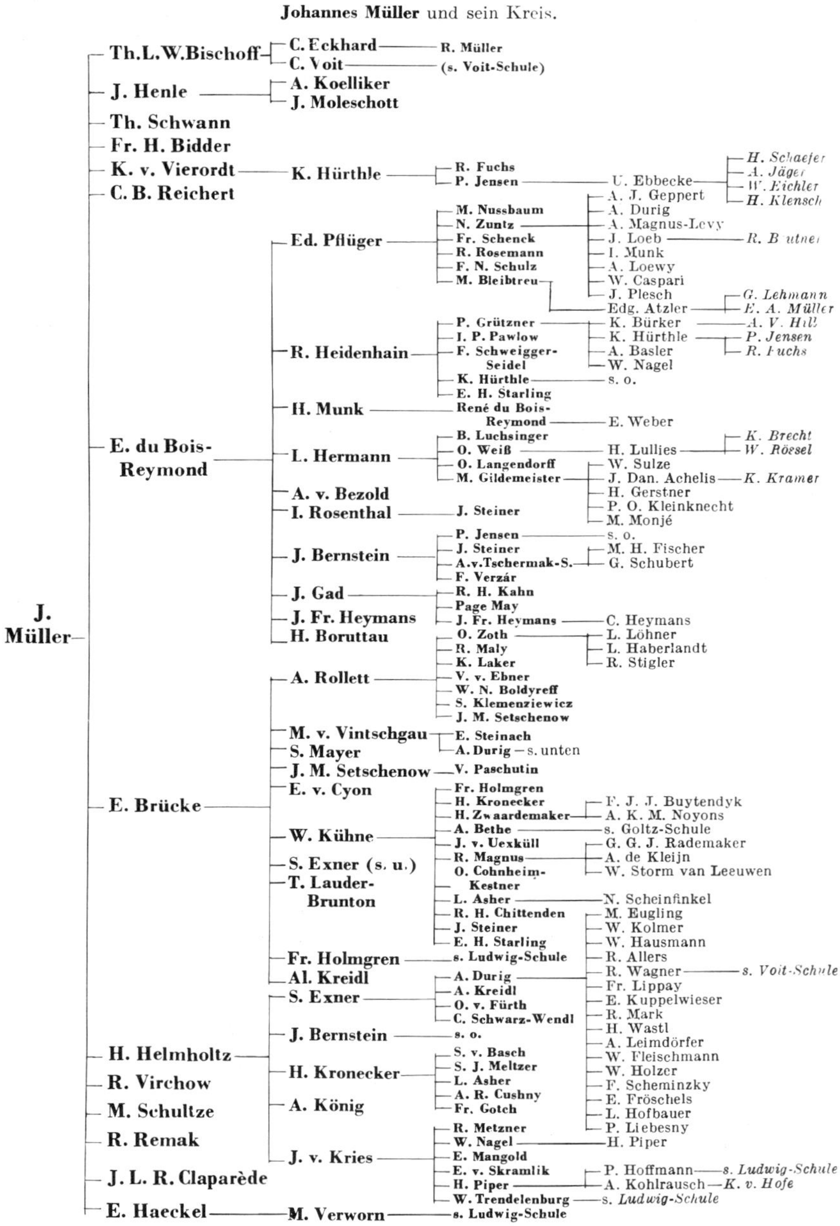

Figure 5. The Müller School intellectual pedigree lists the names of students of Johannes Müller (1801–1858) in Berlin. German students predominate as in the Ludwig School. Interestingly, E. H. Starling, a close associate of A. R. Cushny, was one of Heidenhain's students. [From Rothschuh (33)].

(17) in 1883, he took the occasion to attack the Ludwig hypothesis in his chapter "Excretion of Solutes in the Urine." A careful reading of his contribution reveals that in raising arguments designed to ridicule Ludwig's reasoning, he used the clearance formulation to obtain an estimate of the glomerular filtration rate. His presentation reads as follows:

Doubts Regarding Ludwig's Theory

Ludwig's theory of urinary excretion not only transfers water excretion to the glomeruli but also makes all the solid material in the urine pass with water in dilute solution, to be given up during slow passage down the tubule to the bathing fluid [lymph] *thus gradually to attain the concentration of the secretion emerging from the papillae. If one follows the consequences of this view a few difficulties arise at the very outset.*

1.) An adult on the usual mixed diet excretes approximately 35 grams of urea in 24 hours. The blood contains, taking the highest value obtained by the inexact method of Gscheiden, 25 mg%. From the urea content of the filtrate on the basis of the concept that it is a question of physical filtration, and there is hardly reason to suppose it is fundamentally anything else than the blood content, but (since there are data suggesting an increased concentration of solids in filtrates formed from protein-containing fluids) we will agree to a similar increase in glomerular filtrate so that the filtrate urea concentration therefore would come to 50 mg%—surely a generous concession.

On these assumptions, not less than 70000 ml fluid must be filtered by both kidneys in 24 hours in order to account for the daily output of urea and from this monstrous stream of water taking into account a daily urinary output of 2000 ml, 68000 ml must be reabsorbed by the tubules!

2.) This implication, in itself unbelievable, becomes even more so on the following inferences. The total blood volume of a 75 kg man comes in round numbers to 6 L. In each minute, perhaps three complete circulations of this volume occurs so that in 24 hours 4320 (3 × 60 × 24) circuits of the blood volume would occur or 6 × 4320 = 25920 L of blood flow through the whole body in 24 hours.

The weight of the kidney amounts to 1/20 of the total body weight. On the assumption of uniform distribution of total blood flow through the body, 25920/200 = 130 L blood flow through the kidney in 24 hours. The blood, however, on the calculation above, would yield in the glomerulus 70 L fluid, that is, more than half the weight of total renal blood flow in the glomerular tuft as water. Its paradoxicality loses nothing in the numbers indicating that the greater part of the water returns to the blood and even less if one supposes that a much greater blood flow passes through the kidneys than merely an amount proportional to their weight. So long as one keeps within reasonable limits with these assumptions even more unbelievable numbers emerge for the relationships between the glomerular filtrate and the perfusing blood volume.

If one wants to escape the above mentioned undesirable consequences while maintaining the Ludwig hypothesis nothing remains but to accept the assumption that the urea concentration of glomerular filtrate is extraordinarily much higher than that of the blood.

In the calculation of the quantity of glomerular filtration set out by Heidenhain, it may be noted that he employed the following formulation. Assuming that urea output in the urine per minute is equal to the total urea filtered per minute and that urea undergoes neither reabsorption nor secretion by the tubules, although this results in a higher concentration of urea in urine (U) than in blood (B) as a result of water reabsorption, then using the urine flow per minute (V) to calculate urea output, it is found that

$$\text{filtration rate} = UV/B \tag{6}$$

Here Heidenhain employed the formulation that was later called the maximal urea clearance by Van Slyke and his associates. It may be argued therefore that Heindenhain used the expression to calculate filtration rate without recognizing the possibilities inherent in what was to him an obviously reasonable and commonplace computation. He was much more interested in holding the Ludwig hypothesis up to ridicule. Although there are obviously serious flaws in Heidenhain's argument when considered in the light of modern knowledge of renal and cardiac function and in many other points raised elsewhere in his chapter, his contentions seemed overwhelmingly acceptable to his contemporaries and, though disputed by some, remained dominant until the appearance of A. R. Cushny's (see Fig. 4) monograph *The Secretion of Urine* (9) in 1917 and its revised edition in 1926.

Although further discussion of the rights and wrongs of Heidenhain's attempt to discredit Ludwig's theory of urine formation is not germane to the central theme of this chapter, it does seem appropriate to consider briefly the accusation usually leveled against him, namely, that his argument for active tubular secretion as a basis for urine formation is "vitalistic." Heidenhain did have his training in an environment in which vitalism was not completely rejected but was certainly not encouraged. In his writings Heidenhain was quite firm in denying a vitalistic attitude (16), stating as early as 1874:

In the course of this presentation I have avoided up to this point a question the relevance of which cannot be denied although its solution remains hopeless at this time—the question: What physical and chemical processes occurring in the cells account for the excretion of indigo carmine [soluble indigo blue, disodium 5,5′-indigotin disulfonate]? *As long as the words "the life of the cell" are only an expression indicating the totality of unknown physical and chemical processes occurring in the cells, one cannot hope to define more precisely the activity of excreting cells. The following discussion can only point to leads for further investigation.*

In this clearly expressed attitude, Heidenhain has obviously distanced himself from the view of "vital activity" of the cells as an often arbitrary but teleological element that would be expected to defy analysis in strictly physical terms. Unfortunately, of course, his own caution could not prevent others from using his data and speculations to support vitalist views. It is really this phenomenon against which Cushny leveled his attack on the vitalism implicit in Heidenhain's thesis that urine is formed solely by active tubulocellular secretion in a manner resembling the production of salivary, gastric, and pancreatic secretion or bile, dismissing glomerular filtration as an absurdity. Cushny's success in demolishing Heidenhain's physiological arguments, however, opened up a new era in the history of renal physiology and clearance conceptualization.

Cushny Era

Arthur R. Cushny (Fig. 4) was commonly regarded at the time of his death as the leading pharmacologist of Great Britain and indeed foremost in his profession throughout the world (10). A Scot educated in Aberdeen, he was trained first at the Institute of Physiology in Berne (1889–1890) in physiological methodology by Hugo Kronecker (1839–1914), a former close associate of Ludwig in Leipzig, and then in Strassburg (1891–1893) (at that time a German city) in the new scientific approach to pharmacology by Oswald Schmiedeberg (1838–1921) its greatest pioneer and exponent. There in 1893 he was recruited by J. J. Abel to take the Chair in Pharmacology at the University of Michigan, which Abel was leaving in order to go to the Johns Hopkins Medical School. At the University of Michigan (from 1893 to 1905), at University College London (a new Chair in Experimental Pharmacology) (from 1905 to 1918), and finally at the University of Edinburgh (from 1918 until his death), Cushny's industry and intellectual brilliance were manifested in a series of important publications on digitalis, cardiac arrhythmias, the actions of senecio and other poisons, and optical isomers. In 1899 he published the first systematic textbook of pharmacology, which won worldwide fame and use during many editions. His 1917 monograph *The Secretion of Urine* (9), embodying much of his own work and "*importing a new conception into Ludwig's theory of the process*" as H. H. Dale (10) put it, "*had a great influence on recent speculation and research.*" In reviewing the debate between supporters of Ludwig and Heidenhain, Cushny rejected many of the claims of both and put forward his own "modern view" in which glomerular filtration was described as a simple physical process followed by tubular reabsorption of a modified "optimal" solution from the filtrate. He was particularly vehement in attacking Heidenhain's "vital activity" as a basis for tubular secretion, though he found it necessary to use the expression himself with respect to reabsorptive processes. A feature of Cushny's argument that is important to the subject of this essay is its use of Heidenhain's computation to show that the volume of filtrate necessary in urine formation is not so monstrously large as Heidenhain had considered it (9). Nevertheless he points out (9) that:

> *Heidenhain's figures are certainly striking, and his argument has been sufficient to prejudice superficial readers against the theory he attacks. Let us analyse them a little further, or rather let us examine the same problem in the cat, in which more details are ascertainable than in man. A cat fed on meat only passed on an average 100 c.c. of urine per day containing 12 per cent of urea. The blood-flow through the kidneys, measured by Barcroft and Brodie's method, amounted to 40 c.c. per minute, and the blood contained 0.1 per cent of urea, that is, the 100 c.c. of urine contained as much urea as 12 litres of plasma. The modern view demands that 12 litres of fluid were filtered through the capsules, and that no less than 11.9 litres were absorbed in the tubules, much higher figures in proportion to the relative weights of the cat and man than are calculated by Heidenhain. Each kidney of the cat contains about 16000 glomeruli and tubules, so that the amount of fluid filtered by each glomerulus in the twenty-four hours in my observation was 12000/32000 c.c. = 0.375 c.c., or on the average about 0.015 c.c. per hour. Of this more than 0.014 c.c. was absorbed in its passage along about 3 cm of tubule, leaving less than 1 mg per hour from each capsule to finally enter the collecting tubule. When the immense number of tubules in the kidney is taken into account, the argument of Heidenhain is thus seen not to be so fatal as has been supposed, for 0.015 c.c. per hour cannot be regarded as a very severe task for the capsule, and the absorption of 0.014 c.c. of water per hour would seem to be well within the capacity of the epithelium of a tubule 3 cm. in length.*

In working out his "modern view" of urine formation, Cushny totally eliminated active tubular secretion from consideration and introduced a new concept of "*threshold and no-threshold bodies*," which he defined as substances that enter the tubules in the glomerular filtrate. This notion was derived from Ambard's suggestion in 1910 that substances like glucose appear in the urine only after their plasma concentrations exceed a certain "threshold" (3). Cushny believed that threshold bodies undergo complete reabsorption by the tubules up to the threshold level and that the excess at higher values is excreted in the urine. As a result a changing blood-urine concentration ratio would be observed under different loading conditions. All no-threshold bodies, in contrast, were held to undergo concentration in the urine to the same extent, as a result of tubular water reabsorption, so that their concentration ratios would be expected to be identical and higher than those of threshold products. Mayrs (21),[1] working in Cushny's laboratory in Edinburgh, found that creatinine, sulfate, and phosphate were all concentrated to the same extent in the urine of rabbits while urea was not (21). He concluded that urea is a threshold substance and that the others are not. From these observations Mayrs and Watt (22) deduced that any of the three non-threshold substances could be used to obtain "*evidence of the proportion of plasma which comes into direct contact with renal cells*" and therefore, since tubular secretion could be ruled out, to measure GFR.

CLEARANCE CONCEPT

"*To measure the amount of glomerular filtrate in terms of the total plasma circulating through the kidney,*" they used sulfate because one "*may suppose that filtration through Bowman's capsule does not alter the concentration of sulfate* [in the filtrate], *and that all the sulfate which is filtered appears in the urine.*

Hence

$$\frac{\textit{Glomerular filtrate}}{\textit{Total amount of plasma in kidney}} = \frac{\textit{Sulfate excreted}}{\textit{Sulfate in plasma in kidney}}$$

Since Mayrs and Watt took the "*total amount of plasma in kidney*" as the renal plasma flow in a given time period and "*sulfate in plasma in kidney*" as the "*total amount of sulfate contained in this plasma,*" i.e., plasma concentration of sulfate (P), it may be seen that the GFR values computed for studies of 11 anesthetized rabbits were obtained by the formulation

$$\text{GFR} = \frac{\text{UV (sulfate)}}{\text{P (sulfate)}} \qquad (7)$$

which is essentially that still used today to measure GFR. Mayrs's use of the plasma concentration was evidently suggested by Cushny's computations and served to focus the attention of subsequent workers on the fact that filtrate is derived from the plasma. The same approach was developed for use in human subjects four years later by Poul Brandt Rehberg (1886–1985) in Copenhagen in a series of papers published in the *Biochemical Journal* in 1926.

Rehberg (30) chose creatinine rather than sulfate as a marker of glomerular filtrate, and to overcome the analytical problem posed by low concentrations of creatinine normally found in the plasma, he decided to raise its concentration, using himself as an experimental subject, by ingesting it. He reasoned (without reference to Mayrs and Watt) as follows:

The calculation of the amount of filtrate is possible if we have a substance filtered out through the glomeruli, none of which is reabsorbed during passage through the tubules. Suppose it to be a substance *of this kind and F to be the amount of filtrate formed in the capsules, U the amount of the urine, A_P% the percentage of the substance A present in the plasma in diffusible state, and A_U% the percentage in the urine, then*

$$(1) \qquad \frac{F \times A_P\%}{100} = \frac{U \times A_U\%}{100}$$

This gives

$$(2) \qquad F = \frac{A_U\%}{A_P\%} \times U = C \times U$$

$$\textit{when} \qquad \frac{A_U\%}{A_P\%} = C(\textit{index of concentration})$$

If R is the amount of fluid reabsorbed, then

$$R = F - U = C \times U - U = (C - 1)U.$$

Rehberg's results yielded values for filtration rates up to 200 ml/min, an amount that seemed wholly reasonable in view of his evaluation of evidence adduced by others regarding the number and surface area of the glomerular population for filtration, the rate of renal blood flow, and the reabsorptive area of the tubules. In redefining Cushny's hypothesized "threshold, no-threshold" substances, Rehberg made an important distinction between active reabsorption and simple backdiffusion, arguing that these processes could affect different substances in differing proportion thus producing differences in apparent active reabsorption. To examine this proposition, he measured reabsorption of urea and chloride in himself under various loading conditions, using creatinine to quantify filtered loads and rates of tubular reabsorption. He was thus the first to use measured GFR in evaluating tubular function. He obtained results consistent with tubular uptake of urea solely as a result of backdiffusion and tubular uptake of chloride as a mixture of rapid backdiffusion with high loads and active reabsorption when plasma chloride levels fell below 370 mg%. During the summer of 1930, Rehberg (31) reviewed his experience with this new and promising approach at a meeting in Minneapolis under the leadership of Hilding Berglund and Grace Medes that was organized to discuss the behavior of the kidney in health and disease in light of current advances. At that time Rehberg had little to add regarding the use of his method to explore many physiological problems in greater depth but rather stressed the value of his procedure in clinical studies, presenting considerable data to support his view that the measurement might be helpful in the diagnosis of renal disease. In fact what had come to be called the "Rehberg Test" was widely employed for this purpose and continued to be popular for many years. A concerted effort to find an appropriate substance for measuring GFR was reported at this conference by Rehberg's contemporary, Homer W. Smith (see Fig. 6), who was to advance the use of the clearance approach in studying renal physiology by many ingenious applications during the next thirty years.

Beginning of the Smithean Era

With Smith's entry into the field after Goldring's encounter with Van Slyke at the Rockefeller Institute Hospital in 1928, the New York University Physiological Laboratories bubbled with activity centered on the development and extension of the new concept as a tool for the exploration of renal function in humans and experimental animals. The success of Smith's laboratory in exploiting the new technology between World War I and World War II opened up a new era in renal physiology that Robert F. Pitts [Fig. 6 *bottom*; (29)], a major contributor in clearance methodology (28), was to call the "Smithean era." With the explosion of scientific growth after World War II, students streamed into Smith's laboratory from all over the world to learn the new methodology and above all to profit from Smith's exciting intellectual stimulus and leadership.

He was a tall, thin, lively but reticent man, well aware of his powers but paradoxically shy and somewhat inhibited despite the ebullience and sparkle of his writings and teaching. Born in 1895, the last of six children, he grew up motherless in Cripple Creek, Colorado; he was fascinated by the ambience of a mushroom "gold-mining camp" and driven by an overwhelming scientific curiosity that was nurtured by his family, as he tells us in a short biographical sketch appended to a study of religious thought, *Man and His Gods* (45). After graduation from the University of Denver in 1917, he entered the armed forces with the advent of war to serve as a chemist in the Chemical Warfare Laboratory at American University in Washington, DC. After demobilization in 1919, he earned a doctorate in science under the direction of the physiologist William H. Howell at the Johns Hopkins University in Baltimore, MD, where he continued his friendship with Marshall, whom he had met at the Chemical Warfare Station and who was already established as an important figure in renal physiology. After two years as a fellow with Walter B. Cannon in Physiology at Harvard, he devoted himself to studies of water regulation in fish and in particular to investigation of the role played by the high urea concentrations in body fluids and tissues of elasmobranch fishes.

These studies took him to Siam to examine the osmoregulatory adjustments of urea levels in sharks during seasonal migration from the ocean to fresh water; he also went to Africa to study adaptation by lungfish. These experiences and the time that travel provided for contemplation in those slower paced days gave him the material for a best-selling novel *Kamongo, the Lung Fish and the Padre* in which he manifested what was to be an abiding interest in the implications

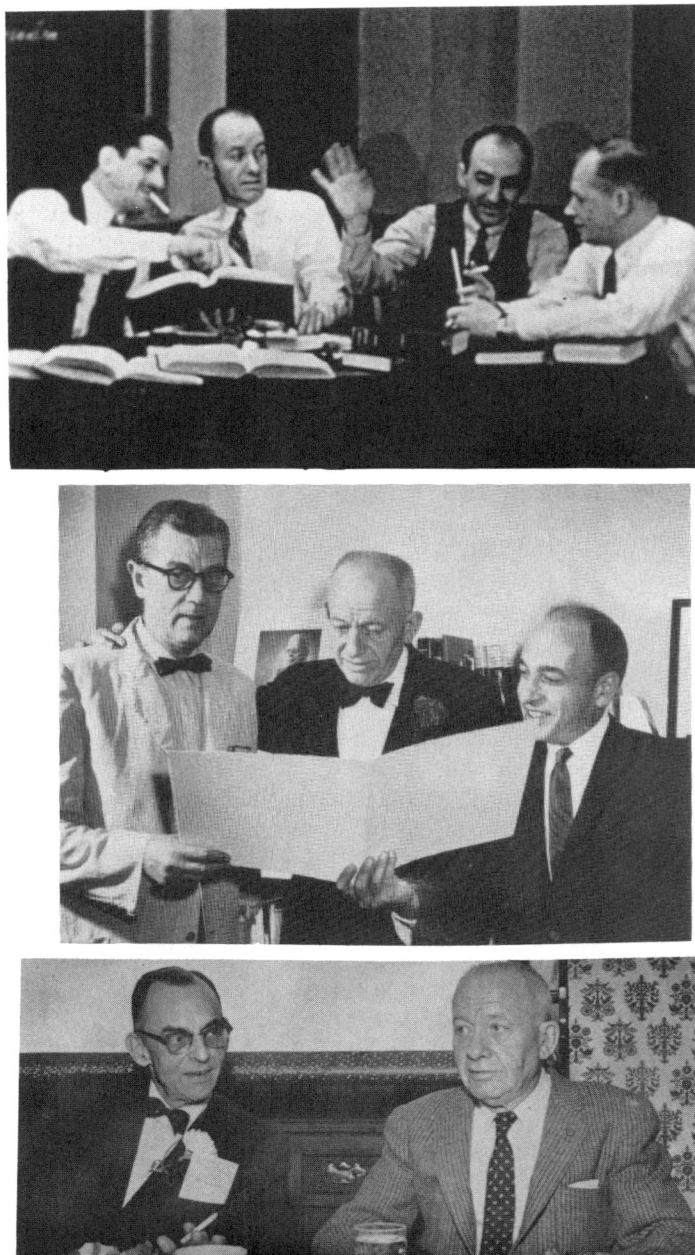

Figure 6. Homer W. Smith (1895–1962) and his associates over three decades. *Top:* Smith's team during an animated planning session during their work on inulin clearance (ca. 1935). From left to right: William Goldring, Smith, Herbert Chasis, and H. A. Ranges. *Middle:* Smith (*center*) at the National Institutes of Health (ca. 1955). James A. Shannon (*left*), and Robert W. Berliner (*right*) are also present. *Bottom:* Smith (*right*) at a dinner in his honor on 6 February 1962. Robert F. Pitts (*left*) had just received the New York University Alumni Association Scientific Achievement Award. [From Chasis and Goldring (8a)].

of religious thought. Owing to these investigations, he was to dig deeply into the problems of evolutionary change in renal adaptations to environmental stress, a foundation that gave all his work with the kidney a depth and color that together with his base in physical chemistry and his skill in communication made his writing unusually effective. In 1928, after three years as Chairman of the Department of Physiology at the University of Virginia, he accepted an appointment as Professor of Physiology and Director of the Physiological Laboratories at the New York University College of Medicine. He continued his work on marine animals during summers at the Mt. Desert Island Biological Laboratory (MDIBL) in Salsbury Cove, ME, and in New York he embarked with his close clinical associates and friends William Goldring and Herbert Chasis (Fig. 6, *top*), on a lifelong investigation of the basic mechanisms of urine formation in both humans and animals.

Renal Clearances as Measures of Fluid Flows

Glomerular Filtration Rate

By the time Smith participated in the Minneapolis conference of 1930, he was already well launched on the search for a suitable substance to use for measurement for GFR. The initial effort in 1928 was focused on the implication of Van Slyke's clearance that it measured a volume flow that could be more sharply defined and quantified by use of appropriate markers. It soon became evident that measurement of both filtration and renal blood flow could now be approached by an inherently noninvasive technique that was suitable for use in studies of kidney function in humans during health and disease as well as in unanesthetized animals under easily controlled conditions. In finding an appropriate marker for use in measuring GFR by the clearance technique, Smith was impressed by Marshall's discovery at MDIBL that the aglomerular fish (*Opsanus tau* and *Lophius piscatorius*) cannot excrete glucose, suggesting that the renal tubules of vertebrates may lack a mechanism by which such a valuable nutrient might be lost by tubular secretion and that all related nonmetabolizable compounds would similarly escape uptake from the tubular urine.

Smith and his colleagues therefore turned their attention to an examination of the excretion of a variety of nonmetabolized carbohydrates by a wide range of vertebrate forms, from the dogfish shark to men and women (39). These investigations led to the discovery that inulin, a complex polysaccharide composed of 32 hexose molecules (chiefly fructose), with a molecular weight of 5,200, was the ideal substance. Inulin had been simultaneously and independently identified by A. N. Richards and his associates at the University of Pennsylvania. Both groups had used the approach of comparing simultaneous excretory rates of exogenous creatinine and of various carbohydrates, including xylose, inulin, sorbitol, and mannitol. The urine-plasma concentration ratios for the latter three were found to be identical in humans and dogs, that of xylose was lower in both, and that of creatinine was higher in humans than in dogs. It was concluded that xylose and creatinine could not be relied upon in human subjects, the former because of tubular reabsorption and the latter because of active tubular secretion. (Creatinine proved entirely suitable, however, in dogs.) It was for this reason that creatinine clearance was rejected as a means of measuring renal function in people despite Rehberg's continued and unsuccessful advocacy. A diagram from Smith's Porter Lectures (1939) [Fig. 7; (41)] summarizes the evidence available at that time supporting the view that inulin is a reliable marker of GFR in men and women. Interference with tubular glucose reabsorption by excess loading to produce hyperglycemia or during the action of phlorizin resulted in the close identity of sucrose and xylose clearances with those of inulin, so that the clearance ratios closely approached unity. Creatinine behaved differently, showing a decline in its clearance as its loading was increased (Fig. 7, *left panel*) and falling to identity with inulin clearance after phlorizin administration. Inulin's lack of toxicity (providing that contaminating pyrogen is removed), its almost complete recovery in urine without evidence of metabolism, and its relative ease of measurement have made it a universally accepted standard for measuring GFR.

Throughout most of the studies of clearance applications in Smith's department during the 1930s, James A. Shannon (Fig. 6, *middle*) made essential contributions in every sphere owing both to his enormous energy, industry, and skill as an experimenter and to the cogency of his thinking. He left the department just before the

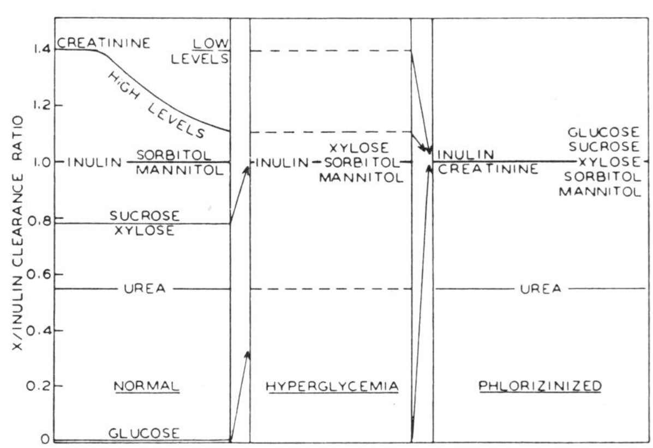

Figure 7. Diagrammatic summary of the evidence available in 1939 based on clearance ratios indicating that inulin clearance is at the level of glomerular filtration in humans. [From Smith (41).]

United States entered World War II to direct the Research Service of the Department of Medicine at Goldwater Memorial Hospital on Welfare Island in the East River in the shadow of the Queensborough Bridge. He continued to work actively in collaborative studies, but with the war he was called away to conduct a clinical investigation of antimalarial drugs. His leadership and the staff he brought together at Goldwater produced major breakthroughs not only in therapy but also in fashioning the quantitative basis for the future field of clinical pharmacology. He went from success in this task to administer, to staff, and in fact to create the National Institutes of Health in Bethesda, MD.

Throughout these studies, which led to the acceptance of inulin, was an obvious concern with active tubular secretion (e.g., with creatinine in men and women) or reabsorption (e.g., for glucose). Thus it was evident from early on that, once established (as Rehberg had already shown), a reliable measure of GFR could serve as a means not only of quantifying filtrate flow but also of determining active transport into and out of the tubular cells. The New York workers were not slow in exploiting this possibility. Their search had been almost exclusively concerned with problems of reabsorption but (as in the case of creatinine) secretion was also evident, and in order to examine the relationship between secretion and loading by the perfusate, a means of measuring renal blood flow is necessary. In addition the self-evident dependence of filtration on intrarenal vascular flows and pressures required information regarding renal hemodynamics. Ideally the clearance of any substance completely extracted by the kidney from its perfusate but not metabolized by or stored in renal cells was seen as the goal toward which to move in finding another adequate marker, this time for renal blood flow. In contrast to a marker for GFR, for which tubular cellular uptake or excretion must be excluded, a reliable marker for renal blood flow would require completely efficient tubular transport from blood to excreted urine.

Renal Blood Flow

Success by Marshall and others in proving conclusively that active tubular excretory transport is a reality opened up the way to the development of a method of measuring renal blood flow. An increasingly critical and objective approach to physiological problems during the last half of the nineteenth century had effectively ousted vitalism as a factor to be considered seriously in any biological context. As Smith pointed out in his 1937 monograph *The Physiology of the Kidney* (40)—a trailblazing work in the history of modern renal physiology—Cushny's

exclusion of tubular excretion was based in no small measure upon the belief that such a process must readmit "vitalism" with its uncon-

trolled and inexplicable forces, into the domain of renal physiology. In retrospect, we see that this fear was quite unjustified. Tubular excretion, viewed as a consequence of the physico-chemical organization of the tubule cells, can be looked upon as mechanistic as filtration itself. In fact, in the absence of any knowledge of how the tubules could absorb the "optimal" fluid, Cushny was forced to ascribe this process to vital activity, even though this activity was reduced to attractively constant and definable proportions.

Nevertheless Cushny's strictures upon tubular secretion may well have played a role, on the one hand, in inhibiting Rehberg's extension of his use of the clearance concept to the measurement of renal blood flow or, on the other, in Van Slyke's failure to use the clearance approach even when he employed urea clearance as a basis for developing an indirect method of determining renal blood flow in dogs.

For this purpose, in 1934 Van Slyke turned to studies of trained dogs in which one kidney had been mobilized and brought into the flank on the same side under the skin where renal venous blood could be easily sampled without recourse to surgical manipulation or anesthesia. Van Slyke, Rhoads, Hiller, and Alving (50) were thus able to obtain simultaneous samples of femoral arterial and renal venous blood painlessly by transepidermal needle puncture. Measurements were made of urea and oxygen concentrations in blood flowing into and out of the kidney under steady-state conditions of fasting and water diuresis in 16 animals (in 8 animals a week or more after unilateral nephrectomy and in 8 animals with 2 kidneys) with and without urea loading. Urine was collected continuously by bladder catheterization and sampled with bladder washout at hourly intervals. Renal blood flow was computed as

$$F = UuV/(A - V_R) \qquad (8)$$

where F is flow (ml/min), UuV is urinary excretion of urea (mg/min), A is arterial blood urea nitrogen content (mg/ml), and V_R is renal venous blood urea nitrogen content (mg/ml). It can be seen that the Fick principle was used in this procedure (without mention) and furthermore that, because

$$UuV = (A - V_R)F \qquad (9)$$

and

$$Cu = UuV/A = [(A - V_R)/A]F \qquad (10)$$

where Cu is Van Slyke's maximal clearance of urea, it follows that

$$Cu = FE \qquad (11)$$

where E is the renal extraction ratio of urea $[(A - V_R)/A]$. These conclusions depend of course on three assumptions: *1*) that a steady-state distribution of urea obtains in the body, 2) that neither intrarenal storage nor production of urea occurs during the period of measurement, and 3) that renal extraction remains constant throughout the hour-long period of urine collection.

CLEARANCE CONCEPT

It is curious that Van Slyke seems to have overlooked or ignored the implications of the method (apparently used for the first time) developed for this difficult and time-consuming study, which was designed primarily for the examination of urinary urea excretion in relation to renal blood flow, oxygen uptake, and a reduction in total renal mass (by unilateral nephrectomy). There is no evidence in this study nor in others that followed that Van Slyke realized that this approach or a method based on it could be used to evaluate renal hemodynamics in connection both with the interrelationships between intrarenal and systemic circulatory adjustments and with urine formation and regulation of body fluid volume and composition.

In contrast, Smith, Goldring, and Chasis (48) seem to have been much more impressed by the view of clearance as the "*volume of plasma required to supply the quantity of 'some substance' excreted in the urine in one minute's time.*" This vision of a clearance as equivalent to flow of a fluid volume differed sharply from Van Slyke's tendency to consider it merely an index, specifically, of urea elimination by the kidneys. The New York University approach led therefore to examination of a variety of foreign nontoxic nonmetabolized substances, the clearances of which clearly exceeded GFR and were thus dependent on active transport from blood to glomerular filtrate in the tubules. In the course of the excretion of one of these, phenol red, in men and women, dogs, rabbits, and chickens [reviewed by Shannon (37)], the clearance level achieved a maximal value (averaging 3.3 times the simultaneously measured GFR) at relatively low plasma concentrations (<1.0 mg% in human subjects), but it was noted that with progressively higher concentrations clearance values fell (self-depression) to levels lower than the simultaneously measured GFR, thus confirming an earlier observation by Marshall and Crane (19).

In an effort to find compounds with clearances higher than those for phenol red, attention turned to radiopaque organic iodine–containing compounds that had proved useful as contrast media in pyelography because of the high urinary concentrations that could be achieved with them. Among these, iodopyracet (Diodrast) and *o*-iodohippurate sodium (Hippuran) were found to be cleared at rates almost two times higher than phenol red and seemed to satisfy the criteria laid down by Smith, Goldring, and Chasis (48) for a suitable marker:

a. The substance, X, should be selected upon the basis of having the highest possible clearance, since the highest clearance must approach most nearly the true blood flow.

b. The plasma concentrations of X must be kept below the level where the clearance is significantly self-depressed.

c. It must be ascertained whether other solutes in the plasma, and particularly substances which are themselves excreted by the tubules, can interfere with the tubular excretion of X.

d. It must be shown that X is concurrently transferred to the urine.

Careful examination and testing of their findings in terms of these considerations and other possibilities such as erythrocyte uptake, intrarenal storage, and destruction gave the work an authority that resulted in almost immediate acceptance. The difficulty of measuring organic iodine in the determination of Diodrast and Hippuran concentrations in blood and urine stimulated a further search for a better marker, which soon yielded sodium *p*-aminohippurate (PAH), which proved to be removed by the kidney from its perfusate as efficiently as Hippuran and much more easily measured colorimetrically.

The close collaboration during these investigations between the Department of Physiology and other departments at New York University School of Medicine has been eloquently described by Herbert Chasis (8). Joining Smith's group as a second-year medical student in 1928, Chasis (b. 1904) contributed significantly for many years in applying the new methods he had helped to develop in studies of renal function in normal humans and in patients with renal and hypertensive disease. Smith and his associates in the Department of Physiology were able to carry out their studies of human kidney function chiefly as a result of the enthusiastic participation of Goldring and Chasis. Both men were keen, highly critical, and committed co-workers with remarkable ability to grasp quickly the essence of each problem on which they worked, to contribute constructively in formulating and solving it, and to insist effectively on the highest standard of medical care and ethical conduct in clinical investigation. This close and friendly collegiality within the New York University faculty was extended to other services in Bellevue Hospital in the course of testing the value of clearances in studies of renal circulation.

The use of Diodrast or PAH clearance for studies of renal blood flow was necessarily predicated on the belief that renal extraction of the marker is close to 100%, a belief that was soon corroborated by direct measurements of renal PAH extraction made possible by the introduction of venous catheterization in 1940 by A. Cournand and D. W. Richards, members of Columbia University's First Medical Service at Bellevue Hospital, just across the street from New York University Physiological Laboratories. Smith had been helpful in making this advance possible and, with the outbreak of World War II in 1941, he and his associates embarked with the Columbia team on a combined study of hemodynamic and renal functional alterations observed in patients during traumatic shock. Workers from this group succeeded in sampling right renal venous blood (left renal venous blood is mixed with nonrenal venous blood from the left spermatic or ovarian vein) during constant PAH infusion in a combined study of 51 normal human subjects (43). They obtained extraction values ranging from 0.81 to 1.0 (with only 1 value <0.88 and a mean value of 0.924). The clearance method could therefore be relied on to yield meaningful values for renal blood flow [calculated in practice as the plasma clearance of PAH or Diodrast divided by (1 − hematocrit)] in unanesthetized dogs and human subjects. The method was quickly applied in studies that demonstrated the remarkable responsivity of renal circulation to stressful states such as anger, fever, and trauma as well as its role in overall cardiocirculatory dynamics. The fraction of renal plasma flow undergoing glomerular filtration could be determined as the ratio between simultaneously measured inulin and PAH (or Diodrast) clearances (C_I/C_{PAH}) and used to appraise glomerulodynamics. The need to maintain relatively low levels of Diodrast or PAH in order to avoid self-depression of clearance values in association with a fall in extraction had also been closely examined in both human subjects and experimental animals; these studies yielded new insights and a better understanding of the mechanisms of tubulocellular transport.

Active Tubular Transport From Filtrate and Perfusate

Success in devising noninvasive and accurate measurements of GFR and renal plasma flow provided for the first time an approach to quantitative evaluation of tubulocellular function in the elaboration of urine under physiological conditions and after injury. The concept of a renal "threshold" (seuil) set out by Ambard and elaborated by Cushny implied the operation of limited tubular transport systems for the reabsorption of glucose from filtrate and secretion of substances like Diodrast and PAH. In Cushny's view glycosuria resulted from a limitation of tubular reabsorption, whereas Heidenhain and his supporters considered it a result of either an injurious "sickening" effect on the normally impermeable glomerular membrane or a stimulus to tubular glucose secretion. The triumph of the filtration-reabsorption theory focused attention on the properties of the reabsorptive system.

The method applied was essentially that introduced by Rehberg (30) to demonstrate passive backdiffusion of urea. Although he had also examined glucose reabsorption in dogs, using the creatinine clearance to measure GFR (27), Rehberg failed [presumably because of analytical difficulties and failure to measure arterial (rather than venous) plasma concentrations] to observe the "saturation phenomenon" convincingly demonstrated in later investigations by Smith, Shannon, and their associates (37, 38, 49). In the formulation devised by these workers, who used inulin clearance (C_I) to measure GFR, tubular reabsorption of glucose (T_G) was computed as the difference between the filtered load [C_I multiplied by the arterial plasma glucose content (P_G) (mg/ml)] and the output in the urine [urinary glucose content (U_G) (mg/ml) multiplied by urine flow (V) (ml/min)]

$$T_G = P_G C_I - U_G V \qquad (12)$$

It was found that gradual elevation of the plasma glucose level

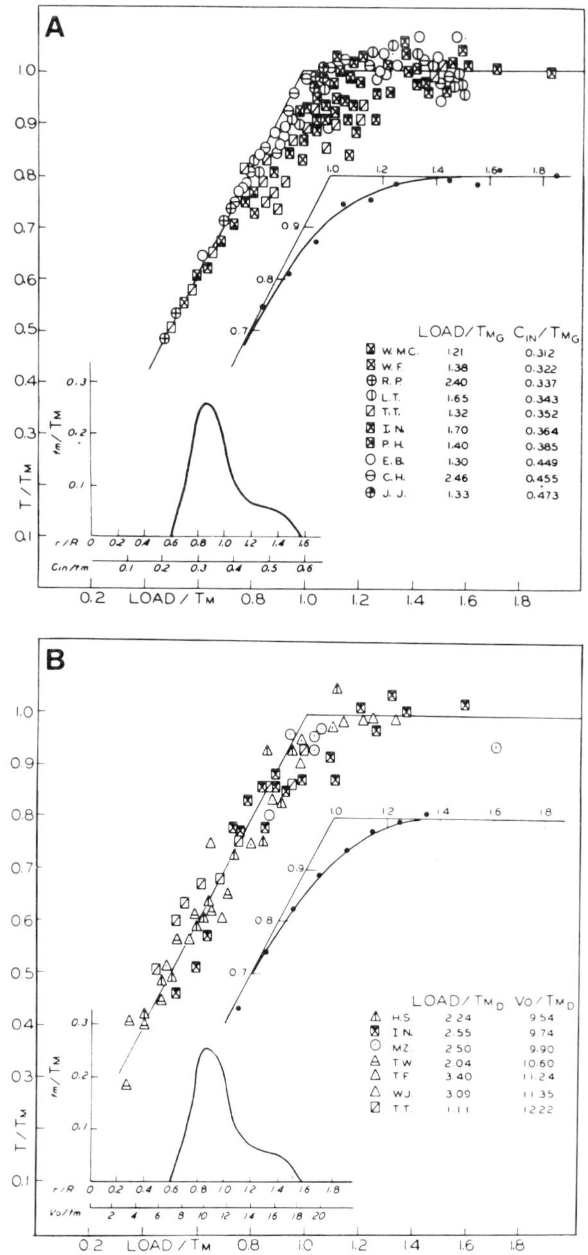

(glucose titration) was associated with reabsorption of the total filtered load as it was increased up to a point at which tubular reabsorption attained a constant maximal rate ("saturation") of glucose reabsorption (Tm_G). When this response was plotted in terms of Tm_G [as in data from human subjects (49) shown in Fig. 8*A*)], the saturation phenomenon for glucose reabsorption was strikingly evident.

A similar response was found when tubular secretion was followed during titration with (for example) Diodrast. In this instance graduated loading was imposed by Diodrast titration and the amount of Diodrast excreted by the tubule cells (T_D) was computed as the quantity appearing in the urine each minute (U_DV) less the amount that had been filtered

$$T_D = U_DV - P_DC_IFW \quad (13)$$

where the amount filtered is calculated as the plasma concentration of Diodrast (P_D) multiplied by the filtration rate and a correction factor—the product of the fraction (F) of Diodrast that is freely dispersed and not protein bound in plasma water and the fraction of plasma water (W) that is fully filterable. Tubular excretion calculated from clearance data in this way was found to rise with plasma concentration to a maximal value that remained constant over a wide range of higher concentrations. This maximal value was designated Tm_D and referred to as an "index of the quantity of functional tubular tissue" or a hypothetical "tubular excretory mass." Mutual interference observed between excretion of phenol red, Diodrast, and Hippuran was regarded as evidence that all shared a common tubular cellular transport mechanism. Smith was to give up the concept of excretory Tm as a measure of tubular excretory mass in a wry footnote many years later in his magistral text *The Kidney: Structure and Function in Health and Disease* (43), in which he wrote:

Seeking some expression to convey the implication that functional measurements made under conditions of saturation represent the total quantity of tissue involved, the writer and his colleagues used the

Figure 8. Normal dispersion of glomerular activity and tubular perfusion in human subjects. *A:* mass plot of data from glucose titrations in 10 normal subjects. Tubular reabsorption of glucose (T) at each point divided by maximal glucose reabsorption rate (T_{M_G}) for the subject under study plotted against load relative to the pertinent Tm. The frequency distribution curve (*inset*) was constructed from averages of these values for increments in load (i.e., Δ load/T_M = 0.1) and plotted against the ratios of relative glomerular activity (r/R) at each level. C_{in}, inulin clearance. *B:* mass plot of data from Diodrast titrations in 7 normal subjects. Data were treated as in *A*, with average Diodrast clearances at low Diodrast plasma levels as a measure of renal plasma flow in each study and assuming constancy thereafter at saturation levels. T_{M_D}, maximal tubular reabsorption of Diodrast; Vo, nephron perfusion. [From Smith et al. (49).]

rather inept expressions "tubular excretory mass" and "tubular reabsorption mass." Happily, the expressions have never come into wide use and are abandoned without regret.

The term Tm, however, continues to be used to denote a transfer maximum both for glucose reabsorption and Diodrast or PAH excretion, although it must be admitted that what that designation in turn may precisely imply still remains debated.

Shannon considered this problem at length in a paper (37) that appeared in *Physiological Reviews* in 1939 just a few months after the paper by Smith, Goldring, and Chasis (48) on Diodrast Tm (Tm_D). By this time Shannon and Fisher (38) had already (1938) dealt briefly with the problem in discussing data indicating a reabsorptive Tm (glucose Tm) in dogs, concluding that glucose may *"enter into reversible combination with some element in the tubule cells, present in constant but limited amount, and that subsequent decomposition of this complex limits the rate of glucose transfer from tubular urine to the blood."* On this initial hypothesis, Shannon (37) adduced equations based on the law of mass action to obtain curves that fitted the clearance data for both reabsorptive and excretory processes. In doing so he found it necessary to assume zero-order kinetics for the first reaction (combination of glucose or Diodrast with the hypothetical intracellular transporter) and first-order kinetics for the second (decomposition of the posited intracellular complex). Shannon's argument was flawed not only as a result of lack of knowledge of the complexities of reabsorptive and excretory activities demonstrated much later in micropuncture studies of segmental function in the tubule but also by the assumption that the kidney may be conceptualized as a single representative nephron. Nevertheless modern and more sophisticated methodologies indicate that the kinetic factors first evaluated by Shannon may well play a dominating role in determining the character of response to solute-titration loading of tubular reabsorptive and excretory processes.

Smith, in contrast to Shannon, sought to explain the singularities of the "titration curve" in terms of the properties of nephron populational dispersion by using the clearance approach to devise a method of defining the nephron population in functional terms. The close agreement between load [reabsorptive = P_GC_I, or excretory = (P_DC_D), minus the quantity filtered] and the amount of each marker undergoing uptake or excretion, respectively, up to the point of saturation, with little or no "splay" in dogs or rats and relatively little in humans (Fig. 8*A*, *B*), a fact that is particularly difficult to explain kinetically, was accounted for by Smith et al. (49) as a result of a functional glomerulotubular balance for reabsorptive activity and "uniformity" of tubular perfusion for excretory activity. In this view the relationship between loading and individual nephron function must be construed only in terms of the sum of the relationships between glomerular filtration in each individual nephron (c_{in}) and the reabsorptive capacity of the tubule (t_{mg}) attached to it or between the individual nephron perfusion (v_o) and its excretory capacity (t_{md}), i.e., c_{in}/t_{mg} or v_o/t_{md}, respectively. Data obtained during glucose or Diodrast titration reflect the sums of glomerular activities (c_{in}/t_{mg}) or tubular perfusions (v_o/t_{md}). The configuration of the titration curve observed in normal human subjects could be interpreted therefore as indicating operation of the nephron population as a whole in urine formation in association with uniformity in single-nephron glomerulotubular integration and perfusion. Smith et al. further inferred *1*) that the concepts of "glomerular intermittency" and "glomerular reserve" derived from studies of the amphibian kidney do not apply to rats, dogs, or human subjects; *2*) that since the rate of glomerular filtration relative to reabsorptive capacity varies within narrow limits at rest, a structural balance obtains (i.e., large glomeruli are attached to large tubules, small ones to small tubules, and so on in proportion); and *3*) that perfusate is delivered uniformly throughout the normal kidney in proportion to the functional capabilities of each nephron.

In the mass plots of normal data obtained in these studies of normal human subjects, it can be seen how frequency-distribution curves of glomerular activity (Fig. 8*A*) and tubular perfusion (Fig. 8*B*) were calculated from averages at successive values observed for increments of the appropriate Δ(load/Tm) = 0.1 as the loads of glucose or Diodrast were increased. To express the calculated points in more general terms, the frequency distributions were evaluated as percentile saturation of nephron mass at each loading level (tm/Tm) relative to glomerular activity or tubular perfusion in the nephron population as a whole (r/R). The reproducibility of such curves and the constancy of the relationships between the variables over a period of several hours in each study indicates convincingly a quasi–steady-state persistence of filtration and perfusion, which is quite incompatible with moment-to-moment glomerular intermittency or perfusional shifts. The remarkable tendency observed in some individuals for saturation of the total nephron population to occur at almost identical loads, with little deviation (splay) from the straight lines, is obscured in the mass plot of all studies. The potential power of the clearance approach as a means of exploring populational dynamics is evident in these findings, but the technical difficulties of such studies, coupled with uncertainty regarding the complexities of tubular segmental activity, gravely cloud interpretation and continue to impede investigation of nephrons en masse.

Closing Perspective

The hiatus in basic research activity imposed by the outbreak of World War II in Europe and later in Asia serves as a fitting point at which to close this discussion of the origin, development, and early applications of renal clearance methodologies. Before doing so, however, it is necessary to consider briefly certain implications of the seemingly contradictory routes by which the final clearance formulation was achieved. The triumph of the physiological approach with its flow-oriented emphasis during the period between the wars seemed to dismiss the solute-oriented views of workers like Ambard, McLean, Addis, and Van Slyke as irrelevant, even wrongheaded. Certainly major advances in understanding water and electrolyte excretion, renal acid-base regulations, output of organic molecules, and other aspects of renal function have continued to emerge during the decades since World War II from flow-focused clearance methodologies that have been fully discussed in recent well-balanced, critical, and erudite reviews (26, 36, 52). In Smith's opinion clearances could be best employed in studies of this kind as mediating means of estimating the quantity of solute brought to or away from tubule cells in filtrate or blood. In this insistence on clearance defined and dimensioned as flow, however, an intrinsic duality in the clearance concept is disregarded. Clearance may be defined, as pointed out in connection with the studies of Van Slyke et al., (e.g., ref. 50) as a product of two variables: a flow (F) and a dimensionless extraction fraction (E) of a solute (x)

$$C_x = FE_x \tag{14}$$

It is quite appropriate, therefore, to express clearance as the quantity of some substance that is moved across a barrier relative to its concentration in the fluid phase from which it moves. The introduction of concepts like whole-body clearance, metabolic clearance, and intrinsic clearance must be predicated on a solute-oriented clearance formulation as an approach to definition of molecular movement per se rather than to a definable flow of fluid. In addition solute clearances can be employed for purposes other than the measurement of either fluid flow or behavior of marker molecules as such. In studies of urinary plasma protein or macromolecular excretion, for example, by such workers as P. P. Lambert in Brussels or B. M. Brenner in Boston, clearances of the solute are dealt with in relative terms to obtain values not of fluid flows but of the dimensions of transglomerular membrane routes. It is evident, then, that both clinical and physiological pathways to clearance conceptualization have opened up new realms of thought and have given us many novel and effective modalities for enriching our knowledge of renal physiology.

I am deeply grateful to R. Steiner (Berne) and C. M. LaRuffa (New York) for their skillful and unfailingly cheerful cooperation in preparing this manuscript. I wish also to express heartfelt thanks to Dr. R. Preisig (Director, Institut für Klinische Pharmakologie, University of Berne) for his encouragement and support, to Dr. U. Boschung (Director, Medizinhistorisches Institut, Berne) and his associates for their gracious hospitality and assistance in using the resources of the institute; to Dr. H. A. Adam (Edinburgh) for sharing his knowledge of A. R. Cushny; to Dr. L. G. Wesson, Jr. (Philadelphia) for calling attention to R. Heidenhain's contribution; and to Dr. L. V. Hanks (Brookhaven) for providing the photograph of D. D. Van Slyke.

This work was supported in part by a grant from the Swiss National Science Foundation.

NOTE

[1] It should be noted that E. Brice C. Mayrs (1891–1964) deserves full credit for his feat in successfully formulating and applying a suitable clearance for the measurement of glomerular filtration in an experimental animal for the first time. Although Cushny was a dynamic and inspiring leader, he was so deeply involved in teaching the course in pharmacology at Edinburgh, in revising his popular textbook, and in many tasks to which he was called outside his department that he could have had little time to participate importantly in Mayrs's studies. In fact he is said to have been very annoyed on learning Mayrs's conclusion that tubular resorbate is not the "optimal" solution required by the "modern view" (46). Nonetheless Mayrs did very little thereafter in renal physiology. He returned in 1923 as Lecturer in Materia Medica at Queens University in Belfast where he had received medical training that led to an MD with honors in 1920. Mayrs had turned to pharmacology after the loss of his left arm during active service with the Royal Army Medical Corps in 1916. He occupied the chair in Pharmacology at Queens from 1928 to his retirement in 1957. He was described in an obituary in the *British Medical Journal* (4/34/64) as the "*most modest and retiring of dons,* [a] *remarkable character* [with whom] *passed an era of University life more leisurely, rather more eccentric, and certainly more individualistic*" than his survivors would ever know.

BIBLIOGRAPHY

1. ADDIS, T. The renal lesion in chronic Bright's disease. *Am. J. Med.* 176: 617–637, 1928.
2. ADDIS, T., and C. K. WATANABE. The rate of urea excretion—first paper. A criticism of Ambard and Weill's laws of urea excretion. *J. Biol. Chem.* 24: 203–220, 1916.
3. AMBARD, L. Lois numériques de la sécrétion de l'urée. *J. Physiol. Pathol. Gen.* 12: 209–219, 1910.
4. AMBARD, L., and A. WEILL. Les lois numériques de la sécrétion rénale de l'urée et du chlorure de sodium. *J. Physiol. Pathol. Gen.* 14: 753–765, 1912.
5. AUSTIN, J. H., E. STILLMAN, and D. D. VAN SLYKE. Factors governing the excretion rate of urea. *J. Biol. Chem.* 46: 91–112, 1921.
6. BEER, J. Trois figures médicales de Strasbourg. *Aesculape* 29: 117–119, 1939.
7. BRIGHT, R. Cases and observations, illustrative of renal disease accompanied with the secretion of albuminous urine. In: *Original Papers of Richard Bright on Renal Disease*, edited by A. R. Osman. London: Oxford Univ. Press, 1937, p. 93–131.

8. Chasis, H. History of collaboration by Department of Physiology at New York University School of Medicine. *Physiologist* 26: 64–70, 1983.

8a. Chasis, H., and W. Goldring (editors). *Homer William Smith, Sc.D.: His Scientific and Literary Achievements*. New York: New York Univ. Press, 1965.

9. Cushny, A. R. *The Secretion of Urine*. London: Longmans, Green, 1917, p. 54.

10. Dale, H. H. Arthur Robertson Cushny, 1866–1926. *Proc. R. Soc. Lond. B Biol. Sci.* 100: xix–xxvii, 1926.

11. Fick, A. *Compendium der Physiologie des Menschen* (3rd ed.). Vienna: Braumuller, 1882, p. 283.

12. Folin, O., and W. Denis. New methods for the determination of total non-protein nitrogen, urea and ammonium in blood. *J. Biol. Chem.* 11: 527–536, 1912.

13. Frey, M. von. Adolf Fick—Gedächtnisrede mit einem Verzeichnis von Adolf Ficks Schriften. *Sitzungsber. Phys. Med. Wuerzburg* 5: 65–80, 1901.

14. Grützner, P. Zum Andenken an Rudolf Heidenhain. *Pfluegers Arch. Gesamte Physiol. Menschen Tiere* 72: 221–265, 1898.

14a. Hamilton, W. F., and D. W. Richards. The output of the heart. In: *Circulation of the Blood: Men and Ideas*, edited by A. P. Fishman and D. W. Richards. New York: Oxford Univ. Press, 1964, p. 96.

15. Hastings, A. B. Donald Dexter Van Slyke, 1883–1971, Managing Editor 1914–1925. *J. Biol. Chem.* 247: 1635–1640, 1972.

16. Heidenhain, R. Versuche über den Vorgang der Harnabsonderung. *Pfluegers Arch. Gesamte Physiol. Menschen Tiere* 9: 1–27, 1874.

17. Heidenhain, R. Absonderungsvorgaenge. Sechster Abschnitt. Die Harnabsonderung (Viertes Capitel. Die Absonderung der festen Harnbestandteile). In: *Handbuch der Physiologie. Fünfter Teil*, edited by L. Hermann. Leipzig, Germany: Vogel, 1883, p. 341–343.

18. Marshall, E. K., Jr. A rapid clinical method for the estimation of urea in urine. *J. Biol. Chem.* 14: 283–296, 1913.

19. Marshall, E. K., Jr., and M. M. Crane. The secretory function of the renal tubules. *Am. J. Physiol.* 70: 465–488, 1924.

20. Marshall, E. K., Jr., and D. M. Davis. Urea: its distribution in and elimination from the body. *J. Biol. Chem.* 18: 53–80, 1914.

21. Mayrs, E. B. The relative excretion of urea and some other constituents of the urine. *J. Physiol. Lond.* 56: 58–68, 1922.

22. Mayrs, E. B., and J. M. Watt. Renal blood-flow and glomerular filtration. *J. Physiol. Lond.* 56: 120–124, 1922.

23. McLean, F. C. The numerical laws governing the rate of excretion of urea and chlorides in man. I. An index of urea excretion and the normal excretion of urea and chlorides. *J. Exp. Med.* 22: 212–236, 1915.

24. McLean, F. C. Physiology and medicine: a transition period. *Annu. Rev. Physiol.* 22: 1–16, 1960.

25. Moeller, E., J. F. McIntosh, and D. D. Van Slyke. Studies of urea excretion. II. Relationship between urine volume and the rate of urea excretion by normal adults. *J. Clin. Invest.* 6: 427–465, 1928.

26. Mudge, G. H., W. O. Berndt, and H. Valtin. Tubular transport of urea, glucose, phosphate, uric acid, sulfate, and thiosulfate. In: *Handbook of Physiology. Renal Physiology*, edited by J. Orloff and R. W. Berliner.

Washington, DC: Am. Physiol. Soc., 1973, sect. 8, chapt. 19, p. 587–652.
27. Ni, T.-G., and P. B. Rehberg. On the mechanism of sugar excretion. I. Glucose. *Biochem. J.* 24: 1039–1046, 1930.
28. Pitts, R. F. *Physiology of the Kidney and Body Fluids.* Chicago, IL: Year Book, 1963.
29. Pitts, R. F. Homer William Smith—January 2, 1895–March 25, 1962. *Biogr. Mem. Natl. Acad. Sci.* 39: 445–470, 1967.
30. Rehberg, P. B. Studies on kidney function. I. The rate of filtration and reabsorption in the human kidney. *Biochem. J.* 20: 447–460, 1926.
31. Rehberg, P. B. The filtration reabsorption theory of kidney function and its use in the clinic. In: *The Kidney in Health and Disease*, edited by H. Berglund and G. Medes. Philadelphia, PA: Lea & Febiger, 1935, p. 73–91.
33. Rothschuh, K. E. *Geschichte der Physiologie.* Berlin: Springer-Verlag, 1953, p. 124.
34. Rothschuh, K. E. *Geschichte der Physiologie.* Berlin: Springer-Verlag, 1953, p. 150.
35. Rothschuh, K. E. *Geschichte der Physiologie.* Berlin: Springer-Verlag, 1953, p. 151.
36. Schuster, V. L., and D. W. Seldin. Renal clearance. In: *The Kidney*, edited by D. W. Seldin and G. Giebisch. New York: Raven, 1985, p. 365–395.
37. Shannon, J. A. Renal tubular excretion. *Physiol. Rev.* 19: 63–93, 1939.
38. Shannon, J. A., and S. Fisher. Renal tubular reabsorption of glucose in the normal dog. *Am. J. Physiol.* 122: 765–774, 1938.
39. Smith, H. W. The excretion of the non-metabolized sugars in the dogfish, the dog, and man. In: *The Kidney in Health and Disease*, edited by H. Berglund and G. Medes. Philadelphia, PA: Lea & Febiger, 1935, p. 92–110.
40. Smith, H. W. *The Physiology of the Kidney.* New York: Oxford Univ. Press, 1937, p. 25.
41. Smith, H. W. Newer methods of study of renal function in man. In: *Lectures on the Kidney.* Lawrence, KS: Univ. of Kansas, Extension Div., 1943, p. 39.
42. Smith, H. W. Renal physiology between two wars. In: *Lectures on the Kidney.* Lawrence, KS: Univ. of Kansas, Extension Div., 1943, p. 63–82.
43. Smith, H. W. *The Kidney: Structure and Function in Health and Disease.* New York: Oxford Univ. Press, 1951.
44. Smith, H. W. *The Kidney: Structure and Function in Health and Disease.* New York: Oxford Univ. Press, 1951, p. 149.
45. Smith, H. W. *Man and His Gods.* Boston, MA: Little, Brown, 1955, p. 445–485.
46. Smith, H. W. Renal physiology. In: *Circulation of the Blood: Men and Ideas*, edited by A. F. Fishman and D. W. Richards. New York: Oxford Univ. Press, 1964, p. 545–606.
47. Smith, H. W. *Homer William Smith, ScD—His Scientific and Literary Achievements*, edited by H. Chasis and W. Goldring. New York: New York Univ. Press, 1965, plates 1, 4, and 16.
48. Smith, H. W., W. Goldring, and H. Chasis. The measurement of the

tubular excretory mass, effective blood flow and filtration rate in the normal human kidney. *J. Clin. Invest.* 17: 263–278, 1938.

49. Smith, H. W., W. Goldring, H. Chasis, H. A. Ranges, and S. E. Bradley. The application of saturation methods to the study of glomerular and tubular function in the human kidney. *J. Mt. Sinai Hosp.* 10: 59–108, 1943.

50. Van Slyke, D. D., C. P. Rhoads, A. Hiller, and A. S. Alving. Relationships between urea excretion, renal blood flow, renal oxygen consumption, and diuresis. The mechanism of urea excretion. *Am. J. Physiol.* 109: 336–374, 1934.

51. Vaughan, V. C. *A Doctor's Memories.* Indianapolis, IN: Bobbs-Merrill, 1926, p. 212.

52. Weiner, I. M. Transport of weak acids and bases. In: *Handbook of Physiology. Renal Physiology*, edited by J. Orloff and R. W. Berliner. Washington, DC: Am. Physiol. Soc., 1973, sect. 8, chapt. 17, p. 521–554.

IV

Micropuncture and Microperfusion

ERICH E. WINDHAGER

THE method of in vivo micropuncture of renal glomeruli, tubuli, and blood vessels has been used by physiologists and nephrologists for the past sixty-five years. The history of micropuncture studies shows that for the first two decades one group of investigators working at the University of Pennsylvania in the laboratory of A. Newton Richards (Fig. 1) dominated the field almost exclusively. These studies therefore constitute a coherent self-contained endeavor. There followed a gap in time, a full decade, before others started, afresh and in many directions, where the previous group had ended. It is because of this particular course of events that one can look upon the history of this field as consisting of two stages, one before and the other after World War II.

MICROPUNCTURE AND MICROPERFUSION

Developments Before 1945

By the end of World War I, Arthur R. Cushny (10) had just summarized the literature on kidney function then available, struggling with the two competing hypotheses of his time, which he tried to consolidate by "the modern view." However, penetrating as Cushny's analysis certainly was, the time was ripe for new technical approaches capable of giving decisive results. Two scientists played the critical role during the first half of our century in developing such approaches and in putting them to use on the right questions at the right time: Joseph T. Wearn (Fig. 2) and Richards.

Richards described the events that led to the introduction of kidney micropuncture in a letter to Paul Weiss (24), President of the Harvey Society, when Carl W. Gottschalk (see Fig. 7) in his Harvey Lecture (23) of December 1962 presented some of the accomplishments of the new wave of kidney micropuncturers. The letter is reprinted in part in the following:

Warfield Longcope was president of the Harvey Society during the year 1919–1920. He invited me to give one of the lectures of the following season. I accepted, having done some perfusion experiments on the rabbit kidney in collaboration with Cecil Drinker and Oscar Plant, which led to the belief that the efferent arteriole was a contractile structure and could take part in the regulation of glomerular capillary pressure. I thought that a description of those experiments might serve as a nucleus of a Harvey Lecture.

During the months preceding the proposed date of the lecture I read August Krogh's work on the capillaries of the frog's tongue, and the thought occurred, if Krogh could see the minute vessels in the tongue, perhaps if I tried, I could see the small vessels in the frog's kidney. Carl Schmidt and I tried and found that the blood vessels of that kidney could quite easily be visualized, and some of our work supported the view that the efferent vessel contracts when subjected to minute concentrations of adrenalin.

I gave the lecture in January 1921 and included in it a description of the behaviour of the frog's glomerular capillaries.

In April of that year I saw Robert Chambers puncture erythrocytes and imagined that I might, with one of his pipettes, apply a little adrenalin to an exposed efferent vessel. In September of that year, Joseph T. Wearn came to work in my laboratory. After he had learned how to expose a living frog's kidney for direct microscopic study and had come to realize its possibilities, I suggested that we make some capillary pipettes and try to apply adrenalin to an efferent vessel and see what happened. He countered with the suggestion, why not puncture a glomerular capsule with the pipette, get some glomerular fluid and find out what was in it. He went back to work, succeeded, and this experiment gave the first direct proof of reabsorption of glucose and chloride from the tubule and pointed to the identity of glomerular fluid with protein-free plasma. Then followed a long series of quantitative studies of plasma, glomerular and tubular urine of amphibia, culminating in the work of Walker, Bott, Oliver and MacDowell (1939–41) which gave similar quantitative information concerning the composition of fluid taken from different levels of the mammalian nephron. The war necessitated stoppage of the work and neither Walker nor I could take it up again.

The work was exceedingly difficult because of the crudity of the apparatus, all of which we had to make ourselves. Many days in 1921–1922 elapsed before Wearn succeeded in withdrawing uncontaminated glomerular urine from a frog.

In a historical vignette published in *The Physiologist* in 1980, only four years before he died at the age of ninety-one, Wearn gave a memorable account of his role in the development and application

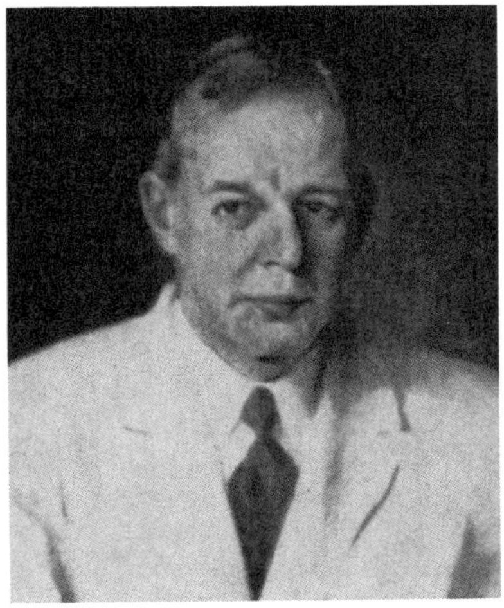

Figure 1. Alfred Newton Richards (1876–1966). This portrait was painted by Joseph C. Johansen in 1933 when Richards was 57 years old and at the height of his scientific career.

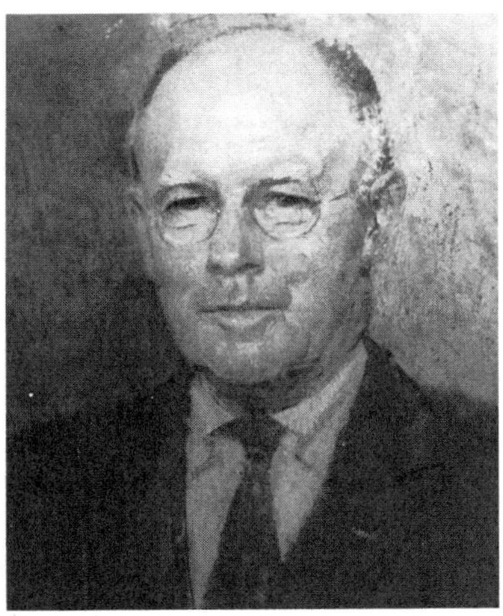

Figure 2. Joseph Treloar Wearn (1893–1984).

of renal micropuncture studies (66). His detailed and fascinating account of the work included the initial success referred to in Richards's letter.

After a good deal of practice I could, with reasonable certainty, insert a pipette into a glomerulus without touching the capillary tuft or the wall of the capsule. Then, early one afternoon, I prepared a frog and inserted the pipette into the glomerulus without touching the capillary tuft or interrupting the blood flow in it. In a little less than an hour's time, the end of the pipette began to show fluid below the mercury. The circulation of the glomerular tuft was rapid and the fluid in the pipette rose steadily. Richards and I literally tiptoed around the laboratory lest we shake the preparation. It was our first sight of such a "copious" amount of glomerular fluid. Late in the afternoon I terminated the collection, transferred the fluid successfully to a capillary tube, and then by dividing the fluid, ended up with four samples of glomerular fluid for testing. We stored the tubes in the refrigerator, adjourned to Richards' house, had a couple of cocktails and then went to a burlesque show.

The next morning we performed tests on all the samples.

The first publication (67), containing descriptions of the methods (Fig. 3) and presenting the new results by Wearn and Richards, appeared in the December 1924 issue of the *American Journal of Physiology.* It was entitled "Observations on the Composition of Glomerular Urine With Particular Reference to the Problem of Reabsorption in the Renal Tubules." The authors' discussion of their data at the time of the publication of these landmark experiments is still entirely valid:

Extended discussion of the results here presented is unnecessary. Direct testing of the fluid eliminated by the frog's glomerulus proves the assumption which was made by the earliest of the modern students of renal physiology, that a protein-free, watery fluid is separated from the blood stream as it passes through the glomerular capillaries....

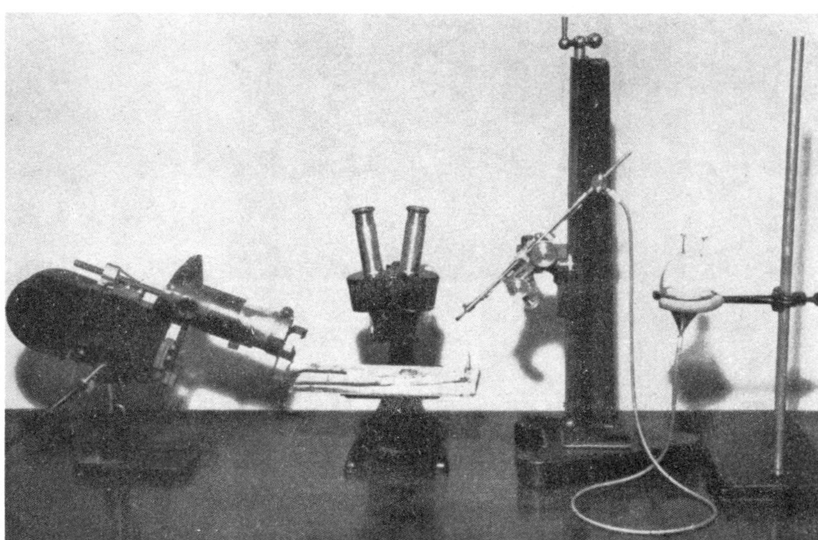

Figure 3. Apparatus used by Richards and his pupils for visualizing frog kidney circulation and for micropuncturing glomeruli and tubuli. *Left* to *right*: arc light for transillumination, binocular microscope with frog board, micropipette holder in Palmer stand, and mercury-leveling board.

The discovery that two substances, sodium chloride and glucose, both of which are normal constituents of blood plasma, are not to be found in bladder urine under the conditions of these experiments, but are to be found in considerable concentration in the fluid taken directly from the glomerulus, proves beyond doubt that reabsorption of these substances must take place in the renal tubules. . . . The conception of differential reabsorption in the tubules therefore receives support of the most direct character. . . . The experiments do not contain direct evidence concerning the nature of the process by which protein-free fluid is separated from the blood in the glomerulus . . . (the results) may be regarded as indirect evidence that the process in the glomerulus is physical and since the most conspicuous physical force demonstrable in the glomerulus is the blood pressure, it may be regarded as evidence in favor of the filtration hypothesis. . . . It will be objected that the observations here reported were made on the frog's kidney which is a mesonephros, and hence is different in the details of its structure from that of mammals; . . . there is no guarantee that these observations are applicable to events in the mammalian kidney. That there is a striking similarity of structure between the glomerulus of the frog and that of mammals no one will deny; that the mesonephros of the frog serves that animal in the same fashion and as effectively as the kidney serves the higher mammals is also hardly open to contradiction. Until observations of similar directness have been made upon mammalian kidney, with contrary results, it is believed that the inferences drawn from these experiments may be extended to the mammalian kidney.

The chemical analysis of the minute fluid samples collected by micropuncture posed severe problems. Radioisotope-labeled compounds, used extensively in later years, were unavailable, of course, to Richards and his colleagues, and they had to develop chemical and physical techniques for the ultramicroanalysis of their samples. As a first step, they attempted to measure the chloride concentration of glomerular fluid but encountered numerous difficulties. Their results on fluid collected from amphibians were published in three papers (14, 68, 71) over a period of ten years. All reported different results.

It was not until after the report by the Swedish investigator Gösta Ekehorn (13) that the chloride concentrations of plasma and glomerular fluid are equal, that Westfall, Findley, and Richards (14), using still another ultramicrochemical method to measure chloride concentrations of glomerular urine and blood plasma in frogs and necturi, felt confident to conclude:

The chloride concentrations of the two fluids were approximately equal. The slight concentration difference, consistent in sign, found in most of the experiments was approximately that which could be expected to result from the operation of the Gibbs-Donnan law of membrane equilibrium. The results, regarded as more trustworthy than those previously obtained in this laboratory by the nephelometric analytical method, confirm those of Ekehorn.

From 1930 to 1935, they obtained data relating to the pH and total solute, total electrolyte, chloride, phosphate, glucose, urea, uric acid, creatinine, phenol red, and inulin concentrations that "*provide a fairly comprehensive picture of the quantitative likeness of the glomerular urine and the blood plasma or an ultrafiltrate from it. . . . The distribution of the values of glomerular urine in relation to those of blood plasma is such as to leave no doubt concerning identity of composition of the two fluids*" (6). Their measurements of inulin concentration were of particular importance because they provided unequivocal evidence that inulin is completely filtrable at the glomerulus, the first criterion for a substance to be used as a measure of the glomerular filtration rate (GFR).

Their next major project was to describe quantitatively the process of tubular reabsorption and to assess the importance of the several segments of the nephron in the process. In 1937 Richards and Arthur M. Walker (47) published a paper entitled "Methods of Collecting Fluid From Known Regions of the Renal Tubules of Amphibia and of Perfusing the Lumen of a Single Tubule." The five succeeding papers (42, 61–64) in the same issue of the *American Journal of Physiology* described the total molecular and chloride concentrations, the reabsorption of glucose and the action of phlorizin on it, the site of acidification of urine, and the role of the tubule in excretion of urea and of inorganic phosphates. This was a remarkable achievement and provided most of our present knowledge of the magnitude and localization of reabsorptive processes in the amphibian kidney.

Walker joined the Richards group in 1926 after internship at Massachusetts General Hospital (MGH). He developed unusual and unique skills in glomerular and tubular micropuncture and made a most important contribution to Richards's research program. His military service was prolonged in both World Wars. He was severely wounded leading an attack in World War I, and after World War II ill health greatly handicapped his career.

He also played a key role in the development of micropuncture techniques in mammalian kidneys, the culminating achievement of Richards's team. Gottschalk, who still knew most of the members of the group personally, gave the following account of this period (24).

Richards and his colleagues recognized that it was highly desirable to have similar studies on the mammalian kidney, but because of the technical difficulties involved—the smaller tubules, the absence of glomeruli on the surface of the kidney, the added problems imposed by respiratory and pulsatile movement of the kidney, etc.—[they] *postponed work on the mammalian kidney until the last. They also recognized that establishing the site of micropuncture was a more*

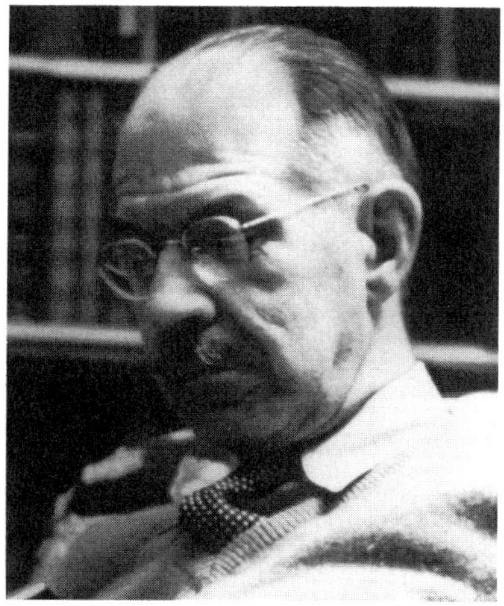

Figure 4. Jean Redman Oliver (1889–1976).

formidable process in the mammalian than in the amphibian kidney and that their methods would not be adaptable for this purpose. Fortunately they were able to obtain the collaboration of Dr. Jean Oliver [Fig. 4], *then in the Department of Pathology, Long Island College of Medicine, a world authority in studying the structure of individual nephrons by microdissection.*

This collaboration of physiologists and morphologists resulted in two landmark papers, published in the October issue of the *American Journal of Physiology* in 1941. The first, by Walker and Oliver (65), was entitled "Methods for the Collection of Fluid From Single Glomeruli and Tubules of the Mammalian Kidney." The second, by Walker, Bott, Oliver, and MacDowell (60), was entitled "The Collection and Analysis of Fluid From Single Nephrons of the Mammalian Kidney."[1] For the next decade, this latter paper was the sole source of direct and quantitative information concerning the function of individual glomeruli and tubular segments in the mammalian kidney:

The analyses indicate that glomerular fluid, entirely or nearly free of protein, contains reducing substances and creatinine in concentrations similar to those existing in plasma water. Within the proximal convolution, all of the reducing substances and at least two-thirds of the fluid are reabsorbed. This fluid reabsorption is an isosmotic process, accomplished without producing any increase in osmotic pressure of the fluid remaining within the tubule; it is not, however, a purely passive reabsorption of unchanged glomerular fluid, for the chloride concentration of tubule fluid increases to a level 1.4 times that obtaining in blood plasma. The existence of this increased chloride concentration apparently requires that bicarbonate be preferentially reabsorbed by the proximal tubule, but the point has not yet been directly examined. The tentative conclusions, drawn from a small number of experiments with distal tubule fluid, are stated in the body of the paper.

These two publications reported the last micropuncture studies performed in Richards's laboratory. World War II had erupted in Europe, and Richards and his colleagues were diverted from their studies of renal physiology to provide important advice and direction for medical research relevant to the war effort.

Developments After 1945

By the end of World War II, micropuncture of single nephrons in vivo had become recognized as the most powerful approach to studying renal function. Fundamental questions that had remained open for nearly a century had been answered unambiguously during the previous two decades by the studies of Richards and his collaborators. Their results had demonstrated that ultrafiltration of plasma is the mechanism of glomerular filtrate formation and that two-thirds of the filtrate is reabsorbed isosmotically in the proximal tubule. Tubular function had been shown to consist of epithelial transport of sodium chloride, bicarbonate, and glucose from tubular lumen to blood and also of the transport of some organic solutes in the secretory direction, that is, from blood to tubular lumen. High chloride concentrations found in the proximal tubules of mammalian kidneys suggested that this nephron segment might play an important role in the acid-base balance of the body. In addition there was some preliminary evidence that distal tubule fluid remains hyposmotic compared to systemic plasma, thereby leading the way to studies of the concentrating and diluting mechanism of the kidney.

Only slowly and in isolated laboratories did the scientific world react to the availability of this powerful new approach to studies of renal function. Considering the large number of unsolved problems in renal physiology, one might have expected that research centers throughout the world would rush to make use of this new opportunity. This was by no means the case. More than ten years elapsed between the 1941 study by Walker, Bott, Oliver, and MacDowell (60) and the publication of the next renal micropuncture study in a critically reviewed journal (79). One can only speculate about the reasons for this apparent inertia of the scientific world. One consideration was certainly the ease with which indirect information on renal function could be deduced from clearance experiments. Knowledge of the function of the whole kidney was still limited, and important results could be collected by the much less demanding approach of urine and plasma collection and chemical analyses on relatively large volumes of biological fluids. However, the major factor was clearly the extraordinary difficulty of the techniques of puncture, microdissection, and ultramicroanalysis of the collected fluid samples. Richards in fact discouraged young investigators who expressed a desire to develop the technique of micropuncture in their own laboratories (24). He feared that newcomers might not always be sufficiently skilled or critical enough to avoid the many potential pitfalls of the technique. The obvious remedy for these fears, the training of new investigators in Richards's laboratory under close supervision by the experienced masters, was no longer possible. His micropuncture laboratory at the University of Philadelphia had ceased to exist because its members, including Richards, had become senior administrators and academicans or had given up academic pursuits. Phyllis Bott (Fig. 5) remained as the sole torchbearer of the new approach. Although perfectly familiar with all aspects of micropuncture, her forte had been the chemical and physical analysis of fluid samples rather than the surgical preparation of mammalian kidneys in vivo for micropuncture and the collection of fluid from glomeruli and tubules. Furthermore, Bott soon became chairperson of the biochemistry department of Women's Medical College in Philadelphia—an activity that obviously must have curtailed her time in the laboratory.

There were probably other reasons for the delay in using micropuncture techniques. After the war the number of investigators working in physiologically oriented laboratories was still very small. In fact, the United States, the main reservoir of academic personnel in the world in 1945, did not initiate its large-scale financial-support program for biomedical research until the early 1950s, while many European countries had lost a whole generation of potential investigators and had to channel all their efforts at recovering from the devastating effects of World War II. It is therefore not surprising

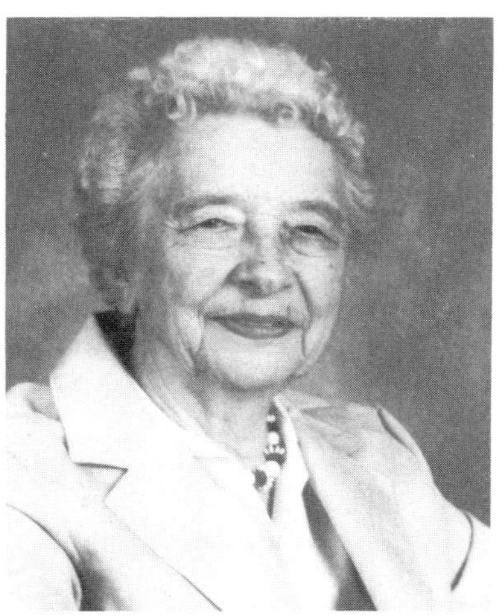

Figure 5. Phyllis A. Bott (b. 1899).

that a citizen of a neutral European country with sufficient imagination, means, courage, and skill was to become the first person after World War II to perform a micropuncture study on mammalian kidneys in vivo (78).

After developing techniques to puncture vasa recta in the renal papilla of golden hamsters in vivo and to measure the osmolality of collected microsamples of blood in his laboratory at the Department of Physiology at the University of Basel, Switzerland, Heinrich Wirz (Fig. 6) journeyed to Bott's laboratory in Philadelphia to learn tubular micropuncture. He did this primarily in the hope of eventually testing whether the concept of countercurrent multiplication, developed by Werner Kuhn on theoretical grounds, was indeed applicable to the process of urine concentration in mammalian kidneys. Wirz's unique contribution to science was that he correctly identified the two most important developments in renal physiology of his time, one a theoretical concept, the other a methodological innovation, and then committed himself to act upon this realization. Prior to his stay in Bott's laboratory, Wirz (78) had already reported that blood samples obtained by vascular micropuncture of vasa recta in the surgically exposed renal papilla of hamsters were hyperosmotic to systemic blood. After his return from Philadelphia, he performed tubular micropuncture experiments on rat kidneys. In his first study, Wirz described the hydrostatic pressure profile along the nephron. This was quickly followed by a paper in which he showed that "early" distal tubule fluid remains hyposmotic to systemic plasma even in highly concentrating kidneys; osmotic equilibration occurs

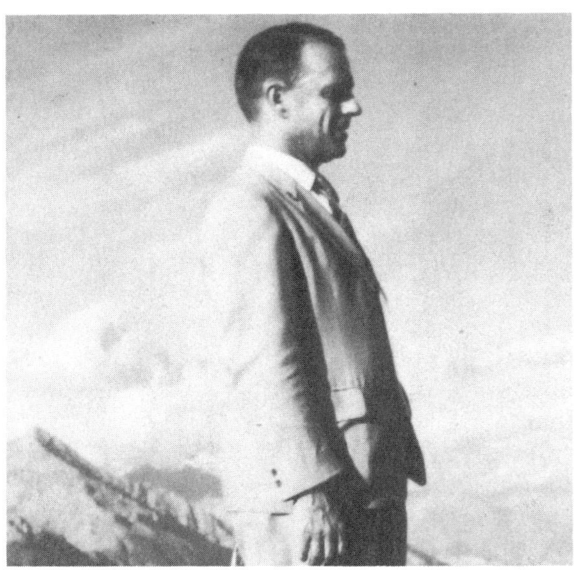

Figure 6. Heinrich A. Wirz (b. 1914).

in the "late" distal tubule but only when the osmolality of the final urine is high. The fact that osmotic equilibration failed to occur during experimentally induced water diuresis, that is, in the absence of antidiuretic hormone, indicates that the physiological role of this hormone is to increase the osmotic water permeability of the late distal nephron.

Wirz's findings that vasa recta blood from the tip of the renal papilla is always hyperosmotic, whereas tubule fluid emerging from the ascending limb of Henle's loop into the early distal tubule is always hyposmotic, were of utmost importance. They lent strong support to Kuhn's hypothesis that countercurrent flow in the loop of Henle and in vasa recta with multiplication of small transmural osmotic gradients is responsible for the concentrating ability of mammalian kidneys.

Two other young investigators, Carl W. Gottschalk (Fig. 7) and Gerhard H. Giebisch (see Fig. 8), started to apply micropuncture techniques soon after Wirz had visited Bott's laboratory. Both had MD degrees and were postdoctoral fellows in physiology departments. At this time Giebisch was still an Austrian exchange visitor at Cornell University Medical College, planning to return to the Department of Pharmacology at the University of Vienna. Gottschalk had been an intern in Internal Medicine at MGH and had then spent two years in the US armed forces in the Canadian Arctic where he had participated in studies of human adaptation to a cold climate. Subsequently he began his research training in the physiology department of Harvard Medical School under the guidance of Eugene M. Landis.

Both Giebisch and Gottschalk were clearly influenced in their choice of research problems by the scientific orientation of these departments. At Harvard Gottschalk found an environment in which cardiovascular function was in the mainstream of interest of several senior members of the Department of Physiology, Landis being the master experimentalist who, many years earlier, had validated Starling's hypothesis of capillary fluid exchange by direct micropuncture. Gottschalk was interested in the pathophysiology of congestive heart failure and in hypertension. For a considerable portion of his fellowship, he was involved in studies on the effect of renal denervation on renal function, a topic that he returned to as a mature scientist several decades later. He also became interested in measuring the hydrostatic pressure within the renal interstitium in normal and hypertensive dogs, using a modification of Landis's technique (38). The movement of a stained Ringer's solution into or out of the tip of a glass micropipette was taken as an index of hydrostatic pressure in the original Landis method and in the modified method used by Gottschalk. However, the pipettes used in Gottschalk's interstitial pressure experiment were much larger; they were approximately 100 microns in diameter, and the pressures measured were only a

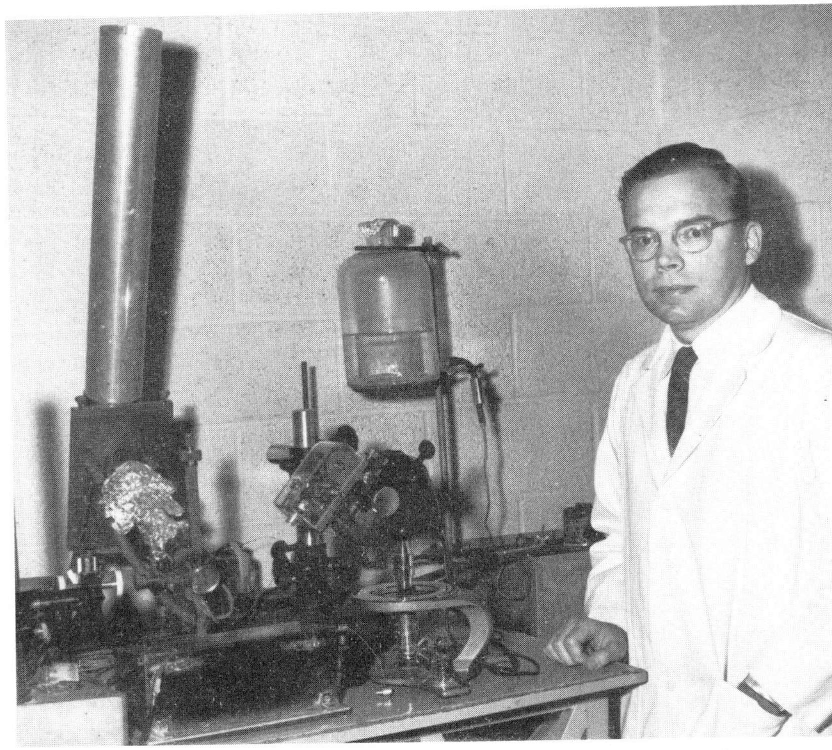

Figure 7. Carl W. Gottschalk (b. 1922) standing next to mammalian micropuncture equipment in his laboratory in the middle 1950s. *Left* to *right*: Knisely quartz-rod illuminator, heated animal board, and modified de Fonbrune micromanipulator.

relative index of interstitial pressure "contaminated" by the unavoidable damage to the vascular compartment. Gottschalk undoubtedly gained considerable practice in preparing kidneys for direct microscopic manipulation, which later facilitated his full-fledged micropuncture studies in rats. While still at Harvard and using some equipment borrowed from Landis, he actually measured intratubular hydrostatic pressure using micropipettes. This activity was forcefully stopped by Landis, who pointed out that such studies would need a minimum time commitment of two years—which at this point were no longer available to Gottschalk because he had to start completing his residency training at MGH. Nevertheless, a clear goal was established and important skills had been acquired. During the next two years as a medical resident, Gottschalk was planning and dreaming of establishing his own micropuncture laboratory as soon as possible after accepting an appointment in the Department of Medicine at the University of North Carolina at Chapel Hill. With these plans he succeeded splendidly in 1954 and was able to recruit Margaret Mylle, who was to become one of the most skilled micropuncturists in the world. During 1954 Gottschalk obtained a large number of observations on the hydrostatic pressure profile along the mammalian nephron, including measurements of hydrostatic pressure in the distal convoluted tubule. He reported these findings in two papers (27, 28) in the *American Journal of Physiology* in 1956 and 1957. With these studies Gottschalk had demonstrated to the many doubtful members of the scientific establishment that micropuncture of mammalian kidneys could be done successfully by someone other than a member of the old group of Richards. This was important because it helped to remove the resistance to granting agencies and department chairmen to supporting young individuals who wished to enter this field of research.

At Cornell, Robert F. Pitts had established himself as the world's leading authority on kidney acid-base metabolism and had made problems of renal tubule ion transport the center of attention in nearly all laboratories of his department. The role of electrical potential gradients as driving forces for ion movement was then widely recognized among renal physiologists, mainly due to the publications of Hans H. Ussing. Also, by the end of the 1940s, microelectrodes with tip diameters less than one micron had been introduced into electrophysiological studies of excitable tissues by Ling and Gerard (24). Giebisch's plan was eventually to combine micropuncture techniques with the newly available method of defining voltages across the tubular wall and across the individual cell membranes of tubular epithelium in vivo. However, the important initial stimulus for getting actively involved in micropuncture was provided by a chance visit to Cornell by the Viennese Internist Erwin Deutsch, who expressed the wish to observe tubular micropuncture. A demonstration of tubular microdissection—not micropuncture—was duly arranged for Giebisch and Deutsch in Oliver's laboratory. On this occasion, Giebisch first realized that only Bott could teach tubular micropuncture. With Pitts's blessing, Giebisch approached Bott, who agreed to accept him as a trainee in 1955, provided that he was willing to reexamine the question of whether the chloride concentration of proximal tubule fluid in *Necturus maculosus* kidney was higher than that of plasma. For Bott this project was important to reevaluate the method of measuring chloride concentrations in ultramicrosamples of deproteinized fluid and to shed light on the apparent incongruity of finding elevated tubular chloride concentrations (64) with no difference in pH across the wall of *Necturus* proximal tubule (42). As it turned out, in this amphibian species there was neither a chloride nor a pH gradient across the proximal tubular epithelium (17). This result validated the pH measurements of Montgomery and Pierce (42) and delegated tubular fluid acidification to the distal nephron of the amphibian kidney. For a few years afterward, many renal physiologists erroneously extrapolated these conclusions to the mammalian proximal tubule, an error that was

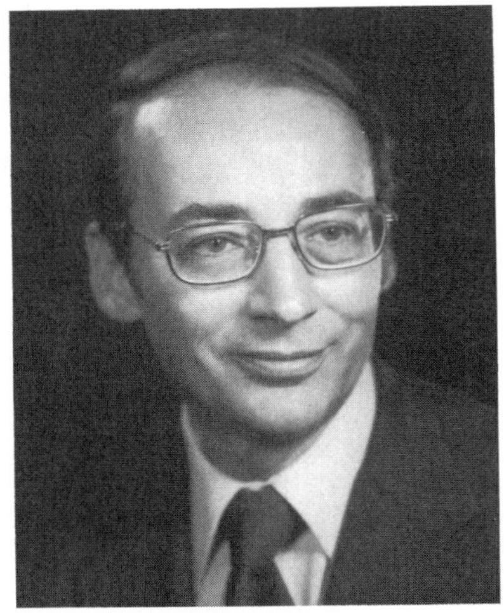

Figure 8. Gerhard H. Giebisch (b. 1927).

only corrected by Gottschalk, Lassiter, and Mylle (25) in micropuncture studies of rat proximal tubules several years later.

On his return to his own laboratory at Cornell in New York City, Gerhard Giebisch (Fig. 8) concentrated all his efforts on defining the electrical driving forces acting on ions in their movement across the tubule wall by measuring the transepithelial as well as the transmembrane voltage in proximal tubules of *Necturus* kidney (18). Although Wilbrandt (75) had measured transepithelial voltages in amphibian kidney tubules in the past, the use of the Ling-Gerard–type microelectrode provided a vast improvement regarding leakage artifacts and, for the first time, offered the opportunity of defining the electrical gradient across the cell membranes proper. This study was greatly facilitated by the description of a microelectrode puller by Alexander and Nastuk (1), which made it much easier to manufacture small-tip microelectrodes than it had been previously when "pulling by hand" was the only known method of producing microelectrode tips for intracellular impalements. In this study Giebisch established that the tubular lumen is electrically negative to the peritubular fluid compartment and that the basolateral cell membrane potential is about −70 mV. These results strengthened the view that sodium is actively reabsorbed and were in agreement with Sidney Solomon's findings (52) in rat kidneys in vivo. Solomon had also used Ling-Gerard–type microelectrodes and had arrived at similar values for the basolateral membrane voltage and the transepithelial electrical potential gradient (−20 mV). However, the problem of accurate localization of the microelectrode tip within the tubule lumen was more problematic in the small mammalian tubules and was to haunt a large number of electrophysiologists working on the kidney in the next two decades.

While Wirz in Switzerland was in the initial stages of his studies of the osmotic composition of vasa recta blood in the hamster papilla and while Gottschalk was slowly crystallizing his eventual research goals, Bott reinvestigated the single-nephron filtration rate in *Necturus* kidneys in which a new ultramicroanalysis for creatinine was described (3). Importantly, in this study latex was used for the first time. Bott injected it into the punctured nephron where it solidified as a luminal cast of the filled portion of the nephron and clearly showed the site of puncture by the appearance of a mushroom-like structure on the tubular cast through the puncture hole. When the excised kidney was placed into acid, the surrounding tissue dissolved while a relatively firm tubular cast remained. With one stroke the need for localizing the puncture site by dissecting the one punctured nephron out of the surrounding thirty thousand intact nephrons was removed. From then on the effort in micropuncture was effectively halved, and the required skills were significantly decreased by the introduction of the "neoprene technique." This was undoubtedly one of the most important technical advances in the entire history of micropuncture development.

Bott continued to maintain a micropuncture laboratory until the early 1960s. After developing the first flame photometer for the ultramicroanalysis of sodium and potassium (4), she published, in collaboration with the newly trained investigator Judith Litchfield, a micropuncture study on the reabsorption of water, potassium, and sodium chloride in rat kidneys (40).

Besides Bott, Wirz, Gottschalk, and Giebisch, a whole group of persons entered the field of micropuncture in one laboratory—all of whom were recruited by A. K. Solomon during the years 1953–1966. Trained as a physical chemist at Harvard, he received his second PhD degree in physics at the Cavendish Laboratory in Cambridge. After wartime service in the British Admiralty, Solomon had developed a keen interest in the biological use of radioactive isotopes. Upon his return from England to the United States, he was recruited by A. Baird Hastings into Harvard's Department of Biochemistry to organize and head a central facility for the use and distribution of radioisotopes in clinical and nonclinical research at Harvard Medical School.

From this facility evolved the Biophysical Laboratory of Harvard Medical School, which became a center of research for membrane transport and permeability under the long-lasting, distinguished leadership of its founder. A. K. Solomon wished to apply isotope techniques to studies of membrane transport in as many organs as there was a reasonable likelihood of obtaining meaningful results, including red blood cells, stomach, intestine, and (last but not least) kidney. His main interest was the ion and water permeability of erythrocytes, but in addition he personally initiated most of the other projects in the laboratory. With respect to the study of ion and water transport in renal tubules, he could initially rely on the advice of John Pappenheimer, who had been actively interested in kidney function for some time (43), and on the microsurgery and vascular micropuncture experience of Landis; both were located in the nearby Harvard physiology department. His own areas of expertise were the mathematical treatment of isotope movement across membranes, radioanalysis, and instrument design.

Because of the emphasis on epithelial (rather than organ) function, an amphibian kidney that had been studied extensively by Richards and his collaborators (45) became the object of all micropuncture studies in A. K. Solomon's laboratory. Qualitatively the kidney of *Necturus* had been shown to be endowed with most of the functions of mammalian kidneys, including glomerular filtration and isosmotic reabsorption of filtered fluid by its proximal tubule. Technically this amphibian kidney offered great advantages over the use of mammalian preparations: luminal diameters five to six times larger, surface localization and hence accessibility of the entire length of the proximal and distal tubules, and the absence of respiratory and pulsatile movements during micropuncture. Because of the advantageous topography of the proximal tubule, this nephron segment could be perfused with artificial solutions of known composition and the collected fluid then analyzed for the concentration of various solutes. Richards and Walker had given a detailed description of this approach as early as 1937 (47). However, despite several years of trial, the autodidactic efforts of the "new generation" at Harvard were never fully successful, as indicated by the fact that the perfused tubules stubbornly refused to show any indication of water reabsorption. In the end, Hans Schatzmann and I arrived at the so-called "stopped-flow" microperfusion technique, in which a fluid droplet isolated from the rest of the tubular contents by oil columns was left stationary in the lumen for twenty minutes and then removed for analysis. This technique was described in a paper that summarized the methodological achievements of all the individuals who had worked on the project from 1953 to 1957 (50). A seemingly minor, but actually very important, contribution had been made by Tom Kennedy at the National Institutes of Health (NIH), who noticed that heavy mineral oil could be stained intensely with Sudan black B and was then easily visible when injected as a small column into the lumen. This obviated the use of metallic mercury droplets as mechanical blocks between the injected intraluminal perfusate and the physiological fluid normally present within the tubule lumen. The use of mercury had been a continuous source of frustration, as very high pressure was required to force it through the small openings of the micropipettes. This injection system was difficult to control: frequently the entire nephron instead of the desired short tubule segment filled with mercury, one of the numerous seals of the pipette connections burst, or other mishaps occurred. Sudan black B was subsequently adopted by most other micropuncture laboratories.

MICROPUNCTURE AND MICROPERFUSION

The stopped-flow microperfusion technique was then used to characterize the mode of proximal tubular transport of sodium and water. Based on whole kidney–clearance experiments, Wesson and Anslow (69) originally presented indirect arguments for the view that in mannitol diuresis sodium was reabsorbed against its concentration gradient across the wall of the proximal tubule. This hypothesis could now be approached directly, and in addition the effect of the transepithelial electrical-potential gradient could be evaluated with Ling-Gerard–type microelectrodes. These studies were facilitated by the introduction of methods for the ultramicroanalysis of various radioactively labeled compounds, particularly inulin and sodium isotopes. By 1958 evidence for the passive reabsorption of water and the active nature of sodium transport in the proximal tubule of the amphibian kidney had been established unequivocally (72, 77). A. K. Solomon then published the first compartmental analysis of transepithelial ion movement as it applied to the renal tubule (51), and subsequent work at Harvard extended such studies to the distal tubule of the amphibian kidney (41).

Some of the research fellows in A. K. Solomon's laboratory who had worked there on *Necturus* kidney continued to study renal function during their subsequent careers, for instance, Donald Oken at Harvard, Guillermo Whittembury in Caracas, Venezuela, Carl Bentzel in Buffalo, and me at Cornell. Others never returned to renal physiology, for instance, Schatzmann, who had greatly contributed to getting the entire project under way and who later added the discovery of the ATP-driven calcium pump in the plasma membrane of red blood cells to his many other scientific achievements.

In the middle 1950s, a nucleus of interest in direct renal-function studies began to crystallize at the Department of Physiology of the University of Göttingen. This department had recently become vacant because of the tragic mountaineering accident of its chairman Opitz, in which he and two of his staff members had lost their lives. Kurt Kramer, previously chairman at Marburg, was then appointed as Opitz's successor at Göttingen. With him came Karl J. Ullrich, who after receiving his medical degree had shown keen interest in the physiology of the renal concentrating and diluting operation. Under still-rather-restricted economic circumstances, Ullrich set up his laboratory in which he first carried out electrolyte analyses on renal medullary slices, the results of which strongly supported Wirz's views of renal medullary function. He then developed the highly original technique of cannulating in vivo single terminal collecting tubules in rat kidney for sampling tubular fluid by means of hand-drawn ultrathin polyethylene capillaries and a number of chemical ultramicroanalyses for urinary constituents, in particular, urea (35) and ammonium ions (58).

At Cornell I had joined Giebisch's laboratory in Pitts's department in 1958. Giebisch had spent the academic year 1956–1957 in the Department of Pharmacology at the University of Vienna, partly to keep a promise he had made to Hans Bruecke before leaving Austria and also to fulfill a requirement of the US Immigration and Naturalization Service. While in Vienna he designed and executed an electrophysiological study of the potassium permeability in rat skeletal muscle, a project that was of considerable physiological interest and that greatly enhanced his skills of working with microelectrodes. In the following year he collaborated with Pitts on what have since become classic studies on acid-base balance in dogs. The idea that I might join Giebisch in a common effort to establish a micropuncture laboratory had been under discussion for several years. It was a logical development in view of a friendship that dated back to our time at the University of Vienna as well as our strong interest in kidney function, and it received the active support of Pitts. Our aim was to study sodium reabsorption in the mammalian kidney, to evaluate chloride transport in *Necturus* proximal tubules using the methods developed in A. K. Solomon's laboratory, and (for Giebisch) to combine the long-described method of double perfusion of amphibian kidneys with measurements of electrical membrane potentials using ion substitutions for the characterization of membrane permeabilities.

This collaboration yielded proof of the ability of mammalian proximal tubules to transport sodium against an electrochemical potential gradient and confirmed (76) in principle the views previously derived from indirect evidence by Wesson, Anslow, and Homer W. Smith (70). The study on bidirectional chloride fluxes gave the first indication of a component of mediated chloride transport in proximal tubules (21), and in another micropuncture study the stopped-flow microperfusion technique was adapted to the rat proximal tubule (20). Giebisch's microelectrode study on the doubly perfused *Necturus* kidney (19) provided the first cell model for ion transport across renal tubular epithelium, in which sodium and potassium membrane permeabilities and the sodium-potassium pump were visualized in the polarized arrangement now generally accepted. The same conclusions had simultaneously been reached by Whittembury, Sugino, and A. K. Solomon (73) in microelectrode studies on kidney slices. Both of these studies rested conceptually on the cell model of sodium transport across frog skin epithelium that had recently been proposed by Koefoed-Johnsen and Ussing (36).

While these studies were in progress, Gottschalk had advanced his micropuncture techniques to the highest possible degree of perfection. With Mylle (29, 30) he provided the first information on the osmolality of fluid collected from the tip of Henle's loop and of adjacent papillary collecting ducts, in both antidiuresis and water diuresis. They were the first to expose and illuminate the renal papilla of hamsters and of desert rodents in such a way that single thin limbs of Henle's loop could be visualized under the stereomicroscope. The use of desert rodents such as *Psammomys obesus* or kangaroo rat was important because of the exceptional ability of these animals to concentrate their urine. It was also known that the renal papillae of these rodents extend far into the renal pelvis, a circumstance that permits transmural puncture of loops of Henle, vasa recta, and collecting tubules over much longer distances from the tip of the papilla than was possible in hamsters. The results obtained in these studies clearly demonstrated that a countercurrent mechanism is responsible for the concentrating operation of mammalian kidneys and were a milestone in the history of micropuncture studies. It was only under the impact of these direct micropuncture results obtained on samples from the loop of Henle that Smith at last relented in his reluctance to accept the countercurrent model of renal medullary function. Of nearly equal importance was Gottschalk's study of tubular acidification in rats, in collaboration with William E. Lassiter and Mylle, in which the transepithelial pH gradients along the proximal and distal tubules were described (25). These data indicated that, in contrast to the amphibian, bicarbonate was preferentially reabsorbed over chloride by rat proximal tubule and that large pH gradients could be maintained across the wall of the distal convoluted tubule. Lassiter had been a resident in medicine at MGH before joining Gottschalk. He and Gottschalk formed a team that has remained active in micropuncture until the present time.

In a workshop on renal physiology organized by Bodil Schmidt-Nielsen in Göttingen in 1959, personal contact was first established among some of the key investigators, particularly Giebisch, Gottschalk, Ullrich, and Wirz. One immediate result of this interaction was that Ullrich and his excellent technician Pehling followed Schmidt-Nielsen's invitation to spend a sabbatical year in North Carolina. A collaborative study was then undertaken in which, initially, the animal experiments were carried out at Chapel Hill in Gottschalk's laboratory and the collected samples were then analyzed in Durham in Schmidt-Nielsen's laboratory at Duke University, a mere ten miles away. Obviously both teams were able to contribute special expertise to this collaboration. Gottschalk and Mylle provided the know-how of transmural micropuncture of cortical and medullary nephron segments in vivo, whereas Ullrich and Pehling provided their expertise in the chemical ultramicroanalyses of some of the major solutes present in tubule fluid. Lassiter provided the radioisotope expertise, and Schmidt-Nielsen, in addition to acting as an important catalyzer in bringing Ullrich to North Carolina, actively participated in this collaboration with her technician O'Dell. The outcome of this combined effort was a description of sodium and water transport by the proximal and distal convoluted tubules of rats in nondiuretic conditions and in mannitol diuresis (59), supporting the notion of active sodium transport by proximal and distal tubules. In a second paper (26), this team published their results on the composition of fluid collected from Henle's loop and the collecting ducts of hamsters and *Psammomys*, providing irrefutable evidence for the countercurrent hypothesis. Their results also provided evidence that sodium transport out of the ascending limb, rather than water movement into this nephron segment, constitutes the so-called "single effect" of multiplier in the renal medulla. The importance of these and previous studies at Chapel Hill was recognized by the American Physiological Society and the Harvey Society by inviting Gottschalk to deliver two highly prestigious lectures, the Bowditch Lecture in 1961 (22) and the Harvey Lecture in 1962 (23).

On his return to Germany, Ullrich persuaded Karl Heinz Gertz, a physicist in the Department of Physiology at Göttingen, to shift his interest from respiratory to renal physiology and, in particular, to micropuncture studies. Gertz was highly imaginative, mathematically inclined, and a good experimentalist. With Ullrich's invaluable input, Gertz designed an ingenious method to measure transepithelial fluxes of water and solutes in mammalian kidneys in vivo. The approach was essentially the same as the stopped-flow microperfusion that had been used in A. K. Solomon's laboratory in amphibians. However, instead of analyzing the inulin concentration of the collected sample as an index of water reabsorption, the decrease in volume of the injected droplet was recorded by time-lapse photography. This approach, named the *split-droplet technique*, provided data on transport and permeability properties of the renal tubular epithelium (16). With Eberhart Frömter, at that time still a medical student, Ullrich started electrophysiological studies on mammalian nephrons. After years of controversy and meticulous experimentation, Frömter was able to provide conclusive data on the magnitude and polarity of the transepithelial voltage in the proximal tubule of rat kidneys (15). All other investigators had previously reported lumen-negative voltages of about 20 mV, the value most commonly observed in random puncture of surface proximal tubules. Changes in tip potentials of the microelectrodes after insertion into the tubule lumen, touching the tubule wall with the electrode tip, and recording shunted intracellular voltages may all have contributed to false measurements. It was Frömter's great contribution to renal physiology to develop, over the course of nearly ten years, methods and rigid criteria for the measurement of transepithelial electrical-potential measurements.

At about the time that Ullrich and Pehling were working at North Carolina, Michael Steinhausen, a young investigator at the University of Heidelberg, was diligently working on the in vivo microphotography of rat kidney cortex. In his search for a dye that is filtered by glomeruli and appears in sufficient concentration in tubule fluid to be visible on microphotographs taken in vivo, he arrived at lissamine green as a suitable candidate. Steinhausen demonstrated that intravenous injection of a bolus of lissamine green was followed by the appearance of sequential, easily visible dye columns in convolutions of proximal and distal tubules at time intervals that corresponded to the velocity of flow of tubular fluid (54). The time of appearance of the front of the moving dye column at a given puncture site could then be used as a good approximation for localizing the point of fluid collection in terms of relative proximal or distal tubule length. From a technical point of view, this was another major advance in micropuncture because it greatly facilitated the task of localizing the site of tubular puncture.

Besides Ullrich and Gertz, other members of Kramer's Department of Physiology at Göttingen became active in renal micropuncture studies. Klaus Thurau (55) and Peter Deetjen worked on renal blood flow (11); with Kurt Kramer they worked on the countercurrent exchange function of vasa recta (56) in Göttingen. These two investigators later established their own highly productive teams. Thurau and Jürgen Schnermann developed the concept that a tubuloglomerular feedback mechanism, involving the juxtaglomerular apparatus, regulates the rate of glomerular filtration (57).

At about the same time, Floyd Rector and James Clapp in Donald Seldin's Department of Internal Medicine in the University of Texas at Dallas began micropuncture studies on problems of acid-base balance and the tubular transport of chloride ions (44). Clapp then moved to NIH, but the team of Rector and Seldin continued to function as one of the foremost centers of research on nephron function and tubular acidification. They were joined by Norman Carter, who was the first to apply H^+-selective glass microelectrodes for measurements of tubule fluid pH. The history of these studies is described by Rector in another chapter of this volume.

In the early 1960s, Robert W. Berliner, who was then director of the Laboratory of Kidney and Electrolyte Metabolism at NIH, succeeded in recruiting a group of outstanding young investigators, most of whom eventually became leaders in the field of micropuncture. Among the earliest in this group were Clapp, James F. Watson, and James H. Dirks, who developed the techniques needed for applying micropuncture methods to dog kidney (9, 12). This step was of major importance inasmuch as it permitted, for the first time, a direct comparison of tubule-puncture data with the mass of information that had accumulated on canine kidney. In later years Clapp concentrated his efforts mainly on renal chloride transport and on the mechanism of action of diuretics, whereas Dirks provided much of the information on tubular handling of divalent cations. Watson's highly promising career ended tragically when he and his wife lost their lives in a head-on car collision while driving from Buffalo, where he had started to establish his own laboratory, to Atlantic City to present his newest results at the FASEB Spring Meeting of the American Physiological Society in 1966.

Other members of Berliner's micropuncture team who later became internationally recognized leaders in renal physiology were Fuminori Sakai and Rex Jamison. While at NIH they succeeded in surgically splitting part of the cortex of rat kidneys in vivo in such a way as to permit transmural micropuncture of collecting ducts (49). Sakai subsequently returned to Japan where he was instrumental in developing a group of outstanding renal physiologists, among them Takeshi Hoshi, who performed pioneering studies on the cotransport of sodium and organic compounds in the renal tubule of the Japanese newt (33). Jamison became the acknowledged expert in micropuncture of medullary structures of the exposed renal papillae of rat kidneys, first at NIH, then at Washington University in St. Louis, and eventually at Stanford. Renal medullary structures in vitro were the subject of micropuncture studies by the Australian investigator Trefor Morgan. Berliner's laboratory was also the training ground for Frank Knox, Fred Wright, and Barry Brenner. They contributed a vast body of information on renal tubular transport, obtained first at NIH and later at the Mayo Clinic (Knox), at Yale (Wright), and the University of San Francisco and Harvard (Brenner). Brenner soon concentrated on problems of glomerular filtration. He was the first to introduce Wiederhielm's method (74) of measuring capillary hydrostatic pressure to studies of glomerular function by direct puncture in Munich-Wistar rats and to estimate the colloid osmotic pressure of blood in postglomerular arterioles from measurements of protein concentration. It was on the basis of these technical advances that he proposed his quantitative description of the balance of driving forces for filtration at the level of the single glomerulus in vivo (5).

Besides introducing new surgical procedures necessary for micropuncture work on dog and monkey kidneys and for exposing collecting ducts in rat renal medulla, many new analytical approaches were introduced at NIH, most of them based on the ingenuity of Robert Bowman and Gerald Vurek in the Laboratory of Technical Development of the National Heart, Lung, and Blood Institute.

Classic micropuncture of single nephrons in vivo is limited by the fact that only those tubule segments that are located on the kidney surface (cortex or exposed renal papilla) are available for the collection of fluid. The first attempt to obtain information on the function of nephrons located deep within the kidneys was made by the pathologist Odd E. Hanssen working at the University of Oslo in Norway. As early as 1958, Hanssen had devised a histochemical method for visualization of filtered ferrocyanide in mouse nephrons by microdissection. Later, during an NIH-sponsored research fellowship at the State University of New York in Brooklyn, ^{14}C-labeled ferrocyanide became available to him. This allowed Hanssen to quantify the amount of ferrocyanide present within the proximal tubules and, by comparing it with its concentration in plasma, to calculate the relative rates of glomerular filtration in single nephrons. In this report to the Second International Congress of Nephrology in Prague in 1963, Hanssen (32) was able to show that the single-nephron GFR of inner cortical nephrons is roughly twice that of nephrons located within the outer cortex. This was the first direct proof of the existence of nephron heterogeneity, a concept that later became the topic of numerous studies. Hanssen's technique was further modified and improved by de Rouffignac (48) and Baines (2) and their respective collaborators to allow measurement of single-nephron GFR in absolute rather than relative terms.

However, the decisive breakthrough to overcome the limitations imposed by the fact that only nephron segments on the kidney surface are available for micropuncture was achieved at the Laboratory of Kidney and Electrolyte Metabolism at NIH where Maurice Burg and Jack Orloff developed methods for microperfusion of isolated tubule segments in vitro. Burg has written a fascinating description of the development of this technique (6). Although the principle of this approach is quite simple, consisting in the isolation of a known nephron segment, its perfusion with a solution of known composition, its placement in an equally well-defined bathing solution, and the analysis of the collected perfusate, the actual development of the method was made possible only by exceptional ingenuity in apparatus design, dexterity, persistence, and sound judgement. Burg had begun to consider the possibility of perfusing tubule segments during his fellowship at NIH (1957–1959) and as a resident in internal medicine (1959–1960). He devoted all of his efforts to the project when he returned to the Kidney and Electrolyte Laboratory as a junior staff member the following year. The task was formidable because every step in the procedure had to be newly designed. Almost none of the well-established techniques used in in vivo micropuncture could be applied to the in vitro perfusion project. The selection of a method for obtaining nephron segments for perfusion posed major problems. After some work on tubular suspensions, it soon became clear that meaningful results could be obtained only if the identity of the perfused tubule segment had been established exactly after its isolation by careful microdissection under microscopic observation. Ivar Sperber (Fig. 9), with his vast experience in microdissection and knowledge of comparative renal microanatomy (53), played a critical role in this respect by teaching Burg and his collaborators how to identify and microdissect, freehand, specific nephron segments.

In 1964 Jared Grantham joined Burg and Orloff and succeeded in collecting fluid from a perfused tubule of a rabbit kidney. The first publication of results obtained on an isolated perfused renal tubule appeared in 1966 (7). It contained data on the maintenance of

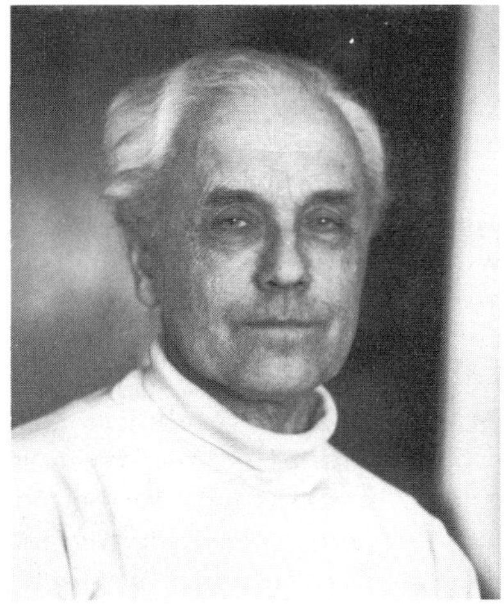

Figure 9. Ivar Sperber (b. 1914). His extensive microdissection of kidneys of different animal species was helpful in designing the early micropuncture studies of the concentrating and diluting mechanism. Sperber's work included the description of the renal portal vein system in chickens, thereby providing a novel approach to studying tubular transport in nonmammalian endothermic animals.

cellular ion gradients in nonperfused tubules and of fluid absorption and *p*-aminohippurate secretion by perfused tubules. This was the beginning of a long series of penetrating studies of renal tubule function at NIH and elsewhere that have provided information not easily obtainable by any other means than by this new technique. Among these major achievements, one might single out the unequivocal demonstration of a small lumen-negative transepithelial voltage in proximal tubules perfused with an ultrafiltrate of plasma (8), the characterization of the permeability characteristics of the thin limbs of Henle's loop (3, 34), and the demonstration of (secondary) active chloride transport by the thick ascending limb of Henle's loop (31). Perfusion of isolated renal tubules has provided information on the transport characteristics of all nephron segments and, in addition, offered a route by which biophysical, biochemical, and cell biological approaches can be correlated with tubular transport and morphology.

Looking back over the past sixty-five years and scanning the information on renal function accumulated during this time, it seems that micropuncture and microperfusion of single nephrons have answered many, if not all, of the most important physiological questions posed in this period. Clearly, these techniques were and remain powerful tools in the hands of skilled investigators. Yet, like all methods in biological science, their yield in terms of the significance for understanding function, was and always will be a reflection of the importance of the hypotheses tested.

I am greatly indebted to Dr. Carl W. Gottschalk for his editorial comments and for extensive advice in writing the history of the development of micropuncture before 1945.

NOTE

[1] The original article (60) cites the authors as Arthur M. Walker and Phyllis A. Bott; Jean Oliver and Muriel C. MacDowell. This indicates that the two separate groups worked in collaboration, the first at the University of Pennsylvania Medical School and the second at the Long Island College of Medicine. (MacDowell was a skilled technician who assisted Oliver with the microdissections.)

BIBLIOGRAPHY

1. ALEXANDER, J. T., and M. L. NASTUK. An instrument for the production of microelectrodes used in electrophysiological studies. *Rev. Sci. Instrum.* 24: 528–531, 1953.
2. BAINES, A. D., C. I. BAINES, and C. DE ROUFFIGNAC. Functional heterogeneity of nephrons. I. Intraluminal flow velocities. *Pfluegers Arch.* 308: 244–259, 1969.
3. BOTT, P. A. Renal excretion of creatinine in *Necturus.* A reinvestigation by direct analysis of glomerular and tubular fluid for creatinine and inulin. *Am. J. Physiol.* 168: 107–113, 1952.
4. BOTT, P. A. The determination of Na and K in biological fluids with the dual-channel ultramicroflame photometer. *Anal. Biochem.* 1: 17–22, 1960.
5. BRENNER, B. M., J. L. TROY, and T. M. DAUGHARTY. The dynamics of glomerular ultrafiltration in the rat. *J. Clin. Invest.* 50: 1776–1780, 1971.
6. BURG, M. B. Introduction: background and development of microperfusion technique. *Kidney Int.* 22: 417–425, 1982.
7. BURG, M., J. GRANTHAM, M. ABRAMOW, and J. ORLOFF. Preparation and study of fragments of single rabbit nephrons. *Am. J. Physiol.* 210: 1293–1298, 1966.
8. BURG, M. B., and J. ORLOFF. Electrical potential difference across proximal convoluted tubules. *Am. J. Physiol.* 219: 1714–1716, 1970.
9. CLAPP, J. R., J. F. WATSON, and R. W. BERLINER. Osmolality, bicarbonate concentration, and water reabsorption in proximal tubule of the dog nephron. *Am. J. Physiol.* 205: 273–280, 1963.
10. CUSHNY, A. R. *The Secretion of Urine.* London: Longmans Green, 1917.
11. DEETJEN, P., and H. BRECHTELSBAUER. Untersuchungen zur cortcalen Durchblutung der Rattenniere bei Mikropunktionsexperimenten (Abstract). *Pfluegers Arch. Gesamte Physiol. Menchen Tierre* 218: 26, 1964.
12. DIRKS, J. H., J. CLAPP, and R. W. BERLINER. The protein concentration in the proximal tubule of the dog. *J. Clin. Invest.* 43: 916–921, 1964.
13. EKEHORN, G. On the principles of renal function. *Acta Med. Scand. Suppl.* 36: 3–717, 1931.
14. FREEMAN, B., A. E. LIVINGSTON, and A. N. RICHARDS. A second series of

quantitative estimations of the concentration of chlorides in glomerular urine from frogs. *J. Biol. Chem.* 87: 467–477, 1930.
15. Frömter, E. Viewing the kidney through microelectrodes. *Am. J. Physiol.* 247 (*Renal Fluid Electrolyte Physiol.* 16): F695–F705, 1984.
16. Gertz, K. H. Transtubuläre Natriumchloridflüsse und Permeabilität für Nichtelektrolyte im proximalen und distalen Konvolut der Rattenniere. *Pfluegers Arch. Gesamte Physiol. Menchen Tierre* 276: 336–356, 1963.

17. Giebisch, G. Measurements of pH, chloride, and inulin concentrations in proximal tubule fluid of *Necturus*. *Am. J. Physiol.* 185: 171–174, 1956.
18. Giebisch, G. Electrical potential measurement on single nephrons of *Necturus*. *J. Cell. Comp. Physiol.* 51: 221–240, 1958.
19. Giebisch, G. Measurement of electrical potential difference on single nephrons of the perfused *Necturus* kidney. *J. Gen. Physiol.* 44: 659–678, 1961.
20. Giebisch, G., R. M. Klose, G. Malnic, W. J. Sullivan, and E. E. Windhager. Sodium movement across single perfused proximal tubules of rat kidneys. *J. Gen. Physiol.* 47: 1175–1196, 1964.
21. Giebisch, G., and E. E. Windhager. Measurement of chloride movement across single proximal tubules of *Necturus* kidney. *Am. J. Physiol.* 204: 387–391, 1963.
22. Gottschalk, C. W. Micropuncture studies of tubular function in the mammalian kidney. *Physiologist* 4(1): 35–55, 1961.
23. Gottschalk, C. W. Renal tubular function: lessons from micropuncture. *Harvey Lect.* 58: 99–124, 1962–1963.
24. Gottschalk, C. W. Dr. A. N. Richards and kidney micropuncture. *Ann. Intern. Med.* 71: 28–37, 1969.
25. Gottschalk, C. W., W. E. Lassiter, and M. Mylle. Localization of urine acidification in the mammalian kidney. *Am. J. Physiol.* 198: 581–585, 1960.
26. Gottschalk, C. W., W. E. Lassiter, M. Mylle, K. J. Ullrich, B. Schmidt-Nielsen, R. O'Dell, and G. Pehling. Micropuncture study of composition of loop of Henle fluid in desert rodents. *Am. J. Physiol.* 204: 532–535, 1963.
27. Gottschalk, C. W., and M. Mylle. Micropuncture study of pressures in proximal tubules and peritubular capillaries of the rat kidney and their relation to ureteral and renal venous pressures. *Am. J. Physiol.* 185: 430–439, 1956.
28. Gottschalk, C. W., and M. Mylle. Micropuncture study of pressures in proximal and distal tubules and peritubular capillaries of the rat kidney during osmotic diuresis. *Am. J. Physiol.* 189: 323–328, 1957.
29. Gottschalk, C. W., and M. Mylle. Evidence that the mammalian nephron functions as a countercurrent multiplier system. *Science Wash. DC* 128: 594, 1958.
30. Gottschalk, C. W., and M. Mylle. Micropuncture study of the mammalian urinary concentrating mechanism: evidence for the countercurrent hypothesis. *Am. J. Physiol.* 196: 927–936, 1959.
31. Greger, R., E. Schlatter, and F. Lang. Evidence for electroneutral sodium chloride cotransport in the cortical thick ascending limb of Henle's loop of rabbit kidney. *Pfluegers Arch.* 396: 308–314, 1983.
32. Hanssen, O. E. Method of glomerular filtration in individual rat neph-

rons. In: *Proc. Second Int. Congr. Nephrol., Prague, 1963.* Amsterdam: Excerpta Med., 1964, p. 527–529.
33. Hoshi, T., and Y. Kikuta. Effects of organic solute-sodium co-transport on the transmembrane potentials and resistance parameters of the proximal tubule of *Triturus* kidney. In: *Electrophysiology of the Nephron*, edited by T. Anagnostopoulos. Paris: INSERM, 1977, vol. 67, p. 135–160.
34. Imai, M. Function of the thin ascending limb of Henle of rats and hamsters perfused in vitro. *Am. J. Physiol.* 232 (*Renal Fluid Electrolyte Physiol.* 1): F201–F209, 1977.
35. Klümper, J., K. Ullrich, and H. Hilger. Das Verhalten des Harnstoffs in den Sammelrohren der Saügetierniere. *Pfluegers Arch. Gesamte Physiol. Menchen Tierre* 267: 238–243, 1958.
36. Koefoed-Johnsen, V., and H. H. Ussing. The nature of the frog skin potential. *Acta Physiol. Scand.* 42: 298–308, 1958.
37. Kokko, J. Sodium chloride and water transport in the descending limb of Henle. *J. Clin. Invest.* 49: 1838–1846, 1970.
38. Landis, E. M. Capillary pressure and capillary permeability. *Physiol. Rev.* 14: 404–481, 1934.
39. Ling, G., and R. W. Gerard. The membrane potentials and metabolism of muscle fibers. *J. Cell. Comp. Physiol.* 34: 413–438, 1949.
40. Litchfield, J. B., and P. A. Bott. Micropuncture study of renal excretion of water, K, Na, and Cl in the rat. *Am. J. Physiol.* 203: 667–670, 1962.
41. Maude, D. L., I. Shehadeh, and A. K. Solomon. Sodium and water transport in single perfused distal tubules of *Necturus* kidney. *Am. J. Physiol.* 211: 1043–1049, 1966.
42. Montgomery, H., and J. A. Pierce. The site of acidification of the urine within the renal tubule in amphibia. *Am. J. Physiol.* 118: 144–152, 1937.
43. Pappenheimer, J. R. Über die Permeabilität der Glomerulummembranen der Niere. *Klin. Wochenschr.* 33: 362–365, 1955.
44. Rector, F. C., Jr., and J. R. Clapp. Evidence for active chloride reabsorption in the distal renal tubule of the rat. *J. Clin. Invest.* 41: 101–107, 1962.
45. Richards, A. N. Urine formation in the amphibian kidney. *Harvey Lect.* Ser. 30, 93–118, 1934–1935.
46. Richards, A. N. The Croonian Lecture. Processes of urine formation. *Proc. R. Soc. Lond. B Biol. Sci.* 126: 398–432, 1938.
47. Richards, A. N., and A. M. Walker. Methods of collecting fluid from known regions of the renal tubules of amphibia and of perfusing the lumen of a single tubule. *Am. J. Physiol.* 118: 111–120, 1937.
48. Rouffignac, C. de, S. Deiss, and J. P. Bonvalet. Détermination du taux individuel de filtration glomérulaire des néphrons accessibles et inaccessibles à la microponction. *Pfluegers Arch.* 315: 273–290, 1970.
49. Sakai, F., R. L. Jamison, and R. W. Berliner. A method for exposing the rat renal medulla in vivo: micropuncture of the collecting duct. *Am. J. Physiol.* 209: 663–668, 1965.
50. Shipp, J. C., I. B. Hanenson, E. E. Windhager, H. J. Schatzmann, G. Whittembury, H. Yoshimura, and A. K. Solomon. Single proximal tubules of the *Necturus* kidney. Methods for micropuncture and microperfusion. *Am. J. Physiol.* 195: 563–569, 1958.

51. SOLOMON, A. K. Single proximal tubules of *Necturus* kidney. VII. Ion fluxes across individual faces of cell. *Am. J. Physiol.* 204: 381–386, 1963.
52. SOLOMON, S. Transtubular potential differences of rat kidney. *J. Cell. Comp. Physiol.* 49: 351–365, 1957.
53. SPERBER, I. Studies on the mammalian kidney. *Zool. Bidr. Uppsala* 20: 249–431, 1944.
54. STEINHAUSEN, M. Eine Methode zur Differenzierung proximaler und distaler Tubuli der Nierenrinde von Ratten in vivo und ihre Anwendung zur Bestimmung tubulärer Strömungsgeschwindigkeiten. *Pfluegers Arch. Gesamte Physiol. Menchen Tierre* 277:23–35, 1963.
55. THURAU, K. W. Renal hemodynamics. *Am. J. Med.* 36: 609–719, 1964.
56. THURAU, K., P. DEETJEN, and K. KRAMER. Hämodynamik des Nierenmarks (II). Weschselbeziehung zwischen vasculärem und tubulärem Gegenstromsystem bei arteriellen Drucksteigerungen, Wasserdiurese und osmotischer Diurese. *Pfluegers Arch. Gesamte Physiol. Menchen Tierre* 270: 270–285, 1960.
57. THURAU, K., and J. SCHNERMANN. Die Natrium Konzentration an den Macula densa-Zellen als regulierender Faktor für das Glomerulumfiltrat (Mikropunktionsversuche). *Klin. Wochenschr.* 43: 410–413, 1965.
58. ULLRICH, K., H. HILGER, and J. KLÜMPER. Sekretion von Ammoniumionen in den Sammelrohren der Saugetierniere. *Pfluegers Arch. Gesamte Physiol. Menchen Tierre* 267: 244–250, 1958.
59. ULLRICH, K. J., B. SCHMIDT-NIELSEN, R. O'DELL, G. PEHLING, C. W. GOTTSCHALK, W. E. LASSITER, and M. MYLLE. Micropuncture study of composition of proximal and distal tubular fluid in rat kidney. *Am. J. Physiol.* 204: 527–531, 1963.
60. WALKER, A. M., P. A. BOTT, J. OLIVER, and M. C. MACDOWELL. The collection and analysis of fluid from single nephrons of the mammalian kidney. *Am. J. Physiol.* 134: 580–595, 1941.
61. WALKER, A. M., and C. L. HUDSON. The reabsorption of glucose from the renal tubule in amphibia and the action of phlorhizin upon it. *Am. J. Physiol.* 118: 130–143, 1937.
62. WALKER, A. M., and C. L. HUDSON. The role of the tubule in the excretion of urea by the amphibian kidney. *Am. J. Physiol.* 118: 153–166, 1937.
63. WALKER, A. M., and C. L. HUDSON. The role of the tubule in the excretion of inorganic phosphates by the amphibian kidney. *Am. J. Physiol.* 118: 167–173, 1937.
64. WALKER, A. M., C. L. HUDSON, T. FINDLEY, JR., and A. N. RICHARDS. The total molecular concentration and the chloride concentration of fluid from different segments of the renal tubule of amphibia. *Am. J. Physiol.* 118: 121–129, 1937.
65. WALKER, A. M., and J. OLIVER. Methods for the collection of fluid from single glomeruli and tubules of the mammalian kidney. *Am. J. Physiol.* 134: 562–579, 1941.
66. WEARN, J. T. Composition of glomerular urine with conclusive evidence of reabsorption in the renal tubules. *Physiologist* 23(5): 1–4, 1980.
67. WEARN, J. T., and A. N. RICHARDS. Observations on the composition of glomerular urine, with particular reference to the problem of reabsorption in the renal tubules. *Am. J. Physiol.* 71: 209–227, 1924.
68. WEARN, J. T., and A. N. RICHARDS. The concentration of chlorides in the

glomerular urine of frogs. *J. Biol. Chem.* 66: 247–273, 1925.
69. Wesson, L. G., Jr., and W. P. Anslow, Jr. Excretion of sodium and water during osmotic diuresis in the dog. *Am. J. Physiol.* 153: 465–474, 1948.
70. Wesson, L. G., Jr., W. P. Anslow, Jr., and H. W. Smith. The excretion of strong electrolytes. *Bull. NY Acad. Med.* 24: 586–606, 1948.
71. Westfall, B. B., T. Findley, and A. N. Richards. Quantitative studies of the composition of glomerular urine. XII. The concentration of chloride in glomerular urine of frogs and necturi. *J. Biol. Chem.* 107: 661–672, 1934.
72. Whittembury, G., D. E. Oken, E. E. Windhager, and A. K. Solomon. Single proximal tubules in *Necturus* kidney. IV. Dependence of H_2O movement on osmotic gradients. *Am. J. Physiol.* 197: 1121–1127, 1959.
73. Whittembury, G., N. Sugino, and A. K. Solomon. Ionic permeability and electrical potential differences in *Necturus* kidney cells. *J. Gen. Physiol.* 44: 689–712, 1961.
74. Wiederhielm, C. A., J. W. Woodbury, S. Kirk, and R. F. Rushmer. Pulsatile pressures in the microcirculation of frog's mesentery. *Am. J. Physiol.* 207: 173–176, 1964.
75. Wilbrandt, W. Electrical potential differences across the wall of kidney tubules of *Necturus. J. Cell. Comp. Physiol.* 11: 425–431, 1938.
76. Windhager, E. E., and G. Giebisch. Micropuncture study of renal tubular transfer of sodium chloride in the rat. *Am. J. Physiol.* 200: 581–590, 1961.
77. Windhager, E. E., G. Whittembury, D. E. Oken, H. J. Schatzmann, and A. K. Solomon. Single proximal tubules of the *Necturus* kidney. III. Dependence of H_2O movement on NaCl concentration. *Am. J. Physiol.* 197: 313–318, 1959.
78. Wirz, H. Der osmotische Druck des Blutes in der Nierenpapille. *Helv. Physiol. Pharmacol. Acta* 11: 20–29, 1953.
79. Wirz, H., and P. A. Bott. Potassium and reducing substances in proximal tubule fluid of the rat kidney. *Proc. Soc. Exp. Biol. Med.* 87: 405–407, 1954.

V

From Renal Tissue Slices to Membrane Vesicles

ARNOST KLEINZELLER

THIS chapter appraises the development of investigative approaches for the dissection of renal function at the cellular level by experimentation in vitro. Such analysis cannot be separated from the nature of the questions asked and reflects the imagination of the investigators involved. The basic criterion for this evaluation has been set by Otto Warburg et al. [(113); translated by me from the German]:

TISSUE SLICES TO MEMBRANE VESICLES

There can be no argument about the unconditional priority of experiments in vivo. If manometric [e.g., in vitro] *and in vivo experimentation are consistent, this offers the possibility of carrying out studies under simplified conditions. If, however, there is no consistence*[1]*, then experiments in vitro are biologically worthless.*

The choice of the experimental approach for in vitro studies is determined by the nature of the question addressed.

Tissue Slices

Concepts and Applications

The tissue-slice technique was introduced in 1923 by Otto Warburg [Fig. 1; (112)] to enable in vitro measurements of tissue gas (O_2 and CO_2) exchange with the Warburg manometer (Fig. 2). Such tissue preparation had to satisfy two essential conditions: a minimum of damaged cells, and a sufficiently rapid diffusion of gases and substrates from the suspending physiological medium into the tissue and of metabolic products from the tissue into the medium. Only when these conditions are satisfied does the diffusion of gases, substrates, and/or metabolic products cease to be rate limiting, and

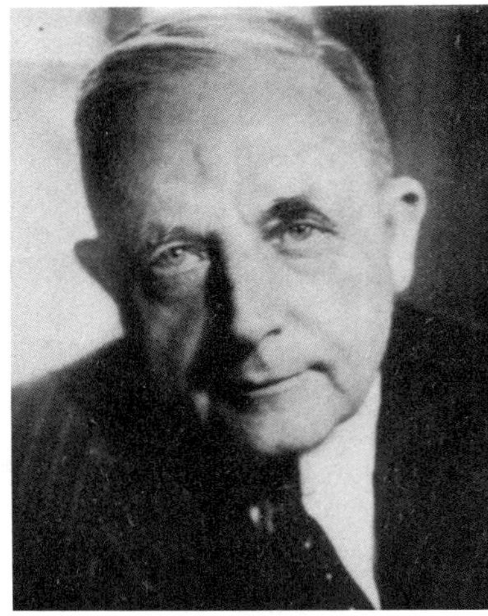

Figure 1. Otto Heinrich Warburg (1883–1970). [From Krebs (67).]

hence valid data are obtained. The limiting thickness (d) of the tissue for O_2 uptake was defined as that thickness at which, under existing experimental conditions, the O_2 pressure in the geometric center of the slice is 0 (see note 2), that is

$$d = \sqrt{8c \cdot D/A}$$

where c is the pressure of the measured gas in the manometric vessel (in atm) in equilibrium with the aqueous suspending medium, D is Krogh's diffusion coefficient of the gas in the tissue (in ml/cm^2), and A is utilization of the gas (in ml $\cdot$ ml tissue^{-1} $\cdot$ min^{-1}). Given the relatively high O_2 uptake by the mammalian renal cortex, the limiting thickness is of the order of 0.3–0.4 mm when the slice is incubated at 38°C with O_2 in the gaseous phase. Warburg also initiated experiments providing evidence that sliced tissue in effect survives prolonged experimentation in vitro: sterile tumor slices incubated for 48 h in vitro (with glucose as substrate) maintain their capacity for growth when transplanted back into rats (90).

The method for preparing slices freehand is simple, particularly as improved by Deutsch (21), and is superior to many efforts for mechanization of the procedure in that the proportion of damaged cells is lower. In addition, renal cortical slices are a remarkably resilient preparation: they can be maintained at 0°C–4°C in a balanced suspending medium for 48 h without a decrease in the rate of O_2 uptake (66) or amino acid accumulation (75). Slices from any species are easily handled and analyzed. Moreover slices withstand more drastic experimental conditions (e.g., replacement of Na^+ in the suspending medium by Li^+ or choline) than do suspensions of tubules or isolated cells. These factors contributed to the fact that

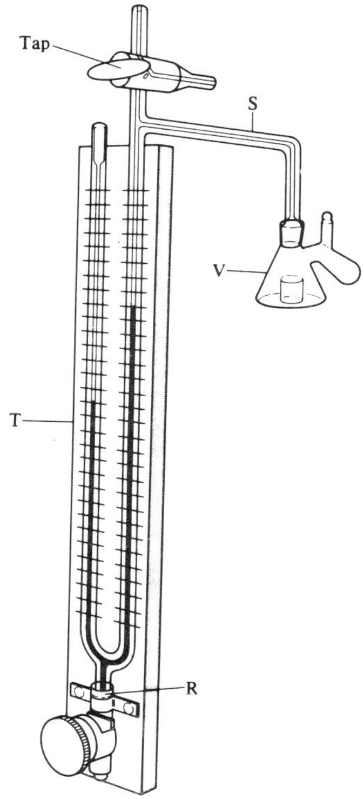

Figure 2. The Warburg manometer: T, U-shaped manometer proper with graduated scale; R, rubber fluid reservoir with Brodie's manometric fluid (adjustment of screw clamp alters the level of fluid in the manometer); Tap, three-way stopcock; S, sidearm; V, vessel with center well (for absorption of CO_2 with KOH) and sidearm for addition of substrate.

for forty years renal slices were the standard technique for the exploration of renal metabolism in vitro. Table 1 summarizes some major metabolic and transport processes analyzed by this technique. Not included in that table are studies aimed at elucidating cell-volume control. Under in vivo conditions the "cloudy swelling" of tissues known to pathologists was later related to an impairment of the mechanisms controlling cell volume. In vitro cell-volume control was vigorously investigated after the pioneering studies of Mudge (82), Wilson (117), and Leaf (71) pointed the way. Early studies also established major differences in the metabolic rates of slices from renal cortex and medulla (36, 72) [despite Warburg's misgivings (113)]. Such observations represented a clear indication that the kidney is characterized by both structural and metabolic heterogeneity.

Table 1 shows that in the early 1930s Hans A. Krebs (Fig. 3) (at Freiburg, Germany, then Sheffield, and finally at Oxford, England) established modern renal biochemistry by using renal (cortical)

TABLE 1
Renal Physiological Processes and Their Correlates Investigated in Cortical Slices

Metabolic properties and functions in vivo	Processes studied in vitro with slices	Ref.
Ammoniagenesis	Ammonia formation from amino acids	64, 65
Gluconeogenesis	Gluconeogenesis	68
Short-chain fatty acids as primary metabolic fuel	Acetoacetate and fatty acids as primary metabolic substrate	116
Ammoniagenesis in acidosis	Ammonia formation from amino acids	93
Adaptation in renal taurine handling	Adaptive changes in taurine accumulation	98
Na^+ and K^+ reabsorption	Na^+ and K^+ transport	82
Hexose reabsorption	Hexose accumulation	58
Amino acid reabsorption	Amino acid accumulation	97
Organic acid (PAH) secretion	Organic acid accumulation	28, 19
Uric acid excretion	Uric acid accumulation	91
Hypoxanthine excretion	Hypoxanthine accumulation	7
SO_4^{2-} reabsorption	SO_4^{2-} accumulation	22
Organic cation excretion	Organic cation accumulation	42
Water-soluble vitamin reabsorption	Ascorbic acid and nicotinic acid accumulation	96a

PAH, *p*-aminohippuric acid.

slices, with emphasis on substrate uptake, transformation, and the regulation thereof. Subsequently, in 1948, the pioneering work of Roy P. Forster [Fig. 4; (28)] at Dartmouth and the Mount Desert Island Biological Laboratory showed that renal slices could also be used to explore the transport process at the cellular level by relating tissue, and later cellular, accumulation or extrusion of solutes to absorption or secretion. This exploration was extended particularly by John V. Taggart (at Columbia, later at Dartmouth) and Gilbert M. Mudge (at Johns Hopkins, later at Dartmouth). An in vitro analysis of the nature of the driving forces for transcellular transport was thus initiated (cf. refs. 28, 29, 31).

A correlation between the metabolism of the kidney and studies of metabolic processes in slices is mostly straightforward. On the other hand, the correlation of cellular uptake (or extrusion) of a solute in vitro (e.g., in slices) with absorption or secretion in vivo is limited by the loss of the physiological geometry of the system. In

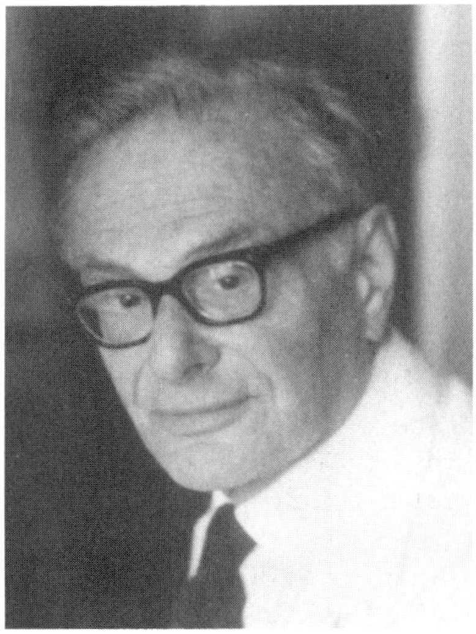

Figure 3. Hans Adolph Krebs (1900–1982). (Photograph taken in 1975.)

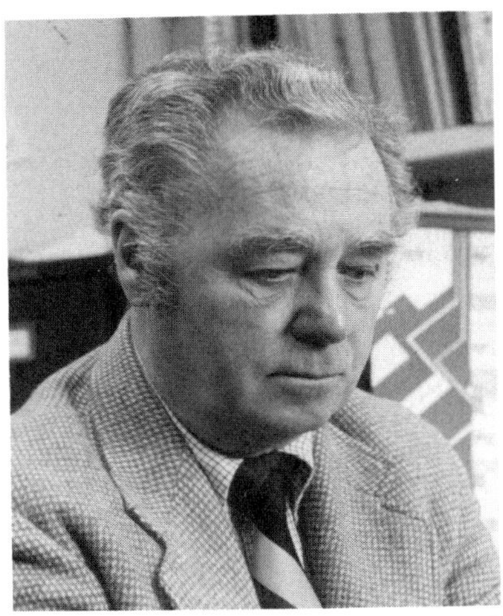

Figure 4. Roy Philip Forster (b. 1911). (Photograph taken in 1976, courtesy of R. P. Forster.)

vivo (or in perfused tubules in vitro) secretion or absorption denotes the movement of a solute (and solvent) across a cellular sheet from one compartment to another. In slices this geometry is lost and only the cellular uptake (or extrusion) of a solute can be followed. It is assumed (simplistically, see Limitations of Tissue Slices, p. 137) that the cells are bathed at both faces by the external medium, and hence changes in the concentration profile between the cells and their environment (i.e., concentration gradient) are determined. Obviously the contribution of the intercellular pathway to the secretory or absorptive process is lost in slices. Knowledge of the vector or the transepithelial process and of the concentration profile of the analyzed solute may lead to a valuable indication of the cellular localization of the uphill step (30, 31). Figure 5 shows the underlying concepts of a transport vector for solute S from the luminal to the serosal (antiluminal) cell side: localization of the uphill process at the luminal side produces the concentration step at this membrane ("push mechanism," Fig. 5*A*). Alternatively, for an uphill process at the basolateral cell membrane ("pull mechanism," Fig. 5*B*), the predicted concentration of S in the cells would be close to that bathing the luminal cell membrane. Thus the knowledge that in vivo *p*-aminohippuric acid (PAH) is secreted into the urine and that in the course of this process a cellular accumulation of this compound takes place can be directly related to the cellular accumulation of PAH in slices (or renal tubules). These observations permit the suggestion (but not proof) that the accumulation step is localized at the basolateral cell membrane (30). The information summarized in Table 1 helps to localize the transport processes. However, in addition to all the limitations given for slices or suspensions of tubules (see TISSUE GEOMETRY, p. 137), closer analysis reveals additional caveats because each of the depicted transport steps is in effect the composite of two rate constants. Additional rate constants must be considered if solute S is metabolizable. Hence the analysis is far from simple.

Table 1 also shows that renal (cortical) slices satisfy Warburg's stringent criterion for the qualitative consistence of experimentation in vivo and in vitro. Quantitative aspects of the criterion are discussed in the next section.

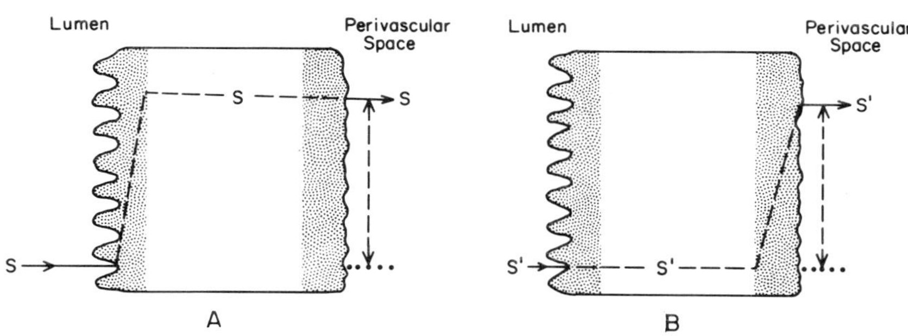

Figure 5. Cellular localization of active (uphill) transport of solute S from the luminal to the peritubular space (absorption). *A*: push mechanism. Active step at the luminal membrane raises the intracellular concentration of S; substrate then exits passively at the basolateral membrane. *B*: pull mechanism. S′ passes through the luminal cell membrane by a passive (equilibrating) mechanism; hence intracellular S′ concentration is close to or lower than that in the luminal space. Active (uphill) mechanism at the basolateral membrane actually extrudes S′ against its concentration gradient from the cell into the peritubular space.

Limitations of Tissue Slices

Cellular Homogeneity

Slices are as homogeneous as the tissue from which they are prepared. Thus some 75% of renal cortical slices consist of proximal convoluted tubules, some distal tubules, and glomeruli. Measured metabolic rates are therefore the mean of those of the cellular components.

Tissue Geometry

The limiting thickness was originally defined for the special case of gas-exchange measurements. However, the diffusion of substrates and/or metabolic products in tissue is considerably lower than that of O_2 (or CO_2); hence *d* represents an upper limit (73). On the other hand, because slicing of necessity damages a portion of the cells, the investigator must balance the desire of working with slices thinner than *d* with the resulting increase in the proportion of damaged (cut) cells. To some extent this predicament can be obviated by decreasing the experimental temperature, thereby increasing *d* on two counts: the increased solubility of O_2 in the suspending medium and the decreased rate of O_2 utilization.

In addition, the diffusion pathway for substrates in the slices is considerably longer than the several micrometers from the supplying capillaries to the cells. This fact alone may severely limit quantitative comparisons between metabolic rates in vivo and in vitro. The microscopic organization of renal tissue further contributes to lengthening the diffusion pathway. This in effect creates an unstirred layer that may also affect the apparent concentration of solutes in this "extracellular space." Therefore the assumption that both faces of cells in a slice are bathed by the incubating medium is an oversimplification.

These points require a pragmatic reevaluation of the limiting thickness for a given process and thus an appraisal of the criteria for the functional integrity of the tissue. Since O_2 uptake alone cannot suffice (the destruction of cell integrity does not necessarily impair O_2 uptake), it appears reasonable to chose as a criterion an energy-requiring metabolic process and seek optimal values. Measurement of cell K^+ has proved to be a sensitive indicator because any impairment of oxygenation in the central portion of the slice immediately results in a decrease in cell K^+. For this criterion, slices of rabbit renal cortex 0.3 mm thick at 25°C were metabolically satisfactory; the K^+ tissue concentration was identical in vivo and in vitro (57, 82). Other equally suitable criteria include gluconeogenesis, the cellular accumulation of a nonmetabolizable substrate, and the ATP/ADP ratio.

Substrate Accessibility at Cellular Sites

The subject of substrate accessibility, particularly in transport studies with renal (cortical) slices, was raised because of microscopic observations that tubular lumina appear to be occluded or collapsed (9, 114). Kinetic data also indicated that in contrast to the basolateral membrane the luminal (brush-border) membrane was not freely accessible to substrates. Thus it was concluded that the slice technique is of limited value because the basolateral membrane is preferentially exposed to substrate in the incubation media (cf. 4, 87). There is ample evidence that the (secondarily) active transport step for a variety of solutes (e.g., the nonmetabolizable glucose analogue methyl-α-D-glucoside) is localized at the brush-border membrane, and slices are known to accumulate this sugar to the same level as tissue in vivo (A. Kleinzeller, unpublished observations) and as renal cortical tubules (with a more accessible brush-border membrane) in suspensions. A close inspection of available experimental data permits a resolution of these divergent views. First, in some of the previously mentioned studies, the realistic limiting thickness was apparently exceeded by incubating tissue at 37°C, and hence cells in the center of the slices showed evidence of anoxia [e.g., swelling and loss of K^+ (cf. ref. 115)]. Morphological changes are considerably smaller at 23°C–25°C (79). Second, as pointed out, the diffusion pathway for a substrate will of necessity be longer through the narrow, often collapsed lumina of the tubular components of the slice, and hence differences in substrate accessibility along the nephron and concentration gradients within the lumen are established. This explains why the transport of methyl-α-D-glucoside is faster in a tubular suspension than in slices (58). The diffusion pathway also favors the basolateral membrane. However, although there are quantitative differences in the accessibility of the cell faces and therefore in the cellular response, qualitatively the results obtained with slices reflect processes in vivo (Table 1). This problem does represent another limitation, and the wary investigator will seek additional techniques for deciding pertinent questions.

Appraisal of the Use (and Misuse) of the Tissue-Slice Technique

The limitations discussed in the previous section led many investigators to reject the slice technique. It appears, however, that such summary judgment is not warranted. Slices of renal tissue represent the simplest in vitro technique for gaining a qualitative overview of correlates of physiological processes (Table 1) and for describing their phenomenology under controlled conditions. The easy handling of the tissue, particularly when rapid changes of media are required, represents an additional advantage. Thus the Na^+ dependence of sugar (59) and amino acid (32) accumulation in the cells was defined in slices, and all pertinent points were then confirmed and extended by more recent specific techniques, such as the use of membrane vesicles. A comparison of the uptake of L-ascorbic acid and nicotinic acid by slices, isolated tubules, and brush-border membrane vesicles (96a) provides clear evidence of this point. A detailed definition of the involved mechanisms may have to be derived by the use of some of the techniques discussed in subsequent sections. Attempts to relate quantitative aspects of the studied phenomena in vitro to the physiological process in vivo are at best difficult for any method, and slices are not an exception. Finally, slices are a rather poor model for studies of the cellular localization of a process unless studied in conjunction with information obtained by other techniques.

TISSUE SLICES TO MEMBRANE VESICLES

Isolated Nephron Segments

The search for methods for preparing defined nephron segments appears to be the direct way of dealing with the vexing problems of cellular heterogeneity in kidney. Development in the last twenty-three years was preceded by other ingenious approaches. In the early 1930s, Robert Chambers (Fig. 6) and his collaborators (16) showed that fragments of chick mesonephros cultured in vitro produce microscopic cysts capable of secreting organic anionic dyes (e.g., phenol red) into the lumina. These pioneering studies proved to be seminal in two respects. The secretion of anionic dyes into the lumina of the tubular cysts inspired later work on the secretion of these compounds into the lumina of teased flounder tubules (see Teased Flounder Tubules, p. 140) and their accumulation (including PAH) in slices of renal cortex (see Concepts and Application, p. 131). Although Chambers's use of the tissue-culture technique did

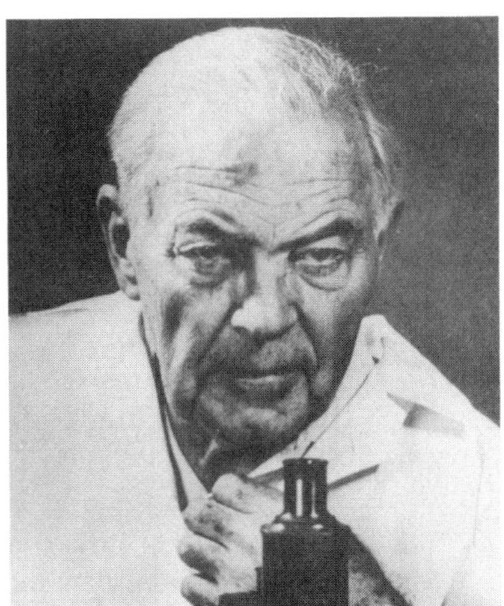

Figure 6. Robert Chambers (1881–1957). [From Chambers and Chambers (15).]

not directly lead to the development of an experimental tool for renal function studies under defined conditions, it did show the way to one of the most recent developments: the use of renal epithelial cells cultured in vitro (see RENAL EPITHELIAL CELLS CULTURED IN VITRO, p. 146). However, the tissue-culture technique enabled Cameron and Chambers (14) to make the unexpected observation that renal tubules in 3.5-mo-old human embryo are able to function by secreting dyes into their lumina and acidifying the secretions.

Some other techniques for preparing isolated segments of nephron have found wide acceptance. Two approaches are used: the mechanical separation of nephron segments and partial digestion of the tissue with proteases followed by separation of component tissue fragments (proximal and distal renal tubules and glomeruli). Both techniques help to respond to the need for preparations that suffer neither from the manipulative disadvantages of whole organs nor from the diffusion limitations of slices.

Teased Flounder Tubules

CONCEPTS AND APPLICATIONS

In 1948 Forster (28) first described the use of teased renal tubules from teleost fish for the study of dye secretion.[4] When fresh flounder kidney is diced into small pieces (~2 mm diam) and, while immersed in a teleost Ringer's solution, the adhering hematopoietic tissue is removed by gentle teasing with blunt dissecting needles, one obtains a mesh of twisted tubules. These tubules close at the cut (torn) ends and thus form elongated cysts with the peritubular face of the tubular epithelium on the outside. The inner (luminal) face is virtually not accessible to the incubating medium. Such tubules secrete organic anionic dyes (e.g., chlorophenol red) into the lumina against concentration gradients of several orders of magnitude [Fig. 7; (53)]. The preparation is remarkedly resilient and easy to handle. Several species have been successfully used for this preparation (31, 54). The species of choice is the winter flounder (*Pseudopleuronectes americanus*). The summer flounder (*Paralichthys lethostigma*), sculpin (*Myoxocephalus octodecimspinosus*), killifish (*Fundulus heteroclitus*), freshwater catfish (*Ameriurus nebulosus*), rainbow trout (*Salmo gairdneri*), and goldfish (*Carassius auratus*) yield somewhat smaller amounts of tubules. The majority of teleost tubules (particularly of marine species) correspond to the proximal tubules of mammalian kidneys; the structure of catfish kidneys permits the separate preparation of proximal and distal segments (31).

This preparation represents a simple tool for studying transport processes localized at the basolateral face of renal epithelial cells in a defined segment of the renal tubule and has been successfully applied for characterizing such transport processes for proteins (77), sugars (60), calcium (95), sulfate (96), and taurine (51).

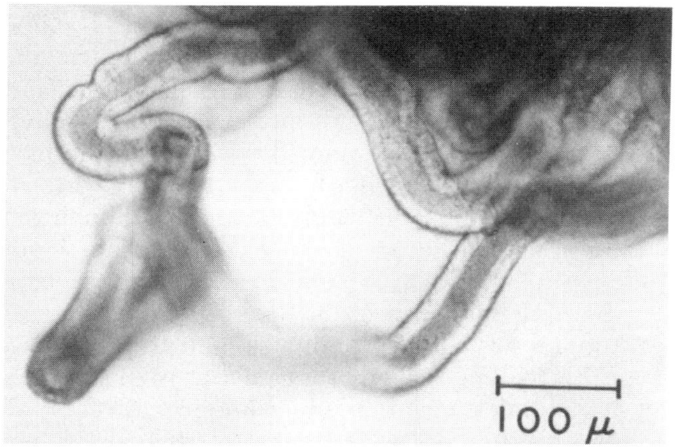

Figure 7. Photomicrograph of flounder tubule with steady-state luminal concentrations of chlorophenol red. Medium contained 25 μM dye. [From Kinter (53).]

Limitations of Teased-Tubule Method

With the teased-tubule method, the vexing problem of a long diffusion pathway to the cellular transport site is avoided. However, the lumina of the cysts represent a distinct extracellular compartment that is not accessible to conventional probes, such as inulin or polyethylene glycol. This prevents a reliable assessment of the apparent intracellular solute concentrations unless other techniques are used in conjunction (60).

Another point of concern relates to the fact that occasionally some teased tubules do not appear to close (31) and hence substrates from the medium may also reach the apical (brush-border) cell membrane. When working with methyl-α-D-glucoside, which enters the cells at the basolateral cell face rather poorly, open tubules may result in an unusual cellular accumulation of this hexose. This same phenomenon is seen when the permeability of intercellular junctions is significantly increased by calcium-free media.

Suspensions of Isolated Renal Cortical Tubules

Concepts and Applications

In 1962 Maurice Burg and Jack Orloff (13) were the first to describe the preparation of a metabolically active suspension of separated renal cortical tubules. In this study collagenase was used to digest the connective tissue that participates in the maintenance of the structural integrity of renal cortex. Their procedure has been widely accepted, with only minor modifications by individual investigators. Significant modifications concerned the now-general acceptance of a combination of collagenase plus hyaluronidase for connective tissue digestion and tubule fragmentation. Gentle centrifugation of the crude suspension sediments tubule fragments and permits removal of cellular debris derived from damaged cells; filtration of the suspension through layers of gauze removes larger particles. It would appear that minor differences in the preparative procedure, and possibly also in the species used, determine the metabolic properties of the preparation. Thus, although the preparation of Burg and Orloff, and its more recent minor modification (35), is not resilient to experimental procedures such as major changes in the ionic composition of the suspending medium when rat cortical tubules are used (92), in a similar preparation of rabbit renal cortex the basement membrane of the tubules is essentially intact and the tubules maintain their integrity even in Na^+-free media. Also the duration of the collagenase plus hyaluronidase treatment appears to affect the degree of fragmentation of the tubules (20).

Several criteria have been suggested (cf. ref. 20) for evaluating the degree of intactness (functional integrity) of cells in tissue fragments prepared by any method, namely: *1*) cell structure (determined by phase-contrast and electron microscopy), *2*) the ability to exclude some dyes (e.g., trypan blue), *3*) respiratory activity in an appropriate balanced medium, and *4*) the ability of the cells to perform integrated metabolic functions normally characteristic of the intact organ.

Of these criteria the first two are of limited value because they do not permit disclosure of relatively minor changes in the properties of the cell membrane or other cellular organelles that may greatly affect the metabolism of the preparation. This point has been clearly demonstrated in isolated hepatocytes (70). As for the third criterion, damage to the cell membrane does not necessarily impair O_2 uptake (see TISSUE GEOMETRY, p. 137); on the other hand, some metabolic poisons such as uncouplers in fact increase O_2 uptake. The most valuable and comprehensive criterion is the fourth. Based on these criteria, the renal tubule preparation does indeed meet stringent demands. Thus Burg and Orloff (13) showed that at steady state the suspension of rabbit renal cortical tubules and intact renal cortex had identical values for tissue Na^+, K^+, H_2O, and extracellular (inulin) space. Moreover suspensions of cortical tubules accumulated PAH approximately three times faster than slices did (Fig. 8); the steady-state level of PAH accumulation ratio was significantly higher in tubule preparations than in slices. Also, tubules had a higher O_2 uptake than did slices and showed a significant response to substrates such as glucose or lactate. These observations were taken as evidence that the shorter diffusion pathways in tubule preparation avoids some of the rate-limiting factors besetting work with slices.

Burg and Orloff recognized that the preparation of renal tubules, as described, suffers from some cellular heterogeneity. In particular,

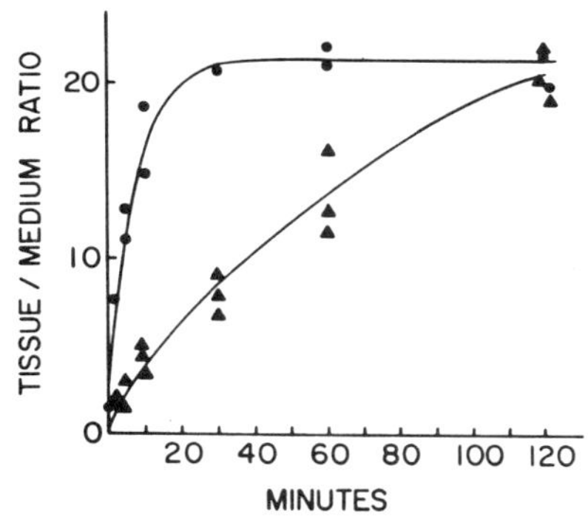

Figure 8. Comparative rates of *p*-aminohippuric acid (PAH) accumulation by tubule suspensions (●) and slices (▲) of rabbit renal cortex. *Abscissa*, established PAH gradient tissue expressed in relative terms (tissue/medium ratio) at 0.075 mM external PAH. [From Burg and Orloff (13).]

portions of distal tubules and glomeruli were present. More recently efforts have been made to remedy this shortcoming by centrifugation of crude suspensions of rat renal cortical tubules on a Percoll density gradient (103, 111). In particular, the preparation by Vinay et al. (111) permits the actual separation of proximal (gluconeogenic) convoluted tubules from fragments of distal (glycolytic) tubules.

Limitations of the Technique

Preparations of renal tubules, even when highly purified, do not completely eliminate problems stemming from the fact that the diffusion pathway to the basolateral membrane is considerably shorter than that to the luminal membrane sites of all component cells. This point of necessity affects the interpretation of kinetic data of processes involving both cell membranes. Obviously the length of the intraluminal diffusion pathway decreases with increasing fragmentation of the tubule, which in turn reflects the duration of the collagenase plus hyaluronidase digestion.

Another possible point of concern relates to the effects of the proteases used in the preparative procedure on the subsequent metabolism of the cells. Although other proteases (e.g., trypsin) have been shown to affect membrane permeability by removing proteins and glycoproteins from the cell surface (cf. refs. 39, 47), no such effects have been reported concerning collagenase treatment.

Finally, there is convincing evidence that isolated tubules are still heterogeneous with respect to cell morphology and function (118).

Appraisal of Renal Cortical Tubule Suspensions

In the previous section, the usefulness of working with suspensions of renal cortical tubules was demonstrated. The advantages of the technique stem from the relative ease of handling and from the ability to prepare tubules in amounts sufficient for biochemical studies of their metabolism. Whenever studied qualitatively, it is remarkable that observations in slices and in tubules were identical[5], notwithstanding the recognized limitations of slices (see Limitations of Tissue Slices, p. 137); quantitatively the rates of transport or metabolism were found to be faster in tubules. The preparation is also much more sensitive to handling than are slices. Finally, purified tubule preparations represent a step forward in defining metabolic processes in terms of the function of specific cells.

Glomeruli

A good yield of isolated glomeruli in suspension can be obtained by mechanically mincing renal cortical tissue into small fragments and then subjecting it to repeated centrifugation or sieving (26). Relatively few studies on this portion of the nephron are available (25, 27).

Suspensions of Isolated Nephron Cells

Defining the metabolic properties of cells derived from specific portions of the nephron appears to be the next major step in the analytical approach to renal physiology. Such direction implies the promise to relate more closely the structural and metabolic properties of the many types of cellular components of the nephron. Hepatocyte suspensions, in which the rates of metabolism of isolated cells closely approximate those found in the liver perfused in vitro, have successfully served as a model for this effort (69).

Concepts and Applications

The required homogeneity of cell suspensions from different portions of the nephron calls for considerable levels of technical accomplishment on several counts:

1. A macroscopic separation of reasonably homogeneous portions of the mammalian kidney cannot be achieved. Purified preparations of portions of the nephron, for example, proximal tubules (see Suspensions of Isolated Renal Cortical Tubules, p. 141), are not homogeneous as to component cells, as convincingly demonstrated by Woodhall et al. (118).

2. Isolated cells (and clumps of cells) can be obtained only by dispersing nonhomogeneous pieces of tissue by extending the digestion of the tissue with proteases (usually collagenase plus hyaluronidase) or by the removal of calcium from the intercellular proteins (e.g., by using citrate as a chelating agent); subsequently a more homogeneous cell preparation may be obtained by density-gradient centrifugation. This procedure requires identification of specific cell types based on their structure and metabolic properties. A novel

technique of isolating specific types of renal cells with monoclonal antibodies (106) may represent progress.

3. The preparation must meet the stringent requirements regarding preservation of functional integrity (see Concepts and Applications, p. 141).

It is immediately apparent that when cellular preparations are used it is not possible to address two crucial aspects of renal (epithelial) function: *1*) The contribution of the intercellular pathway to solute transport across the epithelial sheet is eliminated by the isolation procedure. *2*) The preparation does not permit distinction of the different properties of the luminal and basolateral cell membranes; moreover, the isolation process per se may lead to a rapid loss of (morphological) polarity of the cells, as established with tissue cultures. Several preparations are available.

Suspensions of Chick Kidney Cells

This preparation was developed primarily in order to study the effect of vitamin D [1,25-$(OH)_2D_3$] on phosphate transport in the kidney of a species known to respond well to vitamin D deficiency. The available data show that essential metabolic processes are intact (74).

Renal Cortical Cells

Several methods of obtaining suspensions of renal proximal tubular cells have been described, including free-flow electrophoresis after dispersing cells in a citrate medium (39) and collagenase treatment (48).

Renal Papilla Cells

The medulla contains six or seven cell types. Several methods of obtaining reasonably pure preparations of two of these types have been described. The exsanguinated medulla is excised, diced, and digested with collagenase plus hyaluronidase. The resulting suspension of tubules is then digested further.

Cells of Thick Ascending Limb of Henle's Loop

The crude suspension of papillary tubules is subjected to further digestion with trypsin, and the dispersed cells (6 or 7 cell types) are separated on a Ficoll density gradient (24). The structure and enzymatic activities of the cells in the densest fraction correspond to those of the thick ascending limb, and the criteria of functional integrity are met. This preparation extended our knowledge of the metabolic and transport properties of this portion of the nephron, thus complementing information obtained from perfusion of this nephron segment.

Renal Papillary Collecting Duct Cells

Repeated digestion of papillary tubules with collagenase plus hyaluronidase has been reported to yield a 90% pure suspension of the cells (23). This preparation may actually be identical with one of the lighter cellular fractions found in the density gradient described in the previous section.

Appraisal

The considerable morphological and functional heterogeneity of the nephron represents the basic limitation for obtaining cellular preparations in sufficient amounts for experimentation and for meeting all stringent criteria. This may be why the results obtained thus far with suspensions of cells from specific regions of the nephron have not contributed in a major way to the information obtained by other techniques. In particular the ingenious method developed by Schmidt and Dubach (102) permits an analysis of component enzymes in very small, morphologically defined nephron segments.

Renal Epithelial Cells Cultured In Vitro

Recognition of the morphological and functional heterogeneity of the nephron prompted yet another experimental approach to the cellular aspects of renal function, that is, the use of renal epithelial cells cultured in vitro. The potential for such an approach appears to have first been indicated by the observations by Chambers and Kempton (16) (see Isolated Nephron Segments, p. 139). Renal epithelial cell cultures were acknowledged as an experimental tool for the exploration of renal function when it was found that contrary to widely held views, epithelial cell cultures can display functional and structural polarity corresponding to differentiated structures (38).[6]

Concepts and Applications

Several established renal epithelial cell lines [MDCK (probably derived from the distal portion of canine nephron) (89), LLC-PK_1 (from pig kidney cortex), and A_6 (from toad kidney)] as well as primary cell cultures are now extensively used for the study of specific renal functions. Table 2 summarizes the properties of these cell cultures. Information available in 1984 in this field is summarized in *Tissue Culture of Epithelial Cells*, edited by M. Taub (108).

The immediately apparent advantages of renal epithelial cell cultures, particularly for the study of transport processes, are as follows:

1. The cultured cells form monolayers of apparently homogeneous cell types. The cells display morphological (apical microvilli) and functional polarity; the latter is evidenced by the formation of "domes" (hemicysts) when the cells reach confluence on solid supports (1, 107). Dome formation characterizes epithelial cell cultures

TABLE 2
Processes Studied in Renal Epithelial Cell Cultures

Cell type	Observed process
MDCK	Active Na^+ transport
	Na^+-K^+-2Cl^- cotransport
	Cl^- secretion
	Na^+-H^+ exchange
	Hormonal receptors and effects:
	Catecholamine stimulation
	Cytoplasmic mineralocorticoid receptor
LLC-PK_1	Active Na^+ transport
	Na^+-hexose cotransport
	Na^+-amino acid transport
	Phosphate transport*
	Hormonal receptors and effects:
	Vasopressin receptor
	Calcitonin effect
	1,25-Dihydroxy vitamin D_3 receptor
	Catecholamine stimulation
A_6	Active Na^+ transport
	Hormonal receptors and effects:
	Aldosterone effect, binding
	Insulin effect
	Vasopressin effect
	Adenosine receptor
Proximal tubules	Hydroxylation of 25-hydroxy vitamin D_3†
Primary culture	Na^+-hexose cotransport‡

MDCK, Madin-Darby canine kidney; LLC-PK_1, pig kidney; A_6, toad kidney. * Data from Brown et al. (12) and Rabito (94). † Data from Henry (41). ‡ Data from Sakhrani et al. (101).

grown on solid support. There is consensus that the formation of domes reflects the involvement of a unidirectional net flow of Na^+ and Cl^- (and H_2O) across the cells that is produced by operation of the Na^+–K^+–ATPase at the basolateral cell face, hence a transcellular potential difference is established. The presence of occluding intercellular junctions then permits the establishment of a hydrostatic pressure gradient that lifts a portion of the cells off the impermeable surface, thus forming domes. With cells grown on porous membranes, the hydrostatic pressure gradient dissipates and no domes form.

2. In principle, cell cultures offer the possibility of preparing unlimited amounts of the apparently homogeneous material, particularly if the technique of growing cells on microcarrier beads is adopted (12). This then allows the use of the cells for both transport and metabolic studies, and functional vesicles of microvillous membranes have been successfully prepared (12, 81).

3. The cell monolayers form a sheet that offers the distinct advantages of a simple geometry for studying the sidedness of transport (and metabolism) in the cells, as compared with the complex techniques required for such studies with intact renal tubules.

4. The cells display growth-dependent changes in their properties. On confluence, the cells differentiate morphologically (microvilli formation) and functionally (e.g., methyl-α-D-glucoside accumulation in LLC-PK_1 cells and dome formation) (85). These properties thus offer a unique possibility of studying factors involved in the development of renal cell structure and function.

Limitations of the Preparations

A more detailed analysis of available information limits to some extent noncritical enthusiasm.

First, the existence of an established cell line is not per se sufficient evidence for cellular homogeneity. This point is borne out by observations that monolayers of MDCK cells can display either high (8 $k\Omega/cm^2$) or low (0.08–0.10 $k\Omega/cm^2$) transcellular resistances (105) and two cell clones are postulated (99).

Second, the monolayers of cloned cell lines may show differences in the level of differentiation of individual cells. It has been shown in our laboratory that mitoses occur at both the subconfluent and the postconfluent stages and are also seen in domes (84). There appear to be distinct morphological and functional differences in these types of mitotic cells. Moreover major differences in cell structure and function may be observed on prolonged incubation (A. Kleinzeller, unpublished observations): while at confluence the LLC-PK_1 cells form a simple monolayer with one type of microvilli, one to two weeks after confluence at least two different types of microvilli are seen, the culture loses the character of a monolayer (strands of cells), the activity of some microvillous enzymes (e.g., alkaline phosphatase) increases severalfold as does the capacity for methyl-α-D-glucoside accumulation, and the capacity for the accumulation of amino acids decreases (2). Thus the properties of the cell cultures at each stage represent the mean of a preparation that is heterogeneous as to cell function. No information is available about whether a somewhat more uniform preparation might be obtained by synchronizing the cells when the culture is seeded.

Third, given the functional asymmetry of epithelia, the leakiness of the intercellular junction restricts an analysis of kinetic data. In particular, a recapture of methyl-α-D-glucoside at the apical membrane was seen when the substrate was applied to the medium bathing the basolateral cell face, and it diffused through the leaky "tight" junction (83).

Appraisal of Renal Tissue Culture Technique

Renal epithelial cells cultured in vitro represent an important novel tool for the study of specific processes of renal physiology. New information thus obtained reflects the properties of the given cell population under the established experimental conditions (including past history of the culture and culture media) but does not directly yield any insight into the function of the kidney or even a particular portion of the nephron from which the cells may have been derived. In terms of Warburg's criteria (p. 131), if a particular process characterizing renal function can be demonstrated in a culture of renal epithelial cells, we have the tool for an in-depth study of its specific mechanism, sidedness, regulation, development (to some extent), and we have the potential of looking into the genetic aspects governing the process. This technique, at present only in the initial stages of its development, promises to open new sources of information concerning the cellular biology of renal epithelia (3) and the nature of regulatory mechanisms in cell function.

Membrane Vesicles

The recognition of the dominant role of membrane-transport processes in renal physiology raised questions concerning their actual mechanisms and cellular localizations. Efforts to approach such questions experimentally were greatly stimulated by developments in allied fields. Hans H. Ussing and Valborg Koefoed-Johnsen first experimentally documented the concept of a transcellular transport process reflecting the functional asymmetry of epithelial cells, that is, an arrangement of membranes with various properties in a series array (61).[7] An additional insight was offered when it was found that in the mucosal sheet of the small intestine the properties associated with some transport processes appeared to be localized in the brush border, consistent with the morphological polarity of epithelial cells (80). Thus experimental problems of the sidedness of transport processes in renal cells gained momentum with the promise to proceed beyond the phenomenological level. The study of sidedness of transport processes can be attacked in a variety of ways.

1. Choice of material: Renal tubules are technically more difficult to handle than is the functionally related intestinal mucosa. However, teased tubules of some fish species (see Teased Flounder Tubules, p. 146) and sheets of renal epithelial cells grown in vitro (see Renal Epithelial Cells Cultured in Vitro, p. 136) were found to be convenient experimental tools.
2. Analysis of concentration profile: (See Tissue Slices, p. 131).
3. Biochemical dissection of the experimental material: This approach is based on a detailed knowledge of the transport properties localized in the various membranes. The experience gained in the

study of the hexose transport system may serve as an illustration. Although the Na^+-glucose cotransport system (in microvilli) is sensitive to phlorizin, the uptake of some other sugars was found to be inhibited more by phloretin than by phlorizin (56) and two separate transport pathways for sugars were postulated. It is immediately obvious that such an approach is rather indirect and requires considerable prior information on the processes to be studied.

4. Membrane vesicles: This is the most direct approach to the problem, and hence it quickly found wide appeal when it was shown that such preparations can be obtained in good yield with a satisfactory degree of purity and that technology for measuring the transport process is readily available (for review see ref. 86).

Concepts and Application

The basic steps for obtaining membrane vesicles of renal epithelia are shared by various laboratories: the tissue (e.g., renal cortex) is first homogenized in several steps, thus breaking up cells into membranes (microvillous and basolateral) and other cellular organelles; differential centrifugation then allows separation of soluble cell components and definition of the fractions representing the desired membranes. The combination of electrical and gravitational fields for the separation of membranes by free-flow electrophoresis (40) represented a major new step in isolating and characterizing the membranes according to origin (microvillous and basolateral) and distribution of membrane marker enzymes. This rather tedious procedure is now generally replaced by separation of membrane fractions in a Percoll density gradient (78) or by the precipitation of protein fractions, including the basolateral membranes, by divalent cations (Mg^{2+}, Ca^{2+}, or Mn^{2+}) (10), thus leaving purified microvillous vesicles in suspension to be subsequently collected by centrifugation.[8] A further purification (e.g., enrichment in membrane marker enzymes) may be obtained by a thiocyanate treatment of the microvillous vesicles (44).

There is now a reasonable consensus among investigators regarding the desirable properties of the membrane fractions. Compared with the original homogenate, microvillous membranes are characterized by a sizable enrichment of brush-border marker enzymes, that is, a variety of hydrolases (50). On the other hand, basolateral membranes are enriched in Na^+-K^+-ATPase, impoverished in brush-border hydrolases, and deficient in the enzymes characteristic of mitochondria or lysosomes. The two preparations also differ in their transport capabilities. As shown in Figure 9, when microvillous membrane vesicles prepared in a mannitol medium are placed in a medium containing Na^+ and D-glucose, the sugar rapidly enters the vesicles causing an "overshoot"; after some minutes, glucose that has accumulated in the vesicles against an apparent concentration gradient exits and reaches an equilibrium value identical with that found

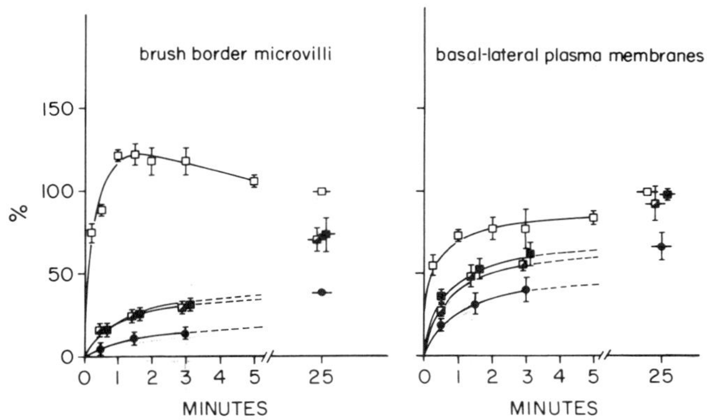

Figure 9. Percent uptake of 1 mM glucose by membrane vesicles of renal cortical cells. D-Glucose with 100 mM NaCl (□), 100 mM KCl (■), or 100 mM NaCl and 0.1 mM phlorizin (◪); and L-glucose with 100 mM NaCl (●). [From Kinne (52).]

TISSUE SLICES TO MEMBRANE VESICLES

when Na^+ is absent or when glucose entry is blocked by phlorizin (52). This overshoot phenomenon is not seen with L-glucose but is consistent with the concept of the Na^+-glucose cotransport system in that the downhill gradient of Na^+ drives glucose uphill into the vesicles; this driving force ceases to act when the Na^+ gradient across the vesicle membrane dissipates, and therefore glucose exits. On the other hand, D-glucose enters the basolateral membrane vesicles via an equilibrating system, only slightly stimulated by Na^+ and mildly sensitive to phlorizin; however, the stereospecificity of glucose transport is evident. Similar results were obtained with amino acids and other transported solutes.

In order to satisfy experimental demands, membrane vesicles must meet several criteria. First, it is crucial to ascertain whether the orientation of the membrane vesicles is identical with that normally found in the cells (i.e., right side out) and the accessibility of substrates, inhibitors (37), or monoclonal antibodies (49) to membrane sites is used as a test. This criterion appears to be met by microvillous membrane vesicles in which the presence of the central actin core actually prevents reversal of the membrane orientation. On the other hand, reports on the basolateral membrane indicate random orientation, judging by the accessibility of the Na^+-K^+-ATPase to external ATP. More recent data (11) claim a more uniform preparation (90% right side out). In this respect the choice of animal species for the preparation of membrane vesicles may be important. Second, the study of any transport process, whether accumulation into or exit from vesicles, requires an intact vesicle structure. This point is usually tested by demonstrating a linear relationship between the uptake of a solute, and the reciprocal of external osmolarity. However, this test does not reveal the proportion of intact vesicles in a given preparation; there are reports indicating that only one in four to six brush-border vesicles is sealed (34). It should be noted that this finding does not per se detract from the validity of data obtained with vesicles. Finally, the criterion of homogeneity is a tenuous one. Ideally the membranes of interest should also be defined according to the cell type from which they originate. Given the cellular heterogeneity of the nephron, this criterion is difficult to meet (see ref. 62). In this respect the preparation of membrane vesicles from renal epithelial cells grown in vitro (12, 81) may be promising, provided that the conditions of growing the cells and of timing their harvest are rigidly uniform.

Another aspect of heterogeneity concerns the fact that in a given preparation the vesicles may differ considerably as to size and possibly as to other properties as well.[9] No solution to this problem is in sight.

The advantages of the preparation are immediately apparent.

1. By breaking up the cells and working with membrane preparations, the student of transport processes avoids major problems relating to intracellular metabolism of the studied solute; thus it is possible to separate experimentally membrane events from cytoplasmic events.

2. The technique allows a rigorous control of both external and intravesicular experimental conditions. A wealth of new information was gained by modifying the ionic composition of the extra- and intravesicular compartments and changing the membrane conductive pathways (e.g., with ionophores). One major advance was the demonstration of the postulated electrogenic nature of the Na^+-glucose cotransport system (5). Such experimentation permits a more detailed description of the kinetic properties of the studied systems and clarification of the thermodynamic driving forces.

3. The preparation can be maintained for prolonged periods in the frozen state (−70°C), thus allowing multiple experiments on the same material and hence reducing biological variability.

4. New and more detailed knowledge of the specific transport systems opened the door to a more molecular approach, with the aim of isolating the transport proteins and eventually reconstituting the system in artificial membranes, as initiated by Crane et al. (18).

The review by Murer and Kinne (86) should be consulted for an extensive list of transport processes and their physiological correlates studied with membrane vesicles. More recently the transport of anionic metabolic substrates has been extensively studied, particularly by Ernest M. Wright and his group (88, 119).

Limitations of Membrane Vesicles

The technology for studying transport phenomena with membrane vesicles has now reached a high level. As with any other experimental technique, its limitations must be considered.

Homogeneity

As pointed out in Concepts and Applications, p. 150, problems of homogeneity persist despite the refined techniques of separating membrane vesicles. Two sources of error must be considered here (43): possible contamination by other cellular membranes known to have a transport system different from the investigated one and several independent pathways for a given solute through the vesicle membrane (109). These problems may have to be assessed separately in every study. Other aspects of heterogeneity concern the differences in vesicle size and properties within a given preparation.

Interpretation of Results

Transport-process measurements are usually expressed in units of solute taken up per milligram of protein in the preparation. It is generally assumed that the intravesicular volume is constant during the experimental procedure. However, particularly for the experimental conditions shown in Figure 9, volume changes may be sizable because there are major differences between the permeabilities of mannitol and the given ionic species. Hence the analysis of an uptake transport process requires particular attention to possible volume changes.

Membrane Vesicles and Cell Function

Vesicles are only one piece of the puzzle (86). Experiments with vesicles are performed under artificial conditions different from those found in cellular preparations. Conclusions must be closely correlated with information obtained from biologically more intact systems.

Appraisal of Membrane Vesicle Technique

The use of membrane vesicles from renal epithelial cells has already proven to be a powerful tool in the study of the biochemical mechanism of specific transport processes involved in renal physiology and has opened the door to an investigation of these particular processes at a molecular level.

Role of Methodological Advances on Concepts in Renal Physiology

The evaluation of the methodology presented in preceding sections provides cogent evidence in favor of the analytical approach to renal physiology. A review of advances made in the last sixty years concerning the renal reabsorption of glucose may serve as an illustration of how progress in methodology is inseparably related to the development of new concepts.

Unequivocal evidence for the reabsorption of glucose from the glomerular filtrate has been provided by A. Newton Richards's micropuncture experiments on frog nephrons. Thus the transport vector for this solute, produced by the proximal renal tubular cells, was established. However, it was the simple clearance technique (see the chapter by Bradley in this volume), dominating the field for about twenty years, that provided evidence for the saturability of the reabsorptive mechanism and some indications of its specificity, including competition of substrates, hence Shannon's concept (104) of an enzymelike reaction of cellular components involved in glucose reabsorption or PAH excretion.

The next major step was the demonstration that renal cortical slices are capable of accumulating free sugar (galactose) against a distinct concentration gradient (63), indicating that the observed transport process is "active." This transport system was subsequently shown to have properties (59) compatible with the newly advanced concept of coupling between Na^+ and glucose transport (17); also, the accumulation process was proven to be active transport (as opposed to the possibility of an involvement of a metabolic event such as phosphorylation) by the observation that the nonmetabolizable glucose analogue methyl-α-D-glucoside was accumulated by the slices against sizable concentration gradients (58). The available information, derived from both in vivo and in vitro studies suggested localization of the glucose-transport system in the renal proximal tubule. Moreover (analogous to intestinal mucosal cells) the involvement of the brush-border membrane in uphill sugar transport was indicated. The techniques used could not per se prove the postulated mechanism. Also, the possibility of the existence of this glucose-transport system in other portions of the nephron was not investigated.[10] Some apparent anomalies observed for sugar transport in slices, particularly the Na^+-independent accumulation of 2-deoxyhexoses (58), raised the possibility of several transport pathways for glucose; clear evidence for the involvement of the basolateral membrane in Na^+-independent glucose (and 2-deoxyglucose) transport was then provided by studies with teased flounder renal tubules (60).

The important role of information obtained by perfusing renal tubules in vivo and in vitro should be emphasized here. Such studies, particularly those of Karl Ullrich and his group (110), provided direct measurements of rates of transcellular sugar fluxes, clinched the Na^+-dependence of the apical uptake of glucose, and more recently proved directly the electrogenic nature of the coupling of glucose and Na^+ fluxes (33).

Unequivocal evidence for the postulated Na^+-glucose cotransport system in brush-border vesicles of renal cortical cells was first supplied by Kinne (52) by demonstrating an uphill flux of free glucose driven by the downhill electrochemical gradient of Na^+ (Fig. 9); the electrogenic nature of the process (the involvement of both Na^+ and K^+ electrochemical gradients) was then proved (5). Moreover the functional polarity of the renal epithelial cells with respect to the predominant pathways of glucose transport in the microvillous and basolateral cell membranes was also conclusively established with the vesicle technique.

TISSUE SLICES TO MEMBRANE VESICLES

The outlined progress cannot be dissociated from the application of improved and new analytical techniques. In the field analyzed in this chapter, the application of specific, enzymatic, analytical micro- and ultramicromethods developed by Lowry and Passonneau (76) and the use of labeled substrates were essential.

These stages in the analysis of the physiology of glucose handling by the kidney represent a gradual change of emphasis from studies of the function of the whole kidney toward analysis of the detailed mechanism of the function of the cellular (and subcellular) level, that is, kidney → renal slices → tubular segments → isolated cells → cell membranes. This methodological progression reflects changes in the specific questions addressed by investigators, and pertinent hypotheses advanced: the demonstration of a reabsorptive mechanism for glucose in the nephron raised the question of the involved driving forces, which was gradually resolved by the demonstration of the Na^+-glucose cotransport system, driven by the operation of the Na^+ pump. At each stage new experimental tools had to be employed in order to transcend the limitations of techniques that yielded results on which the original questions were based and thus to falsify [or substantiate, cf. Huxley (45)] advanced hypotheses.

An analysis of the progress achieved shows that all experimental approaches play unique roles in solving the puzzle. Observations made with any experimental approach are valid only to the extent given by the limitations of the methods employed. In this context it becomes clear that shifting the emphasis for the whole kidney to the cellular (and subcellular) level restricts the scope of the answers to only small pieces of the puzzle; thus information obtained at the cellular level must be reintegrated in order to perceive a better understanding of the physiological phenomenon. Warburg's challenge to investigators studying biological phenomena under simplified, in vitro conditions is appropriate in that answers obtained by in vitro studies at any level of biological organization must be constantly correlated with physiological (in vivo) observation.

Valuable comments on the use of experimental techniques were received from Drs. M. Bergeron, R. P. Forster, S. K. Hong, P. Lund, A. D. C. Macknight, J. B. Pritchard, B. Ross, C. R. Scriver, K. J. Ullrich, and E. M. Wright. Helpful suggestions from Drs. R. W. Berliner, R. E. Davies, L. Goldstein, C. W. Gottschalk, R. Kinne, and J. B. Pritchard are particularly appreciated.

This study was supported in part by National Institutes of Health Grant AM-12619.

NOTES

[1] The term *consistence* (in original: "*dazu stimmen*") implies a judgment as to the nature of the postulated correlation. The burden of proof rests on the shoulders of the investigator.

[2] This particular assumption was justified by Warburg's experimental evidence that the O_2 affinity of the "respiratory enzyme" (cytochrome oxidase) was high enough to make tissue respiration virtually independent of O_2 even at very low O_2 partial pressures. The present value for the operative Michaelis constant (K_m) of cytochrome oxidase is about 0.1 μM, which compares to 200 μM O_2 in an aqueous solution at 37°C in equilibrium with air.

[3] In the light of present knowledge, it is appropriate to specify the actual physiological process as net absorption or net secretion. This reflects the observations that the measured net flux of solute and fluid across an epithelial sheet is the resultant of sometimes opposite fluxes through cell membranes, with a contribution from the intercellular pathway. The view that individual epithelial cells either secrete or absorb does not necessarily hold (6).

[4] This discovery is due to the observation by R. P. Forster (personal communication) that slices of flounder kidney largely disintegrated on incubation in vitro; microscopic examination then showed that the floating tubules were sealed at both ends, resembling cysts seen by Chambers et al. (16).

[5] To my knowledge, the only major difference in observations made with slices and suspensions of renal cortical tubules concerns the pathways of cystine transport (cf. ref. 46). Other differences such as the more direct demonstration of cAMP effects on methyl-α-D-glucoside or of α-aminoisobutyric acid uptake in tubules as compared with slices (55) may relate to an impaired accessibility of cAMP to the actual site(s) of action.

[6] The term *differentiation* is ill defined. In most established lines of renal epithelial cells, microvilli and distinct intercellular junctions appear on confluence of the culture; however, morphologically the cells differ markedly from cells of the renal proximal tubule with dense microvilli (85). Moreover there is clear morphological development of LLC-PK_1 (but not MDCK) cells when the culture is prolonged for several weeks after confluence has been reached. Finally, it should be emphasized that specific functional properties of cells grown in vitro may differ from those found in renal cells derived from adult (differentiated) kidney. This is borne out, for example, by studies on the localization of the furosemide-sensitive Na^+-K^+-$2Cl^-$ cotransport system in MDCK and LLC-PK_1 cells (100).

[7] As early as 1939, Shannon (104) put forward the hypothesis that transcellular active transport in the kidney (reabsorption or excretion of solutes) is brought about by the renal tubular cells having two membranes with different properties, only one of them containing the cellular component with which the solute interacts; the question of the mechanism by which metabolic energy is utilized in the process was left open. The contribution of Forster and Hong (30) was also crucial.

[8] Microvillous membrane vesicles prepared by the Mg^{2+} precipitation technique are considerably "tighter" than those obtained by the Ca^{2+} precipitation method.

[9] Membrane vesicles, particularly those derived from microvilli, are not

spherical. Hence, questions relating to the surface-volume ratio may affect the analysis of transport in the preparation.

[10] Recent evidence suggests that distal portions of the nephron are also capable of reabsorbing glucose and thus play a role in the physiological and pathological renal handling of glucose (8).

BIBLIOGRAPHY

1. ABAZA, N., J. LEIGHTON, and S. G. SCHULTZ. Effects of ouabain on the function and structure of a cell line MDCK derived from canine kidney. *In Vitro* 10: 172–183, 1974.
2. AMSLER, K., and J. S. COOK. Development of Na^+-dependent hexose transport in a cultured line of porcine kidney cells. *Am. J. Physiol.* 242 (*Cell Physiol.* 11): C94–C101, 1982.
3. AMSLER, K., C. SHAFFER, and J. S. COOK. Growth-dependent AIB and meAIB uptake in LLC-PK_1 cells: effects of differentiation inducers and of TPA. *J. Cell. Physiol.* 114: 184–190, 1983.
4. ARTHUS, M.-F., M. BERGERON, and C. R. SCHRIVER. Topology of membrane exposure in the renal cortex slice. Studies of glutathione and maltose cleavage. *Biochim. Biophys. Acta* 692: 371–376, 1981.
5. BECK, J. C., and B. SACKTOR. The sodium electrochemical potential-mediated uphill transport of D-glucose in renal brush border membrane vesicles. *J. Biol. Chem.* 253: 5531–5535, 1978.
6. BERGLUND, F., C.-G. HELANDER, and R. B. HOWE. Inorganic sulfate and thiosulfate: transport and competition in renal tubules of the dog. *Am. J. Physiol.* 198: 586–594, 1960.
7. BERNDT, W. O. The accumulation of ^{14}C-hypoxanthine by slices of rabbit kidney cortex. *Biochem. Pharmacol.* 17: 605–615, 1968.
8. BISHOP, J. H. V., and R. GREEN. Glucose handling by distal portions of the nephron during pregnancy in the rat. *J. Physiol. Lond.* 336: 131–142, 1983.
9. BOJESEN, E., and P. P. LEYSSAC. The kidney cortex slice technique as a model for sodium transport in vivo. A quantitative evaluation. *Acta Physiol. Scand.* 65: 20–32, 1965.
10. BOOTH, A. G., and A. J. KENNY. A rapid method for the preparation of microvilli from rabbit kidney. *Biochem. J.* 142: 575–581, 1974.
11. BOUMENDIL-PODEVIN, E. F., and R. A. PODEVIN. Isolation of baso-lateral and brush-border membranes from rabbit kidney cortex. Vesicle integrity and membrane sidedness of the baso-lateral fraction. *Biochim. Biophys. Acta* 735: 86–94, 1983.
12. BROWN, C. D. A., M. BODMER, J. BIBER, and H. MURER. Sodium-dependent phosphate transport by apical membrane vesicles from a cultured renal epithelial cell line (LLC-PK_1). *Biochim. Biophys. Acta* 769: 471–478, 1984.
13. BURG, M. B., and J. ORLOFF. Oxygen consumption and active transport in separated renal tubules. *Am. J. Physiol.* 203: 327–330, 1962.
14. CAMERON, G., and R. CHAMBERS. Direct evidence of function in kidney of an early human fetus. *Am. J. Physiol.* 123: 482–485, 1938.
15. CHAMBERS, R., and E. L. CHAMBERS. *Explorations Into the Nature of the Living Cell.* Cambridge, MA: Harvard Univ. Press, 1961.
16. CHAMBERS, R., and R. T. KEMPTON. Indications of function of the chick

mesonephros in tissue culture with phenol red. *J. Cell. Comp. Physiol.* 3: 131–167, 1933.

17. CRANE, R. K. Intestinal absorption of sugars. *Physiol. Rev.* 40: 794–825, 1960.
18. CRANE, R. K., P. MALATHI, H. PREISER, and P. FAIRCLOUGH. Some characteristics of kidney Na^+-dependent glucose carrier reconstituted into sonicated liposomes. *Am. J. Physiol.* 234 (*Endocrinol. Metab. Gastrointest. Physiol.* 3): E1–E5, 1978.
19. CROSS, R. J., and J. V. TAGGART. Renal tubular transport: accumulation of *p*-aminohippurate by rabbit kidney slices. *Am. J. Physiol.* 161: 181–190, 1950.
20. DAWSON, A. G. Preparation and some properties of a suspension of fragmented tubules from rat kidney. *Biochem. J.* 130: 525–532, 1972.
21. DEUTSCH, W. An improvement of Warburg's method for cutting tissue slices for respiratory experiments (Abstract). *J. Physiol. Lond.* 87: 56P–57P, 1936.
22. DEYRUP, I. J., and R. E. DAVIES. The effect of temperature on the uptake of radiosulfate by rat renal tissue from radiosulfate containing solutions in vitro. *J. Gen. Physiol.* 44: 555–569, 1961.
23. DWORZAK, D. L., and J. J. GRANTHAM. Preparation of renal papillary collection duct cells for study in vitro. *Kidney Int.* 8: 191–194, 1975.
24. EVELOFF, J., W. HAASE, and R. KINNE. Separation of renal medullary cells: isolation of cells from the thick ascending limb of Henle's loop. *J. Cell Biol.* 87: 672–681, 1980.
25. FOLKERT, V. W., and D. SCHLONDORFF. Altered prostaglandin synthesis by glomeruli from rats with unilateral ureteral ligation. *Am. J. Physiol.* 241 (*Renal Fluid Electrolyte Physiol.* 10): F289–F299, 1981.
26. FONG, J. S. C., and K. N. DRUMMOND. Method for preparation of glomeruli for metabolic studies. *J. Lab. Clin. Med.* 71: 1034–1039, 1968.
27. FONG, J. S. C., and K. N. DRUMMOND. Glomerular metabolism. Glucose and palmitic acid oxidation in normal and nephrotoxic nephritic rats. *Lab. Invest.* 20: 512–515, 1969.
28. FORSTER, R. P. Use of thin kidney slices and isolated renal tubules for direct study of cellular transport kinetics. *Science Wash. DC* 108: 65–67, 1948.
29. FORSTER, R. P., and J. H. COPENHAVER, JR. Intracellular accumulation as an active process in a mammalian renal transport system in vitro. Energy dependence and competitive phenomena. *Am. J. Physiol.* 186: 167–171, 1956.
30. FORSTER, R. P., and S. K. HONG. In vitro transport of dyes by isolated renal tubules of the flounder as disclosed by direct visualization. Intracellular accumulation and transcellular movement. *J. Cell. Comp. Physiol.* 51: 259–272, 1956.
31. FORSTER, R. P., and J. V. TAGGART. Use of isolated renal tubules for the examination of metabolic processes associated with active cellular transport. *J. Cell. Comp. Physiol.* 36: 251–270, 1950.
32. FOX, M., S. THIER, L. ROSENBERG, and S. SEGAL. Ionic requirements for amino acid transport in the rat kidney cortex slices. I. Influence of extracellular ions. *Biochim. Biophys. Acta* 79: 167–176, 1964.
33. FRÖMTER, E. Electrophysiological analysis of rat renal sugar and amino

acid transport. I. Basic phenomena. *Pfluegers Arch.* 393: 179–189, 1982.

34. Gaines, N., and H. Hauser. Leakiness of brush-border vesicles. *Biochim. Biophys. Acta* 772: 161–166, 1984.
35. Guder, W. G., W. Wiesner, B. Stakowski, and O. Wieland. Metabolism of isolated kidney tubules. *Hoppe-Seyler's Z. Physiol. Chem.* 352: 1319–1328, 1971.
36. György, P., W. Keller, and T. Brehme. Nierenstoffwechsel und Nierenentwicklung. *Biochem. Z.* 220: 356–366, 1928.
37. Haase, W., A. Schäfer, H. Murer, and R. Kinne. Studies on the orientation of brush-border membrane vesicles. *Biochem. J.* 172: 57–62, 1978.
38. Handler, J. S., F. M. Perkins, and J. P. Johnson. Studies of renal cell function using cell culture techniques. *Am. J. Physiol.* 238 (*Renal Fluid Electrolyte Physiol.* 7): F1–F9, 1980.
39. Heidrich, H. G., and M. E. Dew. Homogeneous cell populations from rabbit kidney cortex. Proximal, distal tubule, and renin-active cells isolated by free-flow electrophoresis. *J. Cell Biol.* 74: 780–788, 1977.
40. Heidrich, H. G., R. Kinne, E. Kinne-Saffran, and K. Hannig. The polarity of the proximal tubule cell in rat kidney. Different surface charges for the brush-border microvilli and plasma membranes from the basal infoldings. *J. Cell Biol.* 54: 232–245, 1972.
41. Henry, H. L. Regulation of the hydroxylation of 25-hydroxyvitamin D_3 in vivo and in primary cultures of chick kidney cells. *J. Biol. Chem.* 254: 2722–2729, 1979.
42. Holm, J. In vitro studies on the uptake of ^{14}C-labeled tetraethylammonium in mouse kidney. *Acta Pharmacol. Toxicol.* 31: 129–137, 1972.
43. Hopfer, U. Kinetic criteria for carrier-mediated transport mechanisms in membrane vesicles. *Federation Proc.* 40: 2480–2485, 1981.
44. Hopfer, U., T. D. Crowe, and B. Tandler. Purification of brush-border membrane by thiocyanate treatment. *Anal. Biochem.* 131: 447–452, 1983.
45. Huxley, A. F. Discovery: accident or design? The Florey lecture. *Proc. R. Soc. Lond. B Biol. Sci.* 216: 253–266, 1982.
46. Hwang, S. M., J. Foreman, and S. Segal. Developmental pattern of cystine transport in isolated rat renal tubules. *Biochim. Biophys. Acta* 690: 145–153, 1982.
47. Johnson, P. A., and R. M. Johnstone. Alterations in membrane permeability with trypsin treatment. *Can. J. Biochem.* 59: 668–675, 1981.
48. Jones, D. P., G.-B. Sundby, K. Ormstad, and S. Orrenius. Use of isolated kidney cells for the study of drug metabolism. *Biochem. Pharmacol.* 28: 929–935, 1979.
49. Kashgarian, M. Use of monoclonal antibodies in the study of renal function. *Am. J. Physiol.* 247 (*Renal Fluid Electrolyte Physiol.* 16): F533–F538, 1984.
50. Kenny, A. J., and S. Maroux. Topology of microvillar membrane hydrolases of kidney and intestine. *Physiol. Rev.* 62: 91–128, 1982.
51. King, P. A., K. W. Beyenbach, and L. Goldstein. Taurine transport by isolated flounder renal tubules. *J. Exp. Zool.* 223: 103–114, 1982.
52. Kinne, R. Properties of the glucose transport system in the renal brush border membrane. *Curr. Top. Membr. Transp.* 8: 209–267, 1976.

53. KINTER, W. B. Chlorphenol red influx and efflux: microspectrophotometry of flounder kidney tubules. *Am. J. Physiol.* 211: 1152–1164, 1966.
54. KINTER, W. B. Structure and function of renal tubules isolated from fish kidneys. *Fortschr. Zool.* 23: 223–231, 1975.
55. KIPPEN, I., B. HIRAYAMA, J. R. KLINENBERG, and E. W. WRIGHT. Effects of dibutyryl cyclic AMP on the transport of α-methyl-D-glucoside and α-aminoisobutyric acid in separated tubules and brush border membranes from rabbit kidney. *Biochim. Biophys. Acta* 558: 126–135, 1979.
56. KLEINZELLER, A. The Na-independent transport of sugars in renal tubular cells. In: *Na-Linked Transport of Organic Solutes*, edited by E. Heinz. New York: Springer-Verlag, 1972, p. 109–115.
57. KLEINZELLER, A., and A. KNOTKOVÁ. The steady-state efflux of Na^+, K^+ and Cl^- from kidney cortex slices. *Physiol. Bohemoslov.* 16: 214–226, 1967.
58. KLEINZELLER, A., J. KOLÍNSKÁ, and I. BENEŠ. Transport of monosaccharides in kidney cortex cells. *Biochem. J.* 104: 852–860, 1967.
59. KLEINZELLER, A., and A. KOTYK. Cations and transport of galactose in kidney-cortex slices. *Biochim. Biophys. Acta* 54: 367–369, 1961.
60. KLEINZELLER, A., and E. M. MCAVOY. Sugar transport across the peritubular face of renal cells of the flounder. *J. Gen. Physiol.* 62: 169–184, 1973.
61. KOEFOED-JOHNSEN, V., and H. H. USSING. The nature of the frog skin potential. *Acta Physiol. Scand.* 42: 298–308, 1958.
62. KRAGH-HANSEN, V., H. ROIGAARD-PETERSEN, C. JACOBSEN, and M. I. SHEIKH. Tubular localization of Na^+-dependent phenylalanine and glucose transport system. *Biochem. J.* 220: 15–24, 1984.
63. KRANE, S. M., and R. K. CRANE. The accumulation of D-galactose against a concentration gradient by slices of rabbit kidney cortex. *J. Biol. Chem.* 234: 211–219, 1959.
64. KREBS, H. A. Untersuchungen über den Stoffwechsel der Aminosäuren im Tierkorper. *Hoppe Seyler's Z. Physiol. Chem.* 217: 191–227, 1933.
65. KREBS, H. A. The synthesis of glutamine from glutamic acid and ammonia and the enzyme hydrolysis of glutamine in animal tissues. *Biochem. J.* 291: 1951–1969, 1935.
66. KREBS, H. A. Body size and tissue respiration. *Biochim. Biophys. Acta* 4: 249–269, 1950.
67. KREBS, H. A. *Otto Warburg: Cell Physiologist, Biochemist and Eccentric.* Oxford, UK: Clarendon, 1981.
68. KREBS, H. A., D. A. H. BENNETT, P. DE GASQUET, and T. YOSHIDA. Renal gluconeogenesis. The effect of diet in the gluconeogenic capacity of rat-kidney-cortex slices. *Biochem. J.* 86: 22–27, 1963.
69. KREBS, H. A., N. W. CORNELL, P. LUND, and R. HEMS. Isolated liver cells as experimental material. In: *Regulation of Hepatic Metabolism*, edited by F. Lundquist and N. Tygstrup. Copenhagen: Munksgaard, 1974, p. 726–750. (Alfred Benzon Symp. 6.)
70. KREBS, H. A., P. LUND, and M. EDWARDS. Criteria of metabolic competence of isolated hepatocytes. In: *Cell Populations (Methodological Surveys in Biochemistry)*, edited by E. Reid. New York: Wiley, 1979, p. 1–6.

71. LEAF, A. On the mechanism of fluid exchange of tissues in vitro. *Biochem. J.* 62: 241–248, 1956.
72. LEE, J. B., V. K. VANCE, and G. F. CAHILL, JR. Metabolism of C^{14}-labeled substrates by rabbit kidney cortex and medulla. *Am. J. Physiol.* 203: 27–36, 1962.
73. LEUTHARDT, I. Untersuchungen über die Diffusion in Gewebsschnitten. *Biochem. Z.* 299: 281–306, 1938.
74. LIANG, C. T., J. BARNES, L. CHENG, R. BALAKIR, and B. SACKTOR. Effects of 1,25-$(OH)_2D_3$ administered in vivo on phosphate uptake by isolated chick renal cells. *Am. J. Physiol.* 242 (*Cell Physiol.* 11): C312–C318, 1982.
75. LOWENSTEIN, L., K. HUMMELER, I. SMITH, and S. SEGAL. The effect of storage at 4°C on amino acid transport by rat kidney cortex slices. *Biochim. Biophys. Acta* 150: 416–423, 1968.
76. LOWRY, O. H., and J. V. PASSONNEAU. *A Flexible System of Enzymatic Analysis.* New York: Academic, 1972.
77. MAACK, T., and W. B. KINTER. Transport of protein by flounder kidney tubules during long-term incubation. *Am. J. Physiol.* 216: 1034–1043, 1969.
78. MAMELOK, R. D., D. R. MACRAE, L. Z. BENET, and S. B. PRUSINER. Membrane populations of bovine choroid plexus: separation by density gradient centrifugation in modified colloidal silica. *J. Neurochem.* 37: 768–774, 1981.
79. MARTEL-PELLETIER, J., D. GUERETTE, and M. BERGERON. Morphological changes during incubation of renal slices. *Lab. Invest.* 36: 509–518, 1977.
80. MILLER, D., and R. K. CRANE. The digestive function of epithelium of the small intestine. *Biochim. Biophys. Acta* 52: 293–298, 1961.
81. MORAN, A., J. S. HANDLER, and R. J. TURNER. Na^+-dependent hexose transport in vesicles from cultured renal epithelial cell line. *Am. J. Physiol.* 243 (*Cell Physiol.* 12): C293–C298, 1982.
82. MUDGE, G. H. Studies on potassium accumulation by rabbit kidney slices: effect of metabolic activity. *Am. J. Physiol.* 165: 113–127, 1951.
83. MULLIN, J. M., L. FLUK, and A. KLEINZELLER. Basal-lateral transport and transcellular flux of methyl-α-D-glucoside across LLC-PK_1 renal epithelial cells. *Biochim. Biophys. Acta.* 885: 233–239, 1986.
84. MULLIN, J. M, L. FLUK, and T. TCHAO. Mitosis in domes of renal epithelial (LLC-PK_1) cell culture. *J. Mol. Physiol.* 8: 813–828, 1985.
85. MULLIN, J. M., F. WEIBEL, L. DIAMOND, and A. KLEINZELLER. Sugar transport in the LLC-PK_1 renal epithelial cell line: similarity to mammalian kidney and the influence of cell density. *J. Cell. Physiol.* 104: 375–389, 1980.
86. MURER, H., and R. KINNE. The use of isolated membrane vesicles to study epithelial transport processes. *J. Membr. Biol.* 55: 81–95, 1980.
87. MURTHY, L., and E. C. FOULKES. Movement of solutes across luminal cell membranes in kidney tubules of the rabbit. *Nature Lond.* 213: 180–181, 1967.
88. NORD, E. P., S. H. WRIGHT, I. KIPPEN, and E. M. WRIGHT. Specificity of the Na^+-dependent monocarboxylic acid transport pathway in rabbit renal brush border membranes. *J. Membr. Biol.* 72: 213–221, 1983.
89. OJAKIAN, G. K., and D. A. HERZLINGER. Analysis of epithelial cell surface

polarity with monoclonal antibodies. *Federation Proc.* 43: 2208–2216, 1984.
90. Okamoto, Y. Über Anaerobiose von Tumorgewebe. *Biochem. Z.* 160: 52–65, 1925.
91. Platts, M. M., and G. H. Mudge. Accumulation of uric acid by slices of kidney cortex. *Am. J. Physiol.* 200: 387–392, 1961.

92. Podevin, R. A., E. F. Boumendil-Podevin, and C. Priol. Concentrative PAH transport by rabbit kidney slices in the absence of metabolic energy. *Am. J. Physiol.* 235 (*Renal Fluid Electrolyte Physiol.* 4): F278–F285, 1978.
93. Preuss, H. G., S. T. Eastman, O. Vavatsi-Manos, K. Baird, and D. M. Roxe. The regulation of renal ammoniagenesis in the rat by extracellular factors. I. The combined effects of acidosis and physiologic fuels. *Metabolism* 27: 1626–1638, 1978.
94. Rabito, C. A. Phosphate uptake by a kidney cell line ($LLC\text{-}PK_1$). *Am. J. Physiol.* 245 (*Renal Fluid Electrolyte Physiol.* 14): F22–F31, 1983.
95. Renfro, J. L. Calcium transport across peritubular surface of the marine teleost renal tubule. *Am. J. Physiol.* 234 (*Renal Fluid Electrolyte Physiol.* 3): F522–F531, 1978.
96. Renfro, J. L., and J. B. Pritchard. H^+-dependent sulfate secretion in the marine teleost renal tubule. *Am. J. Physiol.* 243 (*Renal Fluid Electrolyte Physiol.* 12): F150–F159, 1982.
96a. Rose, R. C., J. Bianchi, and S. A. Schuette. Effective use of renal cortical slices in transport and metabolic studies. *Biochim. Biophys. Acta* 821: 431–436, 1985.
97. Rosenberg, L. E., A. Blair, and S. Segal. The transport of amino acids in rat kidney cortex slices. *Biochim. Biophys. Acta* 54: 479–488, 1961.
98. Rozen, R., and C. R. Scriver. Renal transport of taurine adapts to perturbed taurine homeostasis. *Proc. Natl. Acad. Sci. USA* 79: 2101–2105, 1982.
99. Rugg, E. L., and N. L. Simmons. Control of cultured epithelial (MDCK) cell transport function: identification of a β-adrenoreceptor coupled to adenylate cyclase. *Q. J. Exp. Physiol.* 69: 339–353, 1984.
100. Saier, M. H. Application of the microbiological approach to the study of passive monovalent salt transport in a kidney epithelial cell line, MDCK. In: *Tissue Culture of Epithelial Cells*, edited by M. Taub. New York: Plenum, 1985, p. 51–66.
101. Sakhrani, L. M., B. Badie-Dezfooly, W. Trizna, N. Mikhail, A. G. Lowe, M. Taub, and L. G. Fine. Transport and metabolism of glucose by renal proximal tubular cells in primary culture. *Am. J. Physiol.* 246 (*Renal Fluid Electrolyte Physiol.* 15): F757–F764, 1984.
102. Schmidt, U., and U. C. Dubach. Differential enzymatic behaviour of single proximal segments of the superficial and juxtamedullary nephron. *Z. Gesamte Exp. Med.* 151: 93–102, 1969.
103. Scholer, D. W., and I. S. Edelman. Isolation of rat kidney cortical tubules enriched in proximal and distal segments. *Am. J. Physiol.* 237 (*Renal Fluid Electrolyte Physiol.* 6): F350–F359, 1979.
104. Shannon, J. A. Renal tubular excretion. *Physiol. Rev.* 19: 63–93, 1939.
105. Simmons, N. L., C. D. A. Brown, and E. L. Rugg. The action of epinephrine on Madin-Darby canine kidney cells. *Federation Proc.* 43: 2225–2229, 1984.

106. SMITH, W. L., and A. GARCIA-PEREZ. Immunodissection: use of monoclonal antibodies to isolate specific types of renal cells. *Am. J. Physiol.* 248 (*Renal Fluid Electrolyte Physiol.* 17): F1–F7, 1985.
107. TANNER, C., D. A. FRAMBACH, and D. S. MISFELDT. Biophysics of domes formed by the renal cell line Madin-Darby canine kidney. *Federation Proc.* 43: 2217–2220, 1984.
108. TAUB, M. (editor). *Tissue Culture of Epithelial Cells.* New York: Plenum, 1985.
109. TURNER, R. J., and A. MORAN. Heterogeneity of sodium-dependent D-glucose transport sites along the proximal tubule: evidence from vesicle studies. *Am. J. Physiol.* 242 (*Renal Fluid Electrolyte Physiol.* 11): F406–F414, 1982.
110. ULLRICH, K. J., G. RUMRICH, and S. KLÖSS. Specificity and sodium dependence of the active sugar transport in the proximal convolution of the rat kidney. *Pfluegers Arch.* 351: 35–48, 1974.
111. VINAY, P., A. GOUGOUX, and G. LEMIEUX. Isolation of a pure suspension of rat proximal tubules. *Am. J. Physiol.* 241 (*Renal Fluid Electrolyte Physiol.* 10): F403–F411, 1981.
112. WARBURG, O. Versuche am überlebendem Carcinomgewebe. *Biochem. Z.* 142: 317–333, 1923.
113. WARBURG, O., K. GAWEHN, and A.-W. GEISSLER. Stoffwechsel von embryonalen Zellen und von Krebszellen. *Z. Naturforsch.* 11b: 657–662, 1956.
114. WEDEEN, R. P., and B. WEINER. The distribution of *p*-aminohippuric acid in rat kidney slices. I. Tubular localization. *Kidney Int.* 3: 205–213, 1973.
115. WEDEEN, R. P., and B. WEINER. The distribution of *p*-aminohippuric acid in rat kidney slices. II. Depth of uptake. *Kidney Int.* 3: 214–221, 1973.
116. WEIDEMANN, M. J., and H. A. KREBS. The fuel of respiration of rat kidney cortex. *Biochem. J.* 112: 149–166, 1969.
117. WILSON, T. H. Ionic permeability and osmotic swelling of cells. *Science Wash. DC* 120: 104–105, 1954.
118. WOODHALL, P. B., C. C. TISHER, C. A. SIMONTON, and R. R. ROBINSON. Relationship between para-aminohippurate secretion and cellular morphology in rabbit proximal tubules. *J. Clin. Invest.* 61: 1320–1329, 1978.
119. WRIGHT, S. H., I. KIPPEN, J. R. KLINENBERG, and E. M. WRIGHT. Specificity of the transport system for tricarboxylic acid cycle intermediates in renal brush borders. *J. Membr. Biol.* 57: 73–82, 1980.

VI

Transport of Electrolytes Across Renal Tubules

GERHARD GIEBISCH

ELECTROLYTE TRANSPORT

BY the 1930s a consensus had been reached that the formation of urine by the kidneys could be accounted for by three processes: filtration of a large amount of fluid in the glomerulus under the hydrostatic pressure generated by the heart, reabsorption of variable amounts of fluid and solutes by the epithelium lining the tubules, and secretion of some substances in the opposite direction from peritubular blood into the tubule fluid.

Filtration in the glomerulus had first been proposed in the pioneering studies by Carl F. Ludwig [Fig. 1; (79, 80)], was further championed by Arthur R. Cushny (32) and was finally proven by A. Newton Richards and Joseph T. Wearn when they punctured single amphibian glomeruli and demonstrated by analysis of the fluid collected from single glomeruli that the filtered fluid was an ultrafiltrate (112, 147, 148).

The second process, reabsorption of solutes and fluid from the filtrate, had already been postulated by Ludwig as a necessary consequence of the high rate at which glomerular filtrate was thought to be formed and to explain the very different composition of urine compared to the filtrate.

It took roughly ten years, from the 1920s to the 1930s, for the third process of urine formation, secretion, to become fully accepted. Strangely, such transport in the direction opposite to reabsorption was at first strongly opposed and later only grudgingly accepted after a series of unambiguous experiments by Eli Marshall and Robert Chambers and their associates (see refs. 28, 85–90). The nature of the mechanisms by which reabsorptive and secretory transport occur and by which such transport is modified remained largely elusive. This early period of renal physiology following World War I was

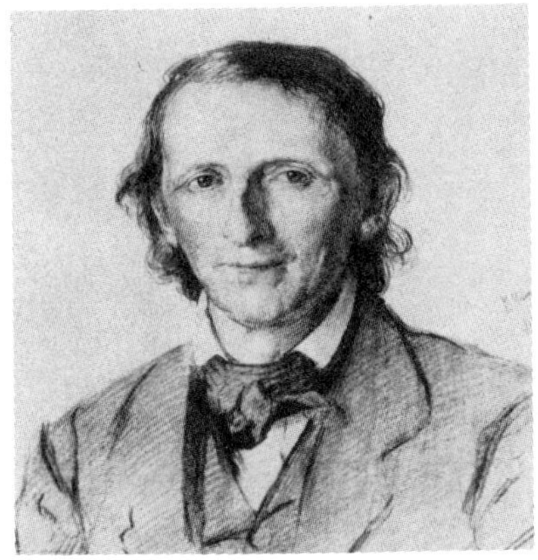

Figure 1. Carl F. Ludwig (1816–1895).

very much concerned with the means to measure filtration rate and to ascertain whether secretion took place. Only later, in the 1930s, did experimentation begin to pinpoint the location of specific transport events within the nephron.

Two developments were particularly important in advancing our understanding of the mechanisms by which solutes and fluid move across the epithelium of renal tubules and by which such transport events are regulated. First, the use of noninvasive clearance techniques allowed the quantitative analysis of the amounts of solutes and fluid filtered, reabsorbed, and secreted. Second, the study of solute and fluid transported in single renal tubules made progress in our understanding of the site and the nature of transport operations possible.

Crucial to the advances in the study of renal fluid and ion transport by noninvasive clearance methods was the introduction by Richards et al. (113), by James A. Shannon (122), and by Shannon and Homer W. Smith (123) of inulin as a substance suitable for measuring filtration rate, although it should be recognized that Poul Brandt-Rehberg's [Fig. 2; (19, 20)] largely intuitive insights on the use of creatinine to obtain a reasonable estimate of glomerular filtration rate preceded the work of Richards and Smith by almost ten years. Brandt-Rehberg, a long-time associate and later the successor of August Krogh in the Zoophysiological Laboratory of Copenhagen, was the first to recognize on theoretical grounds the possibility of measuring glomerular filtration rate by using substances filtered but neither reabsorbed nor secreted. E. Brice C. Mayrs, in Cushny's laboratory, had already drawn attention to the fact that substances such as creatinine and phosphate are highly concentrated in urine and that they are probably only poorly reabsorbed (93). Brandt-Rehberg extended those studies. He chose creatinine clearance as a measure of glomerular filtration rate.

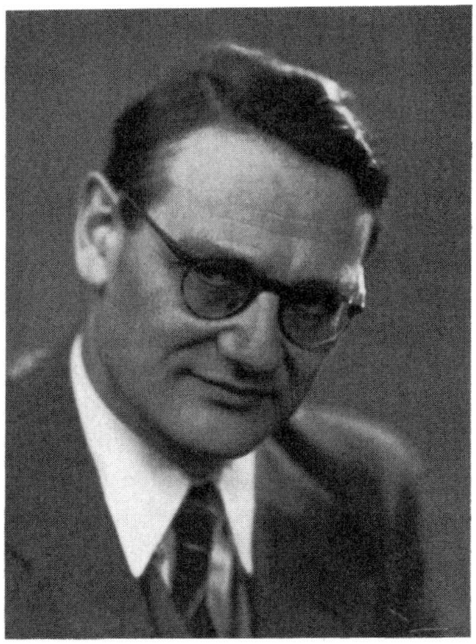

Figure 2. Poul Brandt-Rehberg (1895–1985).

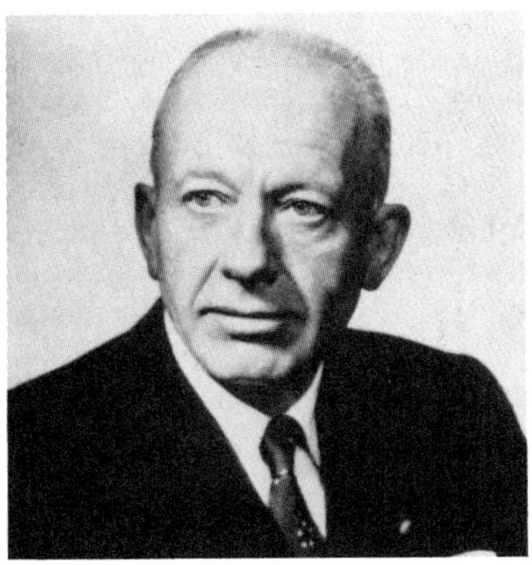

Figure 3. Homer W. Smith (1895–1962).

The development of the flame photometer in the late 1940s was another event that had a profound impact on the direction of research on renal electrolyte transport because it provided a convenient method for the rapid, precise measurement of ions in plasma and urine (6).

It was particularly under the powerful intellectual and personal influence of Homer W. Smith (Fig. 3) and his school in the Physiology Department of the New York University School of Medicine from the 1930s to the early 1960s that clearance methods were introduced to define renal fluid and solute transport in terms of three distinct quantities: filtration at the glomerulus (as measured by inulin clearance), reabsorption (as measured by the difference between amounts filtered and excreted), and secretion (as measured by the difference between amounts excreted and filtered) (125–129). In addition the introduction, again by Smith and his associates, of diodrast and *p*-aminohippurate as substances useful for estimating renal plasma flow broadened the spectrum of tools in renal physiology by making possible the quantitative study of the renal circulation by noninvasive techniques and, in particular, of the effects of hemodynamic changes on water and salt excretion (130). The means thus became available to quantify tubular transport in a wide variety of experimental conditions; to define the effects of experimental manipulations, hormones, and drugs; and to investigate functional disorders in disease states. The ease of study by clearance methods and the possibility of deducing many aspects of renal water and ion transport may have led to the neglect of the powerful but technically much more difficult approach of single-nephron analysis for exploring transport phenomena. Nevertheless the vigorous pursuit of experiments based on the clearance approach provided a firm basis for understanding many key aspects of renal fluid and electrolyte transport. In the United States it was particularly Smith, together with Shannon, Laurence G. Wesson, and W. Parker Anslow, who pioneered the exploration of renal sodium and water transport (127, 153); Robert F. Pitts and Robert S. Alexander at Cornell University, who studied the events underlying renal acidification (107); Robert W. Berliner, Thomas J. Kennedy, and James G. Hilton, first at Columbia and later at the National Institutes of Health, who investigated the renal handling of potassium (9, 10); and Stanley E. Bradley and his co-workers (18) at Columbia University and William Goldring and Herbert Chasis (53) at New York University, who first successfully applied clearance methods to the study of deranged renal function. In Europe François Reubi and his associates at Bern (109) and Claus Brun and his co-workers in Copenhagen (25) also carried out important clearance studies on problems related to hypertension and renal failure.

The pursuit of renal-function studies by the analysis of single-nephron function can be divided into two broad periods. The first period, starting in the early 1920s, was dominated by the towering personality of A. Newton Richards (Fig. 4) in the Pharmacology Department of the University of Pennsylvania. The achievements of Richards and his associates have been well documented (132). The second period started after World War II and led to the rapid development of many new insights into tubule function. Many laboratories started new work on single tubules, and the micropuncture technique has since become a powerful tool that has dramatically broadened our understanding of renal fluid and electrolyte transport.

Richards and Wearn introduced micropuncture in the 1920s, and their first achievement was to prove that the fluid collected from single glomeruli satisfied the filtration theory of Ludwig. The further progress made by Richards, Wearn, Arthur M. Walker, and Phyllis

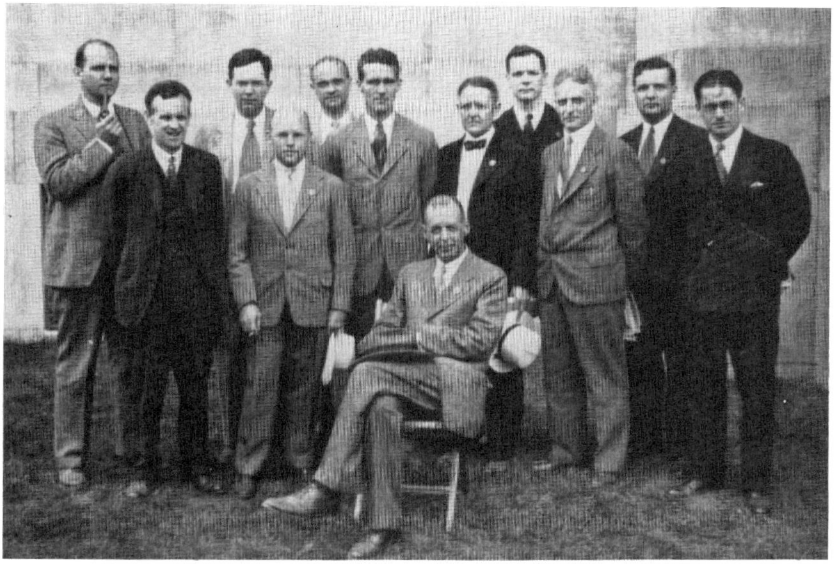

Figure 4. Alfred Newton Richards (seated) and associates in 1929. Standing (*left* to *right*): Walker, Bayliss, Starr, Wearn, Schmidt, Drinker, Plant, Barnwell, Livingston, Hayman, and Florey. [From Starr (132).]

A. Bott during the period from 1925 to 1941 was truly impressive (112). Not only was the ultrafiltrate character of glomerular fluid established beyond reasonable doubt, but painstaking studies on single amphibian tubules also mapped the main sites of transport of a number of solutes. In 1941 these efforts culminated in the landmark paper "The Collection and Analysis of Fluid from Single Nephrons of the Mammalian Kidney," coauthored by Walker, Bott, Jean Oliver, and Muriel C. MacDowell (146; see NOTE in the chapter by Windhager in this volume). Although Richards was not an author of this paper, he can be considered the spiritual father of this important study that represented the culmination of the efforts of his school. The experiments described in the paper dealt not only with the first direct exploration of transport in mammalian nephrons, but it also set the stage for the second phase of single-nephron exploration. By demonstrating the feasibility of studying single mammalian tubules by microtechniques, the way was opened for the extensive study of mammalian nephrons after World War II. The historical development of renal-function studies by micropuncture is the topic of the chapter by Windhager in this volume.

Whereas the early studies of single amphibian and mammalian tubules were largely concerned with the localization of transport events along the nephron, more recent studies have dealt increasingly with mechanisms of electrolyte and fluid transport. In these efforts, renal physiologists received significant stimulation from advances in several areas outside of their own. The definition of active transport as a directly energy-consuming movement of solutes against an electrochemical potential gradient, as contrasted with passive movement along an electrochemical potential gradient (34, 41, 42, 110, 133, 139, 156), led to experiments that specifically addressed this question in single renal tubules. In earlier studies the tubule had been treated as a "black box" without regard to individual cell barriers, and the question of whether a solute moves actively or passively across a specific segment of the whole tubule was asked. With significant advances in microelectrode techniques, including those for measuring cell potentials and ion activities in single tubule cells (15, 44, 50, 137), it became possible to define the electrical properties not only of the tubule as a whole but also of single tubule cells, and it became possible to refine the exploration of transport events by defining the electrochemical driving forces acting on ions as they traverse the apical and basolateral cell membranes. In this connection it is important to stress that the development of the classical two-membrane model of epithelial transport by Valborg Koefoed-Johnsen and Hans H. Ussing (72) also had a profound influence on the study of electrolyte transport in renal tubules. By assigning active- and passive-transport properties to specific cell membranes, it provided a useful conceptual framework for exploring transport phenomena in kidney.

Further refinement of the study of single-nephron function was made possible by a number of other technical advances: the development of techniques for microperfusion of tubules and their peritubular capillaries (137), the introduction of methods for perfusing isolated tubules in vitro (27), the development of highly sensitive methods for analyzing enzyme activities in specified nephron fragments (59, 95, 158), the use of isotopes for measuring permeabilities (100), the development of elemental analysis of single tubule cells by electron-probe analysis (7), and the development of quantitative morphological techniques to correlate transport functions of single tubule cells with ultrastructural alterations (67).

In the following I analyze the evolution of some of the important ideas concerning electrolyte and fluid transport in kidneys since the publication of Cushny's "modern theory" of urine formation in 1917. In this development both clearance and micropuncture experiments were crucial, and only by considering both approaches can we arrive at a full picture of the present state of knowledge of renal electrolyte transport.

Cushny's "Modern Theory"

Arthur R. Cushny (Fig. 5), whose contributions have been amply described (33, 161), holds a unique position in the history of renal physiology. Trained in Aberdeen, Scotland, and doing postgraduate work in Bern and Strasburg, he was appointed at age twenty-seven

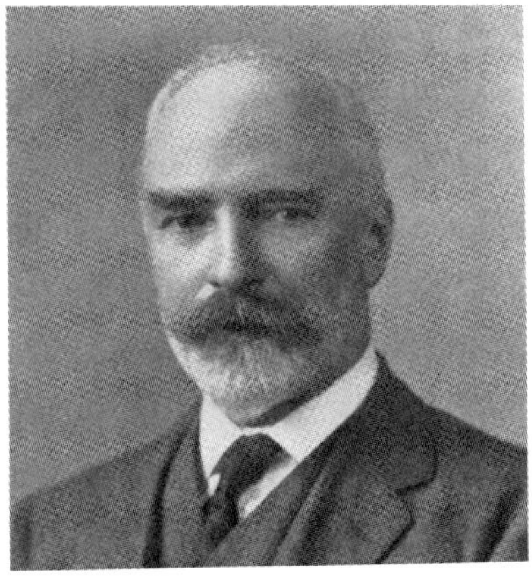

Figure 5. Arthur R. Cushny (1866–1926).

to the Chair of Pharmacology at the University of Michigan in Ann Arbor. His work at that time dealt with important seminal studies on digitalis and cardiac arrhythmias. He returned to England in 1905 and chaired the Department of Pharmacology at University College, London. His career took him back to Scotland in 1918 where he became chairman of Pharmacology at the University of Edinburgh.

Cushny's experimental work on renal function was concerned with the diuretic effect of various anions, particularly chloride, phosphate, and sulfate (32). However, his main contribution was his important monograph on renal function *The Secretion of Urine*. In this book, first published in 1917 and slightly amended in a second edition in 1926, Cushny surveyed the large body of experimental work and proposed a new and quantitative way of thinking in renal physiology. As H. H. Dale put it, Cushny's book brought the then-available evidence dealing with renal function into new focus, and his clear statements and hypotheses on renal function provided for many years the basis for further investigations (33).

Simply stated, Cushny thought that the secretion of urine could be accounted for, in his words, "*by two distinct processes differing not only in site but also in nature. The first of these, the filtration, occurs in the glomerulus, and is purely physical; the second, the reabsorption, occurs in the tubules, and depends on the vital activity of the epithelium.*" He defined the process of filtrate formation very adequately in terms of driving pressures and the characteristics of the glomerular membrane, pointing out that the "osmotic resistance" of the colloids in blood has to be overcome by the blood pressure in the capillaries if filtration is to occur. Clearly his views about glomerular filtration were shown to be correct and they have been amply refined in the years that followed.

Cushny was of course aware that transport activities by the tubules were needed to account for the difference between the compositions of filtrate and urine. He also was aware, for instance, that to explain the excretion of urea by filtration alone, a large volume of filtrate must be formed per minute, and most of the water as well as large fractions of the salts must be reabsorbed during passage through the tubules. To account for such drastic modification of the glomerular filtrate and the selectivity of the reabsorptive process, he proposed that the tubules were endowed with properties to distinguish between "threshold" and "no-threshold" substances. The first group of substances was defined to be taken up by the cells of the tubules and returned to the blood, to be rejected by the tubules and excreted in the urine only when a plasma "threshold" had been reached. "No-threshold" substances, in contrast, were rejected by the tubules at all plasma concentrations and highly concentrated in the final urine by water reabsorption. Cushny clearly recognized the need to endow the tubules with highly discriminatory transport properties, able to return to the blood Locke's fluid, a *"fluid best adapted for the tissues."*

What were the factors thought to be responsible for "regulation" of transport by the tubules? Although Cushny admitted that the absorption of the *"optimal fluid was due to unknown forces and cannot be further analyzed,"* he suggested several factors, among them drugs that increase or decrease the absorbing power of the cells and the presence of unreabsorbable substances that increase the osmotic resistance and impede reabsorption. We note here the nascent idea of osmotic diuresis already expressed and later proven to be essentially correct. Cushny also mentioned that the amount of absorption would depend on and be affected by the time during which the filtrate remained in contact with the cells. Thus, with abundant filtrate formation and rapid fluid passage, absorption by the tubules would be less complete. Although we now consider the effects of "load" on reabsorption more in terms of altered luminal concentrations and solute backflux, washout effects of papillary solutes and the effects of massive osmotic diuresis could be accounted for by Cushny's theory.

It is interesting that Cushny made the suggestion that filtration and reabsorption, although recognized as two independent processes, were nevertheless coordinated by a common blood supply. He proposed that an *"increase in the blood flow through the capsule favors filtration and at the same time increases the blood supply to the tubules and therefore may augment the activity of epithelial cells"* (32). Here is the first mention of glomerulotubular balance, an idea that was later defined by Smith as the increase in sodium chloride and fluid transport by renal tubules in response to an increase in filtration rate and the filtered load of salt and water (127).

There are two aspects of Cushny's "modern theory" that have always caused difficulties. The first is his statement that *"the formation of the glomerular filtrate is due to a blind force, the absorption in the tubules is equally independent of any discrimination, for the fluid is always the same, whatever the needs of the organism at that moment.*" Smith has pointed out that this is a puzzling assertion in view of Cushny's view that the tubules absorb a fluid best adapted for the tissues. Such a process must be subject to regulation and cannot be independent of any discrimination (126, 129).

The second aspect of Cushny's new theory that has not withstood the test of time is his rather strong rejection of secretion by the tubular epithelium. In all fairness, Cushny was aware that it may be necessary to supplement his modern view with secretion by the tubules, but he stated that this possibility should be kept in reserve, to be invoked only if his then-present theory should prove insufficient. It is of interest that even in Cushny's time the view of filtration in glomeruli, reabsorption in tubules, and secretion had already been proposed by Rudolf Metzner (71, 94). This is (as we now know) correct, and Metzner should be given credit for having been one of the first to propose this view.

It is very likely that Cushny's strong support of the view that tubules reabsorb fluid "*independent of any discrimination*" as well as his rejection of secretion had a common cause. Smith pointed out that the early part of this century was a time when quantitative physicochemical principles were progressively applied to biological phenomena and gradually replaced "vitalistic" ideas of cell function (126). He characterized vitalism well: "*multiplicity of function apt to become elastic, even elective, until running riot it would escape from all descriptive rules and become a rule into itself. Such an approach would end in "vitalism," wherein every cell operates in mysterious ways and under its own willful determination to achieve some far-off event.*"

Cushny was strongly influenced by Ernest H. Starling, who had himself advanced the concept of the control of capillary fluid exchange by physical forces — hydrostatic and oncotic pressures. This view influenced Cushny toward accepting Ludwig's thesis of a similar physical process of glomerular filtration (79, 80). Thus it is not surprising that Cushny made every effort to arrive at a "clean," nonvitalistic view of renal function, devoid of murky theories that endowed cells with "vital" forces for performing their functions. However, in the absence of concrete ideas or knowledge of the physical and chemical forces that we now know control transport events, he had to rely on what was then known to be the main driving forces for transport: hydrostatic and colloid oncotic pressures. Ludwig had already faced the same problem when he suggested that reabsorbate was formed by "endosmotic" forces (79, 80). Many years later Cushny realized that selective reabsorption was needed, but not knowing how to account for it by nonvital forces, he remained in an ambiguous position.

His rejection of secretion as one of the functions of the tubules was probably also caused by his strong rejection of vitalism. Rudolph Heidenhain and his associates had proposed secretion as the main function of both glomeruli and tubules (61). Their evidence of tubular secretion was based almost entirely on the presence of dyes that stained lumina and tubule cells, even at a time when blood pressure was too low to sustain glomerular filtration (128). The mechanism of such uptake of dyes was poorly understood and often interpreted as due to the "vital" forces of the cells. Accordingly the process of secretion was suspect to those opposed to vitalism. In hindsight it now seems strange for Cushny to have accepted reabsorption, a "vital" activity of the epithelium, but to exclude secretion by the tubules. However, Cushny's skepticism was certainly a strong challenge to those who thought secretion important. Indeed, evidence supporting the notion of secretion by the tubules was soon forthcoming.

From Cushny's "Modern Theory" to Acceptance of Secretion

As we have seen, Cushny's theory of urine formation had not included secretion as an integrative part, although he had noted the possibility that it might be necessary to supplement his modern view with active secretion.

It was Eli Kennerly Marshall, Jr. (Fig. 6), who provided irrefutable proof of the existence of tubular secretion. He has told well the story of his discoveries in "Two Lectures on Renal Physiology" (88), and two excellent biographical memoirs by Thomas H. Maren on Marshall's activities at Johns Hopkins, where he headed first the Department of Physiology and later the Department of Pharmacology and Experimental Therapeutics, are available (82, 83).

Marshall took as a starting point the fact that the dye phenol red, the rapid urinary excretion of which was the basis of a renal-function

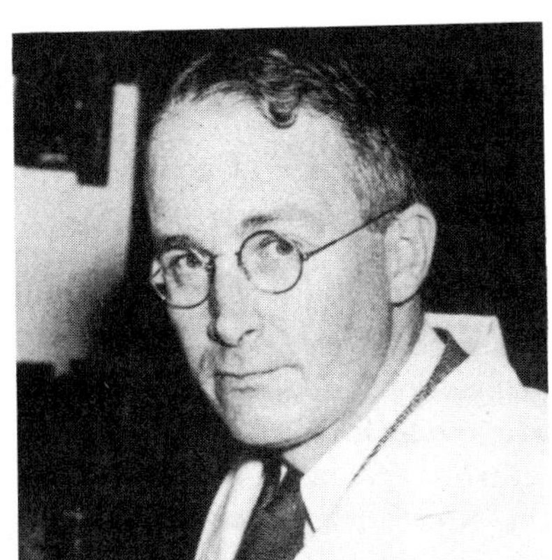

Figure 6. Eli Kennerly Marshall, Jr. (1889–1966).

test introduced by Leonard G. Rowntree (114), was highly concentrated in urine compared to plasma. Phenol red was also accumulated in proximal tubule cells of dogs in which blood pressure had been kept at low levels to abolish glomerular filtration. Most importantly though, Marshall and James L. Vickers showed as early as 1923 that phenol red is tightly bound to blood proteins so that only a small fraction is available for filtration. Given even very generous estimates of filtration rates, Marshall and Vickers could thus demonstrate that the quantity of free and filtrable dye was quite insufficient to account for the relatively high rate of phenol red secretion in kidneys (90). From this observation Marshall and Vickers concluded that secretion must play a role in eliminating substances into the urine.

Marshall's thesis was not immediately accepted (82, 83). A possible weakness—the absence of accurate measurements of glomerular filtration rate to quantify the true amount of phenol red filtered—was circumvented about eight years later by Marshall's demonstration that 70% of phenol red is extracted from the blood perfusing the kidney despite the fact that only about 25% is filtrable (85). Marshall and Marian Crane had earlier provided evidence that secretion must take part in phenol red excretion. They observed, in what might be called one of the first "titration experiments," that urinary excretion rates level off as the level of phenol red is increased, and they remain fairly constant after reaching a maximal value (89). This observation is best explained by filtration of the non-protein bound fraction of phenol red and its secretion, the latter process becoming saturated at high plasma levels of phenol red.

Two earlier but less conclusive bits of evidence had suggested secretion by the renal tubules. First was the observation that aglomerular fish excreted a number of substances including phenol red (85, 87). Clearly, in such fish, urine must be formed by secretion by the tubules. A second observation was that by Chambers, who produced cystlike structures in tissue cultures of chicken kidneys and embryonic human kidneys (28). Phenol red appeared at high concentrations in the lumina of these cysts when it was added to the bathing medium. Interestingly only cysts formed from proximal tubules (not from distal tubules) secreted the dye.

Tubular secretion of uric acid had also been proposed as early as 1924 when Mayrs demonstrated that the quantity of uric acid excreted by chicken kidneys was very much greater than the amount that could have been filtered (91). The argument used to propose urate secretion was the same as that by Marshall: the concentration of uric acid in the blood was much too low to account for the observed excretion rates, given even very high and unrealistic estimates of glomerular filtration rate.

All that was needed for the quantitation of renal transport processes, including secretion, was the introduction of a standard of reference by which filtration rate or (as Smith points out) its corollary, water reabsorption along the tubules, could be reliably measured. It is fair to conclude from these early studies on transport by renal tubules that qualitative evidence for filtration, reabsorption, and secretion was available by the 1930s. However, a quantitative approach to renal transport had to await the introduction of inulin by Richards, Benton B. Westfall, and Bott in 1934 (113) and by Shannon and Smith in 1935 (122, 123).

Early Renal Transport Studies Prior to Inulin

After Marshall's work in the middle 1920s and early 1930s, studies on transport phenomena across renal tubules progressed for several years without the benefit of a precise tool for accurately measuring filtration rate and fluid absorption. Nevertheless a number of advances provided insight into the mechanism of water and salt transport.

A number of interventions were known to inhibit renal transport of electrolytes and fluid. Cushny already had noted that "no-threshold" substances like sulfates and phosphates are not well absorbed by renal tubules. Their rejection by the tubules induces copious urine flows (32). The notion that the osmotic effect of such nonreabsorbable substances induces fluid loss ("catharsis") was thus an early discovery. Similarly the inhibitory action of phlorizin on renal glucose (and fluid and salt) absorption was already well established in the 1920s (92). The diuretic effect of high perfusion pressure in kidneys was also well known at that time (32).

A more biophysical approach to the study of how substances may be transferred into or out of the lumina of renal tubules was that of Rudolf Höber (Fig. 7) and his associates (2). Trained as a general

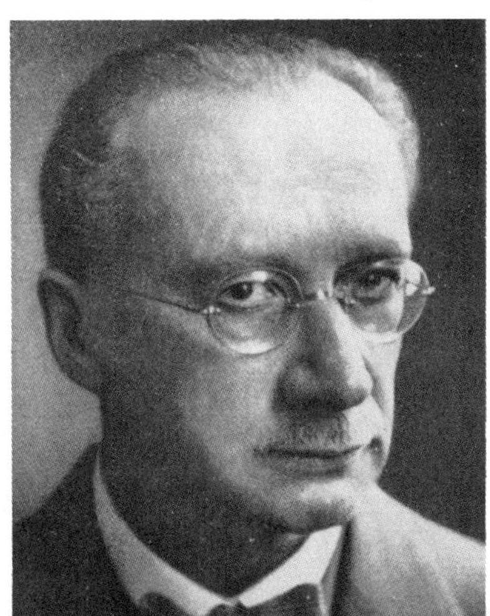

Figure 7. Rudolf Höber (1873–1953).

physiologist with a keen interest in the nature of the biophysics of membrane function, membrane composition, electrical phenomena, and permeability properties, he brought a different outlook to his research that provided novel insights first in Kiel, Germany, where he directed a well-known Department of Physiology from 1915–1933, and later in Philadelphia, where he joined the staff of the Physiology Department of the Medical School of the University of Pennsylvania. The perfused frog kidney preparation had been reintroduced and improved by careful control of the aortic and portal perfusion pressures by Winifred C. Cullis in 1906 (30). Although the functional separation between the two circulations is not absolute, portal fluid does only sparingly reach the glomerular capillaries and aortal perfusion fluid circulates predominantly through glomerular capillaries before mixing with the peritubular blood supply. Using this preparation, Höber was able to examine the effects of ionic substitutions in the aortic and portal fluids and to separate the effects of changes in luminal fluid from those due to changes in the peritubular fluid.

Höber made several discoveries concerning what he called the "unilateral permeability" for chloride ions (63). First he noticed that chloride ions were avidly reabsorbed by the tubules in the perfused kidney so that an almost chloride-free urine was produced. He interpreted these findings as strong evidence for active reabsorption of chloride against a steep concentration gradient. However, when chloride was replaced in the aortic perfusion fluid by sulfate, chloride failed to cross the renal epithelium from the portal perfusion fluid and did not appear in the urine. Höber interpreted these observations correctly by postulating that sulfate (like phosphate and ferrocyanide) is only sparingly permeant. Unable to leave the lumina, its presence prevents chloride entry in exchange for sulfate, rendering the tubules functionally "impermeant" for chloride. We may note that, using the perfused kidney, Höber was one of the first to observe that carbonic anhydrase inhibitors prevent urine acidification.

Höber and his associates extended their studies on perfused frog kidneys to a detailed investigation of dye excretion (65, 66). They observed that, whereas mono or diazo dyes with polar (hydrophilic) character are readily excreted into urine when added to the portal circulation, nonpolar compounds failed to be excreted. They considered the possibility that differences in lipoid solubility might play a role in determining secretion and were able to exclude this as an important factor.

These are the first systematic studies that attempt to establish a structure-function relationship in the analysis of kidney transport processes, taking into account molecular size, chemical structure, and lipoid solubility as possible factors determining transport. Höber deserves credit and recognition for having been one of the first to introduce principles of general and cell physiology and of physical chemistry into renal physiology (64). He demonstrated that principles of diffusion, of apparent active transport, and of permeability can be usefully applied to the study of transport phenomena in kidneys.

Role of Kidney in Maintaining Homeostasis of Body Fluids

Three investigators, Donald Dexter Van Slyke, John P. Peters, and James L. Gamble, have contributed in a major way to our understanding of the role of kidneys in the maintenance of the composition and volume of extracellular fluid. Although they did not primarily address questions and problems related to the mechanisms by which kidneys respond to physiological and pathological stimuli, they helped to develop the methods of studying many biological solutes, and they carefully compared the composition of blood with that of urine so that the central position of the kidney in safeguarding electrolyte and acid-base metabolism became firmly established. They also laid the groundwork for the systematic study of many pathophysiological phenomena, including distortions of the normal pattern of ion composition and abnormalities of the volume and the distribution of body fluids.

Donald Dexter Van Slyke (Fig. 8) had a profound influence on biochemistry and physiology (60). Trained as a chemist (he graduated in 1907 from the University of Michigan), he held the position of chief chemist of the hospital of the Rockefeller Institute in New York.

Van Slyke pioneered the development of many methods for determining the constituents of plasma and other biological fluids. Of his

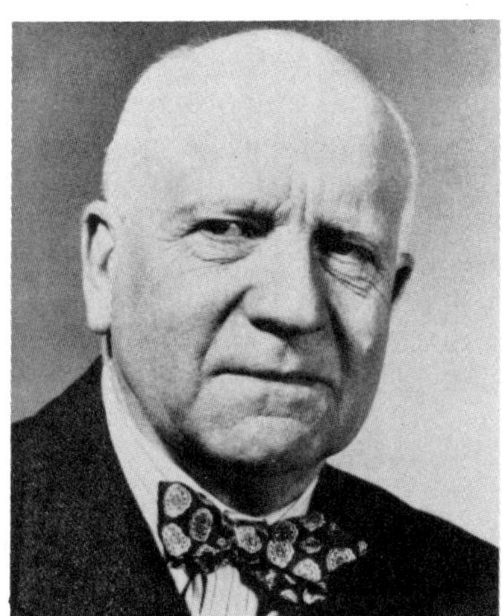

Figure 8. Donald Dexter Van Slyke (1883–1971).

more than three hundred publications, about one hundred are dedicated to the description of methodological advances. To name but a few, Van Slyke's early discovery of gasometric procedures for the measurement of amino acids and urea was followed by a very fundamental physicochemical description of the role of hemoglobin in the transport of oxygen and carbon dioxide, and he provided early and incisive insights into the distribution of anions between plasma and erythrocytes. His contributions to acid-base balance are well known. Van Slyke's contributions also include the design of accurate volumetric and (later) manometric methods for measuring bicarbonate, followed by fundamental and quantitative work on buffers. Defining many basic buffer properties, their interaction with other blood constituents, and their "strength" as defined by the "buffer value," his efforts were crucial to putting the concept of blood and tissue buffering on a sound quantitative basis. In this effort, Franklin C. McLean and Lawrence J. Henderson at Harvard were frequently consulted; this intellectual and noncompetitive exchange between the two laboratories in Boston and New York was most fruitful and productive.

Van Slyke and his associates also devoted considerable efforts to applying their newly developed methods of blood gas and electrolyte analysis to the study of clinical disturbances. Besides establishing the central role of kidneys in urea and ammonium metabolism—it is noteworthy that the study of renal urea excretion led Van Slyke and his colleagues Eggert Møller and John F. McIntosh to introduce the term *urea clearance* in 1928—further work included comprehensive studies of acidosis (twenty-one papers!) and renal failure. Van Slyke's interest in clinical problems also led him to collaborate with his former associate and student John P. Peters to publish a two-volume treatise covering authoritatively what was then known about the chemical methods of analyzing clinical electrolyte derangements (104). This joint venture, entitled *Quantitative Clinical Chemistry*, was immensely successful. The work remained for many years the standard reference of physiologists, biochemists, and clinicians in the area of clinical chemistry. It dealt not only with the physiological and pathophysiological significance of all those compounds in biological fluids for which adequate methods were available, but it also provided a wealth of information on how kidneys respond to changes in plasma composition and body fluid volume. It was also a source of information on electrolyte disturbances in disease. Finally, Van Slyke trained and collaborated with many gifted individuals. His close associations with A. B. Hastings, L. Lundsgaard, A. Hiller, J. Sendroy, J. P. Peters, E. Møller, and J. F. McIntosh were particularly fruitful and productive.

John P. Peters (Fig. 9) worked and spent most of his professional life as the John Slade Ely Professor of Medicine at Yale University in New Haven (103). He was a stimulating and critical internist, who

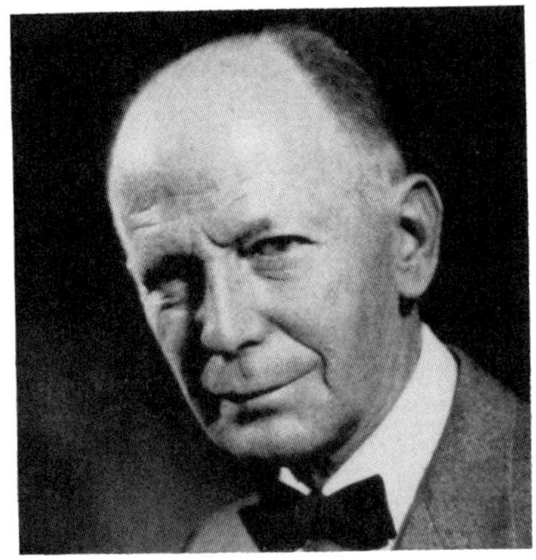

Figure 9. John P. Peters (1887–1955).

maintained throughout his life a profound interest in physiological analysis and interpretation and in biochemical aspects of clinical research, particularly those dealing with abnormalities of electrolyte and acid-base metabolism. His peers and students respected him as an excellent teacher and an inspiring physician.

Peters's bibliography shows a wide interest, and his investigations included studies of electrolyte and water metabolism, of nutritional and endocrine abnormalities, and of renal disease, edema formation, acid-base disorders, and toxemias. From what I have learned from discussions with his former associates, two views of Peters were well known. First, he maintained that as a clinical investigator one ought to study electrolyte and acid-base disturbances in humans. Accordingly he preferred to investigate electrolyte imbalances and renal disturbances in patients, being well aware that such work was harder to do, that experimental settings were more difficult to control, and that interpretations of such work in patients were tenuous. Nevertheless he preferred clinical research to animal experimentation. Second, all who knew him were deeply impressed with how skillfully he applied physiological principles to the study of disease mechanisms. Peters attracted many gifted young investigators. Franklin H. Epstein has well described the special relationship between this outstanding teacher and his students (40). Among them were D. Seldin, L. Welt, T. S. Danowski, P. H. Lavietes, J. Orloff, A. Winkler, and R. J. Elkinton. Their achievements bear witness to Peters's powerful influence.

James L. Gamble [Fig. 10; (see ref. 78)] was a member of the Department of Pediatrics at Harvard Medical School (he was appointed chairman in 1932), and like Peters, he was a physiologically oriented clinician whose insights into fluid and acid-base metabolism left an indelible mark. Trained at Stanford University and at Harvard Medical School, he was drawn to clinical research after an extended

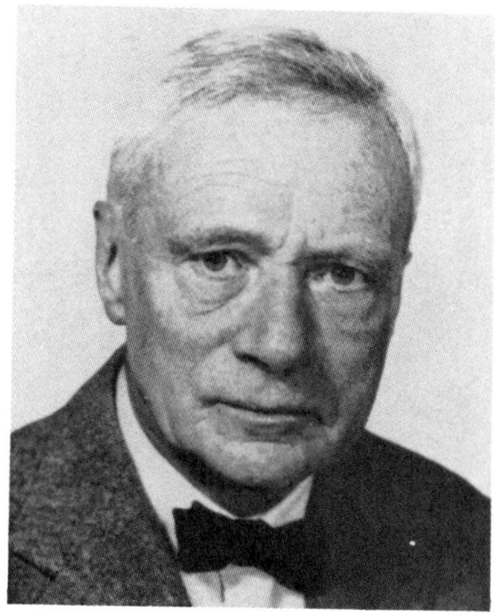

Figure 10. James L. Gamble (1883–1959).

trip to several European Clinics. Robert Loeb has pointed out the lasting influence of Henderson, Professor of Biological Chemistry and Chemistry, in Gamble's career choice and in Gamble's decision to dedicate his life to the study of disease by means of chemistry (78).

Gamble is best known for his extensive analyses of body fluids in terms of their anion and cation composition and for examining not only renal electrolyte patterns but also their relation to shifts of fluid and ions between the main body fluid compartments, the extra- and intracellular fluid (45, 46). Thus he performed extensive balance studies in which the anion and cation compositions of plasma, digestive juices, and urine were correlated. He studied renal adjustments to specific metabolic lesions as they occurred in starvation, dehydration, acid-base abnormalities, and intestinal fluid loss. He drew attention to the fact that both intracellular and extracellular fluid are lost during dehydration, and he noticed that significant urinary potassium loss follows parenteral replacement of intestinal fluid loss with saline-glucose solutions. Gamble's work had significant clinical impact because he emphasized the use of balanced and optimal replacement solutions during the treatment of electrolyte disorders. His work on the unique role of urea in the operation of the urinary concentrating mechanism should also be mentioned. It is discussed in the chapter by Berliner in this volume.

Finally, Gamble also introduced a novel way of presenting and expressing the distribution of electrolytes and fluid in body fluids (45, 46). By juxtaposing anion and cation columns in different body fluid compartments—his "Gamblegrams" are well known to generations of students of electrolyte metabolism—he was able to highlight the quantitative description of basic problems of fluid, acid-

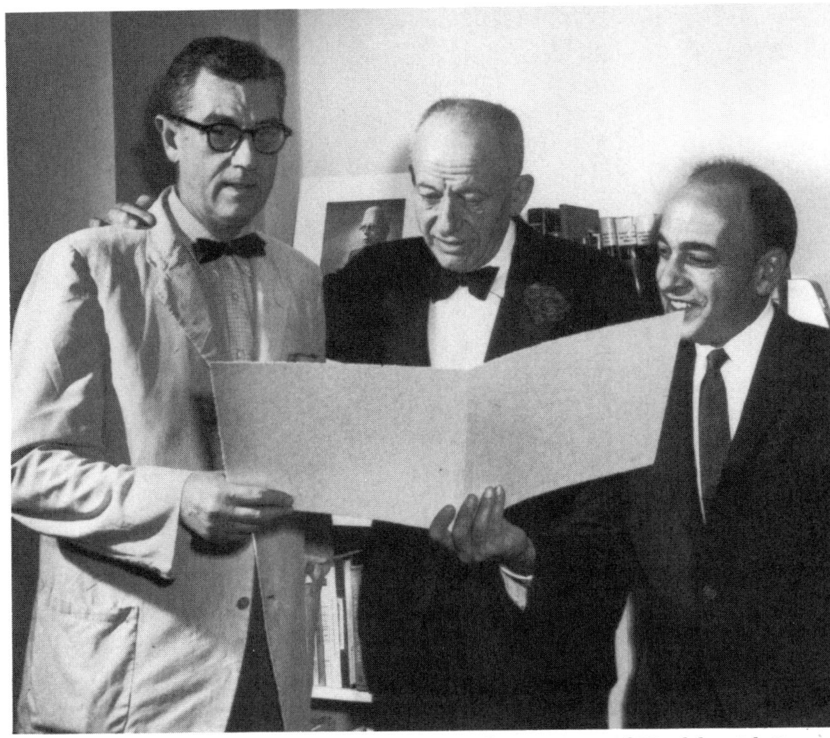

Figure 11. Homer W. Smith at the National Institutes of Health with James A. Shannon (*left*) and Robert W. Berliner (*right*) in 1960.

base, and electrolyte disorders in a didactic manner that has since been generally adopted.

Emergence of Quantitative Methods of Analyzing Renal Electrolyte and Fluid Transport

The introduction of inulin as a reference substance for measuring water movement along the nephron had a powerful impact on renal physiology. With the availability of a reliable tool for the accurate measurement of glomerular filtration rate, methods became available to quantify reabsorption and secretion along the nephron. It has now become possible to approach many questions and problems of renal electrolyte and water transport using quantitative methods. The history of that development has been told well by one of the pioneers in this field, Homer W. Smith (126).

Smith had a major and lasting effect on renal physiology. Pitts, who was a student of Smith's, has written a succinct memoir of him, describing his personal traits and his many contributions to renal physiology (106). I did not know Smith well, and my only memorable encounter with him was on the occasion of a session of the New York Academy of Sciences in 1962, which he chaired. Presenting my first "important" paper, I was probably fortunate that it dealt largely with the electrophysiology of the tubule, not a topic of particular interest to Smith, thus sparing me the type of scrutiny that my less fortunate colleagues of that session did not escape. The presence of the grand old man of renal physiology did not contribute to my tranquility during my presentation.

Those who knew Smith well were deeply impressed by his thorough commitment to renal physiology and his devotion to relentless and logical reasoning, which was apparent during the analysis of data and the design of experiments. He also wrote exceedingly well, and his papers are models of clarity and style.

The beginning of quantitative renal physiology was very much influenced by Smith and his associates. Clearance studies by Smith and his colleagues Wesson and Anslow, by Pitts, and by Berliner, with their associates, laid the groundwork for the body of knowledge of the renal transport of sodium chloride and water, of bicarbonate and acid, and of potassium. However, it should be kept in mind that the evidence then obtained by clearance methods—largely in the late 1940s and throughout the 1950s—was interpreted against the background information provided by the one paper on micropuncture of the mammalian nephron by Walker and his associates (146), which made possible a reasonable account of transport operations in the kidney, including quantitative estimates of electrolyte and fluid movement across individual segments of the nephron.

Figure 12 summarizes the generally accepted views on sodium and fluid transport along the mammalian nephron, as suggested by

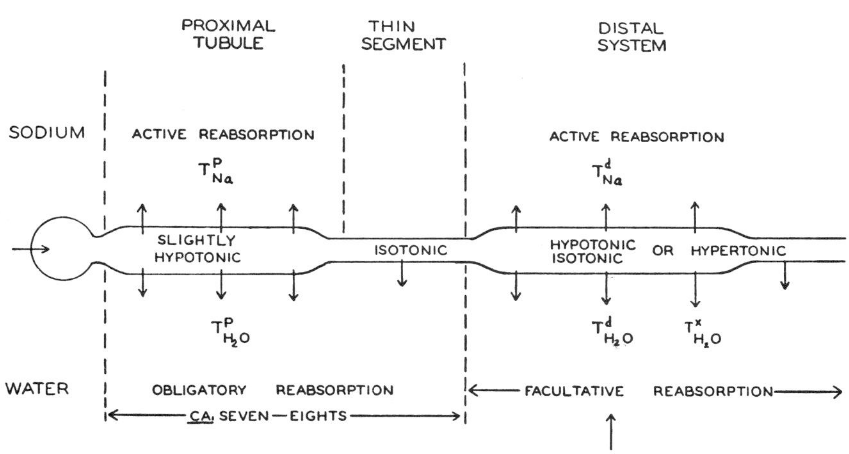

Figure 12. Schematic representation of sodium and water reabsorption. T^p_{Na} and $T^p_{H_2O}$, reabsorption of sodium and water across the proximal tubule epithelium; T^d_{Na} and $T^d_{H_2O}$, reabsorption of sodium and water across the distal tubule; $T^x_{H_2O}$, moiety of water reabsorbed to form an osmotically concentrated urine. [From Smith (125).]

Smith, Wesson, and Anslow in the early 1950s (127, 149, 153), well before the resurgence of micropuncture studies in the later 1950s. Reabsorption of sodium was conceived as taking place in at least two steps. Isosmotic reabsorption in the proximal tubule of about four-fifths of the filtered load was thought to occur by an active process because proximal sodium and water reabsorption are reduced when poorly reabsorbable solutes in the lumina produce a gradient of sodium concentration across the epithelium. The process of proximal salt and fluid transport was viewed as an "obligatory" process, normally destined to retrieve the bulk of the filtrate and not subject to any significant physiological control.

By contrast the distal tubule was seen as a site at which steep concentration gradients could be generated until all but very small amounts of sodium had been reabsorbed from the tubule fluid. Only about one-eighth of the filtrate was thought to be available for distal reabsorption, which was thought to be saturable and intrinsically limited in its capacity. Finally, the distal tubule was thought to be the main site at which sodium reabsorption was susceptible to hormonal control, particularly to adrenal steroids and pituitary hormones. Endowed with considerable flexibility, transport along the distal tubule was thought of as a "facultative" transport process.

We note in passing that the thin segment of Henle's loop was assigned the role of osmotic equilibration, permitting a slightly hypotonic proximal tubule fluid to become isotonic. We now know that this view was wrong and that this segment of the nephron is critically involved in the elaboration of an osmotically concentrated urine (56).

What were the critical experiments that led to the development of Smith's concept of sodium and fluid transport along the nephron? Evidence was already available from micropuncture experiments that proximal tubule fluid was always nearly isosmotic with plasma and that about 80% of the fluid was reabsorbed in this segment (146). This important information, summarized in Figures 13 and 14, was extrapolated to almost all clearance studies, and these micropuncture data provided a convenient subdivision into proximal and distal events. Whenever, in clearance studies, fluid and electrolyte excretion exceeded that fraction of the filtrate thought to be reabsorbed in the distal tubule, a proximal site of involvement was assumed.

Complementary evidence for an unequal distribution of transport between proximal and distal nephron sites was also provided by Wesson and Anslow, who studied sodium chloride and water excretion during extreme osmotic diuresis (151). Massive loading with mannitol, a poorly reabsorbable sugar, led to the excretion of an almost isotonic urine involving large fractions of water (67%) and of sodium (25%). They argued that, under conditions of such massive urine flow, changes in composition of fluid along the distal tubule

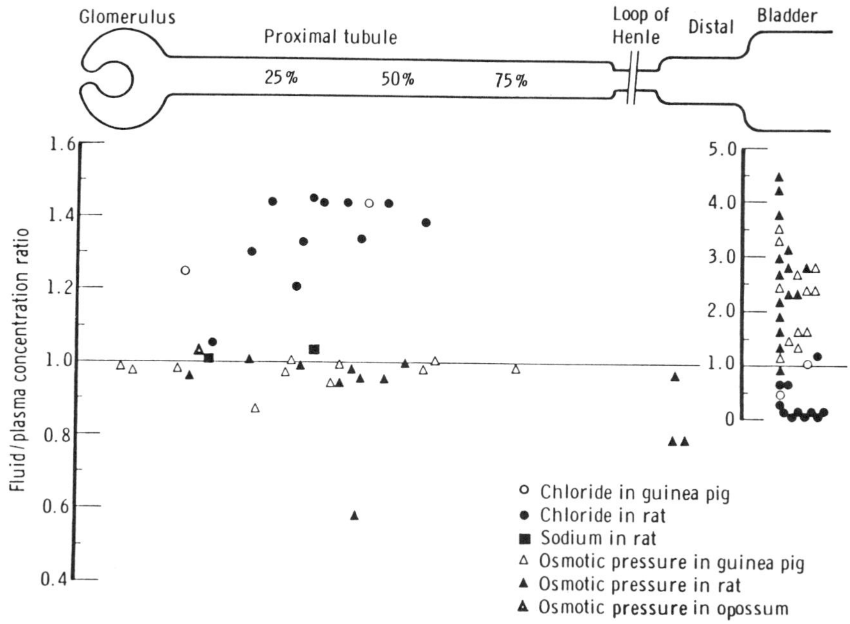

Figure 13. Sodium, chloride, and osmotic concentrations in proximal tubule fluid in rats, guinea pigs, and opossums. Osmotic pressure measurements of the early distal segment and of bladder urine are included. [From Wesson (149) based on data in ref. 146.]

were minor and that the composition of the final urine approached that at the end of the thin limb. Because the concentration gradient of sodium between urine and plasma was sizable, about 60–90 mM, it was argued that movement between tubule fluid and plasma was active in nature.

For many years, the distinction of whether a process was proximal or distal depended on the size of the response. If some intervention led to excretion of an amount of fluid in excess of that assigned to the distal diluting segment, it involved inhibition of proximal transport. If it was smaller, it was thought most likely to be a distal effect, although some mix between proximal and distal effects could never be excluded.

This general schema of topography of salt and fluid reabsorption, persuasively advanced by Smith, Laurence G. Wesson (Fig. 15, *left*), and W. Parker Anslow (Fig. 15, *right*), was generally accepted, and many of its features have been shown to be correct. Several modifications, though, were necessary. We now know that during osmotic diuresis the distal tubule does modify the composition of the fluid emerging from Henle's loop so that the final urine does not precisely represent the fluid emerging from the proximal tubule (158). Also, it is now well established that the function of the loop of Henle is to

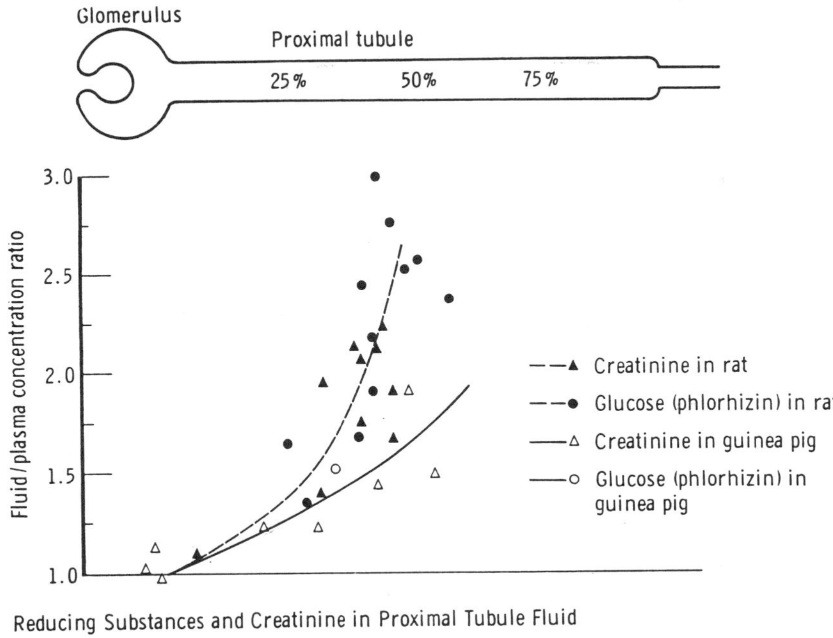

Figure 14. Fluid-plasma concentration ratios of creatinine and of glucose after phlorizin in the proximal tubule of rats and guinea pigs. Extensive water absorption is apparent. [(From Wesson (149) based on data in ref. 146.]

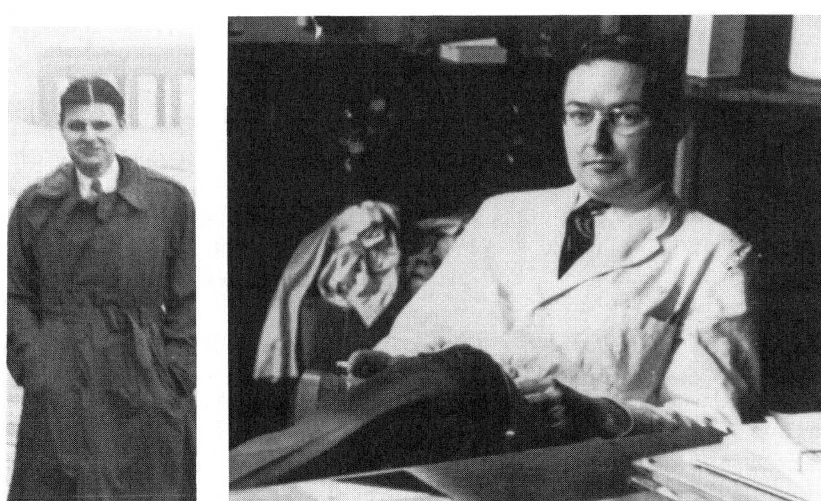

Figure 15. Laurence G. Wesson (b. 1917) (*left*) and W. Parker Anslow, Jr., (1912–1966) (*right*).

dilute the urine, thus having properties other than just allowing osmotic equilibration (56). Nevertheless, given the paucity of direct information on tubular transport and reliance on a good deal of speculation, one is impressed by the intuitive acumen and the insight of this first post-Cushny theory of renal salt and water transport.

Refinements of Original Model of Salt and Fluid Transport

The quantity of sodium chloride that appears in urine is part of the filtered load that escapes reabsorption by the tubules. One of the first questions that attracted attention was whether changes in filtration rate, (i.e., in the filtered load) or changes in reabsorption by the tubules were responsible for the changes in urinary salt excretion that occurred in physiological and pathophysiological settings (150). Resolution of this problem has proved to be difficult.

The problem may be stated briefly in the following way. Given the very large quantities of salt and fluid filtered, only a very small fraction of the filtered sodium chloride normally escapes reabsorption. Accordingly very minor changes in the sodium chloride load, if reabsorption remains more or less constant, could account for very significant relative changes in excretion. Also, because filtration rate cannot be measured very accurately, it becomes difficult to exclude changes in filtered load sufficient to account for a given change in excretion, were reabsorption to be unchanged. This problem has generated a voluminous literature and was reviewed by Wesson (150).

Despite these difficulties, it became apparent that sodium reabsorption by the renal tubules was variable and characterized by impressive adaptability. One of the first to demonstrate such a phenomenon were Wesson and Anslow and their co-workers (151). Important aspects of their experiment are shown in Figure 16. The data were obtained during volume expansion of the extracellular fluid, with solutions carefully prepared to minimize disturbances of the normal plasma composition. From inulin and from plasma and urine sodium determinations, a careful comparison of the filtered sodium load with the excretion rate showed that overall sodium reabsorption could change independently of the filtered sodium load, as seen from the increased reabsorption rates at points of equal filtration.

These experiments were later expanded and clarified by excluding ambiguous changes in filtration rate. The most convincing strategy has been to lower filtration rate artificially during maneuvers designed to increase the excretion of sodium (35). Such a situation simplifies the problem, and in many experimental settings it was possible to provide clearcut evidence for independent changes in the rate at which sodium chloride was reabsorbed. Again, it should be realized that such results do not preclude that a decreased

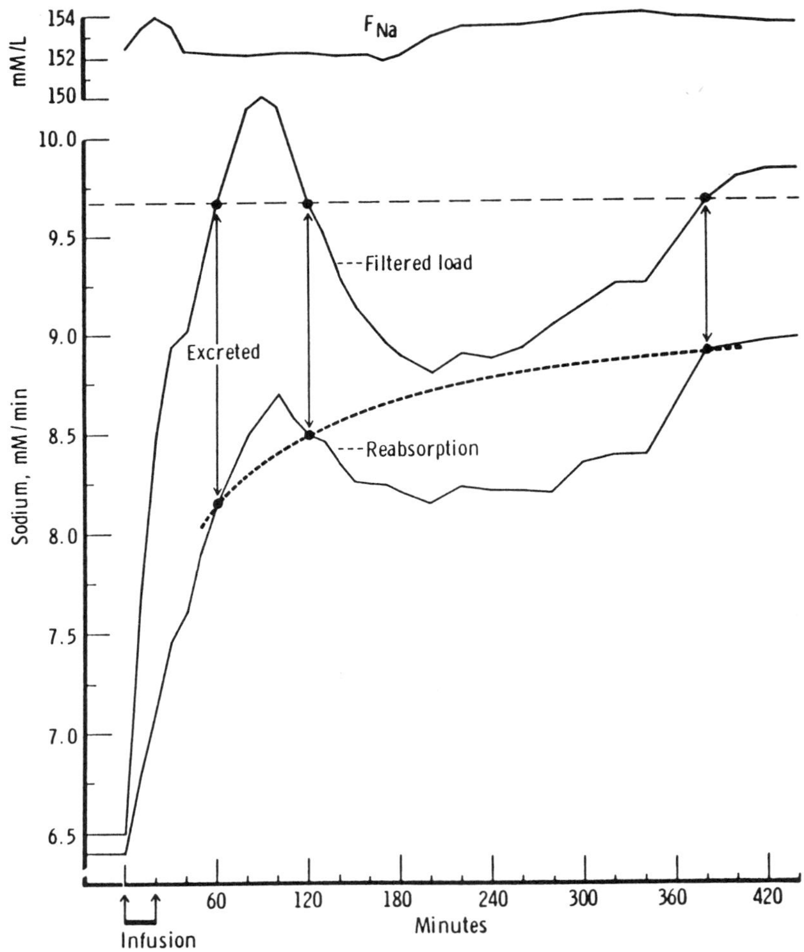

Figure 16. Filtration, excretion, and reabsorption of sodium in unanaesthetized dogs after acute expansion of extracellular fluid by balanced saline solution. Heavy broken line connects points of equal filtration rate. Rising rate of reabsorption is apparent. [From Wesson et al. (152).]

filtration rate, had it occurred, could not have additional effects on sodium handling by the kidneys.

The possibility of measuring changes in sodium chloride reabsorption by the renal tubules with some accuracy generated a large body of literature (see refs. 127, 149, 150). Studies dealt with the effects of infusions of ions other than sodium chloride, of diuretics and adrenocortical steroids, renal nerve stimulation, and the action of sympathomimetic amines and pituitary hormones. The introduction of clearance methods also provided, for the first time, a firm basis for defining glomerular and tubular contributions to altered salt excretion occurring during salt deprivation and salt excess, during changes in posture, and (last but not least) in disease models and clinical situations of abnormal salt retention and salt loss.

Involvement of Sodium in Ion-Exchange Mechanisms

ELECTROLYTE TRANSPORT

Two further developments significantly advanced our state of knowledge of transport events in kidney. Based on a series of clearance experiments, strong evidence became available that sodium ions are not only reabsorbed with chloride as the counterion but that sodium ions during reabsorption also are exchanged for other cations, notably hydrogen and potassium.

The exchange of sodium for hydrogen ions, first postulated by Smith as early as 1937 (125), was put on a firm experimental basis by Robert F. Pitts (Fig. 17) and his associates. Pitts's career was remarkable because he had already made important contributions to physiology as a very young investigator before embarking on the study of urine acidification. In a series of experiments in Stephen W. Ransom and Horace W. Magoun's laboratory in Chicago, at that time one of the most active and innovative centers of central nervous system physiology, Pitts had played a key role in defining, by stereotaxic exploration, the role of pontine, medullary, and spinal substrates for respiratory rhythmicity (107). Having received his doctorate at Hopkins and first having been trained as a neurophysiologist, he later joined Smith's laboratory at the New York University School of Medicine. Recruited as an assistant professor, he worked for a doctorate in medicine while teaching and redirecting his research toward renal physiology. He did his second series of "classical" experiments at Syracuse and at Cornell University Medical College; at both of these institutions he headed respected physiology departments.

The development of the ideas that led Pitts to consider that hydrogen ions are not secreted by the renal tubules with anions but

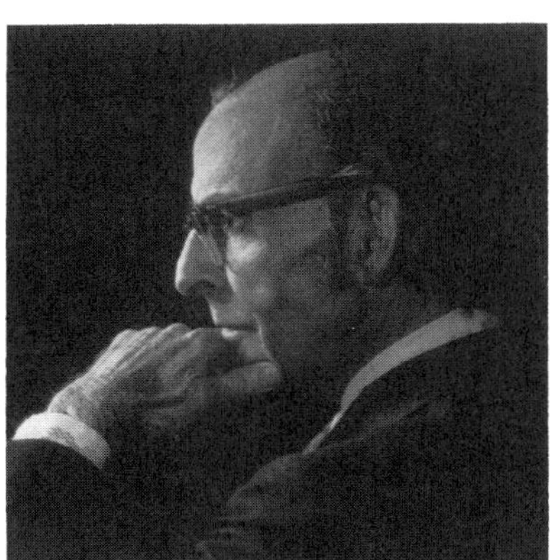

Figure 17. Robert F. Pitts (1908–1977).

are secreted in exchange for a portion of the filtered sodium moiety is described in detail in the chapter by Rector in this volume. For the somewhat humorous and bizarre aspects of Pitts's first paper (with Robert S. Alexander) "The Nature of the Renal Tubular Mechanism for Acidifying the Urine" (107), the reader may consult Alexander's account of the background that led to these experiments. So firmly was Pitts convinced of the outcome of the studies that he wrote the complete paper, minus only the data, prior to the execution of the experiments (1). It was submitted and accepted without change. Based on the observation that the selective reabsorption of filtered alkaline buffers during forced acidification cannot account for the amount of hydrogen ions excreted, Pitts and Alexander correctly concluded that sodium ions must exchange for hydrogen ions and that sodium reabsorption is intimately involved in the renal regulation of acid-base metabolism.

At the same time that sodium ions were implicated in the secretion of hydrogen ions, clearance experiments by Berliner and his associates Kennedy and Hilton demonstrated that sodium ions also exchange for potassium (9, 10). These investigators pioneered the field of renal potassium handling, providing not only data on the mode of renal potassium transport but also presenting a cell model that accounts for the relationship between potassium-, sodium-, and hydrogen-ion translocation across individual cell membranes of tubule cells (8).

Robert W. Berliner (101), after receiving his medical doctorate from Columbia Medical School, worked at Goldwater Memorial Hospital for about eight years before moving to the National Institutes of Health in Bethesda, where he became chief of the Laboratory of Kidney and Electrolyte Metabolism in 1950. He stayed at the National Institutes of Health until 1973. Most of his work on renal potassium transport was done in collaboration with Tom Kennedy and Jack Orloff.

Sporadic evidence had already been available that potassium ions could be secreted by renal tubules, particularly in pathophysiological conditions when filtrate formation, and with it the filtered load of potassium, was abnormally low. However, the physiological role of such sporadically demonstrated net potassium secretion remained at first obscure.

The main contributions of Berliner and his colleagues were *1*) the demonstration that potassium secretion can regularly be induced by potassium loading in the nondiseased kidney, a finding almost simultaneously also reported by Gilbert Mudge and his associates (97); *2*) the important proposal that secretion of potassium is the process responsible for potassium excretion, even under conditions when the amount of potassium in the final urine is only a relatively small fraction (10%–20%) of the filtered potassium load; and *3*) the fact that potassium ions are secreted in exchange for sodium, a cation-exchange process shown to be sensitive to alterations in acid-base balance (8).

The evidence for the potential of kidneys for secreting potassium ions was straightforward: potassium excretion in excess of filtered potassium. That potassium secretion, and not incomplete reabsorption, is responsible for urinary excretion was deduced from the relative constancy of potassium excretion during changes in the filtered load of potassium. This feature of potassium excretion is strikingly different from the exquisite sensitivity of sodium excretion after a fall in the filtered sodium load. Finally, Berliner and his associates also provided convincing evidence that potassium ions are secreted not with anions moving in the same direction but by an exchange process involving sodium. The crucial experiment here showed that large changes in urinary potassium excretion can be induced at a time when nonreabsorbable anions make up most of the urinary anion load and chloride excretion remains unchanged.

The impact of Pitts and Berliner's ideas was striking. I recall the sense of excitement and the anticipation of new developments when I joined the Department of Physiology at Cornell in 1952. Based on the cell models of Pitts and Berliner, cell models that described the transport of sodium, hydrogen, and potassium in terms of specific and interrelated transport processes, it now became possible to design experiments directed towards replacing the empirical "black-box" approach, in which the epithelium of the renal tubule was lumped into one barrier, with cell models in which individual transport events were assigned to specific cell membranes. In retrospect it is interesting how much was deduced from rather indirect experimentation on whole kidney without knowledge of such transport parameters as tubular permeability, driving forces acting on ions across individual transport barriers, or the role of specific active ion pumps in the translocation of individual ions.

The state of the art of this period of renal research dealing with problems of fluid and electrolyte transport largely based on clearance experimentation is well represented in the series of Annual Conferences on Renal Function, held from 1949 to 1953 under the auspices of the Josiah Macy, Jr., Foundation (17), chaired by Pitts and edited by Bradley. These sessions, including extensive discussions by the then-leading experts in the field, provide an excellent insight into the scope of problems, into the great ingenuity of deduction, and into the intuitive and speculative acumen typical of that period of renal research. Careful reading of these conference reports also make it clear that the largely indirect approach of clearance methods to the study of electrolyte transport by renal tubules had its limitation. Clearance experimentation attempted to analyze the nature of specific transport events at specific tubule sites by comparing urinary composition and urinary excretion rates with the composition of solutes in plasma and the rate of their filtration in the glomerulus.

Because they provided information only on the integrated function of many nephron segments with distinctly different functions in series, these studies were often inadequate to directly address questions of transport by the cells of specific tubule segments. Deductive yet indirect reasoning had reached a peak. In order to proceed further, renal research explored and focused on new directions and new methods. New concepts of epithelial transport developed in isolated epithelia also provided a powerful stimulus. This coincided with a renaissance of interest in studying renal transport functions at the single-nephron level.

Impact of the Ussing–Koefoed-Johnsen Model of Salt Transport

In 1958 Koefoed-Johnsen and Ussing published their model of ion transport across frog skin epithelium (72). The work of Hans H. Ussing (Fig. 18) has had great significance for investigators of epithelial and renal electrolyte transport. Trained initially as a marine biologist in Krogh's Zoophysiological Laboratory where he obtained a research professorship in 1951 (Ussing became chairman of the Institute of Biological Chemistry in 1960), he was throughout his career critically involved in advancing the field of ion transport. Early engagement with tracers introduced him to these powerful tools for the study of unidirectional ion movement. He was instrumental in tracer studies of active and passive transport, involved early in seminal studies of sodium exchange diffusion in muscle, and soon focused on detailed studies of ion movement in isolated frog skin, a preparation to which he remained loyal all his life. Krogh had previously shown that frogs take up sodium chloride from very dilute solutions, a phenomenon that lent itself favorably to the study of transport phenomena. Ussing's work, which he summarized well (140), included several incisive discoveries. He was instrumental in

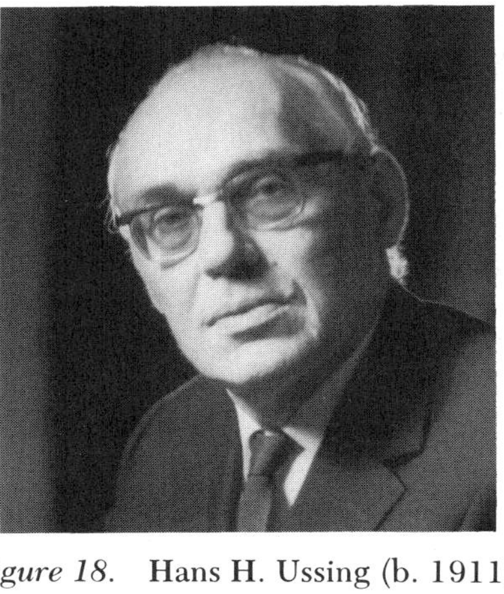

Figure 18. Hans H. Ussing (b. 1911).

describing the flux-ratio equation as a means of distinguishing active and passive transport; he introduced the measurement of the short-circuit current as a means of defining active ion transport; he explored the coupling between solute and solvents and described solvent drag; and in studying the role of active sodium transport, he conceived and produced the two-membrane model for frog skin ion transport. The concepts developed by Ussing and his associates have provided a firm conceptual basis for the study of ion transport, and all of those concerned with exploring ion and fluid movement across renal tubules owe much to his efforts (141).

Ussing and Koefoed-Johnsen's cell model is shown in Figure 19; it incorporates the basic transport mechanisms found in epithelial cells endowed with the ability of vectorial net transport of solutes. Including the same transport mechanisms found in nonpolar cells, namely, active ATP-driven sodium-potassium exchange and passive leak pathways for sodium and potassium, it achieves two important functions of epithelial cells: maintenance of optimal sodium and potassium concentrations and vectorial sodium transport. This is achieved by the strategic placement of active- and passive-transport components into the two cell membranes: the outside ("pond side") and inside ("blood side") of the epithelial cell. Whereas the outside cell membrane is highly permeable to sodium (sodium selective), the

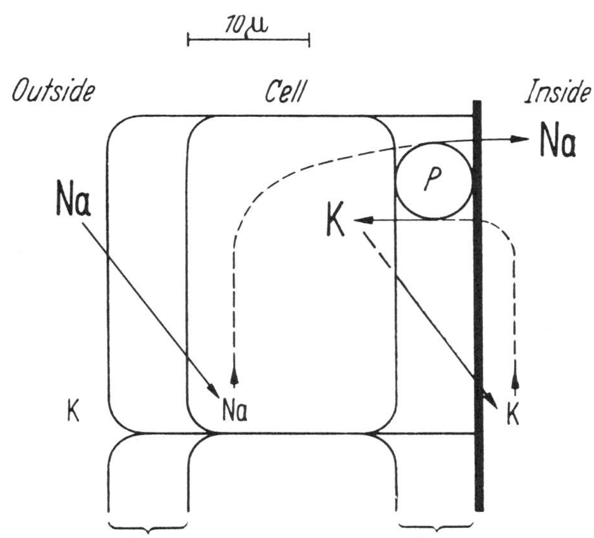

Figure 19. Diagrammatic representation of movements of cations across the outer cell membrane (O.c.m.) and inner cell membrane (I.c.m.) of an epithelial cell. Oblique arrows, passive and highly selective diffusion; P, "pump" with exchange of Na^+ for K^+. Size and level of chemical symbols indicate concentration levels of cations. [From Koefoed-Johnsen and Ussing (72).]

inside membrane is the site of active sodium-potassium exchange (the "sodium pump") and has a high permeability to potassium (potassium selective). The model of the cell accounts satisfactorily for a high potassium and low sodium concentration in the cell, a net sodium transport from the outside to the inside, and a transepithelial difference in electrical potential that is the sum of two diffusion potentials in series: one generated by the sodium selectivity and the appropriate gradient of sodium concentration across the outside membrane and the other similarly generated by the appropriate gradient of potassium concentration across the inner membrane of the cell.

With only three modifications, the two-barrier model of epithelial transport of Ussing and Koefoed-Johnsen accounts for most basic aspects of renal sodium and potassium transport.

First, the entry of sodium ions through the apical membrane is accomplished in tubule cells by a number of co- and countertransport mechanisms (26, 51, 116, 136, 145). Such coupled carrier-mediated transport processes link the energy of the sodium gradient across the apical membrane to the movement of other solutes such as glucose, amino acids, phosphate, and mono- and dicarboxylic acids in the same direction, a process that ultimately achieves the movement of the nontransported solute against a difference of electrochemical potential. Similarly, "downhill" sodium movement across the apical membrane can also be coupled to the movement of hydrogen ions in the opposite direction. Such sodium-hydrogen exchange accounts for acidification of tubule fluid in the proximal nephron.

Sodium movement across the apical membrane of tubule cells can also be coupled to the movement of two other ions in the same direction. Electroneutral transport of sodium with potassium and two chloride ions has been described in some segments of the tubule (58, 99).

Second, in the original model shown in Figure 20, the apical membrane is permeable only to sodium ions. This limits net solute movement to sodium, restricting potassium transport exclusively to recycling across the inside (antiluminal) membrane. In the kidney, however, the apical membrane of cells of the distal nephron have, in addition to a sodium permeability, a significant and variable permeability to potassium. This property endows this segment of the nephron with the capacity to secrete potassium ions into the lumen (164).

Third, in the original Ussing–Koefoed-Johnsen model (Fig. 19), net sodium transport was entirely transcellular. In expanding the original cell model, Ussing and Erich E. Windhager later included an additional, parallel pathway for ion movement, an intercellular shunt pathway that allows passive ion transport between cells (141). Such an extracellular transport route is also present in the renal tubule, particularly in the proximal tubule where the shunt pathway between cells is responsible for the significant "leakiness" to ions of this segment of the nephron (14, 16, 26, 44, 49, 51).

Return to the Nephron: the Second Era of Transport Studies on Single Renal Tubules

In the 1950s a return to micropuncture techniques set the stage for important progress in renal transport physiology. As is so often the case, the success of this period of renal research was due to the opportune coincidence of new conceptual and methodological advances.

As mentioned previously, novel concepts of the functional organization of epithelia provided a challenge to renal physiologists to apply to the kidney the new insights gleaned from the exploration of transport phenomena in "simple" flat epithelia. Thus the early work of Ussing, Huf, Leaf, Orloff, Edelman, and their associates on isolated amphibian epithelia and that of Crane, Curran, Solomon, Schultz, Dietschy, and their colleagues on intestinal epithelia in vitro was concerned with extensive and detailed explorations of transport phenomena, using such new approaches as short-circuit measurements and tracer flux analyses to study permeability and electrical potential and using resistance measurements to gain insight into the driving forces and paths of transport of individual ions.

The challenge posed by these studies on isolated epithelia was to develop renal preparations that allowed a degree of experimental control similar to that achieved in flat epithelia in vitro. The improvement of micropuncture techniques and the evolution of microperfusion techniques, first in vivo and later including the isolation of single tubules and their perfusion in vitro, can be seen as efforts to achieve this aim. The exploration of transport phenomena on single renal tubules was also substantially aided by many methodological advances, among them the development of new methods to measure substances in nanoliter samples, the introduction of tracers, and new electrophysiological techniques that had their origin in neurophysiology.

Localization of Transport Processes Along the Nephron

It may be recalled that the first micropuncture study of Walker, Bott, Oliver, and MacDowell was almost exclusively concerned with measurements of fluid movement, of osmolality, and of chloride concentrations in the proximal tubule (146). Beginning with the micropuncture studies of Heinrich A. Wirz and Bott (163); Bott (13); Carl Gottschalk, William Lassiter, and Margaret Mylle (54, 55); Windhager and Gerhard Giebisch (158); Karl Ullrich, Bodil Schmidt-Nielsen, Gottschalk, Lassiter, and Mylle (138); Claude P. Lechène et al. (76); Gerhard Malnic, Ruth M. Klose, and Giebisch (81); and

John Dirks, James R. Clapp, and Berliner (38), a systematic exploration of the sites within the nephron at which solutes are reabsorbed and secreted was undertaken. It was confirmed that the proximal convoluted tubule is the site of extensive isosmotic retrieval of most of the filtrate, that the loop of Henle elaborates a hypotonic fluid, and that the distal nephron is the site at which further fine tuning of sodium excretion and extensive potassium secretion takes place. Additional studies on solutes such as calcium (75), phosphate (134), urea (74), bicarbonate (56), and ammonium (52) followed. This first phase of new micropuncture studies provided detailed and new information on the segmental localization of transport along the nephron.

The application of these micropuncture techniques in vivo provided information only on those tubule segments that could be approached from the surface, being thus limited to portions of the proximal and distal tubule and portions of the structures at the very tip of exposed renal papillae.

With the introduction of the method of isolating and perfusing single renal tubules in vitro, ion transport could also be studied in subcortical segments of the loop of Henle as well as in cortical and medullary collecting ducts (27). The combination of micropuncture studies in vivo and of microperfusion studies in vitro has by now provided extensive and detailed mapping of solute transport along the nephron, including the localization of hormone actions, of the effects of various drugs and diuretics, and of the pathophysiological modifications of transport in models of kidney disease. The amount of information gained in the last twenty-five years on the localization and magnitude of reabsorptive and secretory transport along the nephron is impressive. It has provided the basic information needed for the study of the cellular mechanisms of solute and fluid transport across the nephron.

Exploration of Transport Mechanisms in Single Renal Tubules

Active Versus Passive Transport

One of the first problems addressed was that of deciding whether active transport is involved in the movement of specific solutes across the tubule. Given the definition of active transport as the energy-consuming movement of a solute against an electrochemical potential gradient (139), it became possible to test directly where active transport takes place.

Two methods in particular found widespread application. One was the quantitative measurement of net solute movement, either by micropuncture or microperfusion methods, at the same time that both the transepithelial concentration and electrical-potential differ-

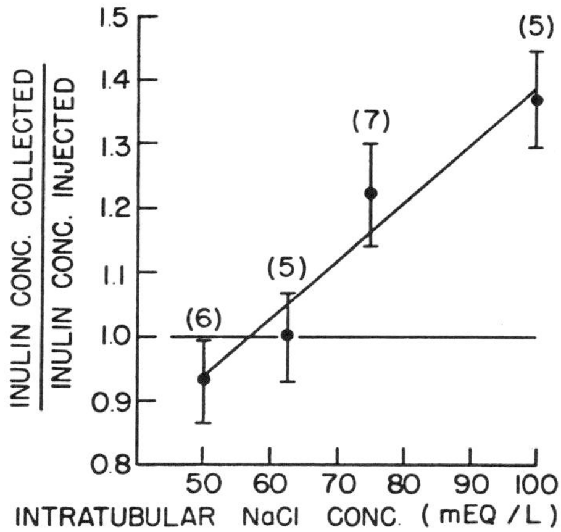

Figure 20. Water absorption as a function of intratubular NaCl concentration. Results are from stationary microperfusion experiments in which mannitol was used to maintain isosmotic conditions. Water movement was measured by changes in inulin concentration. [From Windhager et al. (160).]

ence were also measured. An alternative method consisted in determining the concentration difference across a defined tubule segment when the net flux was zero. For this latter approach, stationary microperfusion methods were particularly useful.

An instructive experiment addressing the problem of sodium transport across the proximal tubule epithelium is summarized in Figure 20 (160). In this important stationary microperfusion ("split-drop") experiment, carried out in Arthur Solomon's Biophysical Laboratory at Harvard Medical School by Windhager, G. Whittembury, D. Oken, and H. J. Schatzman, proximal tubules of *Necturus* were filled with isosmotic solutions of progressively lower sodium concentration, and net movement of fluid was monitored by measuring the change of inulin concentration in the fluid reaspirated from the tubule. The fact that sodium movement takes place against sizeable concentration gradients at a time when the lumen is electrically negative demonstrated the presence of active sodium transport. The establishment of a critical and transport-limiting transepithelial gradient of sodium concentration was also noted. Tracer experiments using $^{22}Na^+$ demonstrated that the measured net movement of sodium ions is the result of much larger unidirectional sodium fluxes and that a large backflux of sodium from the peritubular fluid into the lumina opposes reabsorptive transport (100). Accordingly the observation that sodium transport stops at a transepithelial sodium concentration difference of about 30 mM was explained by a "pump-leak" model in which the net backflux of sodium ions increases as the luminal sodium concentration decreases (owing to a decrease in the passive component of outflux) until the two unidirectional opposing fluxes become equal. These experiments established sodium transport as one of the major active transport operations in the amphibian renal tubule. Active solute sodium transport was also shown to be present in mammalian proximal tubules (51, 73). This pump-leak model of electrolyte transport was the first to be proposed for the kidney, and it opened the way for similar studies with a wide variety of electrically charged and uncharged solutes.

An extensive series of studies on the mechanisms of transport across renal tubules was also pursued by Karl Ullrich (Fig. 21) and his colleagues in the Physiology Institutes of Göttingen and Berlin and the Max Planck Institute of Biophysics in Frankfurt. Ullrich, a student of Kurt Kramer's (the founder of the school of German renal physiologists after World War II) was born in Würzburg, Germany, where he also received his medical training. He began his career as an internist but soon joined Kramer's Physiology Institute in Marburg. He moved with Kramer to Göttingen in 1955 where he headed an active group of young renal physiologists. After a short period as chairman of the department of physiology at the Free University of Berlin, he became head of the Physiological Section of the Max Planck Institute for Biophysics in Frankfurt, a position he still holds.

During his career Ullrich attracted many gifted colleagues, among them Karl Heinz Gertz, Klaus Hierholzer, Peter Deetjen, Harold Sonnenberg, Eberhard Frömter, and more recently Rolf Kinne, Heini Murer, and Gerhard Burckhardt. Karl Sauer, a member of Reinhold Schlogel's Biophysics group at the Max Planck Institute in Frankfurt, also provided important theoretical input for assessing the quantitative concepts of active- and passive-transport components, driving forces, coupling coefficients between individual flux components,

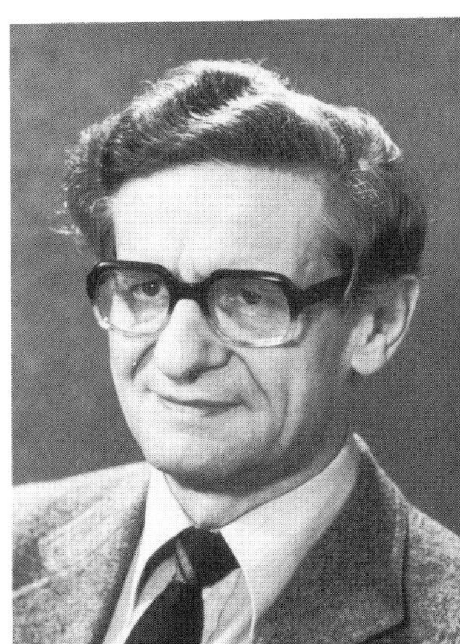

Figure 21. Karl J. Ullrich (b. 1925).

and energy requirements (135). This effort was also importantly stimulated by theoretical work on irreversible thermodynamics. Investigators such as Kedem and Katchalsky (70) and Katchalsky and Curran (69) have made essential contributions to the development of the conceptual background of this approach to the study of transport.

Ullrich and his associates determined the concentration difference across defined tubule segments when fluid movement was suppressed by the addition of poorly reabsorbable solutes, such as mannitol or raffinose, to the perfusion solution. The gradient of solute concentration across the epithelium was measured after steady state had developed. Using these methods, Ullrich and his associates, notably E. Frömter, Michael Kashgarian, and D. Marsh, demonstrated active transport of sodium, potassium, and bicarbonate in the proximal tubule (43, 68, 84). Ullrich and his associates' studies were complemented by those of K. H. Gertz (1920–1979), who used his "shrinking droplet" not only to evaluate the establishment of limiting sodium concentration gradients across the proximal tubule but also to provide evidence that significant net influx of sodium occurs whenever the luminal sodium concentration falls below the critical concentration maintained by active sodium transport (48).

Development of Concepts of Solute-Solvent Coupling

Although the notion that transepithelial fluid movement in kidney is somehow dependent on active sodium chloride transport was implied in the early work of Wesson and Anslow and their colleagues (151, 153), little further progress was made until the problem was studied in single renal tubules. The main question was how solute movement across tubules is coupled to that of fluid.

The dependence of transepithelial fluid movement on sodium reabsorption was evidenced by the demonstration, already referred to and shown in Figure 20, that water movement across the proximal tubule depends on the transepithelial difference of sodium concentration and ceases when net sodium transport is arrested. It is noteworthy that in early micropuncture studies a transepithelial osmotic concentration difference across the proximal tubule had not been detected (56). Because osmosis was strongly implied as the most likely mechanism of solute-solvent coupling, an osmotic pressure difference located somewhere between the two bulk fluid phases, the luminal and the peritubular fluid, was required.

The search for a fluid compartment differing in osmotic pressure from the luminal and peritubular fluid was complemented by the theoretical work of Curran and MacIntosh (31) and Patlak et al. (102). Faced by a similar problem of explaining isosmotic fluid movement across the intestinal epithelium, these authors demonstrated, in a model of epithelial transport, that net fluid movement can occur against a gradient of osmolality under the conditions shown

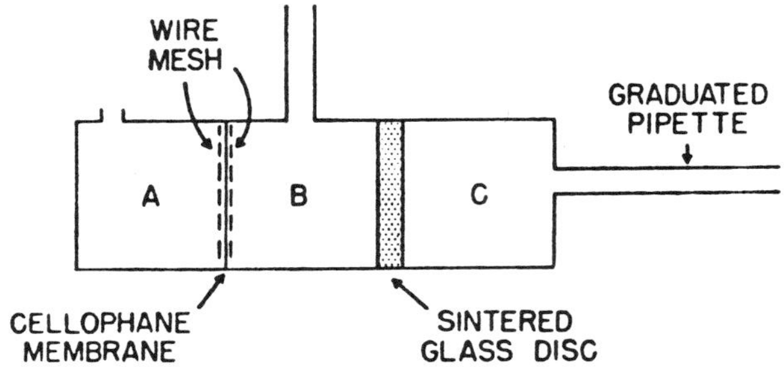

Figure 22. Model system of solute-solvent coupling. Solutions in compartments A and C were well stirred. Compartment B was unstirred and closed. Net volume flow was measured by means of a graduated pipette sealed into compartment C. Permeability to test solute (sucrose) of cellophane membrane was low, that of sintered glass disk was high. [From Curran and Macintosh (31).]

in Figure 22. The model requires a central, intraepithelial fluid compartment that contains a slightly hypertonic fluid and requires that the membranes that separate this compartment from the two bulk phases have different permeabilities to solutes; net fluid movement then takes place through the barrier with low permeability to solute. The feasibility of such a model to account for isosmotic, bulk fluid movement was later explored by Whitlock and Wheeler (154), Diamond (36), Diamond and Bossert (37), and Sackin and Boulpaep (115).

Application of this model to the epithelium of the proximal tubule is shown in Figure 23. The essential features include a "middle" compartment within the epithelium, which is separated from the tubule lumen by the junctional complex that links neighbouring proximal tubule cells and from the peritubular space by the basement membrane. Active sodium transport provides the necessary solute input into the intraepithelial compartment, and incomplete mixing with the fluid in the peritubular space prevents dissipation of the hypertonicity.

Many questions have been raised about this model and the theories developed to explain fluid movement across the proximal tubule. One question asked whether the higher protein concentration in peritubular blood could be an effective driving force for net fluid movement across the proximal tubule. A stimulating effect of an increase in peritubular protein concentration on sodium reabsorption in whole kidney had been a consistent finding in the clearance studies of Vereerstraeten and co-workers (143, 144) and in experiments by Earley, Martino, and Friedler (39). The micropuncture and microperfusion studies of Lewy and Windhager (77), Spitzer and Windhager (131), Brenner and Troy (21), and Green, Windhager, and Giebisch (57) localized this effect to the proximal tubule. It was particularly Windhager and his associates who provided strong evidence that the peritubular oncotic pressure is an important control

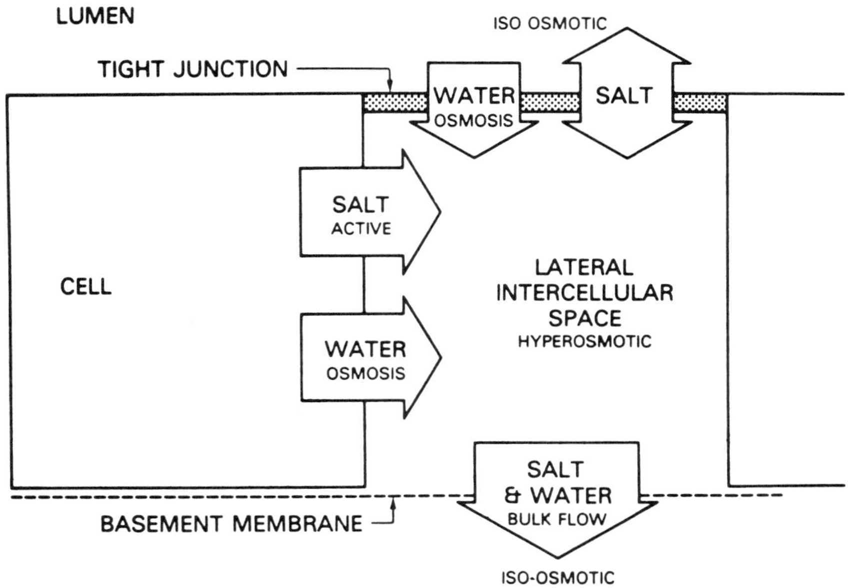

Figure 23. Epithelial cell model of proximal tubule demonstrating coupling of salt and water. Emphasis is placed on osmotic water movement through tight junction, although movement of water through cells also occurs. [From Burg (26).]

factor of proximal fluid transport and that it is the translocation of fluid out of the interspace compartment that is under control by the peritubular protein concentration (77, 131). The suggestion of Ludwig (79, 80) that peritubular oncotic forces across the whole epithelium can directly lead to significant proximal reabsorption was reconsidered by Vander et al. (142) and Bresler (22–24). Quantitative studies on single proximal tubules have confirmed that such a mechanism exists but that it accounts for only a small fraction of the reabsorption of fluid across the proximal tubule (57).

Another question is whether or not other driving forces such as modest luminal hypotonicity and solvent drag are also involved in transepithelial fluid transport and, if so, how much intraepithelial hypertonicity is actually needed to drive fluid transport at physiological rates. The problem of how much fluid moves between cells is also of interest, and the many studies addressing this issue owe their impetus to the cell model shown in Figure 22. The reader is referred to the papers by Berry (11), Whittembury (155), and Andreoli and Schafer (3, 4, 117–120) for discussion of the still-unresolved issues of solute-solvent coupling in the proximal tubule. Clearly the problem is less complex in the distal tubule and in the collecting duct where significant hypo- or hypertonicity develops and where, accordingly, adequate driving forces for the movement of water by osmosis are easily detectable.

Electrophysiological Techniques

The application of electrophysiological techniques has substantially contributed to our understanding of the mechanisms by which ions traverse the epithelium of renal tubules. The measurements of currents carried by ions is a convenient and useful way to examine the movement of charged ionic species, both across the whole epithelium as well as across individual cell barriers. It should be realized that only charged-ion movement, ion movement by electrodiffusion, or that of charged carrier molecules can be assessed by electrophysiological measurements of currents, resistances, and voltages. Electroneutral-ion movement by co- or countertransport escapes electrophysiological detection.

To begin with, early electrophysiological studies explored the direction and magnitude of the transepithelial potential difference along the nephron and thus defined one of the driving forces acting on transepithelial ion movement. Transepithelial electrical-resistance measurements defined the relative electrical "leakiness" of individual tubule segments to ions. Such studies defined the proximal tubule and parts of Henle's loop as a low-resistance epithelium and showed increased "tightness" to passive transepithelial ion movements of the distal nephron (14, 15, 49).

A second approach to the electrophysiological characterization of the renal epithelium had to do with the impalement of single tubule cells by microelectrodes (49). Combined with transepithelial potential measurements, such measurements provided information on the transmembrane potential across individual tubule cell membranes and thus made it possible to measure one of the driving forces acting on ions as they traverse the apical and basolateral cell membrane. This approach was further refined by the introduction of ion-sensitive microelectrodes, which provided information on cytoplasmatic ion activities in single amphibian and mammalian tubule cells. Measuring ion-activity gradients together with electrical potentials across the individual cell membranes of tubule cells became a powerful tool for characterizing ion movement in terms of movement along or against an electrochemical potential gradient and for localizing active and passive transport mechanisms to specific membrane sites within tubule cells. It was particularly the laboratories of Boulpaep and Frömter, together with their associates, who have successfully exploited the electrophysiological approach to the study of electrolyte transport in renal tubule cells (14, 15, 43, 44). An instructive example is the analysis of the proximal tubule.

The relatively high leakiness of the proximal tubule has been established by electrophysiological investigations. Figure 24 summarizes the basic equivalent circuit proposed by E. L. Boulpaep for the proximal tubule cell (14–16, 44, 157). The essential features include ionic batteries in both cell membranes and an important

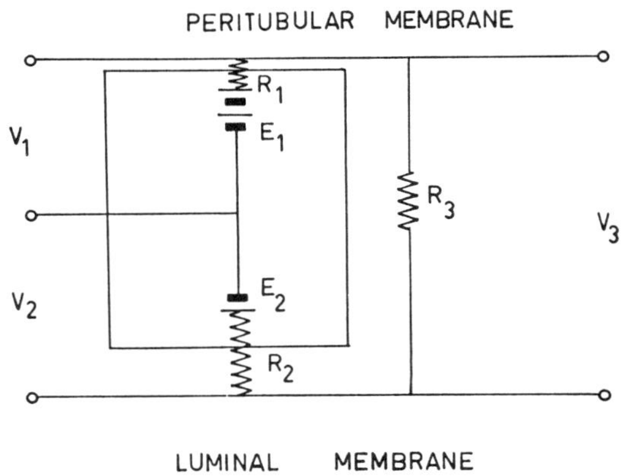

Figure 24. Model of equivalent electrical circuit for proximal tubule cell and overall epithelium. V_1, potential difference across peritubular membrane of cell; E_1, electromotive force of peritubular membrane, which may be of either polarity and is equivalent to combined electromotive forces of diffusional pathways; R_1, resistance of peritubular (and lateral) membrane of diffusion pathway. Same elements are represented for luminal membrane$_2$; V_3, transepithelial potential difference; E_3, paracellular electromotive force (of either polarity) resulting from dissipative leaks; R_3, paracellular resistance. [From Boulpaep (14).]

parallel pathway for ion flux, expressed in Figure 24 as the paracellular shunt resistance. The low shunt resistance in the proximal tubule explains the generation of intraepithelial current flow and the extensive coupling between electrical events in the basolateral and the apical cell membranes. The observation that the transepithelial electrical resistance is much lower than that of the two individual cell membranes in series is also strong supportive evidence for a highly conductive intercellular pathway for current flow. The work of Frömter and his associates on the electrophysiology of mammalian proximal tubules has also been well summarized (44).

Development of Cell Models of Sodium, Chloride, Calcium, and Potassium Transport

Many experiments have dealt with the problem of how solutes move across the renal tubules, not only across the epithelium as a whole but also across individual membranes of the cell and through intercellular spaces. To answer this question, knowledge of the driving forces and ion conductances across each limiting transport barrier is necessary. Although such detailed information is not always available, considerable progress has been made concerning the localization and nature of the transport processes in the apical and basolateral membranes of tubule cells.

Figures 25–27 present diagrammatically some of the pathways of ion transport in the proximal and distal nephron.

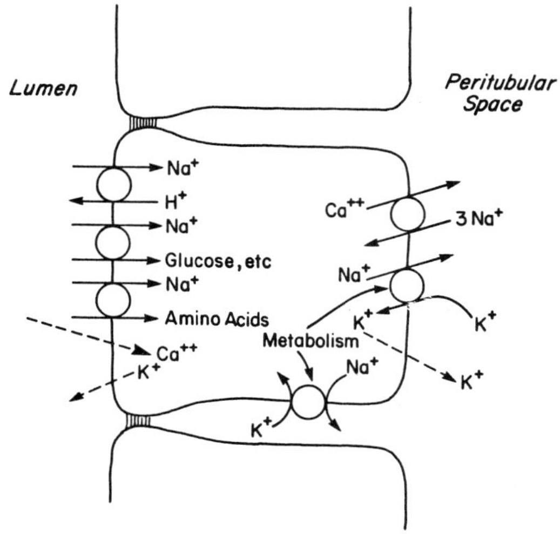

Figure 25. Model of proximal tubule cell. Apical membrane is characterized by Na^+-dependent co- and countertransport mechanisms and diffusion pathways for Ca^{2+} and K^{2+}; the basolateral membrane is characterized by active Na^+-K^+ exchange, Ca^{2+}-Na^+ exchange, and K^+ diffusion. [Adapted from Burg (26) and Giebisch and Aronson (51).]

Figure 25 summarizes the present state of knowledge of ion transport in the proximal tubule. Many laboratories have been involved in providing the information necessary to locate transport to either the apical or basolateral cell membranes of proximal tubule cells [a detailed account of these contributions is not attempted (see refs. 53 and 108 for review)]. The features of the model were elucidated by a wide range of techniques, including luminal and peritubular perfusion, ion substitution, specific blockers of carrier-mediated and passive transport, and electrophysiological procedures such as measurements of transepithelial and cell membrane potentials and measurements of intracellular ion activities with ion-specific electrodes (14, 15, 44).

A few general features of the proximal cell model in Figure 25 should be noted. The basolateral membrane is the site of active, ATP-driven sodium-potassium exchange, of a potassium-conductive pathway, and of a sodium-calcium exchanger (159). It is the sodium-potassium pump that lowers cell sodium and provides the energy for all apical co- and countertransport mechanisms as well as for basolateral sodium-calcium exchange. Whereas the basolateral membrane is largely involved in providing the energy for secondary active transport across the apical cell membrane, the specific transport properties of tubule cells are due to the insertion of specific carriers or leak permeabilities into the apical membrane. In the proximal tubule, these processes involve cotransport of sodium with organic solutes (sugars and amino acids), anions such as phosphate and sulfate, and several mono- and dicarboxylic acids. A countertransport system that exchanges mainly sodium for hydrogen ions is also present (5, 98, 116).

In the diluting segment, the thick ascending limb of Henle and the early distal tubule of amphibia, apical sodium transport is linked to movement of potassium and chloride [Fig. 26; (58, 99)], whereas in the initial and cortical collecting tubule, the main pathway for translocation of sodium from lumen to cell is by electrodiffusion (Fig. 27). Principal cells of the distal nephron are characterized by a high apical potassium permeability. The high permeability to potassium is an essential feature of this segment because it is importantly involved in the process of potassium secretion [Fig. 27; (164)].

It is appropriate to acknowledge the stimulation that physiologists concerned with renal transport have received from studies with many different techniques, sometimes in other tissues. The model of cotransport coupling of sodium to glucose was suggested by Crane

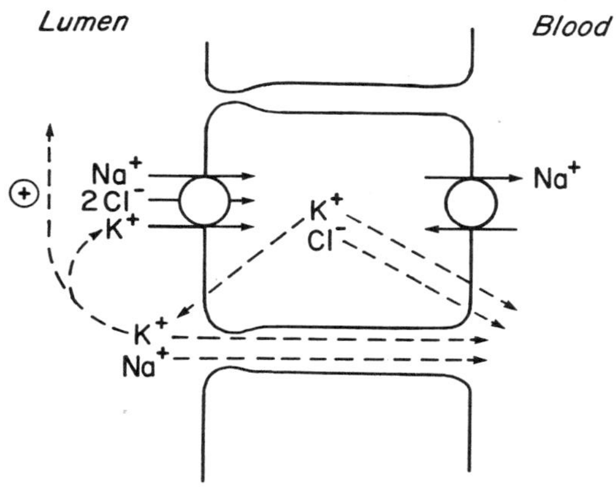

Figure 26. Model of diluting segment cell (mammalian thick ascending limb and amphibian diluting segment). Note Na^+-K^+-$2Cl^-$ cotransport in apical cell membrane. [From Wright and Giebisch (164).]

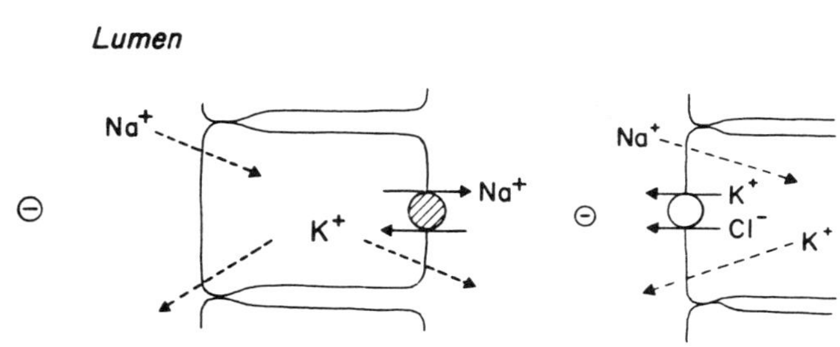

Figure 27. Model of principal cell in initial and cortical collecting tubule. Apical membrane contains diffusion pathways for Na^+ and K^+ and possibly also a KCl cotransport mechanism. [From Wright and Giebisch (164).]

(29) and Schultz and Curran (121); sodium-hydrogen exchange by work on brush-border membrane vesicles by Murer, Hopfer, and Kinne (98) and extended by Aronson (5) and Sacktor (116); and calcium-sodium exchange by Blaustein (12) and Reuter and Seitz (111). Finally, the electrically neutral cotransport of sodium, potassium, and two chloride ions was first discovered in Ehrlich ascites tumor cells by Geck and Heinz and their associates (47). The discovery of ATPase as a key element of active sodium-potassium transport by Skou (124) and the careful mapping of site-specific enzymes and of the substrate sensitivity of transport in defined tubule segments by Guder, Ross, and their associates (59, 162) should also be mentioned.

A biochemically oriented approach to the study of fluid and solute transport has been initiated by François Morel and his school (Fig. 28). Morel was born in Geneva where he received his early training in biology and medicine. Active in France since 1948, he was first associated with the Department of Biology of the Atomic Energy Commission in Saclay before assuming the directorship of the Laboratory of Cell Physiology at the Collége de France. He has trained many of the renal physiologists in France and has had a number of able associates, among them M. Guinnebault, C. Amiel, C. de Rouffignac, S. Jard, M. Bergeron, C. Lechène, N. Roinel, C. Le Grimmelec, and somewhat later, M. Imbert-Theboul, D. Chabardes, and A. Doucet. Besides exploring renal ion transport by a combination of micropuncture and tracer studies, Morel and his associates, in particular Chabardes, Imbert-Theboul, and Doucet, have developed sensitive methods for the localization and study of the mode of hormone action in fragments of kidney tubules (95, 96).

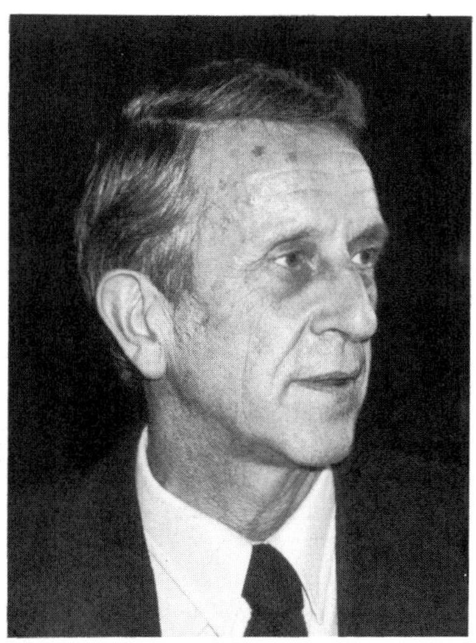

Figure 28. François Morel (b. 1923).

By careful dissection of individual tubule segments and the measurement of cAMP release following addition of known amounts of hormones, Morel and his colleagues were able to provide detailed information on the functional segmentation of the nephron in terms of hormone-related activation of adenylate cyclase. This work has been especially stimulating because it not only provided new information about the target site of many peptide and other hormones, but it also implicated previously unrecognized sites of hormone action in the nephron. Morel's work is representative of the ingenious combination of two approaches: that of assessing transport directly by micropuncture and of carrying out correlated, highly localized "segmental" biochemistry.

Outlook and Conclusion

Recent transport physiology has greatly advanced since Cushny's "modern theory of urine formation." New concepts as well as new and powerful techniques have provided a constant source of stimulating new ideas and the means to test them in kidney. We now have a fairly comprehensive idea of how electrolytes are handled along the nephron and what the main transport processes are. In many instances it is now possible to assign the steps in transport to specific cell membranes of the tubule cells or to the intercellular path of transport.

Continued research dealing with renal transport physiology promises further advance. Recent studies have often used a reductionist approach such as work on isolated cells, cell cultures, isolated membrane vesicles, and excised membrane patches. Also, cell biologic and genetic techniques for the isolation of membrane carriers and membrane channels are being increasingly incorporated into renal research. These powerful tools promise significant advances in our understanding of how the kidney, by a multitude of individual, specific, and localized transport processes, modifies the filtrate and returns to the blood a fluid "*ideally suited to the tissues*" (32).

I am especially indebted to Dr. Robert W. Berliner for help and advice in the preparation of the manuscript. In preparing this chapter, I had the benefit of fruitful discussions with John M. Davis, Carl W. Gottschalk, Arnost Kleinzeller, Donald W. Seldin, Philip Steinmetz, Klaus Thurau, Guillermo Whittembury, and Erich E. Windhager. I am also indebted to Amabel Shih for editorial assistance.

My work has been supported by NIH grant AM17433.

BIBLIOGRAPHY

1. Alexander, R. S. Pitts and urine acidification. *Physiologist* 26: 364–366, 1983.
2. Amberson, W. R. Rudolf Höber: his life and scientific work. *Science Wash. DC* 120: 199–201, 1954.

3. Andreoli, T. E., and J. A. Schafer. Effective luminal hypotonicity: the driving force for isotonic proximal tubular fluid absorption. *Am. J. Physiol.* 236 (*Renal Fluid Electrolyte Physiol.* 5): F89–F96, 1979.
4. Andreoli, T. E., and J. A. Schafer. External solution driving forces for isotonic fluid absorption in proximal tubules. *Federation Proc.* 37: 154–160, 1979.
5. Aronson, P. S. Mechanisms of active H^+ secretion in the proximal tubule. *Am. J. Physiol.* 245 (*Renal Fluid Electrolyte Physiol.* 14): F647–F659, 1983.
6. Barnes, R. B., D. Richardson, J. W. Berry, and R. L. Hood. Flame photometry. A rapid analytical procedure. *Ind. Eng. Chem.* 17: 605–611, 1945. (Analytical Edition.)
7. Beck, F., R. Bauer, U. Bauer, J. Mason, A. Dorge, R. Rick, and K. Thurau. Electron microprobe analysis of intracellular elements in the rat kidney. *Kidney Int.* 17: 756–763, 1980.
8. Berliner, R. W. Renal mechanism for potassium excretion. *Harvey Lect.* 55: 141–171, 1961.
9. Berliner, R. W., and T. J. Kennedy, Jr. Renal tubular secretion of potassium in the dog. *Proc. Soc. Expt. Biol. Med.* 67: 542–545, 1948.
10. Berliner, R. W., T. J. Kennedy, Jr., and J. G. Hilton. Renal mechanisms for excretion of potassium. *Am. J. Physiol.* 162: 348–367, 1950.
11. Berry, C. A. Water permeability and pathways in the proximal tubule. *Am. J. Physiol.* 245 (*Renal Fluid Electrolyte Physiol.* 14): F279–F294, 1983.
12. Blaustein, M. P. The interrelationship between sodium and calcium fluxes across cell membranes. *Rev. Physiol. Biochem. Pharmacol.* 70: 33–82, 1974.
13. Bott, P. A. Micropuncture study of renal excretion of water, K, Na and Cl in *Necturus*. *Am. J. Physiol.* 203: 662–666, 1962.
14. Boulpaep, E. L. Ion permeability of the peritubular and luminal membrane of the renal tubular cell. In: *Transport und Funktion Intracellularer Elektrolyte,* edited by F. Kruck. Munich, FRG: Urban & Schwarzenberg, 1967, p. 98–107.
15. Boulpaep, E. L. Electrophysiology of the kidney. In: *Membrane Transport in Biology,* edited by G. Giebisch, D. C. Tosteson, and H. H. Ussing. Berlin: Springer-Verlag, 1979, p. 97–144.
16. Boulpaep, E. L., and H. Sackin. Equivalent electrical circuit analysis and rheogenic pumps in epithelia. *Federation Proc.* 38: 2030–2036, 1979.
17. Bradley, S. E. *Renal Function.* New York: Josiah Macy, Jr., Found., 1950.
18. Bradley, S. E., H. Chasis, W. Goldring, and H. W. Smith. Hemodynamic alterations in normotensive and hypertensive subjects during the pyrogenic reaction. *J. Clin. Invest.* 24: 749–756, 1945.
19. Brandt-Rehberg, P. Studies on kidney function. I. The rate of filtration and reabsorption in the human kidney. *Biochem. J.* 20: 447–485, 1926.
20. Brandt-Rehberg, P. Über die Bestimmung der Menge des Glomerulusfiltrats mittels Kreatinin als Nierenfunktionsprufung, nebst einigen Bemerkungen über die Theorien der Harnbereitung. *Zentralbl. Inn. Med.* 50: 367–377, 1929.
21. Brenner, B. M., and J. L. Troy. Postglomerular vascular protein con-

centration: evidence for a causal role in governing fluid reabsorption and glomerulotubular balance by the renal proximal tubule. *J. Clin. Invest.* 50: 336–349, 1971.
22. Bresler, E. H. On criteria for active transport. *J. Theor. Biol.* 16: 135–146, 1967.
23. Bresler, E. H. Ludwig's theory of tubular reabsorption: the role of physical factors in tubular reabsorption. *Kidney Int.* 9: 313–322, 1976.
24. Bresler, E. H. A model for transepithelial fluid transport. *Am. J. Physiol.* 235 (*Renal Fluid Electrolyte Physiol.* 4): F626–F637, 1978.
25. Brun, C., E. O. Knudsen, and F. Raaschon. Kidney function and circulatory collapse; post-syncopal oliguria. *J. Clin. Invest.* 25: 568–574, 1946.
26. Burg, M. B. Renal handling of sodium, chloride, water, amino acids, and glucose. In: *The Kidney,* edited by B. Brenner and F. C. Rector. Philadelphia, PA: Saunders, 1981, p. 328–370.
27. Burg, M., J. Grantham, M. Abramow, and J. Orloff. Preparation and study of fragments of single rabbit nephrons. *Am. J. Physiol.* 210: 1293–1298, 1966.
28. Chambers, R., and R. T. Kempton. Modification of function of the chick mesonephros in tissue culture with phenol red. *J. Cell. Comp. Physiol.* 3: 131–166, 1933.
29. Crane, R. K. Na^+-dependent transport in the intestine and other animal tissues. *Federation Proc.* 24: 1000–1006, 1965.
30. Cullis, W. C. On secretion in the frog's kidney. *J. Physiol. Lond.* 34: 250–271, 1906.
31. Curran, P. F., and J. R. Macintosh. A model system for biological water transport. *Nature Lond.* 193: 347–348, 1962.
32. Cushny, A. R. *The Secretion of the Urine* (2nd ed.). London: Longmans Green, 1926.
33. Dale, H. H. Arthur Robertson Cushny (1866–1926). *Proc. R. Soc. Lond. B Biol. Sci.* 100: xix–xxvii, 1926.
34. Dean, R. B. Theories of electrolyte equilibrium in muscle. *Biol. Symp.* 3: 331–348, 1941.
36. Diamond, J. M. The mechanism of isotonic water transport. *J. Gen. Physiol.* 48: 15–42, 1964.
37. Diamond, J. M., and W. H. Bossert. Standing-gradient osmotic flow. A mechanism for coupling of water and solute transport in epithelia. *J. Gen. Physiol.* 50: 2061–2083, 1967.
38. Dirks, J. H., W. J. Cirksena, and R. W. Berliner. The effect of saline infusion on sodium reabsorption by the proximal tubule of the dog. *J. Clin. Invest.* 44: 1160–1170, 1965.
39. Earley, L. E., J. A. Martino, and R. M. Friedler. Factors affecting sodium reabsorption by the proximal tubule as determined during blockade of distal sodium reabsorption. *J. Clin. Invest.* 45: 1668–1684, 1966.
40. Epstein, F. H. Recollections of nephrology: Peters and Seldin. Presentation of the First John P. Peters Award to Donald W. Seldin, 1983. *Semin. Nephrol.* 4: 107–112, 1984.
41. Fenn, W. O. The role of potassium in physiological processes. *Physiol. Rev.* 20: 377–415, 1940.
42. Fenn, W. O., and D. M. Cobb. The potassium equilibrium in muscle. *J. Gen. Physiol.* 17: 629–656, 1934.

43. Frömter, E. Viewing the kidney through microelectrodes. *Am. J. Physiol.* 247 (*Renal Fluid Electrolyte Physiol.* 16): F695–F705, 1984.
44. Frömter, E., G. Rumrich, and K. J. Ullrich. Phenomenologic description of Na^+, Cl^-, and HCO_3^- absorption from proximal tubules of rat kidney. *Pfluegers Arch.* 343: 189–220, 1973.
45. Gamble, J. L. Companionship of water and electrolytes in the organization of body fluids. In: *Lane Medical Lectures.* Stanford, CA: Stanford Univ. Press, 1951, vol. 5, p. 1–90.
46. Gamble, J. L. *Chemical Anatomy, Physiology and Pathology of Extracellular Fluid* (6th ed.). Cambridge, MA: Harvard Univ. Press, 1954. (Lecture Syllabus.)
47. Geck, P., C. Pietrzyk, B.-C. Burckhardt, B. Pfeiffer, and E. Heinz. Electrically silent cotransport of Na^+, K^+, and Cl^- in Ehrlich cells. *Biochim. Biophys. Acta* 600: 432–447, 1980.
48. Gertz, K. H. Transtubuläre Natrium-chloridflüsse and permeabilität für Nichtelektrolyte im proximalen und distalen Konvolut der Rattenniere. *Pfluegers Arch.* 276: 336–356, 1963.
49. Giebisch, G. Measurements of electrical potential difference in perfused single proximal tubules in *Necturus* kidney. *J. Gen. Physiol.* 44: 659–678, 1961.
50. Giebisch, G. Renal potassium transport. In: *Membrane Transport in Biology,* edited by G. Giebisch, D. C. Tosteson, and H. H. Ussing. Berlin: Springer-Verlag, 1979, vol. 4A, p. 215–298.
51. Giebisch, G., and P. S. Aronson. The proximal nephron. In: *Physiology of Membrane Disorders,* edited by T. E. Andreoli, J. F. Hoffman, D. D. Fanestil, and S. G. Schultz. New York: Plenum, 1986, p. 669–700.
52. Glabman, S., R. M. Klose, and G. Giebisch. Micropuncture study of ammonia excretion in the rat. *Am. J. Physiol.* 205: 127–132, 1963.
53. Goldring, W., H. Chasis, A. Ranges, and N. W. Smith. Effective renal blood flow in subjects with essential hypertension. *J. Clin. Invest.* 20: 637–653, 1941.
54. Gottschalk, C. W. Renal tubular function: lessons from micropuncture. *Harvey Lect.* 58: 99–123, 1963.
55. Gottschalk, C. W., W. E. Lassiter, and M. Mylle. Localization of urine acidification in the mammalian kidney. *Am. J. Physiol.* 198: 581–585, 1960.
56. Gottschalk, C. W., and M. Mylle. Micropuncture study of the mammalian urinary concentrating mechanism: evidence for the countercurrent hypothesis. *Am. J. Physiol.* 196: 927–936, 1959.
57. Green, R., E. E. Windhager, and G. Giebisch. Protein oncotic pressure effects on proximal tubular fluid movement in the rat. *Am. J. Physiol.* 226: 265–276, 1974.
58. Greger, R., and E. Schlatter. Properties of the lumen membrane of the cortical thick ascending limb of Henle's loop of rabbit kidney. *Pfluegers Arch.* 396: 315–324, 1983.
59. Guder, W. G., and B. D. Ross. Enzyme distribution along the nephron. *Kidney Int.* 26: 101–111, 1984.
60. Hastings, A. B. Donald Dexter Van Slyke. *Biogr. Mem. Natl. Acad. Sci.* 48:308–360, 1976.
61. Heidenhain, R. Versuche über den Vorgang der Harnabsonderung. *Pfluegers Arch.* 9: 4, 1874.

62. HEINZ, E. Grundmechanismus der Magensaureproduktion und deren Regulation. *Klin. Physiol.* 1: 184–203, 1960.
63. HÖBER, R. The formation of urine. In: *Physical Chemistry of Cells and Tissues,* edited by R. Höber. Philadelphia, PA: Blakiston, 1945, p. 553–579.
64. HÖBER, R. *Physical Chemistry of Cells and Tissues.* Philadelphia, PA: Blakiston, 1945.
65. HÖBER, R., and P. M. BRISCOE-WOOLLEY. Conditions determining the selective secretion of dyestuffs by the isolated frog kidney. *J. Cell. Comp. Physiol.* 15: 35–146, 1940.
66. HÖBER, R., and P. M. BRISCOE-WOOLLEY. Further studies on conditions determining the selective renal secretion of dyestuffs. *J. Cell. Comp. Physiol.* 16: 63–70, 1940.
67. KAISSLING, B., and W. KRIZ. Structure-function correlation in transporting epithelia. In: *The Kidney: Physiology and Pathophysiology,* edited by D. W. Seldin and G. Giebisch. New York: Raven, 1985, p. 307–316.
68. KASHGARIAN, M. H., H. STOECKLE, C. W. GOTTSCHALK, and K. ULLRICH. Transtubular electrochemical potentials of sodium and chloride in proximal and distal renal tubules of rats during antidiuresis and water diuresis (diabetes insipidus). *Pfluegers Arch.* 277: 89–106, 1963.
69. KATCHALSKY, A., and P. F. CURRAN. *Nonequilibrium Thermodynamics in Biophysics.* Cambridge, MA: Harvard Univ. Press, 1967.
70. KEDEM, O., and A. KATCHALSKY. A physical interpretation of the phenomenological coefficients of membrane permeability. *J. Gen. Physiol.* 45: 143–179, 1961.
71. KENNEY, R. A. *The Metzner Theory of Urine Formation.* The Hague: Junk, 1957.
72. KOEFOED-JOHNSEN, V., and H. H. USSING. The nature of the frog skin potential. *Acta Physiol. Scand.* 42: 298–308, 1958.
73. KOKKO, J. P., M. B. BURG, and J. ORLOFF. Characteristics of NaCl and water transport in the renal proximal tubule. *J. Clin. Invest.* 50: 69–76, 1971.
74. LASSITER, W. E., C. W. GOTTSCHALK, and M. MYLLE. Micropuncture study of net transtubular movement of water and urea in nondiuretic mammalian kidney. *Am. J. Physiol.* 200: 1139–1147, 1961.
75. LASSITER, W. E., C. W. GOTTSCHALK, and M. MYLLE. Micropuncture study of renal tubular reabsorption of calcium in normal rodents. *Am. J. Physiol.* 204: 771–775, 1963.
76. LECHÈNE ,C., F. MOREL, M. GUINNEBAULT, and C. DE ROUFFIGNAC. Étude par microponction de l'élaboration de l'urine. I. Chez le rat dans différents états de diurese. *Nephron* 6: 457–477, 1969.
77. LEWY, J. E., and E. E. WINDHAGER. Peritubular control of proximal tubular fluid reabsorption in the rat kidney. *Am. J. Physiol.* 214: 943–954, 1968.
78. LOEB, R. F. James Lawder Gamble. *Biogr. Mem. Natl. Acad. Sci.* 36: 146–160, 1962.
79. LUDWIG, C. *Beitrage zur Lehre vom Mechanismus der Harnsecretion.* Marburg, Germany: Elwert, 1843.
80. LUDWIG, C. *Lehrbuch der Physiologie des Menschen.* Heidelberg, Germany: Wintersche, 1861.

81. Malnic, G., R. M. Klose, and G. Giebisch. Micropuncture study of renal potassium excretion in the rat. *Am. J. Physiol.* 206: 674–686, 1964.
82. Maren, T. H. Eli Kennerly Marshall, Jr. 1889–1966. *Bull. Johns Hopkins Hosp.* 119: 247–254, 1966.
83. Maren, T. H. Eli Kennerly Marshall, Jr. *Biogr. Mem. Natl. Acad. Sci.* 56: 313–354, 1987.
84. Marsh, D. J., K. F. Ullrich, and G. Rumrich. Micropuncture analysis of the behavior of potassium ions on rat cortical tubules. *Pfluegers Arch.* 277: 107–119, 1963.
85. Marshall, E. K., Jr. A comparison of the function of the glomerular and aglomerular kidney. *Am. J. Physiol.* 94: 1–10, 1930.
86. Marshall, E. K., Jr. The secretion of phenol red by the mammalian kidney. *Am. J. Physiol.* 99: 77–86, 1931.
87. Marshall, E. K., Jr. The comparative physiology of the kidney in relation to theories of renal secretion. *Physiol. Rev.* 14: 133–159, 1934.
88. Marshall, E. K., Jr. Two lectures on renal physiology. *Physiologist* 9: 367–384, 1966.
89. Marshall, E. K., Jr., and M. M. Crane. The secretory function of the renal tubules. *Am. J. Physiol.* 70: 465–488, 1924.
90. Marshall, E. K., Jr., and J. L. Vickers. The mechanism of the elimination of phenolsulphonephthalein by the kidney. A proof of secretion by the convoluted tubules. *Bull. Johns Hopkins Hosp.* 34: 1–7, 1923.
91. Mayrs, E. B. The relative excretion of urea and some other constituents of the urine. *J. Physiol. Lond.* 56: 58–68, 1922.
92. Mayrs, E. B. On the action of phlorhizin on the kidney. *J. Physiol. Lond.* 57: 461–466, 1923.
93. Mayrs, E. B. Secretion as factor in elimination by birds. *J. Physiol. Lond.* 58: 276–287, 1924.
94. Metzner, R. Die Absonderung und Herausbeforderung des Harns. *Nagel's Handbuch Physiol. Mens.* 2: 207–258, 1906.
95. Morel, F. Sites of hormone action in the mammalian nephron. *Am. J. Physiol.* 240 (*Renal Fluid Electrolyte Physiol.* 9): F159–F164, 1981.
96. Morel, F., and A. Doucet. Hormonal control of kidney functions at the cell level. *Physiol. Rev.* 66: 377–468, 1986.
97. Mudge, G. H., J. Foulks, and A. Gilman. The renal excretion of potassium. *Proc. Soc. Exp. Biol. Med.* 67: 545–547, 1948.
98. Murer, H., U. Hopfer, and R. Kinne. Sodium/proton antiport in brush-border-membrane vesicles isolated from rat small intestine and kidney. *Biochem. J.* 154: 597–604, 1976.
99. Oberleithner, H., G. Giebisch, F. Lang, and W. Wang. Cellular mechanism of the furosemide sensitive transport system in the kidney. *Klin. Wochenschr.* 60: 1173–1179, 1982.
100. Oken, D. E., G. Whittembury, E. E. Windhager, and A. K. Solomon. Single proximal tubules of *Necturus* kidney. V. Unidirectional sodium movement. *Am. J. Physiol.* 204: 372–376, 1963.
101. Orloff, J. Presentation of the George M. Kober Medal to Robert William Berliner. *Trans. Assoc. Am. Physicians* 97: 147–163, 1984.
102. Patlak, C. S., D. A. Goldstein, and J. F. Hoffman. The flow of solute and solvent across a two-membrane system. *J. Theor. Biol.* 5: 426–442, 1963.

103. Paul, J. R., and C. N. Long. John Punnett Peters. *Biogr. Mem. Natl. Acad. Sci.* 31: 347–375, 1958.
104. Peters, J. P., and D. D. Van Slyke. *Quantitative Clinical Chemistry.* Baltimore, MD: Williams & Wilkins, 1932.
105. Pitts, R. F. Organization of the respiratory center. *Physiol. Rev.* 27: 609–630, 1946.
106. Pitts, R. F. Homer William Smith. *Biogr. Mem. Natl. Acad. Sci.* 39: 445–470, 1967.
107. Pitts, R. F., and R. S. Alexander. The nature of the renal tubular mechanism for acidifying the urine. *Am. J. Physiol.* 144: 239–254, 1945.
108. Rector, F. C., Jr. Sodium, bicarbonate, and chloride absorption by the proximal tubule. *Am. J. Physiol.* 244 (*Renal Fluid Electrolyte Physiol.* 13): F461–F471, 1983.
109. Reubi, F. C., and P. H. Futcher. The effects of histamine on renal function in hypertensive and normotensive subjects. *J. Clin. Invest.* 28: 440–446, 1949.
110. Reuter, H. In memory of Walther Wilbrandt. *J. Membr. Biol.* 57: 83–84, 1980.
111. Reuter, H., and N. Seitz. The dependence of calcium efflux from cardiac muscle on temperature and external ion composition. *J. Physiol. Lond.* 195: 451–470, 1968.
112. Richards, A. N. Processes of urine formation. *Proc. R. Soc. Lond. B Biol. Sci.* 126: 398–432, 1938. (Croonian Lect.)
113. Richards, A. N., B. B. Westfall, and P. A. Bott. Renal excretion of inulin creatinine and xylose in normal dogs. *Proc. Soc. Exp. Biol. Med.* 32: 73–75, 1934.
114. Rowntree, L. A., and J. T. Geraghty. An experimental and clinical study of the functional activity of the kidneys by means of phenolsulphophthalein. *J. Pharmacol. Exp. Ther.* 1: 579–593, 1909.
115. Sackin, H., and E. L. Boulpaep. Models for coupling of salt and water transport: proximal tubular reabsorption in *Necturus* kidney. *J. Gen. Physiol.* 66: 671–733, 1975.
116. Sacktor, B. Transport in membrane vesicles isolated from the mammalian kidney and intestine. In: *Current Topics in Bioenergetics,* edited by R. Sanadi. New York: Academic, 1977, p. 39–81.
117. Schafer, J. A. Mechanisms coupling the absorption of solutes and water in the proximal nephron. *Kidney Int.* 25: 708–716, 1984.
118. Schafer, J. A., C. S. Patlak, and T. E. Andreoli. Fluid absorption and active and passive ion flows in the rabbit superficial pars recta. *Am. J. Physiol.* 233 (*Renal Fluid Electrolyte Physiol.* 2): F154–F167, 1977.
119. Schafer, J. A., S. L. Troutman, and T. E. Andreoli. Volume reabsorption, transepithelial potential differences, and ionic permeability properties in mammalian superficial proximal straight tubules. *J. Gen. Physiol.* 64: 582–607, 1974.
120. Schafer, J. A., S. L. Troutman, M. L. Watkins, and T. E. Andreoli. Flow dependence of fluid transport in the isolated superficial pars recta: evidence that osmotic disequilibrium between external solutions drives isotonic fluid absorption. *Kidney Int.* 20: 588–597, 1981.
121. Schultz, S. G., and P. F. Curran. Coupled transport of sodium and organic solutes. *Physiol. Rev.* 50: 637–718, 1970.

122. SHANNON, J. A. The excretion of inulin by the dog. *Am. J. Physiol.* 112: 405–413, 1935.
123. SHANNON, J. A., and H. W. SMITH. The excretion of inulin, xylose and urea by normal and phlorizinized man. *J. Clin. Invest.* 14: 393–401, 1935.
124. SKOU, J. C. Enzymatic basis for active transport of Na^+ and K^+ across cell membrane. *Physiol. Rev.* 45: 596–617, 1965.
125. SMITH, H. W. *The Physiology of the Kidney.* New York: Oxford Univ. Press, 1937.
126. SMITH, H. W. Renal physiology between the wars. In: *Lectures on the Kidney.* Lawrence, KS: Univ. of Kansas Press, 1943, p. 65–82. (Porter Lectures, series IX.)
127. SMITH, H. W. *The Kidney. Structure and Function in Health and Disease.* New York: Oxford Univ. Press, 1951.
128. SMITH, H. W. Highlights in the history of renal physiology. *Georgetown Med. Bull.* 13: 4–48, 1959.
129. SMITH, H. W. Renal physiology. In: *Circulation of the Blood, Men and Ideas,* edited by A. P. Fishman and D. W. Richards. New York: Oxford Univ. Press, 1964, p. 545–606.
130. SMITH, H. W., N. FINKELSTEIN, L. ALIMINOSA, B. CRAWFORD, and M. GRABER. The renal clearance of substituted hippurine and derivatives and other aromatic acids in dog and man. *J. Clin. Invest.* 24: 388–404, 1945.
131. SPITZER, A., and E. E. WINDHAGER. Effect of peritubular oncotic pressure changes on proximal tubular fluid reabsorption. *Am. J. Physiol.* 218: 1188–1193, 1970.
132. STARR, I. Alfred Newton Richards, scientist and man. *Ann. Intern. Med.* 71: 1–89, 1969.
133. STEINBACH, H. B. Sodium and potassium in frog muscle. *J. Biol. Chem.* 133: 695–701, 1940.
134. STRICKLER, J. C., D. D. THOMPSON, R. M. KLOSE, and G. GIEBISCH. Micropuncture study of inorganic phosphate excretion in the rat. *J. Clin. Invest.* 43: 1596–1607, 1964.
135. ULLRICH, K. J. Permeability characteristics of the mammalian nephron. F. SAUER. *Appendix:* Nonequilibrium thermodynamics of kidney tubule transport. In: *Handbook of Physiology. Renal Physiology,* edited by J. Orloff and R. W. Berliner. Washington, DC: Am. Physiol. Soc., 1973, sect. 8, chapt. 12, p. 377–414.
136. ULLRICH, K. J. Renal tubular mechanisms of organic solute transport. *Kidney Int.* 9: 172–188, 1976.
137. ULLRICH, K. J., and R. GREGER. Approaches to the study of tubule transport functions. In: *The Kidney: Physiology and Pathophysiology,* edited by D. W. Seldin and G. Giebisch. New York: Raven, 1985, p. 427–470.
138. ULLRICH, K. J., B. SCHMIDT-NIELSEN, R. O'DELL, G. PEHLING, C. W. GOTTSCHALK, W. E. LASSITER, and M. MYLLE. Micropuncture study of composition of proximal and distal tubular fluid in rat kidney. *Am. J. Physiol.* 204: 527–531, 1963.
139. USSING, H. H. The alkali metal ions in isolated systems and tissues. In: *Handbook of Experimental Pharmacology,* edited by O. Eichler and A. Farah. Heidelberg: Springer-Verlag, 1960, p. 1–195.

140. Ussing, H. H. Life with tracers. *Annu. Rev. Physiol.* 42: 1–16, 1980.
141. Ussing, H. H., and E. E. Windhager. Nature of shunt path and active sodium transport path through frog skin epithelium. *Acta Physiol. Scand.* 61: 484–504, 1964.
142. Vander, A. J., R. L. Malvin, W. S. Wilde, and L. P. Sullivan. Reexamination of salt and water retention in congestive heart failure. *Am. J. Med.* 25: 497–502, 1958.
143. Vereerstraeten, P., and M. de Myttenaere. Effect of raising transtubular oncotic gradient on sodium excretion in the dog. *Pfluegers Arch.* 302: 1–12, 1968.
144. Vereerstraeten, P., and C. Toussaint. Role of the peritubular oncotic pressure on sodium excretion by avian kidney. *Pfluegers Arch.* 302: 13–23, 1968.
145. Vogel, G., F. Lauterbach, and W. Kroger. Die Bedeutung des Natriums für die renalen Transporte von Glucose und Para-Aminohippursaure. *Pfluegers Arch.* 283: 151–159, 1965.
146. Walker, A. M., P. A. Bott, J. Oliver, and M. C. MacDowell. The collection and analysis of fluid from single nephrons of the mammalian kidney.; *Am. J. Physiol.* 134: 580–595, 1941.
146a. Wardener, de, H. E., I. H. Mills, W. F. Clapham, and C. J. Hayer. Studies on the efferent mechanism of the sodium diuresis which follows the administration of intravenous saline in the dog. *Clin. Sci.* 21: 249–258, 1961.
147. Wearn, J. T. Composition of glomerular urine with conclusive evidence of reabsorption in the renal tubules. A vignette. *Physiologist* 23 (5): 1–4, 1980.
148. Wearn, J. T., and A. N. Richards. Observations on the composition of glomerular urine with particular reference to the problem of reabsorption in the renal tubules. *Am. J. Physiol.* 71: 209–227, 1924.
149. Wesson, L. G., Jr. Glomerular and tubular factors in the renal excretion of sodium chloride. *Medicine* 36: 281–396, 1957.
150. Wesson, L. G., Jr. *Physiology of the Human Kidney.* New York: Grune & Stratton, 1969.
151. Wesson, L. G., Jr., and W. P. Anslow, Jr. Excretion of sodium and water during osmotic diuresis in the dog. *Am. J. Physiol.* 153: 465–474, 1948.
152. Wesson, L. G., Jr., W. P. Anslow, Jr., L. G. Raisz, A. A. Bolomey, and M. Ladd. Effect of sustained expansion of extracellular fluid volume upon filtration rate, renal plasma flow, and electrolyte and water excretion in the dog. *Am. J. Physiol.* 162: 677–686, 1950.
153. Wesson, L. G., Jr., W. P. Anslow, and H. W. Smith. The excretion of strong electrolytes. *Bull. NY Acad. Med.* 24: 586–606, 1948.
154. Whitlock, R. T., and H. O. Wheeler. Coupled transport of solute and water across rabbit gallbladder epithelium. *J. Clin. Invest.* 43: 2249–2265, 1964.
155. Whittembury, G. Mechanisms of epithelial solute-solvent coupling. In: *The Kidney: Physiology and Pathophysiology,* edited by D. Seldin and G. Giebisch. New York: Raven, 1985, p. 199–214.
156. Wilbrandt, W., and T. Rosenberg. The concept of carrier transport and its corollaries in pharmacology. *Pharmacol. Rev.* 13: 109–183, 1961.

157. WINDHAGER, E. E., E. L. BOULPAEP, and G. GIEBISCH. Electrophysiological studies on single nephrons. *Proc. Int. Congr. Nephrol.* 1: 98–107, 1967.
158. WINDHAGER, E. E., and G. GIEBISCH. Micropuncture study of renal tubular transfer of sodium chloride in the rat. *Am. J. Physiol.* 200: 581–590, 1961.
159. WINDHAGER, E. E., A. TAYLOR, T. MAACK, C. O. LEE, and M. LORENZEN. Studies on renal tubular function. In: *Functional Regulation at the Cellular and Molecular Level,* edited by A. Corradino. New York: Elsevier/North-Holland, 1982, p. 299–316.
160. WINDHAGER, E. E., G. WHITTEMBURY, D. E. OKEN, H. J. SCHATZMANN, and A. K. SOLOMON. Single proximal tubules of the *Necturus* kidney. III. Dependence of H_2O movement on NaCl concentration. *Am. J. Physiol.* 197: 313–318, 1959.
161. WINTON, F. R. *Modern Views on the Secretion of Urine.* London: Churchill, 1956. (Cushny Memorial Lect.)
162. WIRTHENSOHN, G., and W. G. GUDER. Renal substrate metabolism. *Physiol. Rev.* 66: 469–497, 1986.
163. WIRZ, H., and P. A. BOTT. Potassium and reducing substances in proximal tubule fluid of the rat kidney. *Proc. Soc. Exp. Biol. Med.* 87: 405–407, 1954.
164. WRIGHT, F. S., and G. GIEBISCH. Regulation of potassium excretion. In: *The Kidney: Physiology and Pathophysiology,* edited by D. W. Seldin and G. Giebisch. New York: Raven, 1985, p. 1223–1249.

VII

Control of Sodium Excretion

HUGH E. DE WARDENER

ONE hundred years ago, it was recognized that renal excretion of salt is related to its dietary intake. Carl F. Ludwig (36) pointed out in 1869:

The proportion of chloride of sodium in the body as a whole is not always the same. It depends on the quantity taken daily, and may be increased or diminished within certain limits. If a definite quantity be taken daily for some time the same quantity will be found in the urine, so that the amount present in the body is constant. If the quantity consumed be now increased, no increase takes place in the excretion for about three days, a storage of salt is taking place in the body. After about three days the quantity excreted in the urine will again be found equal to the quantity daily taken, the amount present in the body remaining constantly at a higher level.

SODIUM EXCRETION

The concept of glomerular filtration was accepted in Ludwig's time, but glomerular filtration rate (GFR) was not measured until 1935 (44). The absence of this measurement permitted a wide variety of suggestions about the intrarenal mechanisms concerned in the formation of urine and the excretion of its various constituents. Ludwig (34, 35) thought that glomerular filtrate was passively reabsorbed by the tubules by the fall in hydrostatic pressure and the increase in plasma oncotic pressure in the postglomerular peritubular vessels. This concept about tubular function was revived in a modified form about 100 years later. In 1909 Ernest Henry Starling [Fig. 1; (50)] suggested that the GFR was ~1.5 liters/day. He calculated:

[If] all urinary constituents were derived from the glomerular transudate (filtration) 30 liters of fluid would have to be filtered through the glomeruli in order to excrete 30 grams of urea, which is the daily output of a man. Of these 30 liters, 28 would have to be reabsorbed in the tubules. Since the amount of blood flowing through the two

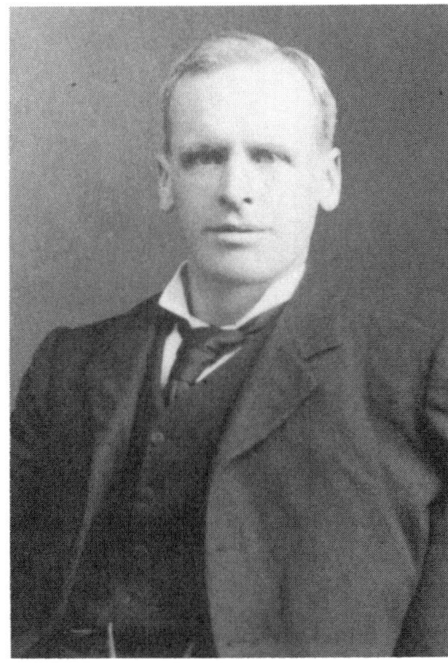

Figure 1. Ernest Henry Starling (1866–1927).

kidneys in a man probably varies between 1,600 and 1,800 liters in the 24 hours, there would be no difficulty in the production of such an amount as 30 liters, which would only represent a concentration in the blood in its passage through the glomeruli of under 2%. The secretion and reabsorption of such large quantities of fluid seems, however, a clumsy way of arriving at a urine, whose composition should be adapted to the needs of the animal, and as we have seen, the occurrence of an actual secretion of urea by the cells of the tubules takes away the necessity of assuming any such wasteful proceeding. It is probable that the actual amount of the glomerular filtrate in the 24 hours may not exceed to any large extent the actual amount of urine formed by the whole kidney in this time.

It was assumed that tubular function was mainly secretory. Barcroft and Straub (5), for instance, regarded it "*as a fair assumption that if urine appears without increased oxidation in the kidney itself, the mechanism which accounts for its appearance is a purely physical one, whereas if there is a marked increase in the metabolism of the kidney a secretory process is called into play.*"

Discussions and theories about the control of sodium excretion were divided into those that were concerned with the afferent system, which stemmed mainly from the contemplation of diseased states in humans, whereas information on efferent control was most often obtained from the isolated kidney or from deeply anesthetized, sometimes eviscerated animals. In many experiments only changes in urine flow were measured. With the benefit of hindsight, however, one can discern the origin of some of those factors that have become established variables in the control of sodium excretion. In early experiments only chloride was measured, and it was assumed that there were parallel changes in sodium excretion. In this chapter the evolution of knowledge of afferent and efferent control of sodium excretion are described separately.

SODIUM EXCRETION

Afferent Control of Sodium Excretion

Starling (50) was the first to put forward the idea that the renal excretion of salt (and water) was conditioned by the volume of body fluids, particularly the blood volume. He was trained in medicine at Guy's Hospital in London and worked with Kuhne at Heidelberg and with Rudolph Heidenhain at Breslau before becoming Professor of Physiology at University College, London. His habit of intermingling normal physiology and illness probably initiated the pathophysiological approach to disease. In addition his faith in the value of exact science to practical medicine and his recurrent conflicting wish to be directly involved in the relief of suffering were so compelling that once, if not twice, he was on the point of leaving physiology for full-time work in the wards. Starling was a large-hearted man and is described as having a "*rare courtesy and a smile of extraordinary charm and attraction.*" At the age of sixty-one he was found drowned in Kingston Harbour, Jamaica. He was buried the following day a few miles away at Halfway Tree Parish Church.

Starling suggested that the sum total of body fluids was so arranged that the blood supply to the brain was maintained at a point just equal to its need. He considered that if the blood volume was increased by a transfusion, the small vessels throughout the body would dilate to accommodate the blood; this in turn would increase filtration through the capillaries, and thus increase lymph flow and glomerular filtration, which would cause an increase in salt and water excretion. The reverse occurred with blood loss. Starling considered that the edema of heart failure was due to renal salt and water retention caused by a hemorrhage because, with a failing heart, "*the vascular bed is bled into the veins and cardiac cavities.*" He recognized therefore that changes in extracellular fluid can control blood volume and that the kidneys control the extracellular fluid volume. Starling clearly had in mind that urinary sodium and water excretion were controlled by changes in the volume of blood contained in the arteries and capillaries, not by the total volume of blood.

In 1935 Peters (38) revived the suggestion that sodium excretion might be related to the volume of circulating blood. "*It may well be that it is the fullness of the blood stream which provokes the diuretic response on the part of the kidneys.*" Again he thought it more likely that it was some change in the distribution of the blood volume that was important, rather than the total blood volume. In 1948 J.G.G. Borst [Fig. 2; (13)] also supported the concept that blood volume and urinary sodium excretion were related via changes in extracel-

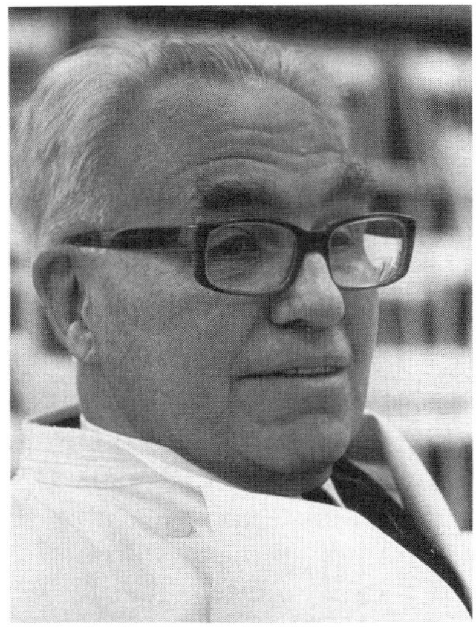

Figure 2. Jacob Geradus Gerbrant Borst (1902–1975).

lular fluid volume. He and his wife Borst de Geus worked in Amsterdam, where he was Professor of Medicine. Much of their work was performed during the occupation of Holland during World War II. They performed meticulous day-to-day electrolyte-balance studies on patients, relating the changes to the variations in jugular venous pressure measured under precise conditions. Their contribution and that of his department to the history of the control of urinary sodium excretion were of the utmost importance. Borst considered that his hypothesis was simply an extension of Starling's. The clearest account of Borst's idea was in a paper entitled *Hypertension explained by Starling: Theory of the Circulation.* Like Guyton after him, he suggested that the rise in the arterial pressure corrected a renal difficulty in excreting sodium. "*Thus a seemingly normal sodium output is maintained at the expense of the hypertension.*"

Borst believed that changes in the volume of blood in the venous circulation were important because they influenced the central venous pressure and thus the cardiac output. Borst also held that it was the cardiac output that controlled urinary sodium excretion, although how it did so was unclear. His prescient suggestions, however, were that "*blood flow in the body or to certain organs might not meet, or exceed certain requirements which would be monitored by receptors transmitting impulses via a nervous pathway, either directly to the kidney, or by the intervention of a hormone or a series of hormones.*"

Since that time there has been general agreement that blood volume, more particularly at some regional site, is an important factor in the afferent control of sodium excretion. Epstein, Post, and McDowell (19) studied patients with substantial posttraumatic arteriovenous aneurysms. Temporary closure of the fistulae by external pressure suddenly increased the blood volume on the arterial side of the circulation and was associated with a rise in urinary sodium excretion. There was no change in GFR, renal blood flow, or renal venous pressure. Therefore it was proposed that "*the renal excretion of sodium may be conditioned by the degree of filling of some portion of the arterial tree.*" However, closure of the arteriovenous fistulae caused a sudden rise in arterial pressure and a fall in heart rate. In light of what is now known about the effect of sudden changes in arterial pressure on tubular reabsorption of sodium, it looks as if the rise in sodium excretion was due, in part, directly to the rise in pressure. The fall in heart rate also demonstrates that there was an associated change in baroreceptor function. It is therefore possible that the rise in sodium excretion was also due, in part, to a change in renal nerve control of tubular sodium excretion because there is now evidence of baroreceptor control of sodium excretion via the renal nerves.

Maurice B. Strauss (Fig. 3) and his colleagues (51) suggested that the effect of posture and congestion of the head on urinary sodium excretion (32) was due to the presence of circulatory volume receptors situated within the cranium. Strauss was a physician and a physiologist who straddled the three Boston medical schools for about forty years with a genial perspicacity. He was a member of the staff of each and of the Boston Veterans Hospital. He was an expert on hematology and diseases of the kidney, and he advanced knowledge in the renal control of salt and water by performing experiments on humans. Strauss in Boston and Peters, Professor of

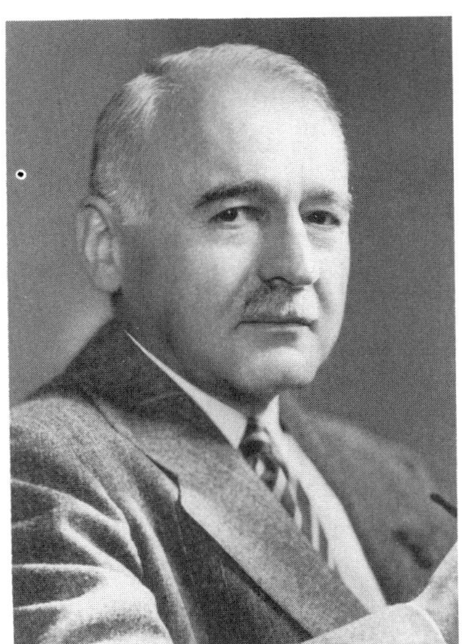

Figure 3. Maurice B. Strauss (1904–1974).

Medicine at Yale, were contemporaries who generated an interest in the control of salt and water, which enthused many of their pupils such as Welt, Seldin, and Papper, who carried on the tradition. Strauss was the subject of many of his own experiments. Collecting his nighttime urine in a plastic container kept in the lavatory made him reflect and comment on the automaticity of human behavior: he observed that often in the middle of the night, having emptied his bladder into the container, he nevertheless found himself, to his own irritation, pulling the chain as he left the lavatory.

Intrathoracic Blood Volume

The prominence of the intrathoracic blood volume in the control of urinary sodium excretion became manifest from the work of Henry et al. (27). They had first become interested in the effect of high positive- and negative-pressure breathing on renal function (18, 47). High positive-pressure breathing, which presumably tends to reduce intrathoracic blood volume, lowers the cardiac output and is associated with a fall in urine flow, sodium excretion, glomerular filtration, and renal blood flow similar to that found with an acute hemorrhage. Negative-pressure breathing, which produces an opposite but lesser effect on cardiac output and is presumably associated with an increase in intrathoracic blood volume, produces a water diuresis. A natriuresis only occurs in special circumstances (37). To locate the intrathoracic vascular receptors, Henry et al. (27) studied the effect of distension of the left auricle by inflating a balloon in the left atrium. This increased the hydrostatic pressures throughout the whole pulmonary vascular bed, including the right ventricle. The effect of this maneuver was compared with the effect of placing snares around the pulmonary veins near the hilus, which had a similar effect on the pulmonary vascular bed and right ventricle but excluded the left auricle. In the initial experiments, it was found that distension of the left auricle induced a water diuresis; sodium excretion was not measured. Subsequently it was shown that in anesthetized animals a water diuresis is usually accompanied by a modest increase in urinary sodium excretion. Later (24, 42) it was demonstrated that the rise in urinary sodium excretion accompanying left auricular distension is much greater in unanesthetized animals, when it can be demonstrated in adrenalectomized animals, even if the renal blood flow is controlled. On the other hand, in the conscious primate an increase in left atrial pressure does not alter urinary sodium excretion (though immersion up to the neck does do so).

Immersion

In 1962 Graveline and Jackson (23), who were interested in the effects of weightlessness in space, were the first to show that immersion of a person up to the neck while in a sitting position for several hours induces a substantial increase in sodium excretion. Immersion shifts blood from the lower parts of the body into the thorax, which distends the intrathoracic blood volume of the subject with his own blood, thus reproducing what occurs in acute volume expansion while avoiding all those extraneous variables, which are inherent in using an exogenous volume expander. The associated brisk rise in urinary sodium excretion has been studied by three main groups (2, 8, 20). Immersion up to the neck increases central blood volume by about 700 ml, of which 180 ml is accommodated in the heart. The central venous pressure rises by about 12–18 cm, and the intrathoracic pressure (in the esophagus) rises by about 4–5 cm. The natriuresis takes place despite the administration of large amounts of deoxycorticosterone acetate. It is important to note that most immersions last several hours and that throughout this time the increased urinary sodium excretion continues uninterruptedly, though total blood volume and extracellular fluid volume must be falling: a striking demonstration that the vascular volume, which influences the urinary excretion of sodium, is not the total blood volume.

Neural Pathways

The results of the experiments performed to delineate the afferent neural pathways that influence urinary sodium excretion following left atrial distension, blood volume expansion, and immersion are difficult to interpret (56). In dogs vagotomy and cardiac denervation abolish the natriuresis of left atrial distension. In rats spinal cord transection at the level of C_8 in one set of experiments abolished the natriuresis of blood volume expansion, whereas in another the natriuresis still occurred. In monkeys bilateral vagotomy or removal of the middle cervical ganglion down to T_6 sympathetic ganglion failed to abolish the natriuresis of immersion, but blood volume expansion after vagotomy, sinoaortic denervation, and thoracic dorsal rhizotomy produced a marked blunting of sodium (and water) excretion (39). This suggests that in anesthetized monkeys there exists a marked redundancy of afferent function. However, some confusion has been caused by failing to consider the efferent limb or limbs through which a particular afferent being studied might act. For instance, immersion is often associated with some rise in arterial pressure but a natriuretic substance also appears in urine (for review see ref. 56). It is not unreasonable to suppose that afferents from the chest might stimulate several efferent natriuretic mechanisms. For instance, it is now palpably obvious that part of the rise in urinary sodium excretion in many of these experiments may be due to the stimulating effect of atrial distension on the release of atrial natriuretic peptide (see Atrial Natriuretic Peptide, p. 220). It is also probable that a long-acting natriuretic substance, which has not yet been characterized (56), is also involved; there are no observations on the precise afferent mechanism involved in its release.

Compliance of Interstitial Space

There have been a few suggestions that urinary sodium excretion may be related to afferents originating from interstitial space, more particularly from within the head (48). These proposals have been difficult to investigate. Nevertheless, because extracellular fluid volume is related to blood volume, any factor that controls the partition of extracellular fluid between plasma and interstitial fluid should be important. The compliance of the interstitial space is one such factor. In 1974 Lucas and Floyer (33) pointed out that the ratio of plasma volume to the total extracellular fluid volume increases more significantly after bilateral nephrectomy than after a unilateral nephrectomy in which the remaining ureter is placed into the inferior vena cava. They suggested that this change may be due to the absence in the bilaterally nephrectomized animals of a substance secreted by the kidney that appears to be independent of the excretory function of the kidney but the rate of release of which is dependent on the amount of renal mass and its effective perfusion with blood. Studies on patients with chronic renal failure (31) have yielded similar results to those obtained in bilaterally nephrectomized animals.

Sodium Concentration in Cerebrospinal Fluid

The afferent mechanisms discussed in the previous sections are those concerned with changes in fluid volumes. There is, in addition, some evidence that changes in the sodium concentration of cerebrospinal fluid and hepatic arterial plasma may have an effect on urinary sodium excretion independent of any direct effect of plasma sodium concentration on the kidney. A significant natriuresis can be induced in a variety of species by experimentally raising the concentration of sodium in the cerebrospinal fluid in the brain (1). Conversely, reductions in cerebrospinal fluid sodium concentrations have an antinatriuretic effect. Unusually, in these experiments, some attempts have been made to distinguish the efferent natriuretic mechanisms involved (7), and in rats the natriuresis appears to be mediated by a hormone other than aldosterone or angiotensin II.

The concept that the liver may play a role in the afferent limb of urinary sodium excretion is based on the observation that infusions of isotonic saline cause a greater rise in urinary sodium excretion when they are given into the portal vein than when they are given into the inferior vena cava (56). There have also been some claims that the liver makes a natriuretic substance that may act as a natriuretic hormone (56). Collectively these observations arouse curiosity but are not compelling.

Efferent Control of Sodium Excretion

Before it was possible to measure glomerular filtration rate, the apparent extravagance of the kidney in filtering and then reabsorbing approximately 180 liters/day of plasma filtrate had not been envisaged. It was assumed that the volume of glomerular filtrate controlled the volume of urine and that therefore the rate of urinary excretion was mainly controlled by changes in filtration rate. The gradual recognition of the overriding importance of tubular reabsorption in the control of sodium excretion began in the early 1960s. It became clear that under physiological conditions, changes in sodium reabsorption in the proximal tubule and loop of Henle have little if any effect on urinary sodium excretion and that the only changes in tubular sodium reabsorption that affect the amount of sodium in urine are those that occur in the collecting duct (55). For instance, the natriuresis of chronic sodium loading is not accompanied by a change in proximal tubule sodium reabsorption and a natriuresis can be induced acutely with small amounts of intravenous saline without a change in proximal tubule reabsorption. It is also possible to administer large infusions of saline, hyperoncotic albumin, or whole blood in such a way that they produce the same fall in proximal tubular sodium reabsorption and yet have very different effects on urinary sodium excretion. The reason that GFR and urinary sodium excretion have so little relationship is that the amount of sodium reabsorbed from the proximal tubule and loop of Henle is directly related to the amount of sodium delivered to these parts of the nephron. In the collecting duct, however, sodium reabsorption is independent of the amount that is delivered. Instead it is related to the needs to maintain sodium balance.

Nevertheless, in an overall sense, little has changed. In the past it was considered that those variables that altered urinary sodium excretion, such as arterial and venous pressures, renal nerve activity, plasma oncotic pressure, and volume expansion, did so by altering GFR. Many of the early experiments that led to these conclusions were made on isolated kidneys (43) or isolated heart-lung-kidney preparations (4) and sometimes in eviscerated animals (10). In some of these experiments, there was no flow of urine unless the blood was diluted with saline, but these experiments demonstrated that certain physical factors do effect the flow of urine and the excretion of salt. One of the principal changes that has occurred since that time is the discovery that these physical factors do not have their effect on sodium excretion by changing GFR but by their effect on the rate of sodium reabsorption by the tubule.

Difficulties in Distinguishing Between Changes in Glomerular Filtration Rate and Changes in Tubular Reabsorption in the Control of Sodium Excretion

Attempts to distinguish between the relative importance of these two mechanisms were hindered by a variety of technical difficulties. For instance, the methods used to alter GFR also alter tubular reabsorption of sodium.

Early experiments in which it was claimed that tubular changes could occur independently of changes in GFR were based on demonstrating an unequivocal change in the excretion rate of some substance despite an unchanging quantity of that substance being filtered into the nephron. Nevertheless, these experiments were repeatedly criticized on the grounds that the techniques used to measure glomerular filtration were not sufficiently accurate to justify such claims. It was pointed out that a small change (3 ml/min) in filtration rate might be undetected but that such a change would produce a rise in filtered sodium of 420 μmol/min, which could explain a rise in sodium excretion of anything less than this. Such warnings might perhaps have been more muted if those who made them had been aware of the nephron's remarkable intrinsic automaticity and seemingly limitless capacity to adjust sodium reabsorption to the filtered load. The kidney of a normal human filters approximately 24,000 mmol of sodium/day, reabsorbs about 23,000, and yet can make a change of 1–2 mmol in the day's urinary sodium excretion. Micropuncture has now established that the bulk of sodium reabsorption occurs in the proximal tubule and ascending loop of Henle, the rate of reabsorption in both areas being instantaneously adjusted to changes in the amount of sodium delivered to them. These two areas of the nephron can therefore be considered as automatic buffers that prevent large fluctuations in the amount of sodium that is finally delivered into the collecting ducts. This facilitates the fine adjustments in sodium reabsorption made in the collecting duct, which ensure that the amount of sodium excreted in urine is that required to maintain sodium balance.

Many experiments were performed that claimed that GFR had little to do with sodium excretion (56). In particular, between 1942 and 1951, White's group showed in a series of experiments in normal and hypophysectomized dogs that the resulting low GFR in hypophysectomized dogs did not cause sodium retention, even if the animal was given deoxycorticosterone acetate in large amounts. Furthermore, raising the GFR to normal or above normal in such animals caused no increase in sodium excretion. Nevertheless, observations of this kind made little impact.

Importance of Tubular Reabsorption in Volume Control of Urinary Sodium Excretion

The point was not resolved until 1961 when we [de Wardener, Mills, Clapham, and Hayter (57)] demonstrated that, in normal dogs receiving large amounts of salt-retaining steroids and vasopressin, an infusion of saline causes a rise in urinary sodium excretion, even when GFR is substantially reduced. This experiment was carried out largely to settle a bet. At that time Ivor H. Mills and I were lecturers in Sharpey Shaeffer's Department of Medicine at St. Thomas's Hospital, London. Mills had just returned from working on aldosterone with Fred Bartter at the National Institutes of Health. Aldosterone was in short supply. Half seriously (over coffee) I suggested that aldosterone probably had little to do with urinary sodium excretion. I had been impressed by the evidence outlined in the previous section and by Relman and Schwartz's experiment in which they had administered aldosterone to normal human subjects and observed the phenomenon that became known as the "aldosterone escape phenomenon." I was also struck by the ability of patients with chronic renal failure to stay in sodium balance, though their GFR was less than 5 ml/min, and they showed no evidence of diminished steroid excretion. Mills was genuinely shocked by my suggestion. As a result we decided to work together to find out if indeed a change in urinary sodium excretion could be demonstrated despite a high concentration of aldosterone and a fall in GFR.

A balloon placed in the thoracic aorta was inflated at the same moment as a saline infusion was begun. The abdominal aortic pressure was thereby lowered to 80 mmHg, and there was an associated fall in GFR of 30 ml/min. There was also some reduction in renal blood flow. Therefore, as the saline infusion was being given, there was a marked reduction in the quantity of sodium filtered through the glomerulus. Nevertheless there was a brisk rise in sodium excretion due to a decrease in tubular reabsorption of sodium. It was clear that this fall in tubular reabsorption of sodium must have occurred because of some mechanism other than a fall in the concentration of a salt-retaining steroid. Subsequently most investigators pursued the possibility that the mechanisms responsible for the increase in sodium excretion were directly related to the dilutional effect of adding saline to the blood. Their aim was to find out if those physical factors that had been shown to have parallel effects on urinary sodium excretion and GFR could also influence tubular reabsorption of sodium.

Relatively few workers looked into the proposal put forward by Mills, Clapham, Hayter, and me (57) that at least part of the fall in tubular sodium reabsorption might be due to a change in the concentration of a circulating substance other than aldosterone. We had considered from the beginning that at least part of the rise in sodium excretion that had occurred in the thoracic balloon–saline infusion experiments must be the result of the dilutional effect of saline on the blood. To determine the importance of this dilutional effect, we performed cross-circulation experiments between a control dog and another receiving a saline infusion. Changes in hematocrit, plasma protein, and plasma sodium concentrations were the same in both dogs, but the donor dog receiving the saline had a much greater natriuresis. This difference could not be explained by differences in arterial pressure, venous pressure, *p*-aminohippuric acid clearance, and glomerular filtration rate. As a result it was proposed that the greater rise in urinary sodium excretion in the dog given saline was due to the release of a circulating substance other than aldosterone.

Volume Expansion with Equilibrated Blood

Similar cross-circulation experiments were performed by others. The results were variable (56), and it became clear that unless volume expansion could be achieved without diluting the blood, the claim that any part of the ensuing natriuresis was due to the plasma acquiring natriuretic properties other than those caused by dilution were less than totally convincing. In order to establish that the natriuretic effect of volume expansion was, at least in part, due to a change in the plasma other than dilution, it was necessary to expand the blood volume without diluting the blood and simultaneously to exclude the effect on the kidneys of alterations in renal nerve activity and arterial pressure. In 1967 these criteria were met by Bahlman et al. (3), who used two techniques to expand the blood volume in dogs without changing the blood composition. The volume-expanded dogs were given deoxycorticosterone acetate and vasopressin before the experiment. In one group of experiments, blood was circulated for at least 75 min in and out of a reservoir that initially contained Hartman's solution and 2.5% albumin. During this time the animal's blood came into equilibrium with the content of the reservoir. Blood from the reservoir was then transfused into the dog. In another group of experiments, cross-circulation between a large dog and a small dog was carried out at a rate of 200–300 ml/min. After 45 min the tube carrying blood from the small dog to the large dog was totally occluded. Blood then flowed from the large dog to the small dog for 5 min, which expanded the latter's blood volume by 40%. One kidney of the small dog had previously been denervated, and a snare had been loosely placed around the aorta above the origin of the renal arteries. As the blood volume was expanded, the aortic snare was tightened to lower abdominal aortic pressure by a few mmHg. Nevertheless there was an immediate increase in urinary sodium excretion accompanied by a rise in *p*-aminohippuric acid clearance and filtered sodium in both the innervated and denervated kidneys. It was concluded that the increase in urinary sodium excretion could not be due to a dilutional effect, a change in renal nerve activity, or a rise in arterial pressure and that thus it was the result of a change in the concentration of a circulating substance that simultaneously increased renal blood flow and GFR. Others demonstrated that the rise in urinary sodium excretion could occur even with a fall in filtered sodium (56) and concluded that the circulating substance might directly affect the capacity of the tubules to transport sodium.

As these experiments were being performed in normal animals, parallel and complimentary observations were being performed by Bricker's group (56) on the plasma of humans and animals suffering from chronic renal failure. They pointed out that in renal failure, although the number of nephrons gradually diminishes, sodium intake usually remains unchanged. Sodium balance therefore has to be maintained by increasing the amount of sodium excreted by each nephron. This is achieved by diminishing the amount of filtered sodium that is reabsorbed. Bricker's group demonstrated that extracts of plasma obtained from volume-expanded animals and from animals and humans with chronic renal failure are natriuretic and inhibit sodium transport by anuran membranes.

Intrinsic Capacity of Kidneys to Respond to a Natriuretic Stimulus

The search for a circulating natriuretic substance revealed the interesting phenomenon that the effect of a natriuretic stimulus is in part related to an alterable capacity of the kidney to respond to the stimulus. This was first demonstrated by Sonnenberg and Pearce in 1962 and then confirmed by some neat experiments by Nizet (56). He found that a transplanted kidney obtained from a sodium-loaded dog had a greater natriuresis when the blood volume of the recipient was expanded than when the kidney was obtained from a sodium-deprived animal. This phenomenon may be related to the interstitial volume of the kidney, for Lameire et al. (56) showed that in a normally fed rat the natriuresis of an acute saline administration can be prevented by lowering the arterial pressure to 70 mmHg. On the other hand, if the rat has previously been chronically salt loaded, reducing the arterial pressure does not abolish the natriuresis of acute saline volume expansion (56).

Short- and Long-Acting Natriuretic Hormones

In the next few years, it was found that acute volume expansion is associated with a change in the concentration of at least two natriuretic substances in the plasma. The effect of one is rapid in onset and of short duration; the other has a slow onset and a prolonged effect. For some years the short-acting natriuretic substance was obtained from extracts of plasma and urine, whereas the long-acting substance was demonstrable in whole plasma and was therefore less likely to be an artifact. The effect of the long-acting substance could be observed by expanding the blood volume of a rat with equilibrated blood (56). Two milliliters of blood were removed at the height of the natriuresis and centrifuged; the resultant 1 ml of plasma was injected into another anesthetized, 300-g dehydrated rat. This caused a small but significant natriuresis that began after 1 h and was still increasing 2 h after injection. That such a small amount of plasma should have this effect suggested that the natriuresis was indeed caused by an increase in the concentration of a potent natriuretic substance, as opposed to a decrease in the concentration of an antinatriuretic substance.

Atrial Natriuretic Peptides

One short-acting natriuretic substance has been extracted from the atria and has been identified and synthesized (56). It had been known since 1964 that atrial muscle cells contain large numbers of specific granules of a type that suggested a secretory role. Marie Guillemot and Hett in 1976 and de Bold in 1979 had noted that the number of granules varies inversely with salt and water intake. In 1981 de Bold, Borenstein, Veress, and Sonnenberg found that the administration of atrial extracts induces a natriuresis of very rapid onset and decay. On 28 December 1983, Flynn, de Bold, and de Bold announced the amino acid sequence of a 23-residue atrial peptide with potent natriuretic properties. Nine days later Currie et al. described the amino acid sequence and synthesis of two atrial natriuretic peptides that contain 21 and 23 amino acids, respectively. A week later Kangawa and Matsuo reported the isolation, amino acid sequence, and synthesis of a 28-amino acid peptide prepared from human atria, which only differs from the rat peptide in that a methionine replaces an isoleucine at position 12 of the molecule. The principal biochemical effect of atrial natriuretic peptides appears to be to stimulate particulate guanylate cyclase activity. The concentration of atrial natriuretic peptide in plasma is raised after one week of high sodium intake, during immersion, in heart failure, in renal failure, during paroxysmal tachycardia, in essential hypertension, and in the spontaneously hypertensive rat and the Dahl hypertensive rat. The cause of the natriuresis is not understood. Atrial natriuretic peptides have no effect on sodium transport in isolated tubules nor do they inhibit Na^+-K^+-ATPase as assayed on purified preparations of Na^+-K^+-ATPase, erythrocyte Na^+-K^+-ATPase, or with cytochemical bioassays. On the other hand they are vascular vasodilators, particularly of the renal medullary vessels. It is possible therefore that the acute natriuresis induced by an acute injection is due to a rise in hydrostatic vascular pressure around the collecting ducts. There are receptors for atrial natriuretic peptide in the glomeruli and collecting duct. If isolated segments of these two sites are incubated in a fluid medium containing natriuretic peptides, they (in contrast with the other parts of the nephron) can be shown to secrete cGMP in increased amounts. However, there is as yet no obvious connection between this phenomenon and sodium reabsorption.

It is possible that in addition to the direct effect of the atrial natriuretic peptide on kidneys, the peptide may be responsible for a natriuresis of slow onset by means of its documented inhibitory effect on renin and aldosterone secretion. The exact physiological role of atrial natriuretic peptide has still to be delineated. There is some confusion about the afferent signal responsible for the increase of atrial natriuretic peptide concentration in plasma. The acute rise in left auricular pressure produced by inflating a balloon within the auricle induces a brisk rise in plasma atrial natriuretic peptide level, whether or not the animal is vagotomized or the heart is denervated, but vagotomy or cardiac denervation prevent a rise in urinary sodium excretion. Perhaps therefore the rise in urinary sodium excretion associated with left auricular distension is not so much related to the effect of atrial natriuretic peptides but to the presence of other natriuretic substances or vagotomy interferes with the kidney's ability to respond to atrial natriuretic peptide.

In addition there are the observations of Linden and his colleagues (56) that left atrial distension in dogs endows the plasma with an ability to inhibit the flow of fluid of the isolated Malpighian tubule from the blood-sucking insect *Rhodnius prolixus*. The excretory organs of this insect consist of four Malpighian tubules in the coelomic cavity that open into the cloaca. After a blood meal, unwanted sodium, potassium, and water (which are absorbed from the gut into the coelomic cavity) are actively secreted from the cavity into the lumina of the Malpighian tubules, and so to the exterior. Thus inhibition of active sodium and potassium transport in the Malpighian tubules of this insect diminishes urine flow and sodium excretion, whereas in the mammalian nephron inhibition of cation transport increases urine flow and sodium excretion. In *Rhodnius prolixus* the active-transport processes in the Malpighian tubules are under the control of a hormone produced by neural tissue in the upper mesothorax. Plasma from dogs undergoing left atrial distension inhibits the active-transport process in isolated Malpighian tubules. This inhibition is due to an increase in the plasma concentration of a humoral agent with a molecular weight below 1,800 daltons (41). It is not known from where it originates. In contrast with the atrial natriuretic peptide, this substance has not been detected in the plasma of vagotomized dogs.

Plasma Na^+-K^+-ATPase Inhibitor

The finding that plasma acquires increased natriuretic properties with volume expansion led to experiments that attempted to demonstrate the presence of a circulating sodium-transport inhibitor in vitro following volume expansion with equilibrated blood. The initial studies were carried out in 1970 by Clarkson et al. and by Buckalew and Lancaster (56). The first group estimated the intracellular sodium and potassium concentrations of renal tubules incubated in fresh whole plasma obtained from dogs before and after expansion of the blood volume with equilibrated blood. There was a rise in intracellular sodium and a fall in intracellular potassium. Buckalew and Lancaster measured the effect on the short-circuit current of toad bladder and of ultrafiltrates and dialysates from plasma obtained from dogs that had escaped the effect of mineralocorticoid administration. Both groups found that plasma taken after either blood-volume expansion or escape from mineralocorticoid inhibits sodium transport.

During the history of the search for the natriuretic hormone, an assumption began to be made that the increase in the ability of plasma to cause a natriuresis and its increased capacity to inhibit sodium transport were due to a change in the concentration of one and the same substance. It stemmed mainly from the fact that in extraction procedures the natriuretic and sodium-transport–inhibitory activities were found in the same fraction. This assumption was so widely accepted that in one published and refereed paper it was stated that the natriuretic capacity of an extract was measured on frog skin. However, in view of the observation that a powerful sodium-transport inhibitor such as ouabain does not cause natriuresis (except in toxic doses), that many workers who have attempted to purify the natriuretic substance only assess the sodium-transport–inhibitory activity of their material, and the recent finding that atrial natriuretic peptides do not inhibit sodium transport, it now seems more prudent not to assume that the hormonal components of the natriuresis that accompanies volume expansion are necessarily due to a change in the concentration of the same hormonal substance as that responsible for the increased sodium-transport–inhibitory activity.

From 1976 onward it was shown that the increased sodium-transport–inhibitory powers of plasma after volume expansion may be due to its capacity to inhibit Na^+-K^+-ATPase as measured with a wide variety of living tissues and purified extracts of Na^+-K^+-ATPase (56). There is some evidence that the plasma Na^+-K^+-ATPase inhibitor may arise from the hypothalamus. Several groups have used a variety of methods to purify and extract such an inhibitor from the hypothalamus. Most groups identify their material by its ability to inhibit red cell Na^+-K^+-ATPase, purified preparations of Na^+-K^+-ATPase, and its capacity to displace ouabain from the surface of red cells, or to cross-react with digoxin antibody. However, a variety of irrelevant endogenous substances have these properties. Such tests therefore cannot distinguish whether the inhibitory substance being extracted from the hypothalamus has any relation to the inhibitor in the plasma. However, one group using a cytochemical bioassay has found that the ability of plasma to inhibit Na^+-K^+-ATPase of fresh guinea pig proximal tubules at 4–6 min has a remarkable selectivity in that many plasma substances that inhibit purified preparations of Na^+-K^+-ATPase (such as vanadate, dehydroepiandrosterone, linoleic acid, and oleic acids) have no effect on fresh guinea pig kidney at 4 and 6 min (21). Moreover the concentration of this cytochemically bioassayable substance in plasma rises with volume expansion and diminishes with sodium depletion. The largest quantity of cytochemically assayable material is present in the hypothalamus, where again the concentration rises with dietary salt loading. The highest quantities are found in the hypothalamus of the spontaneously hypertensive strain of rat. The apparent selectivity of the cytochemical bioassay and the finding that during extraction procedures the substance in the plasma and hypothalamus appears in the same fractions and shares the same properties suggests that the Na^+-K^+-ATPase inhibitor in plasma and the hypothalamic extract are the same. It is not known if the Na^+-K^+-ATPase inhibitor is natriuretic.

Antinatriuretic Hormones

Aldosterone

In 1927 Bauman and Kurland were the first to draw attention to the fall in serum sodium concentration after adrenalectomy in animals; at about the same time it was reported that the administration of sodium chloride to such animals ameliorates their condition (45). A few years later Loeb prolonged the survival of patients with Addison's disease by giving them large quantities of salt by mouth. There was some confusion at first about whether adrenal cortical extracts contained one or two substances, one of which affects carbohydrate and protein metabolism and the other affects sodium and potassium balance. Until 1950 some investigators still considered it unnecessary to hypothesize the existence of two substances. However, after 11-deoxycorticotrophin was synthesized (the sodium-retaining capacity of which was much greater than cortisol), naturally occurring endogenous substances with a similar powerful sodium-retaining effect were sought. In 1950 Deming and Leutscher (15) were the first to demonstrate the presence of increased quantities of a potent sodium-retaining substance in the urine of patients suffering from generalized edema. Subsequently they demonstrated that it was a steroid. Leutscher's group also showed an increased urinary output of this substance in the urine of normal subjects on a low-sodium diet and that it was absent from the urine of patients with Addison's disease. The aldosterone molecule was identified in 1954. By 1970 micropuncture techniques had established that aldosterone increases sodium reabsorption in the distal end of the distal tubule and in the collecting duct, which is why it affects urinary sodium excretion.

Angiotensin II

In 1898 Robert Tigerstedt (Fig. 4) and Bergman (53) were the first to demonstrate that kidneys contain a hypertensive substance. At that time and for many years afterward, this work was unnoticed. Tigerstedt, who came from Finland, was Professor of Physiology at Stockholm and had been a pupil of Ludwig's at Helsingfors. His principle work was on the physiology of muscle and nerve, circulation, and respiration. He died in 1923 many years before the importance of his work was finally recognized. It was not until nearly seventy years after his first experiment that angiotensin was identified and structured. It was soon found that angiotensin II stimulates an increased secretion of aldosterone from the adrenal gland, but at

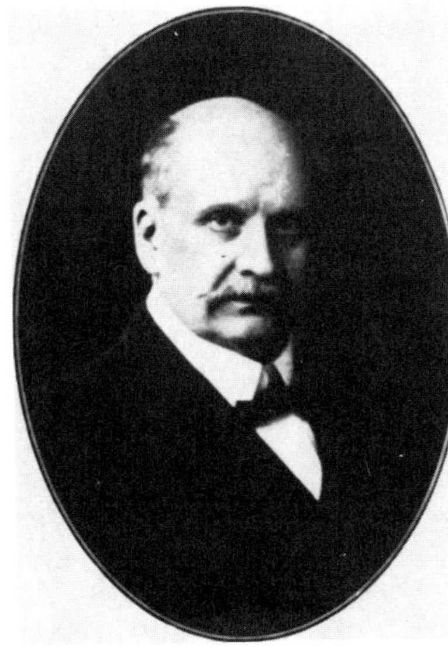

Figure 4. Robert Tigerstedt (1853–1923).

first it was believed that angiotensin II itself was natriuretic. This stemmed from observations made with the administration of pharmacological amounts of angiotensin that induced a brisk rise in arterial pressure. The finding that small infusions of angiotensin lower urinary sodium excretion was thought to be due to the associated fall in renal blood flow and GFR. More recent evidence, however, suggests that angiotensin II does have a direct effect on sodium reabsorption. This has been shown by infusing angiotensin II in sufficiently small amounts to cause diminished sodium excretion with no consistent change in GFR or renal blood flow. It has been shown by Harris and Young (25) that microperfusion with low doses of angiotensin II (10^{-12}–10^{-10} M) of the capillaries around a proximal tubule increases sodium reabsorption from the tubule, though higher doses (3×10^{-7}–10^{-6} M) inhibit sodium reabsorption.

Effect of Intrarenally Produced Substances on Urinary Sodium Excretion

Kinins, prostaglandins, and dopamine are potent local renal vasodilators manufactured by the kidney. In general renal vasodilators are natriuretic. The role of these substances in the normal control of urinary sodium excretion is to set the scene for those factors that do control urinary sodium excretion. Their absence reduces renal blood flow, particularly of the medulla, and reduces the effect of natriuretic stimuli.

Peritubular Physical Factors

The peritubular physical factors include plasma oncotic pressure, peritubular capillary hydrostatic pressure, hematocrit, peritubular interstitial space, and the renal nerves.

Effect of Hydrostatic Pressure on Sodium Excretion

SODIUM EXCRETION

Arterial Pressure

The natriuretic effect of a sudden rise in arterial perfusion pressure to an isolated kidney was a well-recognized phenomenon in 1909 when Starling wrote his monograph *Fluids of the Body* (50). He assumed it to be a self-evident truth that this must be due to a "*rise in pressure in the glomerular capillaries.*" In 1917 Arthur R. Cushny stated, "*No other gland is known to respond so readily to changes in the blood pressure*" (14). Again it was acute changes in pressure that were being described. Blake; Wegria, Ward, and Frank; Shipley and Study; and Selkurt, all of whom controlled the perfusion pressure to a kidney in situ, again demonstrated that urinary sodium excretion is directly related to acute changes in perfusion pressure but that, within the range of pressures that cover circulatory autoregulation of renal blood flow (100–180 mmHg), large changes in sodium excretion appear without any significant change in GFR or renal blood flow (55). Earley and Friedler and their colleagues in the 1960s finally produced evidence unequivocally demonstrating that the acute effect of pressure on sodium excretion was not due to changes in GFR (55). They first induced unilateral vasodilatation by renal artery infusions of acetylcholine or bradykinin, which induced a large increase in renal blood flow and sodium excretion without any consistent change in GFR. Angiotensin or noradrenaline was then infused intravenously to raise the systemic arterial pressure to both kidneys. This rise was accompanied by a further substantial rise in sodium excretion from the vasodilated kidney while the renal blood flow fell and GFR did not change significantly. The other kidney, which was not being infused with a vasodilator, also had a reduction in renal blood flow, no significant change in GFR, and no change in urinary sodium excretion. Earley and Friedler concluded that the rise in urinary sodium excretion in the vasodilated kidney was due to the transmission of hydrostatic pressure to some distal portion of the renal vasculature and that it was this local increase in pressure that causes the fall in tubular reabsorption of sodium. They further suggested that the increase in peritubular capillary pressure probably increases the interstitial volume of the kidney and that it was this effect of the rise in pressure that in some way influences sodium reabsorption. During the 1970s and more recently, it has been established by micropuncture in situ that acute increases in hydrostatic pressure diminish sodium reabsorption in the proximal tubule, the loop of Henle, and the collecting duct.

Earley and Friedler's suggestion that the effect of hydrostatic pressure on tubular sodium reabsorption is due more to its effect on the interstitial space than to a direct effect of the pressure on the tubule has been supported indirectly by Helman et al. (26). They found that in vitro an increase in bath hydrostatic pressure on the cortical collecting duct enhances the transtubular potential difference (and presumably, therefore, active sodium transport). Thus the effect of a change in a peritubular hydrostatic pressure imposed on a tubule in vitro is opposite to the effect found in vivo. Some other unexplained anomalies can be demonstrated with pharmacological agents. The systemic administration of prostaglandin E, acetylcholine, and bradykinin cause a brisk rise in the hydrostatic pressure of the peritubular capillaries of the proximal tubule but no change in sodium reabsorption (30). Nevertheless there is a rise in urinary sodium excretion, another illustration of the insignificance of proximal tubule function in sodium excretion.

A persistent change in arterial pressure, particularly a persistent rise, does not have any evident effect on urinary sodium excretion. In other words, patients with essential hypertension show no evidence of combating a persistent tendency to lose sodium. The explanation is that, in contrast with an acute rise in arterial pressure, a persistent rise in arterial pressure is not transmitted to the peritubular venous capillaries. The most direct evidence of this protective phenomenon is that the renal vein wedge pressure in patients with essential hypertension is not raised (58). The mechanism responsible for this rise in vascular resistance upstream of the peritubular venous capillaries is not understood. It is probable that it is directly due to the rise in arterial pressure, but it cannot be related to circulatory autoregulation, in which an acute rise in arterial pressure induces a rapid increase in vascular resistance as a direct result of the effect of the raised pressure on the vascular smooth muscle. Circulatory autoregulation occurs within a few seconds of an acute rise in pressure, but it does not prevent the rise in urinary sodium excretion that occurs with an acute rise in arterial pressure. There is one mechanism in arterial hypertension that increases vascular resistance but is unrelated to a direct effect of the rise in perfusion pressure. This has been shown in an experiment in which a partially occluding clip is placed on one renal artery while the other kidney is left intact. When the animal became hypertensive, the isolated, unclipped kidney, which had been perfused by the high pressure, had (as expected) a pressure-natriuresis curve that was shifted to the right; that is, a higher perfusion pressure was needed to obtain the same urinary sodium excretion rate as that obtained with lower pressures in a control kidney removed from a normotensive animal (52). Unexpectedly, however, the pressure-natriuresis curve of the isolated clipped kidney that had not been perfused at a high pressure was shifted even farther to the right. Whatever the mechanism responsible, it is clear that a kidney in a hypertensive animal may acquire a right shift of its pressure-natriuresis curve that is independent of a direct effect on the arterial pressure on the kidney.

Renal Venous Pressure

The most important point about the relation of urinary sodium excretion to renal venous pressure is that, because of certain sphincterlike organs in the renal venous system, intrarenal venous pressure is normally about 16–18 mmHg. Hence any rise in central venous pressure to a level less than this has no effect on intrarenal venous pressure.

Earlier experiments demonstrated that a rise in renal venous pressure causes a fall in urinary sodium excretion and that if the rise in pressure is not too great there is no accompanying change in GFR or renal blood flow. In later experiments, however, it was found that a rise in renal venous pressure may diminish sodium reabsorption and cause a rise in urinary sodium excretion despite a fall in GFR and renal blood flow. This remarkable discrepancy was partially explained by Walters and Salhut (30), who found that, whereas a rise in renal venous pressure raises urinary sodium excretion in an oliguric dog, it lowers it in a saline-loaded dog. They pointed out that the earlier experiments were performed in animals given saline presumably to ensure a satisfactory urine flow. The cause of this difference between oliguric and saline-loaded animals is due to a difference in response of the loop of Henle (30) to the rise in venous pressure. In euvolemic rats the rise in pressure decreases sodium reabsorption by the loop, whereas in saline-expanded rats it causes an increase in reabsorption. This increase in sodium reabsorption is apparently due to a rise in the intratubular hydrostatic pressure of the loop of Henle, suggesting that in saline-loaded rats the rise in renal venous pressure obstructs the tubule. In other words, although a rise in renal venous pressure increases peritubular hydrostatic capillary pressure in both oliguric and saline-loaded rats, the diminution in sodium reabsorption that this causes is offset in saline-loaded animals by the obstructive effect of the rise in renal venous pressure on the flow of tubular fluid through the loop of Henle, which increases sodium reabsorption.

Effect of Plasma Oncotic Pressure on Urinary Sodium Excretion

The infusion of hypo- or hyperoncotic solutions systemically or into the renal artery can with few exceptions alter urinary sodium reabsorption and, more particularly, proximal tubular sodium reabsorption. There are also numerous observations that the addition of saline or albumin to the blood flowing to an isolated kidney perfused by a heart-lung preparation or by a pump oxygenator causes a change in the urinary excretion of sodium. These observations span nearly eighty years, starting with those of Barcroft and Straub in 1910 (5). In accordance with their experiments, there have been many observations on the isolated proximal tubule, which on the whole agree that proximal tubule sodium reabsorption is directly related to extratubular oncotic pressure. It is to be noted, however, that the effect of peritubular protein concentration on reabsorption from the proximal tubule perfused in vitro depends on some property of the tubule wall that changes when distension occurs; the effect of oncotic pressure on sodium reabsorption disappears with increasing distension (40).

On the other hand, perfusion of the peritubular capillaries of a proximal tubule in situ does not have any effect on proximal tubule sodium reabsorption. It is true that in the earlier in situ studies performed with various artificial solutions such as Ringer's, which contain bovine albumin, the peritubular oncotic pressure was sometimes found to be directly related to proximal tubule sodium reabsorption. Later in vivo experiments, however, in which it was found that proximal tubule sodium reabsorption was unaffected by changes in peritubular capillary oncotic pressure, were performed with concentrated or protein-free rat plasma. One interesting technical point emerged in these later studies: the osmolality (as opposed to the oncotic pressure) of the peritubular capillary perfusate must be constant because it was found that a change of as little as 10 mosmol/kg H_2O could cause a substantial change in sodium reabsorption (28). There is little evidence of the effect of plasma oncotic pressure on other parts of the nephron except for an important observation by Schwartz and Burg, who observed that the addition of albumin to the bath fluid had no effect on transepithelial voltage or lumen-to-bath sodium transport of the isolated collecting duct (46). If peritubular oncotic pressure in vitro does not influence sodium transport in the collecting duct, it is difficult to envisage why changes in the plasma oncotic pressure of blood in the renal artery should affect urinary sodium excretion in vivo. Overall, these conflicting observations in the proximal tubule and collecting duct are difficult to interpret. It is probable that oncotic pressure does have an effect on the collecting duct in situ and that this is brought about by a change in the periductal interstitial space.

Clinically, changes in plasma oncotic pressure have no detectable effect on overall sodium balance. Large reductions in plasma albumin, which are often associated with large increases in GFR, should cause a tendency to lose sodium, but on the contrary they usually accompany a gross diminution in sodium excretion and the accumulation of much edema. Conversely, as the plasma albumin then rises, which should cause a greater tendency to retain sodium, there is usually a massive natriuresis.

Effect of Changes in Hematocrit on Urinary Sodium Excretion

When changes in hematocrit are induced without a simultaneous change in blood volume or plasma oncotic pressure, most investigators have failed to find any effect of hematocrit on urinary sodium excretion. Schrier and Earley, however, demonstrated an inverse relationship between hematocrit and sodium excretion. They suggested that this is due to changes in blood viscosity, which they considered caused changes in vascular resistance and therefore alterations in peritubular capillary hydrostatic pressure (55).

Effect of Plasma Sodium Concentration on Urinary Sodium Excretion

On the whole the evidence suggests that changes in plasma sodium concentration and urinary sodium excretion are directly related. Blythe and Welt (54) described an ingenious experiment that distinguished this effect from the simultaneous effect of changes in GFR and plasma oncotic pressure, which usually accompany a change in plasma sodium concentration. A 30-min control period, during which a balloon was inflated in the thoracic aorta of a dog, was followed by the release of the balloon. At this point a hypotonic infusion was given intravenously, which made it possible to study the effect on sodium reabsorption of lowering plasma sodium concentration while keeping filtered sodium relatively unchanged. During the hypotonic saline infusion, urinary excretion of sodium decreased and sodium reabsorption rose despite an increase in arterial pressure, an expansion of the extracellular fluid volume, and a slight fall in GFR, all of which would tend to cause a diminution of tubular sodium reabsorption. Thus a low plasma sodium concentration increases sodium reabsorption, a conclusion in agreement with several other workers who have suggested that a high plasma sodium concentration decreases sodium reabsorption. These observations are consistent with those of Holzgreve and Schrier (28), who found that changes of as little as 10 mosmol/kg H_2O in the osmolality of the fluids used to perfuse the peritubular capillaries caused a profound effect on sodium reabsorption from the proximal tubule.

Effect of Renal Nerves

In 1859 Claude Bernard (10) was the first to describe an effect of the renal nerves on urine flow. Having noted that "*le petit splanchnique se rend directement dans le rein en suivant les vaisseaux*," he dissected down to the splanchnic nerve in an anesthetized dog in which no urine was flowing. Urine appeared on cutting the splanchnic nerve.

For the next century the effect of denervation on renal function and sodium excretion was bedeviled by the fact that some workers performed their experiments on anesthetized animals, whereas others worked on conscious animals. Not surprisingly they obtained different results. It was eventually demonstrated that anesthesia induces a renal vasoconstriction and a reduction of urinary sodium excretion, which can be prevented or abolished by renal denervation. It was therefore realized that during anesthesia denervation does not cause a rise in urinary sodium excretion; it reverses a fall (11). As with all the other factors that influence sodium excretion, it was initially believed that the fall in urinary sodium excretion that occurred with anesthetically induced renal nerve stimulation was due to the associated reduction in GFR. Bonjour et al. (12) were the first to demonstrate that the changes in sodium excretion that occur with manipulation of the renal nerves can take place independently of simultaneous changes in filtration rate and therefore that renal nerves might influence tubular reabsorption of sodium directly. Smythe et al. (49) and Gill and Bartter (22), using either norepinephrine infusions or guanethidine blockade, had come to the same conclusion, but it was difficult to decide whether the change in tubular reabsorption was due primarily to some direct action on sodium transport mechanism of the cell or was secondary to a change in renal hemodynamics that alters peritubular hydrostatic pressure. For instance, it was shown that infusions of norepinephrine cause a redistribution of blood flow from the cortex to the outer medulla, and such a redistribution was claimed by Barger (6) to be responsible for changes in sodium excretion. Whatever the merits of this hypothesis, there is now no doubt that catecholamines do have a direct action on sodium transport. This has been demonstrated on frog skin and in isolated proximal tubules (9). Di Bona (16) and colleagues have shown that low-level stimulation applied experimentally to the renal nerves induces significant decreases in urinary sodium excretion without any significant change in glomerular filtration, renal blood flow, or intrarenal distribution of blood flow. Conversely some experiments in which sympathetic nerve activity is reduced by left atrial distension or by stimulation of the stellate ganglion have also been performed. Both procedures increase sodium excretion with no change in filtration rate or renal blood flow. However, now that it is known that atrial distension induces a rise in plasma atrial natriuretic peptide, the first group of these experiments is possibly less relevant than the second.

Overall, therefore, there seems little doubt that renal nerves influence urinary sodium excretion. The fact that a transplanted kidney handles sodium excretion perfectly adequately should not be construed as indicating that renal nerves are not significantly involved in the physiological regulation of sodium balance. In normally innervated kidneys, the reduction of urinary sodium excretion associated with chronic sodium depletion is certainly due in part to the effect of the renal nerves; presumably in their absence, the smooth regulation of sodium excretion is due to the multiplicity of other factors that control sodium excretion.

Influence of Solute Output on Urinary Sodium Excretion

SODIUM EXCRETION

The effect of an increase in solute output on urine flow was first studied by Knowlton (29) and by Dreyer and Verney (17) in the first and second decades of this century; they used sodium sulfate, urea, or phlorizin to block glucose reabsorption in isolated kidneys. It was established that the resultant increase in urine flow is unrelated to a change in renal blood flow. This diuretic and natriuretic phenomenon, which has come to be known as an osmotic diuresis, is now often studied with mannitol as the diuretic agent. The mechanisms whereby an osmotic diuresis influences sodium excretion in the proximal tubule have been unraveled (54), but thereafter they are less clear cut.

In the proximal tubule, the fluid remains isosmotic to plasma under all conditions, including the intravenous infusion of mannitol. In normal circumstances, therefore, the concentration of sodium in the tubular fluid remains the same or just below that of plasma. However, during an infusion of mannitol, the intratubular sodium concentration in the proximal tubule fluid decreases progressively while the osmolality of the fluid remains isosmotic because it contains the unabsorbable mannitol. The active transfer of sodium out of the tubule tends to lower the osmolality of the fluid within the tubule, and because the proximal tubule is unable to sustain an osmotic gradient, water immediately begins to follow the sodium out of the tubule; hence the fluid returns to the isosmotic state. Nevertheless the loss of fluid from the tubule lumen raises the concentration of the unabsorbed mannitol, so isosmolality is now associated with a low sodium concentration. At sodium gradients of 30–50 mM at the end of the proximal tubule, it is probable that no further net transport of sodium out of the fluid can take place. Nevertheless the evidence suggests that sodium continues to be actively pumped out of the tubule lumen into the intercellular canals at a normal rate. However, at high sodium concentration gradients across the tubule wall, diffusion of sodium from intracellular canals back into the tubule lumen (via the tight functions) then equals the active transfer of sodium out of the tubule lumen. At this point net sodium reabsorption from the proximal tubule ceases long before the normal amount of sodium has been removed from the tubule fluid, and the remaining amount of sodium and water in the tubule fluid is delivered into the loop of Henle. Evidence in favor of this sequence of events is that oxygen consumption in dog kidney is the same both before and after mannitol infusion. In all other situations in which there is a change in urinary sodium excretion, sodium reabsorption and oxygen consumption parallel each other. The lack of parallelism between oxygen consumption and apparent sodium reabsorption during an osmotic diuresis suggests strongly, therefore, that true active reabsorption of sodium is unchanged and that the apparent reduction in sodium reabsorption is due to backdiffusion.

Because the descending limb of Henle is freely permeable to water but relatively impermeable to sodium chloride and is surrounded by a hyperosmolar interstitium, some of the excess fluid that is delivered into the descending loop of Henle with an osmotic diuresis diffuses into the interstitial space. However, the fall in the osmolality of the interstitium increases medullary blood flow, which greatly reduces the hyperosmolality of the interstitial space. This in turn reduces the amount of water that diffuses out of the tubule, and thus much of the water and all of the excess sodium that come into the descending loop of Henle pass into the impermeable ascending limb of Henle, the main function of which is to reabsorb chloride and sodium and prevent the resorption of water. During an osmotic diuresis, however, the reabsorption of chloride (and consequently of sodium) is impaired for reasons that are not at all clear. Therefore much of the water and sodium chloride that enter into the ascending limb of Henle travel into the distal tubule and collecting duct as a large flow of hypotonic fluid. This overwhelms the limited reabsorbing capacity of these two sites, which are normally geared to the reabsorption of much smaller amounts of sodium, with the result that large amounts of sodium appear in the urine.

Unidentified Intrarenal Changes That Influence Urinary Sodium Excretion

The fluctuating intrinsic ability of the kidney to respond to a natriuretic stimulus has been discussed earlier. An intrinsic abnormality in the kidney's handling of sodium occurs in the nephrotic syndrome and in essential hypertension. In the nephrotic syndrome, the kidney's increased reabsorption of sodium appears to be due to a local change in the kidney, which may be secondary to the large amounts of protein that are reabsorbed and digested by the tubules. Sodium retention often occurs despite a markedly raised GFR. No specific histological change accompanies this acquired abnormality.

Patients with essential hypertension and rats with hereditary hypertension have a congenital increase in sodium reabsorption in the proximal tubule. In humans this is evident as a low lithium- to creatinine-clearance ratio. Because lithium is only reabsorbed in the proximal tubule, the lower the clearance, the greater the reabsorption. The same genetic abnormality has been demonstrated with micropuncture in the spontaneously hypertensive rat by placing isotopically labeled sodium in the early part of the proximal tubule. Sodium reabsorption was assessed from the amount that appeared in the urine. It was found that when labeled sodium was placed into the distal end of the proximal tubule, the same amount appeared in the urine of the spontaneously hypertensive rat as in the urine of its normotensive control, whereas when the label was placed into the beginning of the proximal tubule significantly less appeared in the urine of the former.

Conclusion

Many mechanisms control the urinary excretion of sodium. The precise way in which even well-known factors such as the arterial pressure, the oncotic pressure, and the renal nerves operate are still under investigation. In addition there are other mechanisms, the presence of which has been detected, but either their nature or their physiological importance is unclear. These include angiotensin II, atrial natriuretic peptide, the long-acting natriuretic hormone, the plasma's ability to inhibit Na^+-K^+-ATPase, those physiologically undetectable intrarenal changes in some renal diseases that cause intense retention of sodium, and the genetic abnormality of the proximal tubule in essential hypertension.

SODIUM EXCRETION

BIBLIOGRAPHY

1. Andersson, B. Regulation of body fluids. *Annu. Rev. Physiol.* 39: 185–200, 1977.
2. Arborelius, M., U. I. Balldin, B. Lilja, and C. E. G. Lundgren. Hemodynamic changes in man during immersion with the head above the water. *Aerospace Med.* 43: 592–598, 1972.
3. Bahlmann, J., S. J. McDonald, M. G. Ventom, and H. E. de Wardener. The effect on urinary sodium excretion of blood volume expansion without changing the composition of the blood in the dog. *Clin. Sci.* 32: 403–413, 1967.
4. Bainbridge, F. A., and C. L. Evans. The heart, lung, kidney preparation. *J. Physiol. Lond.* 48: 278–286, 1914.
5. Barcroft, J., and H. Straub. The secretion of urine. *J. Physiol. Lond.* 41: 145–167, 1910.
6. Barger, A. C. Renal hemodynamic factors in congestive heart failure. *Ann. NY Acad. Sci.* 139: 276–284, 1966.
7. Beasley, D., and R. L. Malvin. Role of natriuretic factor in central nervous system (CNS)-induced natriuresis (42044). *Proc. Soc. Exp. Biol. Med.* 178: 575–579, 1985.
8. Behn, C., O. H. Gauer, K. Kirsch, and P. Eckert. Effects of sustained intrathoracic vascular distension on body fluid distribution and renal excretion in man. *Pfluegers Arch.* 313: 123–135, 1969.
9. Bello-Reuss, E. Effect of catecholamines on fluid reabsorption by the isolated proximal convoluted tubule. *Am. J. Physiol.* 238 (*Renal Fluid Electrolyte Physiol.* 7): F347–F352, 1980.
10. Bernard, C. *Leçons sur les propriétés physiologiques et les altérations pathologiques des liquides de l'organisme.* Paris: J. B. Baillière et Fils, 1859, p. 171–176.
11. Berne, R. M. Hemodynamics and sodium excretion of denervated kidney in anesthetized and unanesthetized dog. *Am. J. Physiol.* 171: 148–158, 1952.
12. Bonjour, J.-P., P. C. Churchill, and R. L. Malvin. Change of tubular reabsorption of sodium and water after renal denervation in the dog. *J. Physiol. Lond.* 204: 571–582, 1969.
13. Borst, J. G. G. The maintenance of an adequate cardiac output by the

regulation of the urinary excretion of water and sodium chloride; an essential factor in the genesis of oedema. *Acta Med. Scand.* 130: Suppl. 207: 1–71, 1948.
14. Cushny, A. R. *The Secretion of Urine.* London: Longmans Green, 1917.
15. Deming, Q. B., and J. A. Leutscher. Bioassay of desoxycorticosterone-like material in urine. *Proc. Soc. Exp. Biol. Med.* 73: 171–175, 1950.

16. Di Bona, G. F. Neural control of renal tubular sodium reabsorption in the dog. *Federation Proc.* 37: 1214–1217, 1978.
17. Dreyer, N. B., and E. B. Verney. The relative importance of the factors concerned in the formation of the urine. *J. Physiol. Lond.* 57: 451–456, 1923.
18. Drury, D. R., J. P. Henry, and J. Goodman. The effects of continuous pressure breathing on kidney function. *J. Clin. Invest.* 26: 945–951, 1947.
19. Epstein, F. H., R. S. Post, and M. McDowell. The effect of an arteriovenous fistula on renal hemodynamics and electrolyte excretion. *J. Clin. Invest.* 32: 233–241, 1953.
20. Epstein, M., and T. Saruta. Effect of water immersion on renin-aldosterone and renal sodium handling in normal man. *J. Appl. Physiol.* 31: 368–374, 1971.
21. Fenton, S., E. M. Clarkson, G. A. MacGregor, J. Alaghband-Zadeh, and H. E. de Wardener. An assay of the capacity of biological fluids to stimulate renal glucose-6-phosphate dehydrogenase activity in vitro as a marker of their ability to inhibit sodium potassium-dependent adenosine triphosphatase activity. *J. Endocrinol.* 94: 99–110, 1982.
22. Gill, J. R., and F. C. Bartter. Adrenergic nervous system in sodium metabolism. II. Effects of guanethidine on the renal response to sodium deprivation in normal man. *N. Engl. J. Med.* 275: 1466–1471, 1966.
23. Graveline, D. E., and M. M. Jackson. Diuresis associated with prolonged water immersion. *J. Appl. Physiol.* 17: 519–524, 1962.
24. Hamilton, W. F., J. O. Davis, D. S. Howell, R. G. Ellison, E. E. Hague, and W. J. Brown, Jr. Experimental mitral stenosis and ascites formation. *Am. J. Physiol.* 190: 500–502, 1957.
25. Harris, P. J., and J. A. Young. Dose-dependent stimulation and inhibition of proximal tubular sodium reabsorption by angiotensin II in the rat kidney. *Pfluegers Arch.* 367: 295–297, 1977.
26. Helman, S. I., J. J. Grantham, and M. B. Burg. Effect of vasopressin on electrical resistance of renal cortical collecting tubules. *Am. J. Physiol.* 220: 1825–1832, 1971.
27. Henry, J. P., O. H. Gauer, and J. L. Reeves. Evidence of the atrial location of receptors influencing urine flow. *Circ. Res.* 4: 85–90, 1956.
28. Holzgreve, H., and R. W. Schrier. Variation of proximal tubular reabsorptive capacity by volume expansion and aortic constriction during constancy of peritubular capillary protein concentration in rat kidney. *Pfluegers Arch.* 356: 73–86, 1975.
29. Knowlton, F. P. The influence of colloids on diuresis. *J. Physiol. Lond.* 43: 219–231, 1911.
30. Knox, F. G., J. I. Mertz, J. C. Burnett, and A. Hapamati. Role of hydrostatic and oncotic pressures in renal sodium reabsorption. *Circ. Res.* 52: 491–500, 1983.
31. Koomans, H. A., J. C. Roos, E. J. Mees, and I. M. K. Delawi. Sodium

balance in renal failure. A comparison of patients with normal subjects under extremes of sodium intake. *Hypertension* 7: 714–721, 1985.
32. LEWIS, J. M., R. M. BUIE, S. M. SEVIER, and T. R. HARRISON. The effect of posture and of congestion of the head on sodium excretion in normal subjects. *Circulation* 2: 822–827, 1950.
33. LUCAS, J., and M. A. FLOYER. Changes in body fluid distribution and interstitial tissue compliance during the development and reversal of experimental renal hypertension in the rat. *Clin. Sci. Mol. Med.* 47: 1–11, 1974.
34. LUDWIG, C. F. W. Nieren und Harnbereitung. In: *Handworterbuch der Physiologie,* edited by R. Wagner. Braunschweig, Germany: Vieweg, 1844, vol. 2, p. 628.
35. LUDWIG, C. F. W. *Lehrbuch der Physiologie des Menschen.* Heidelberg, Germany: Winter, 1861, vol. 2.
36. LUDWIG, C. F. W. Manuscript notes of lectures 1869–1870. In: *A Textbook of Pharmacology, Therapeutics and Materia Medica,* edited by T. L. Brunton. Philadelphia, PA: Lea, 1885, p. 503.
37. PABST, K., and O. H. GAUER. Reflex volume change of sodium excretion in the dog. *Verhande Deutsch. Ges. Kreis.* 25: 263–265, 1959.
38. PETERS, J. P. *Body Water: The Exchange of Fluids in Man.* Springfield, IL: Thomas, 1935.
39. PETERSON, T. V., F. T. FELTS, and N. L. CHASE. Intravascular receptors and renal responses of monkey to volume expansion. *Am. J. Physiol.* 244 (*Heart Circ. Physiol.* 13): H55–H59, 1983.
40. PIRIE, S. C., and D. J. POTTS. The effect of peritubular protein upon fluid reabsorption in rabbit proximal convoluted tubules perfused in vitro. *J. Physiol. Lond.* 337: 429–440, 1983.
41. PITHER, J. M., M. F. KNAPP, R. J. LINDEN, and M. J. PEARSON. Diuresis from stimulation of left atrial receptors in dogs: further purification of the causative agent from plasma. *Q. J. Exp. Physiol.* 68: 167–177, 1983.
42. REINHARDT, H. W., G. KACZMARCZYK, R. MONHAUPT, and B. SIMGEN. The possible mechanism of atrial natriuresis—experiments on chronically instrumented dogs. In: *Hormonal Regulation of Sodium Excretion,* edited by B. Lichardus, R. W. Schrier, and J. Ponec. Amsterdam: Elsevier/North Holland, 1980, p. 63–72.
43. RICHARDS, A. N., and O. H. PLANT. Urine formation in the perfused kidney. I. The influence of alterations in renal blood pressure on the amount and composition of urine. *Am. J. Physiol.* 59: 144–183, 1922.
44. RICHARDS, A. N., B. B. WESTFALL, and P. A. BOTT. Renal excretion of insulin, creatinine and xylose in normal dogs. *Proc. Soc. Exp. Biol. Med.* 32: 73–75, 1934.
45. ROSS, E. J. *Aldosterone and Aldosteronism*, London: Lloyd-Luke, 1975.
46. SCHWARTZ, G. J., and M. B. BURG. Mineralocorticoid effects on cation transport by cortical collecting tubules in vitro. *Am. J. Physiol.* 235 (*Renal Fluid Electrolyte Physiol.* 4): F576–F585, 1978.
47. SIEKER, H. O., O. H. GAUER, and J. P. HENRY. The effect of continuous negative pressure breathing on water and electrolyte excretion by the human kidney. *J. Clin. Invest.* 33: 572–577, 1954.
48. SMITH, H. W. Salt and water volume receptors. *Am. J. Med.* 23: 623–652, 1957.
49. SMYTHE, C. M., J. F. NICKEL, and S. E. BRADLEY. The effect of epinephrine

(USP), L-epinephrine, and L-norepinephrine on glomerular filtration rate, renal plasma flow, and the urinary excretion of sodium, potassium, and water in normal man. *J. Clin. Invest.* 31: 499–506, 1952.

50. STARLING, E. H. *The Fluids of the Body.* London: Constable, 1909.
51. STRAUSS, M. B., R. K. DAVIS, J. D. ROSENBAUM, and E. C. ROSSMEISL. Production of increased renal sodium excretion by hypotonic expansion of extracellular fluid volume in recumbent subjects. *J. Clin. Invest.* 31: 80–86, 1952.
52. THOMPSON, J. M. A., and C. J. DICKINSON. The relation between the excretion of sodium and water and the perfusion pressure in the isolated, blood-perfused, rabbit kidney, with special reference to changes occurring in clip-hypertension. *Clin. Sci. Mol. Med.* 50: 223–236, 1976.
53. TIGERSTEDT, R., and P. G. BERGMAN. Niere und kreislauf. *Skand. Arch. Physiol.* 8: 223–271, 1898.
54. WARDENER, H. E. DE. The control of sodium excretion. In: *Handbook of Physiology. Renal Physiology,* edited by J. Orloff and R. W. Berliner. Washington, DC: 1973, chapt. 21, p. 677–720.
55. WARDENER, H. E. DE. The control of sodium excretion. *Am. J. Physiol.* 235 (*Renal Fluid Electrolyte Physiol.* 4): F163–F173, 1978.
56. WARDENER, H. E. DE, and E. M. CLARKSON. Concept of natriuretic hormone. *Physiol. Rev.* 65: 658–759, 1985.
57. WARDENER, H. E. DE, I. H. MILLS, W. F. CLAPHAM, and C. J. HAYTER. Studies on the efferent mechanism of the sodium diuresis which follows the administration of intravenous saline in the dog. *Clin. Sci.* 21: 249–258, 1961.
58. WILLASEN, Y., and J. OFSTAD. Renal sodium excretion and the peritubular capillary physical factors in essential hypertension. *Hypertension* 2: 771–779, 1980.

VIII

Formation of Concentrated Urine

ROBERT W. BERLINER

IT is now generally agreed that the formation of concentrated urine in the mammalian kidney is effected by the production of a highly concentrated environment around the medullary collecting ducts in which the final concentrating process occurs by osmotic equilibration of the collecting duct contents with the hypertonic surroundings. Only some of the details remain in doubt concerning the processes by which that hypertonic environment is produced.

FORMATION OF URINE

Observations that might have suggested at least the essential features of the concentrating process go back to the early years of this century, but there is nothing to suggest that their significance was appreciated. Instead those observations remained largely forgotten until a half century later when their relevance to our current understanding of the urinary concentrating mechanism became apparent. In the interim, ideas about the concentrating process followed what were at the time more conventional ways of thinking in renal physiology, ways that in this case led to dead ends.

Because the early observations did not lead in any direct way to the views now current but remained submerged for a long time, it is perhaps useful to begin in the middle rather than at the beginning, to consider first some of the ideas and observations that preceded the recognition in the middle 1950s that the conventional approach to renal physiological problems had led, in the case of the concentrating mechanism, to an impasse. Fortunately at that time the essentials of the correct mechanism had already been proposed.

In his book *The Physiology of the Kidney* (52) published in 1937, Homer W. Smith began the chapter "Theories of Renal Function" with the statement: "*All theories of renal function have, of course, been based on the structure of the nephron.*" It is apparent that he was referring largely to the relationship of the glomerulus to its attached tubule. Unfortunately attention to the structure did not go much further. For most renal physiological problems, except the

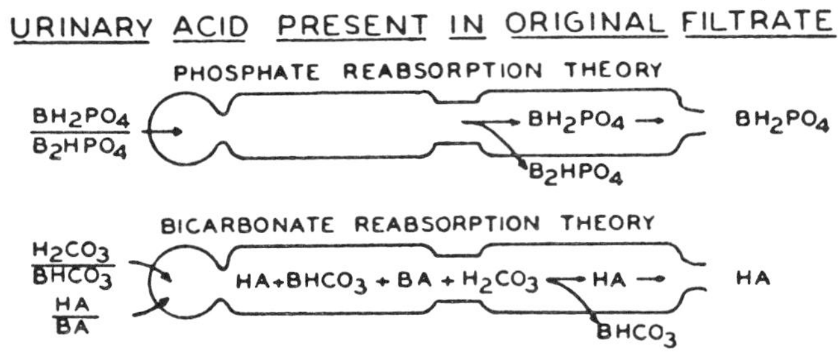

Figure 1. Typical representations of a nephron in the 1940s and 1950s. [From Pitts (48).]

concentrating mechanism (and tubuloglomerular feedback), the conventional picture of the nephron, much as illustrated in Figure 1, could serve quite adequately. This figure from a paper by Robert F. Pitts (48) is not unlike a number of others of that period in showing a glomerulus with the proximal and distal tubules joined together by an insignificant connecting segment. For convenience the whole was pictured as lying in a straight line with regard neither to the convolutions of the tubules nor to the structure and location of the loop of Henle, so that these anatomical features did not readily gain consideration.

Although it was recognized that the effluent from various nephrons was gathered in collecting tubules and collecting ducts, the epithelium of the latter structures was not considered to have significant transport functions. Smith's statement in his 1951 monograph (53) (which, incidentally, repeats almost verbatim a statement in his 1937 book) epitomizes this view: "*The cytology of the collecting tubule does not suggest any specialized function other than service as conduits, and they are so treated by almost all writers.*" He did add that there was some evidence that might be interpreted as indicating that the collecting tubules had a reabsorptive function, particularly for water.

Although the formation of concentrated urine had long drawn the attention of clinicians because it could be used as an indicator for impaired renal function, it was not much studied by renal physiologists until development of the flame photometer directed greatly increased attention to the regulation of salt and water excretion. An explanation for the formation of dilute and concentrated urines became the subject of more general interest. The formation of dilute urine could be accounted for relatively easily; it merely required that salt, the major osmotic constituent of the glomerular filtrate, be removed from the tubule lumen without permitting the escape of the equivalent amount of water. The process required only a relatively low permeability to water in the epithelial lining of the tubule from the point of salt absorption until the urine left the kidney. It was known that vasopressin, the antidiuretic hormone, had the property of increasing the permeability of responsive epithelia to water (6, 31). Thus it was not difficult to explain the excretion of dilute urine in water diuresis or the increase in urine concentration, at least up to the osmotic concentration of the blood, in response to the administration or stimulated release of vasopressin.

At least as early as his 1937 book on the kidney (52), Homer Smith had developed a schema of the distribution of water reabsorption in the nephron. This was based on investigations by clearance techniques, the limited amount of micropuncture information then available (for studies only in amphibians), and observations on the volume and time course of water diuresis. He divided reabsorption into two processes: obligatory reabsorption of about 80% of the filtered volume in the "proximal system" and facultative reabsorption of nearly all of the remaining volume in the "distal system" under the influence of antidiuretic hormone from the pituitary. In 1951 there had been little elaboration of this model when Smith published his monumental monograph *The Kidney: Structure and Function in Health and Disease*:

> *In the current view, the reabsorption of water by the renal tubules involves at least two more or less independent processes: (1) passive water reabsorption in the proximal tubule and thin segment (proximal system) and, under appropriate circumstances, in the distal tubule; and (2) active water reabsorption that is presumably confined to the distal system, i.e., in the distal tubule and possibly in the collecting ducts also. So far as is known only active water reabsorption is under rapidly variable hormonal control.*

(Note the use of the term *active water reabsorption* for the process that yields hypertonic urine, which is discussed later in this chapter.) These ideas are represented in Figure 2 from Smith's later book *Principles of Renal Physiology* (54) published in 1956, in which he wrote:

> *The concentrating operation appears to consist of a continuing constant reabsorptive operation which removes an approximately constant quantity of solute-free water ($T^c_{H_2O}$) from the antecedent isosmotic tubular urine so long as the volume of the latter exceeds the $T^c_{H_2O}$. It is not determined whether this concentrating operation is located in the most distal portion of the distal segment, or in the collecting ducts, though fragmentary evidence favors the latter. Neither is it known whether the concentrating operation is activated by ADH: the induction of antidiuresis by this hormone, by abolishing water diuresis, may simply expose the concentrating operation to view.*

The latter possibility was shortly thereafter shown to be the correct one when Berliner and Davidson (2) and Del Greco and de Wardener (12) demonstrated that hypertonic urine can be produced in the absence of antidiuretic hormone.

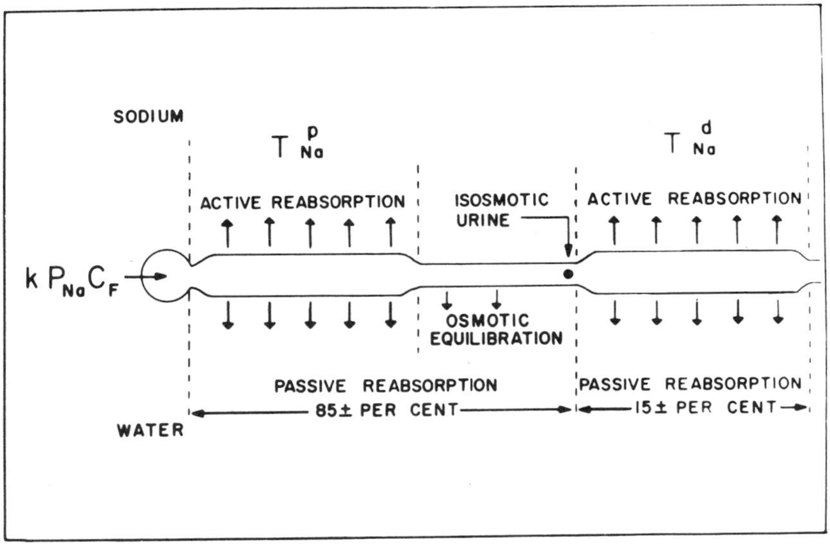

Figure 2. Schema showing reabsorption of sodium and water in the proximal and distal segments. [From Smith (55).]

The introduction by Smith and his colleagues (53, 62) of the concept of $T^c_{H_2O}$ and of its inverse, the free water clearance (C_{H_2O}), the latter presumed to represent the osmotic equivalent of the salt reabsorbed in the distal system, provided the framework for the design and interpretation of most of the studies of salt and water excretion through the 1950s.

The idea of active reabsorption of water, however, presented a serious problem. Certainly there was no established precedent for active transport of water anywhere in the animal kingdom. The alternative to water removal in producing concentrated urine, namely addition of solute, seemed clearly excluded because the concentration of urine is relatively independent of the nature of the solute that it contains. The only solute, the excretion of which varies much with urine concentration, is urea, and in this case the change is in the wrong direction: excretion falls as urine concentration increases. In fact it was the relative independence of the rate of solute excretion from the rate of urine flow that led to the perception that urine must become concentrated in one of the last steps of urine formation, that is, in the collecting system.

The question that required an answer, then, was: What kind of process could transport water against an apparently large gradient of activity from concentrated urine to blood? In other words, what kind of mechanism could effect the active transport of water? Quantitative considerations pose problems in the transport of water that do not exist in the transport of solutes, which can reasonably be considered to combine one molecule or ion at a time to a transporter;

however, water molecules in mammalian fluids outnumber the total of all of the solute particles by a factor of about 200 to 1. It would be difficult to conceive of a carrier sufficiently abundant or turning over rapidly enough to handle such a load, even without consideration of how such a process might be energized.

FORMATION OF URINE

Attention therefore turned to some process that could move water in bulk, the obvious candidate being a process dependent on osmosis. A model of such a process had been proposed by Frank and Mayer (15). The concept was that some solute present in the transporting cells would be involved in a cycle of polymerization and depolymerization. The polymerization at one end of the cell would lower the osmotic pressure at that point; the polymer would diffuse to the opposite end of the cell where it would be broken down into its monomeric constituents, increasing the osmotic pressure in that region accordingly; the monomers would then diffuse back across the cell to be repolymerized. Thus a gradient of osmotic pressure would be produced within the cell and could provide the driving force for water movement. For a time it was believed that some process like the Frank-Mayer model could account for the formation of concentrated urine. This comforting illusion was dispelled, however, when in 1955 William Brodsky and his associates (5) showed on thermodynamic grounds that the process contemplated in the Frank-Mayer model could not generate, within the short distance provided by the thickness of the epithelium lining the renal tubule, a gradient steep enough to generate urine of the concentrations attainable in even the human kidney.

The demonstration that the Frank-Mayer model could not explain the production of hypertonic urine made it apparent that a different way of thinking about the concentrating process was required. Attention was redirected to the loop of Henle and the renal medulla because of the ideas concerning their function that had been offered by Werner Kuhn and his associates (23, 36).

Observations suggesting that the medulla, and specifically the loop of Henle, had some relationship to the formation of concentrated urine go back to the early years of this century. Most often cited in this connection is the contribution of Karl Peter (Fig. 3), who in his 1909 monograph *Investigations Concerning the Structure and Development of the Kidney* (46) described a correspondence among various mammalian species between the length of the loop of Henle and the specific gravity of the urine that each produced.

Peter was born in Frankfurt an der Oder in 1870 and did anatomical work in Freiburg, Breslau, and Würzburg before joining the faculty of the University of Greifswald in 1905. He became a full professor in 1917 and directed the institute there until he became emeritus in 1955. His work dealt with many aspects of embryology and developmental anatomy. He died in Munich in 1955 shortly before his eighty-fifth birthday.

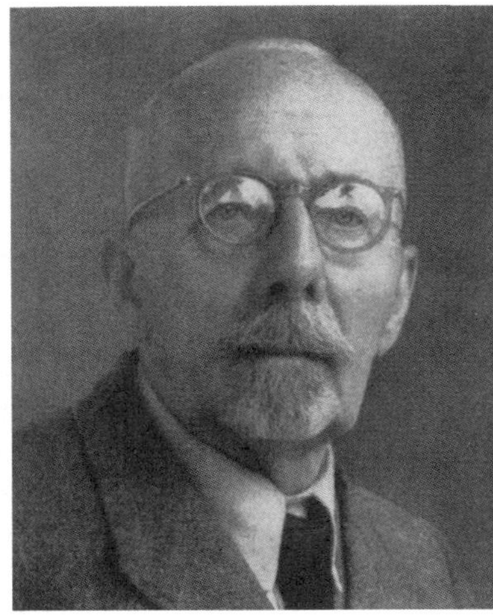

Figure 3. Karl Peter (1870–1955).

Actually there had been even earlier studies that suggested an important role of the medulla in the formation of concentrated urine. In 1902 Filehne and Biberfeld (14) had reported finding that the osmotic pressure of medullary tissue was higher than that of the cortex. The 1908 observations of Hirokawa (25) (translated from German by Carl Gottschalk) were even more to the point:

The urine present in the medulla has a much higher osmotic pressure than that of the convoluted tubules of the cortex; therefore the osmotic pressure of the urine increases considerably during its passage through the loops of Henle and collecting tubules. . . . The osmotic pressure of the medulla is extraordinarily variable; it is almost without exception higher than that of the cortex, and is higher the more concentrated the excreted urine.

It is not clear whether these studies had any influence on the thinking of the time, but if they did it was not apparent until their relevance became manifest with the development of the idea of the countercurrent mechanism of urine concentration. Neither of these papers is among the 2,300 cited in Smith's 1951 book. It is also interesting to note that Peter's obituary (also translated by C. Gottschalk) in the *Münchener Medicinische Wochenschrift* in 1955 states, "*His most famous work concerned the development of the nose and mouth.*" One might venture to guess that the kidney work had achieved greater status a few years later when the role of the loop in urine concentration was given more general acceptance.

For a few years during the 1930s the loop of Henle was widely believed to be the site of urine concentration. This was largely due to a paper published by Burgess, Harvey, and Marshall (8). In examining the effect of Pitressin on representatives of each of the vertebrate classes, they found no effect on urine flow in either catfish or frogs. The effect in the alligator was striking, often with extended anuria, but was discounted because it was associated with what appeared to be a very marked decrease in glomerular filtration. In chickens and dogs, Pitressin produced decreases in urine flow with relatively small changes in the measures of glomerular filtration. On the basis of these observations it was concluded that antidiuretic hormone had its effect on the loop of Henle, the only renal structure present exclusively in birds and mammals, and that the effect was a stimulation of water absorption in the loop. Eli Kennerly Marshall was a leading figure in the study of the kidney and appears repeatedly in this volume for his many important contributions. A. McGee Harvey was a medical student at the time but was later and for many years chairman of the Department of Medicine at Johns Hopkins and a leader of American internal medicine. This particular paper, however, was not up to their usual standards. Only urine flow and an index of glomerular filtration (clearance of xylose or sucrose) were measured. They said nothing about the production of hypertonic urine, although their conclusions have often been interpreted as if they dealt with the formation of concentrated urine. They did not, in fact, make any measurements of osmolality. The possible contribution of dead-space errors to the apparent drop in glomerular filtration rate was not, apparently, considered. And it has subsequently been found that amphibians do respond to vasopressin by producing a less dilute urine (51).

In an earlier paper, "Observations on the Function of the Frog's Kidney" published in 1927, Marian M. Crane (10) had reached the same conclusion concerning the role of the loop of Henle as did Burgess et al. Her inference was, however, more relevant to the concentrating mechanism because it related directly to the formation of concentrated urine rather than only to the effect of pituitary extracts on urine flow. It is the ability to form hypertonic urine, not the ability to respond to antidiuretic hormone, that distinguishes renal function in birds and mammals from that of other vertebrates. [Crane had still earlier (1924) been E. K. Marshall's collaborator in one of the landmark studies in renal physiology: the demonstration that phenol red is secreted into the lumina of the renal tubules (41).] In her 1927 paper (10), Crane reported that the osmotic pressure of frog urine was never greater than that of the blood:

Since the chief anatomical difference between a frog's kidney and that of a mammal is the absence of the loop of Henle in the former, the failure of the frog's tubule to reabsorb water against osmotic pressure suggests that it may be in the loop of Henle that such reabsorption takes place. If such is the case, the power to excrete a hypertonic urine should appear first in those animals in which a loop is first developed. Huber has described a very definite loop in the bird's kidney, so according to this theory the bird should be able to

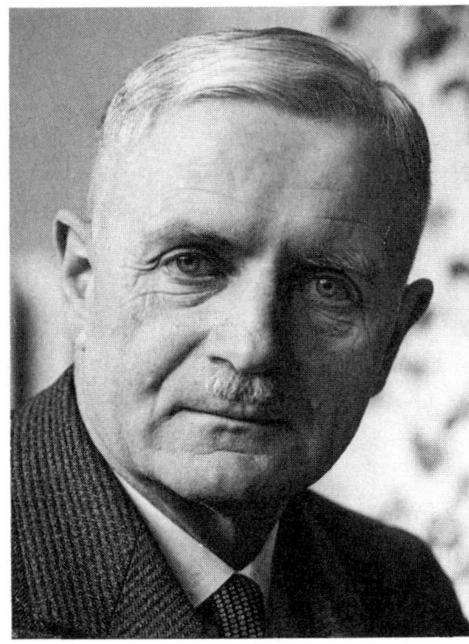

Figure 4. Werner Kuhn (1899–1963).

excrete a urine hypertonic to the blood. d'Errico reports freezing point determinations indicating that the osmotic pressure of the chicken's urine is a little higher than that of the blood.

For these reasons and particularly because of the paper by Burgess, Harvey, and Marshall (8), it was widely believed that the loop of Henle was the site at which the urine was rendered hypertonic. That possibility was shown to be very unlikely by the observation of Walker, Bott, Oliver, and MacDowell (61; see NOTE in the chapter by Windhager in this volume), published in 1941, that fluid in the early distal tubules having already passed through the loop was not hypertonic, in fact was apparently somewhat dilute, in rats producing markedly hypertonic urine. The hypotonicity of fluid in the early distal tubule was not readily interpretable at the time, and because it was found in only two of the total of three samples by a somewhat imprecise method, it received relatively little attention until some years later when Heinrich Wirz (65; see Fig. 6) confirmed and extended this finding and pointed out its probable significance.

By the time that it became apparent that there was no adequate model for the formation of concentrated urine by active transport of water, considerable evidence had been adduced by Wirz to support the idea, first introduced by Werner Kuhn (Fig. 4) and his associates (23, 36), that urine becomes concentrated by water loss from the collecting ducts to an environment made hypertonic by the action of the loop of Henle (64, 68).

Kuhn earned his Ph.D. degree in physical chemistry at the University of Zurich in 1921. He worked for two years as a fellow of the Rockefeller Foundation under Niels Bohr at the Institute of

Theoretical Physics in Copenhagen. The work that he accomplished in Copenhagen was the basis for his appointment in physical chemistry at the University of Zurich in 1927. Following another visit to England, this time with Rutherford at the Cavendish Laboratory in Cambridge, he accepted several academic appointments in Germany—Heidelberg, Karlsruhe, and Kiel—before being made Chairman of the Department of Physical Chemistry at the University of Basel in 1939, a position he held until his death.

Kuhn's work included contributions to several areas. He worked on resonance phenomena of atomic nuclei and gamma rays, elucidated the structural characteristics of optical stereoisomers, and had a strong and lasting interest in the structural analysis of large molecules, particularly those of elongated shape. It was, however, beginning in 1936, in Kiel, that he started to work on the analysis of those processes that provided the basis for the countercurrent principle in the kidney. He studied several separation and concentrating mechanisms that dealt with a wide spectrum of applications, including the separation of isotopes by repeated centrifugation.

Kuhn's achievements were honored by several personal distinctions. He was a member of the Akademia Leopoldina, a foreign honorary member of the American Academy of Arts and Sciences, and he received honorary doctorates in medicine and the natural sciences in Heidelberg and Kiel. He was also a recipient of the Marcel Benoist prize for his contributions to the interpretation of living phenomena, and he received with Wirz the Rudolf Schunk prize in recognition of outstanding achievements in medicine (Fig. 5).

Heinrich Wirz (Fig. 6) received his early education and medical education in Basel where he also became a member of the faculty of the Department of Physiology before accepting a leading position at Ciba (and Ciba-Geigy). During his earlier academic career (1947–1948), he spent time with Homer Smith in the Physiology Department at New York University and became acquainted with micropuncture techniques in Phyllis Bott's laboratory during a six-week period in the early 1950s. He met Kuhn in Basel and began a close and productive collaboration.

Kuhn, having devised the principle of the countercurrent multiplier and having become aware of the hairpin shape of the loop of Henle as well as the fact that some relationship between the loop and the formation of concentrated urine had been suggested, proposed in a paper with K. Ryffel that urine became concentrated as it flowed through the medulla by the action of the loop behaving as a countercurrent multiplier (36). The paper, published in German during World War II, received essentially no attention until the idea was presented again by Hargitay and Kuhn in 1951 with a new system for the operation of the countercurrent multiplier, including a working model (23). At the same time Wirz, along with Hargitay

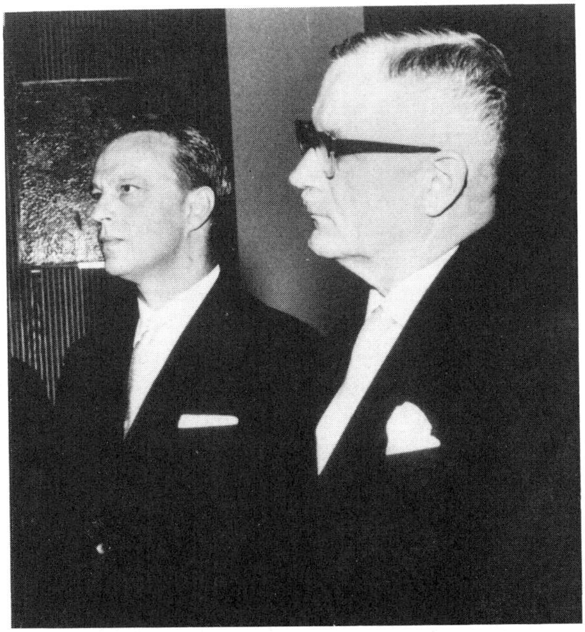

Figure 5. Heinrich Wirz (*left*) and Werner Kuhn (*right*) receiving the Ludwig Schunk award of the Justus Liebig University in Giessen, West Germany, in 1963.

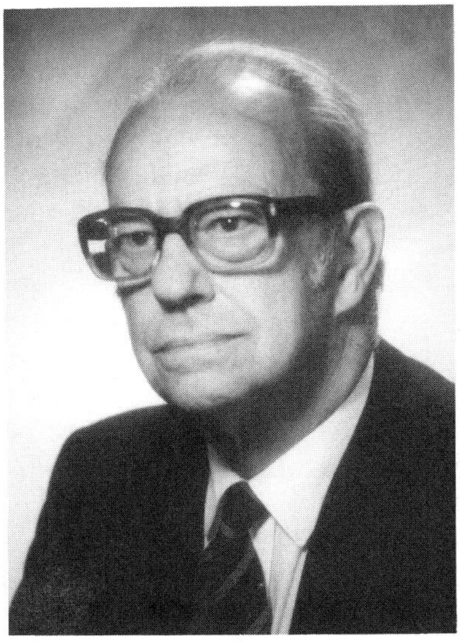

Figure 6. Heinrich Wirz (b. 1914).

and Kuhn, reported a study of the osmolality of medullary structures in rat kidney, in which it was shown that the osmotic pressure (depression of the melting point of the frozen medulla) increases

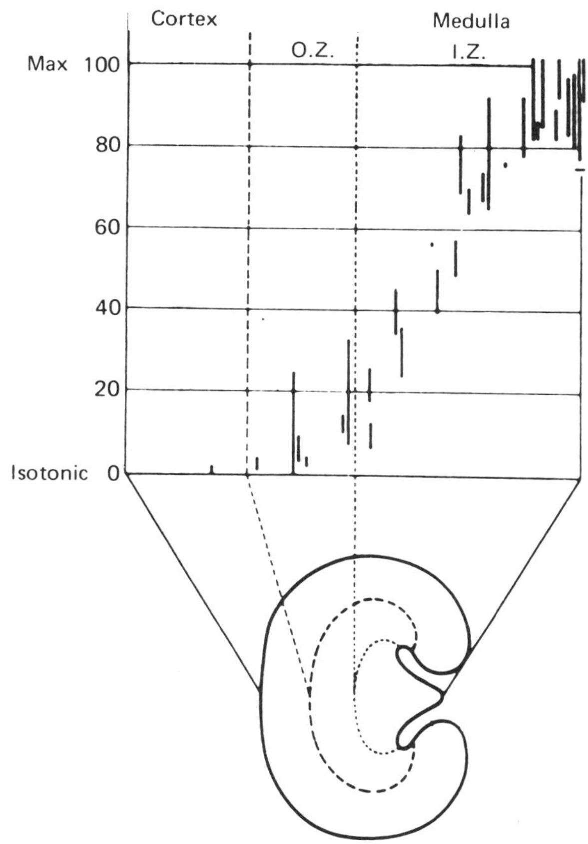

Figure 7. Osmolality (as percentage of maximum) of fluids at various depths in rat kidney. [From Wirz, Hargitay, and Kuhn (68).]

progressively from cortex to papilla and uniformly in all of the structures at any given level [Fig. 7; (68)].

The model of Hargitay and Kuhn depended on hydrostatic pressure to produce the single effect, which was multiplied by the countercurrent flow. In this model (Fig. 8), the inflowing fluid (corresponding to the descending limb of the loop) was separated from the outflowing fluid (ascending limb) by a semipermeable membrane. Hydrostatic pressure applied to the colloid-containing fluid on the inflow side produced the corresponding difference in colloid osmotic pressure between the two limbs. The more concentrated fluid was then distributed between the two limbs, and a new difference was generated by water movement from inflow side to outflow side. As this process is repeated with continuous flow, fluid near the tube connecting inflow to outflow becomes considerably more concentrated than the fluid that could be produced by the single effect alone. To Hargitay and Kuhn, this was a model that demonstrated the validity of the principle, but it could not be

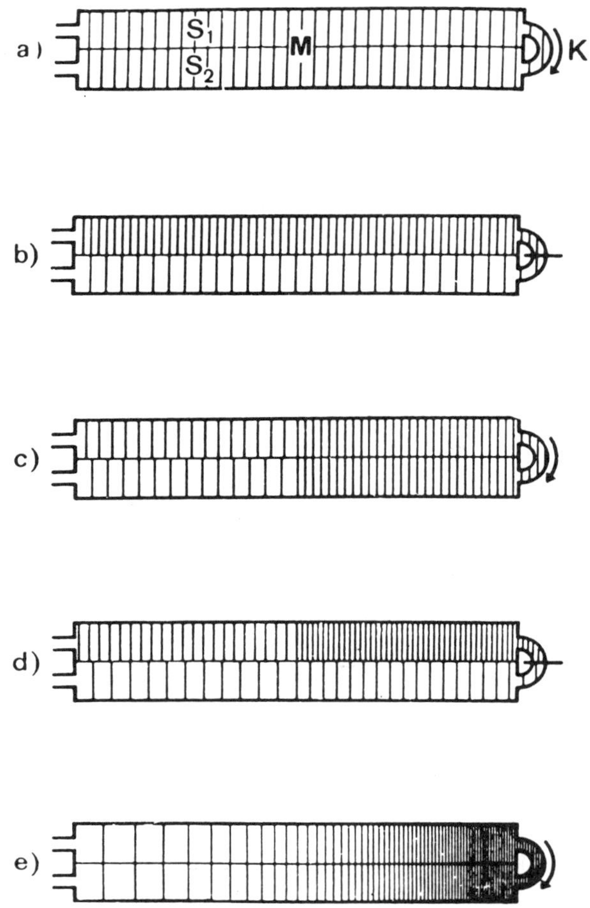

Figure 8. Countercurrent-multiplier model of Hargitay and Kuhn. Increased osmolality represented by more intense hatching. [From Wirz and Dirix (67).]

considered a physical representation of the loop of Henle because the hydrostatic pressure available in the loop of Henle was not sufficient (to say nothing of the fact that the two limbs of the loop are not contiguous). They pointed out that the model could operate equally well on the basis of salt transport in the opposite direction, from ascending limb to descending limb.

The cryoscopic study by Wirz et al. (68) of the various structures in the renal medulla was viewed skeptically by many who, reluctant to reorient their thinking so drastically, adopted Smith's view (55) that the uniformly high osmotic pressure in all of the renal structures at a given level could have been due to diffusion of water vapor from the various structures to the concentrated urine in the collecting ducts. At that time no one pointed out that the fluid in collecting

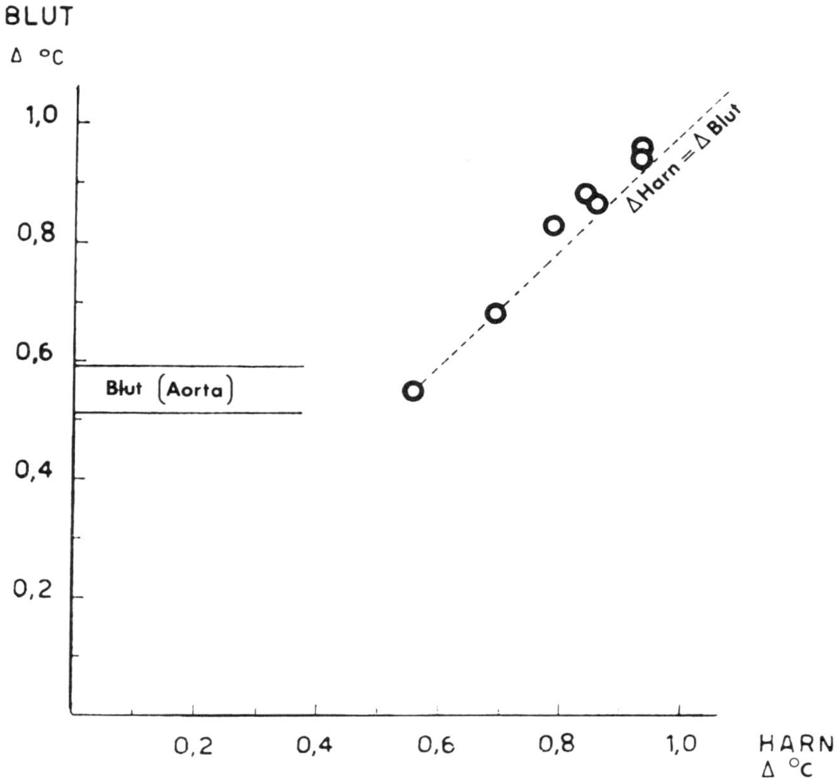

Figure 9. Osmolality (freezing-point depression) of urine (*abscissa*) and blood (*ordinate*) at the tip of the papilla in hamsters. [From Wirz (64).]

ducts is only a small fraction of the fluid in any cross section and that it would require that the urine be many times more concentrated before taking up water from the other structures than it was found to be when measured by Wirz et al. [This point was later made by Wirz (66).] In any case, not discouraged by the skepticism of most renal physiologists, Wirz went on accumulating evidence. In 1953 he demonstrated that blood collected from the vasa recta near the tip of the papilla in golden hamsters had the same high osmotic pressure as the urine obtained at the same time [Fig. 9; (64)]. This not only was in accord with the less direct observations of Wirz et al. (and could not, of course, be explained by postmortem diffusion of water) but also was incompatible with the idea of water reabsorption by an active process from the collecting ducts into a region isotonic with the cortex. This latter would require that the blood draining the collecting ducts be more dilute than systemic blood, albeit to only a small extent if the flow were large relative to the amount of water reabsorbed. However, the blood in the vasa recta could certainly not be more concentrated than peripheral blood.

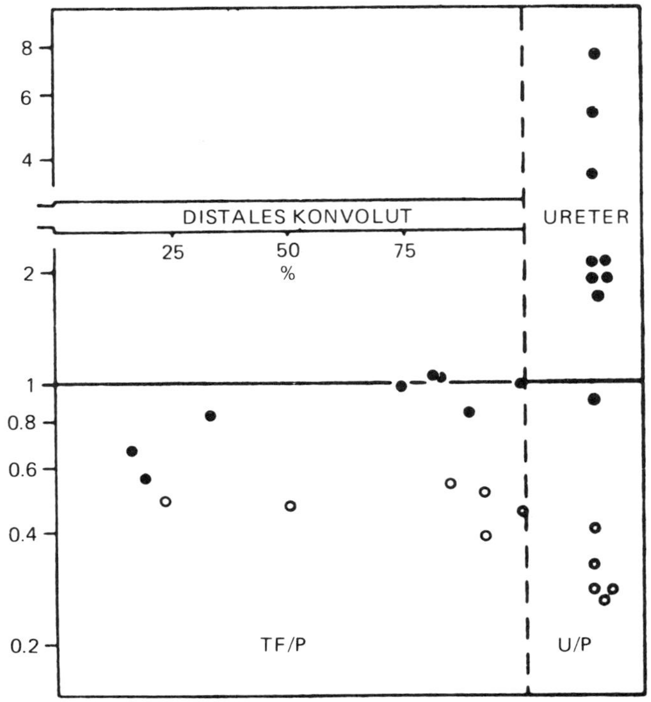

Figure 10. Osmolality of fluid from distal tubules in rats producing dilute (○) and concentrated (●) urine. TF, tubule fluid; P, plasma; U, urine. [From Wirz (65).]

In further support of the role of the loop of Henle in producing the hypertonicity of the renal medulla were the findings reported by Wirz (65) in 1956 from a study of the osmolality of fluid in the proximal and distal tubules in rats producing both dilute and concentrated urine (Fig. 10). In accord with the finding of Walker, Bott, Oliver, and MacDowell (61) and as confirmed many times since, the fluid in the proximal tubule is isosmotic with systemic blood in antidiuresis. For the first time it was shown that the same is true in kidneys undergoing water diuresis. Furthermore, in accord with sketchy earlier findings of Walker, Bott, Oliver, and MacDowell, the fluid in the early distal tubule was hypotonic to blood, whether the urine being formed was dilute or hypertonic. When the urine was dilute, the fluid remained hypotonic throughout the length of the distal tubule; when the urine was concentrated, the fluid attained the same osmotic pressure as the blood before reaching the end of the distal convolution, but it never achieved hypertonicity despite the fact that the urine had much higher osmolalities. These findings made it clear that the collecting system was indeed the site at which the urine acquired its hypertonicity. In addition the dilute character of the fluid emerging from the loop of Henle was quite in accord with the presumption that the loop, behaving as a countercurrent multiplier, was responsible for the high osmolality of the medulla.

Meanwhile new measurements of the osmotic pressure and solute concentrations in the renal medulla were undertaken by Karl Ullrich and his associates (60) to explore the predictions of the Wirz, Hargitay, and Kuhn model. They found, as had Filehne and Biberfeld (14) and Hirokawa (25), that the osmotic pressure of tissue slices from hydropenic dogs, as indicated by their swelling in solutions of various solute concentrations, increased steadily from the outer medulla to the tip of the papilla. They also found that the concentrations of sodium, chloride, and urea rose progressively from the cortex to the papilla. [The high and increasing concentration of chloride in medullary tissue had been reported in the 1940s by Glimstedt (17) and by Ljungberg (37) but had been interpreted in terms of chloride reabsorption without mention of urinary concentration.]

It is clear that by the middle 1950s the evidence for a high osmolality in all of the medullary structures and for a role of the loop of Henle in its production had become very strong indeed. [This coincided with the demonstration by Brodsky et al. (5) of the inadequacy of the Frank-Meyer model.] There remained an unresolved problem concerning just how the loop of Henle figured in the process. All of the models by Kuhn and his associates illustrating the principle of the multiplier involved transport of water from the inflowing limb to the outflowing limb of the model or transport of solute from the outflowing limb to the inflowing limb. The uptake of fluid from a third tube (analogous to the collecting duct) was channeled directly into one of the limbs of the counterflow system (Fig. 11). In attempting to fit such a model to the renal medulla, certain problems arose. Of course the two limbs of the loop are not contiguous, but it is necessary that they be so only for the model driven by hydrostatic pressure, which was never a serious possibility. For the solute-transport model, the two limbs need not be in contact, provided each limb transports solute in the right direction, but the collecting duct cannot be separated from one or the other limb because the models require that water lost from the collecting duct leave the system in the outflow from the ascending limb. In addition, if the water lost from the collecting duct is to enter the loop, the surface through which it moves must be water permeable, whereas the remainder of the surface of the loop must be impermeable to water if water is not to move along with solute from one limb to the other. It is thus difficult to see how a loop behaving in the manner proposed by Kuhn and his associates could act on its surroundings.

Given the evidence for the hypertonicity of medullary structures and for a role of the loop of Henle but unable to fit the Hargitay and Kuhn model to the actual situation, my colleagues and I proposed a different way of looking at the mechanism (3). Rather than concentrating on the possible countercurrent-multiplier function of the

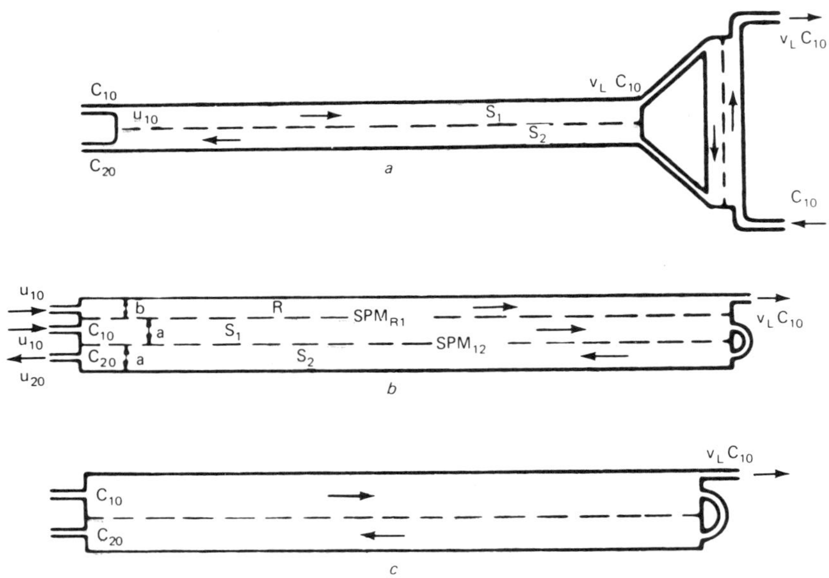

Figure 11. Countercurrent-multiplier models illustrating uptake of water directly into the multiplier itself. Model *b* most closely approximates the renal medulla. Water moving under a hydrostatic pressure head from S_1 (descending limb) and S_2 (ascending limb) across semipermeable membrane SPM_{12} raises osmotic pressure in S_1. The single effect is multiplied by countercurrent flow. Water moves from channel R (collecting duct) into S_1 across semipermeable membrane SPM_{R1}. Water lost from R leaves the system in the outflow from S_2. [From Hargitay and Kuhn (23).]

loop, we proposed that the loop be looked upon as a pump delivering salt without equivalent water deep into the medulla. This would raise the osmotic pressure of the medullary interstitium, and the fluid in the collecting ducts would equilibrate osmotically with this interstitium. The water reabsorbed from the collecting ducts would leave the medulla in the vasa recta rather than the ascending limb. [We were unaware at the time that Wirz, in a paper delivered to a symposium of the Colston Research Society, had also suggested that the water might enter the medullary interstitium and be carried off in the vasa recta (66).] We then went further by suggesting that the whole idea of the countercurrent multiplier be abandoned. We visualized a water-impermeable loop transporting salt from its lumen to the interstitium of the medulla throughout its length. This proposal was not incompatible with anything then known; after all Wirz, Hargitay, and Kuhn had not detected the hypotonicity of the fluid in the ascending limb that Wirz (65) later found. However, our proposal of a dilute fluid in the loop of Henle was shown, even before the paper appeared, to be wrong. Carl Gottschalk (see Fig. 13) and Margaret Mylle collected fluid from loops, vasa recta, and collecting ducts in the hamster papilla and found that they all had

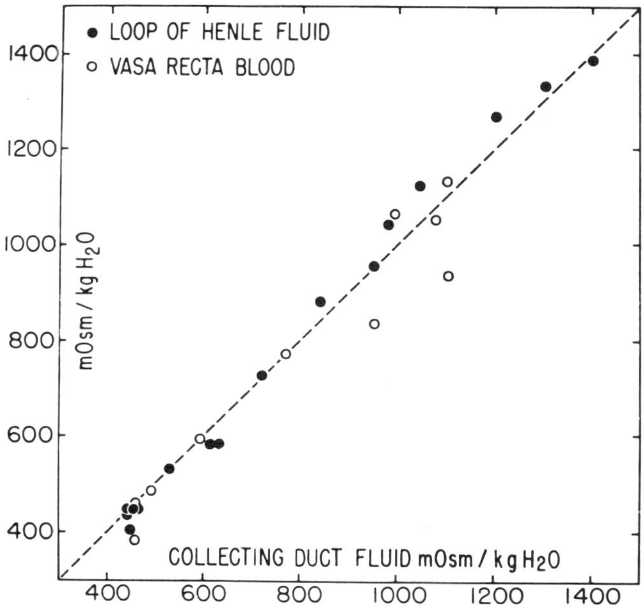

Figure 12. Relation between the osmolality of collecting duct fluid and fluid from loops of Henle and vasa recta blood in 9 hamsters, 1 kangaroo rat, and 1 *Psammomys obesus.* [From Gottschalk and Mylle (21).]

the same high osmolality in animals producing hypertonic urine [Fig. 12; (20)]. The picture of the loop that emerged thus differed from our proposal in the character of the descending limb, which being permeable to water, makes the loop a countercurrent multiplier. Its function can be considered to be to deliver salt to the medullary interstitium at high concentrations without large concentration differences across the epithelium of the loop, rather than to move water or salt between the two limbs.

Our paper also attempted to explain an old observation by Gamble, McKhann, Butler, and Tuthill (16), who in 1934 measured the volume of urine excreted by rats on a low-protein diet after they were fed various solutes alone and in pairs. They found that when the animals were fed pairs of solutes the urine volume was always the sum of that excreted when each solute was administered alone—except when one of the solutes was urea, in which case the volume excreted was less than that when the nonurea solute was given alone. They referred to this phenomenon as "*An economy of water in renal function referable to urea*" (16). The studies of Gamble et al. were subjected to considerable criticism, particularly because their rats had free access to water, but their conclusions have been supported by several studies not subject to similar criticisms (4, 11). In our 1958 paper, we pointed out that, as a consequence of water reabsorption without the equivalent amount of urea in cortical tubules, urea is highly concentrated in the collecting ducts and that a high concentration of urea can be achieved by permitting it to diffuse from the collecting duct into the interstitium in which it is trapped by the countercurrent exchanger formed by the vasa recta. Thus much of the urea in the collecting duct can be osmotically balanced by urea in the interstitium, leaving the salt delivered by the loop of Henle to balance the nonurea solute in the collecting ducts. Such a mechanism might explain why urea might be excreted in water already committed to the excretion of other solutes; it would not explain Gamble's "*economy of water.*" A more important role of urea that would account for "*economy of water*" was later offered by Stephenson (57) and by Kokko and Rector (34).

The observations of Gottschalk and Mylle established once and for all that the loop is indeed a countercurrent multiplier. Since that time studies of the concentrating mechanism have focused largely on attempts to determine how that function is accomplished.

Carl W. Gottschalk (Fig. 13) was born in Salem, Virginia, attended Roanoke College, and in 1945 graduated from the University of Virginia School of Medicine. He served as a house officer at Massachusetts General Hospital and as a research fellow in the Department of Physiology at Harvard Medical School before moving to the University of North Carolina as a fellow in cardiology in 1952. Appointed to the faculty, he became Professor of Medicine and Physiology, he was appointed Career Investigator of the American Heart Association in 1961, and since 1969 has held the title of Kenan Professor of Medicine and Physiology.

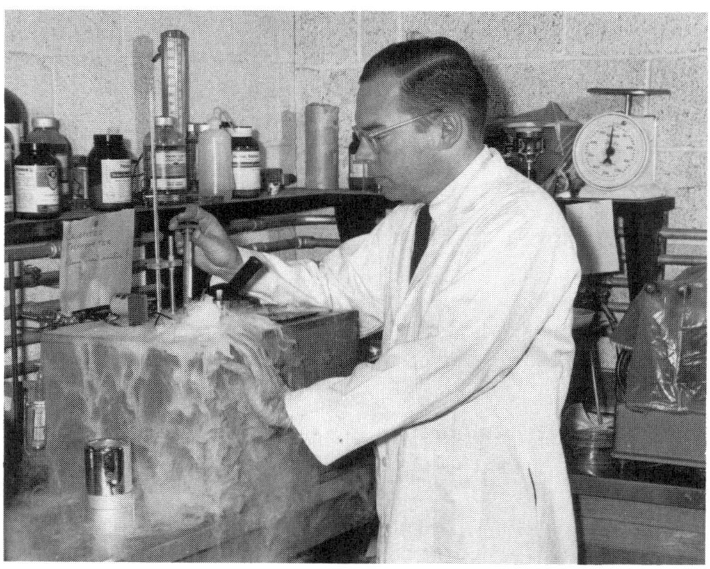

Figure 13. Carl W. Gottschalk (b. 1922) measuring a freezing-point depression of tubule fluid with the Ramsay osmometer (1958).

The observations by Gottschalk and his associates at Chapel Hill relevant to urinary concentration were not limited to the measurements (previously referred to) that documented the equivalent osmolalities in all the papillary structures of animals producing concentrated urine. During 1958 and 1959 they made numerous measurements of the osmolality of fluid collected by micropuncture from proximal and distal tubules, loops, vasa recta, and collecting ducts in rodents of several species (21). These confirmed and greatly extended the observations of Walker, Bott, Oliver, and MacDowell and the more extensive studies of Wirz. Among the observations were: all samples of fluids from proximal tubules were isosmotic within the error of measurement whether the urine was hypertonic or dilute (Fig. 14), fluid in the early distal tubule was dilute whether the final

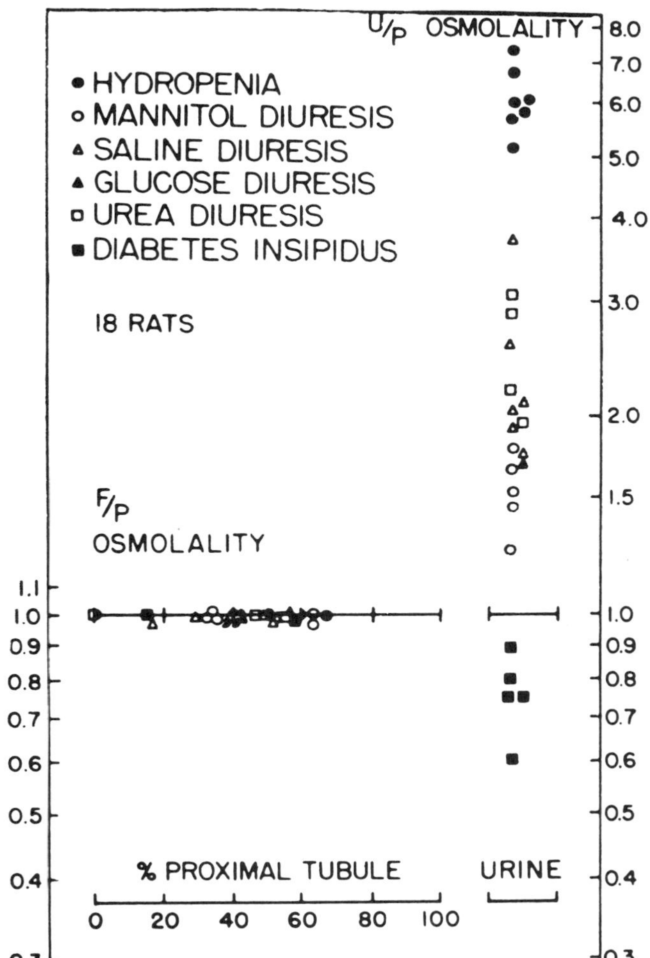

Figure 14. Osmolality of fluid in rat proximal tubule and urine. [From Gottschalk and Mylle (21).]

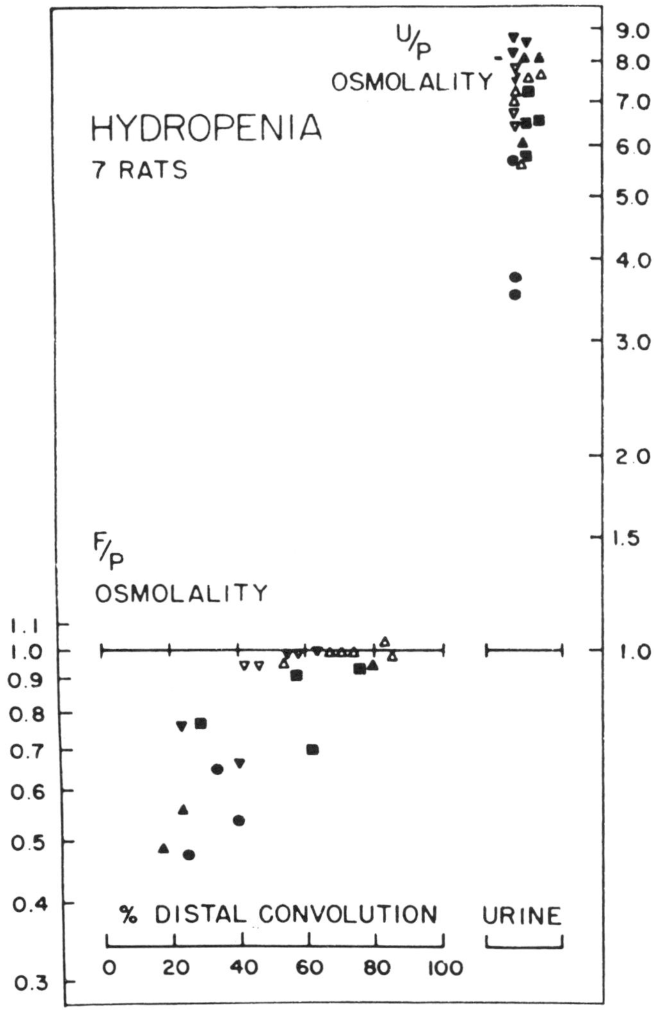

Figure 15. Osmolality of distal convoluted tubule fluid and urine in hydropenic rats. [From Gottschalk and Mylle (21).]

urine was dilute or concentrated (Fig. 15), when the urine was concentrated it achieved the same osmolality as the blood but never became hypertonic before leaving the distal tubule. They also showed that, when fluid colored with nigrosine was injected between oil droplets into descending limbs in hamsters, the fluid was reabsorbed, the dye being rapidly concentrated. When similar injections were made in ascending limbs, the volume remained unchanged, but when the fluid was reaspirated, it was found to have the high osmolality of the renal papilla (19). These results, which demonstrated that the descending limb has a high permeability to water while the ascending limb has a low permeability to water but a high permeability to solute (salt), were presented somewhat hesitantly, but they anticipated by several years other studies that, through the use of more direct measurements, yielded the same conclusion (16, 23, 44).

They also found that in hamsters with diabetes insipidus the fluid in loops of Henle and the blood in vasa recta were hyperosmotic when fluid in the collecting ducts was clearly more dilute than the blood, indicating the low permeability of the collecting ducts in the absence of vasopressin (18). Although the osmolality in loop and vasa recta was distinctly higher than that of systemic blood, it was considerably lower than that often found in animals producing concentrated urine. It is not clear whether the difference was the consequence of greater water loss from the still-dilute collecting system (1, 30), of an effect of vasopressin on salt transport in the thick ascending limb, which has more recently been found, at least in certain rodents (9, 42), or of a very low concentration of urea. Quite probably all of these factors are involved.

Since Wirz and Gottschalk provided the definitive data establishing the validity of the countercurrent-multiplier model, most of the effort has been directed toward determining how the loop of Henle, particularly the thin segments, functions. From the first recognition that the loop behaves as a countercurrent multiplier, questions have been raised as to whether the thin limbs could possibly have the required characteristics. There has never been any doubt concerning the structural suitability of the thick ascending limb for active transport, and the studies of Burg and Green (7) and of Rocha and Kokko (49), demonstrating the active transport of salt by this segment, provided a surprise only in the orientation of the electrical potential, lumen-positive relative to the outside, which suggested that chloride was the actively transported ion. It was subsequently shown by Rainer Greger and his colleagues (22) that the process involves cotransport of sodium, potassium, and chloride and that the driving force is provided by the low sodium concentration in the cells maintained by Na^+-K^+-ATPase.

The thin segments have presented conceptual problems from the start. Homer Smith summarized this (55) when he first declared his acceptance of the countercurrent hypothesis at the New York Academy of Medicine in 1958:

> *Least of all do I like to see the squamous epithelium of the thin segment freely permeable to water (if not to sodium also) in the descending limb, only to acquire water impermeability and active sodium transport at the tip of the loop for no better reason, apparently, than the circumstance that it has turned a corner.*

Two issues are raised here: Is there reason to believe that the characteristics of the two thin limbs differ so markedly? Is it possible that the flat epithelium lining the ascending thin limb, poor in mitochondria and other subcellular structures, has the machinery needed to provide active salt transport at a rate sufficient to account for the salt concentration in the renal medulla?

The first question has clearly been answered in the affirmative. The difference found by Gottschalk (19) between the fates of droplets injected into ascending and descending limbs has already been cited. The much lower permeability to water of ascending thin limbs was confirmed by Trefor Morgan and me (44) when we perfused loops in the excised papillae of rats and even more definitively by Masashi Imai and Juha Kokko (27, 33), who perfused segments of the loop of rabbits in vitro.

The issue of salt transport by the thin ascending limb has been much more difficult to resolve. A number of proposals have been offered that would have relegated the thin segment to a totally passive role, essentially that of a countercurrent exchanger, recognizing salt transport only in the thick ascending limb in the outer medulla. The problem was in explaining the fact that the concentrations of sodium and chloride continue to rise through the inner medulla if the transport of salt is limited to the outer medulla. A proposal suggesting that such a rise in concentration could be effected simply by countercurrent exchange with active salt transport only by the thick ascending limb (47) prompted a mathematical analysis by John Stephenson (56) that proved that in a countercurrent system no concentration greater than that of the inflow can be achieved without an input of energy. Similar conclusions were reached by Kelman, Marsh, and Howard (32). It has sometimes been assumed that the need for an input of energy implies that there must be active transport of salt by the thin limb, but this is not a valid inference, provided some alternative means of supplying energy is available. Models later proposed by Stephenson (57) and by Kokko and Floyd Rector (34) offered that alternative.

Other proposals eliminating the thin segments from the countercurrent-multiplier function were made by Ullrich and his associates (24) and by Marsh (38). In both instances active salt transport was assumed to be performed by the collecting ducts rather than the loops, but it was difficult to see how the urine could be made more concentrated by removing salt from it. In any case, the idea that the thin segments of Henle's loop could behave only as a passive exchanger was eliminated by the study of Jamison, Bennett, and Berliner (29), who took advantage of a technique devised by Fuminori Sakai (50) that exposed for micropuncture in rats a much greater length of the loop than had previously been accessible. When samples from descending limbs were compared with paired samples from ascending limbs at the same level in the papilla, it was found that the osmolality of ascending limb samples was uniformly lower than that of the corresponding descending limb samples and that the difference was largely explained by a difference in sodium (chloride)

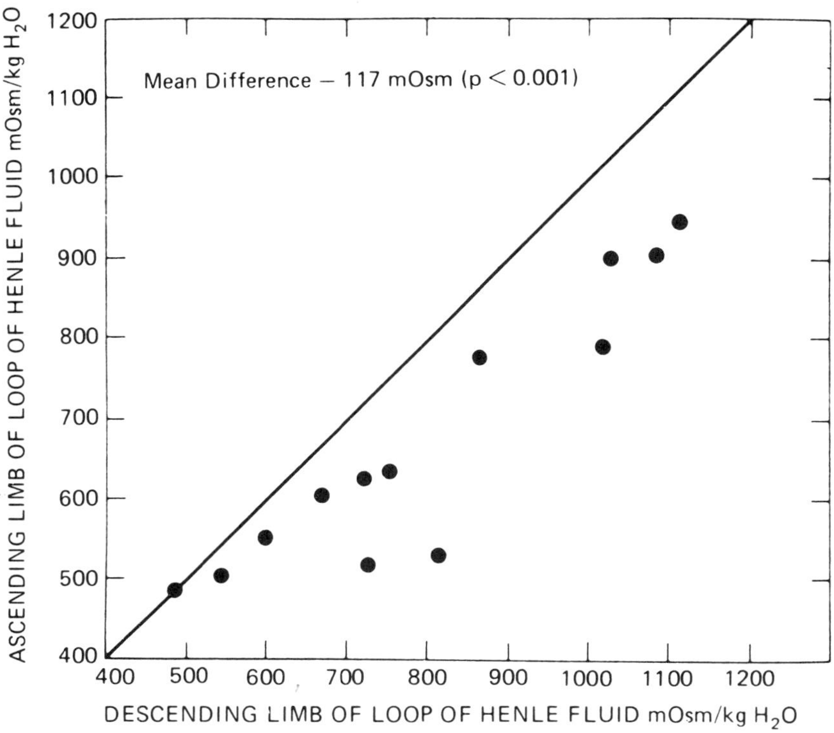

Figure 16. Comparison of osmolalities of fluid from ascending thin limbs and adjacent descending limbs of the loop of Henle. [From Jamison, Bennett, and Berliner (29).]

concentration (Fig. 16). This was not only precisely the opposite of what might be expected of a countercurrent exchanger but clearly showed that the ascending limb was supplying salt to the interstitium as was to be expected for a countercurrent multiplier. [The only alternative, i.e., addition of water to the ascending limb, was excluded by Rex Jamison's later demonstration (28) of a decrease, rather than an increase, in volume between descending and ascending limbs.]

That the thin limb functions as a countercurrent multiplier seemed clear, but there remained problems about its ability to transport salt actively. In addition to the implications of the epithelial structure, it had not been possible to detect unequivocal evidence of salt transport against concentration gradients by the thin ascending limb. Early reports of the development of an electrical potential difference across the epithelium of thin limbs (40, 63) were not confirmed in later studies (27, 33). Although small differences of concentration have been found in some studies (43, 58), no evidence of salt transport could be found in the thin ascending limb of loops in isolated rat papillae or in segments of rabbit loops perfused in vitro (27, 33).

The capacity of the thin ascending limb to deliver salt to the inner medulla need not, however, be dependent on active transport by the lining epithelium if a driving force can be provided by some other input of free energy. Such a mechanism was proposed simultaneously by Kokko and Rector (34) and by Stephenson (57). In their models the free energy is supplied to the inner medulla by the concentrated solution of urea in the collecting ducts. This solution provides for a transfer of energy from the cortex and outer medulla to the inner medulla. In the cortex salt and water are reabsorbed in distal and collecting tubules, leaving in the lumina an isotonic solution containing mostly urea. This solution is further concentrated as it passes through the outer medulla by the movement of water into the interstitium rendered hypertonic by the reabsorption of salt in the thick ascending limb. (Juha Kokko, currently Professor of Medicine at Emory University; Floyd Rector, Professor of Medicine at the University of California, San Francisco; John Stephenson, Professor of Physiology, Cornell Medical School; and Rex Jamison, Professor of Medicine, Stanford University were all at one time associated with the laboratory of Kidney and Electrolyte Metabolism of the National Heart Institute.)

The idea of using a solution of a second solute to yield a concentrating effect, not possible in a single-solute system without active solute transport or a hydrostatic pressure gradient, is to be found in the first paper relating urinary concentration to the countercurrent multiplier (36). The model of Kuhn and Ryffel is illustrated in Figure 17. The late rediscovery of this type of mechanism led Wirz (67) to write, "*It is questionable that this paper was thoroughly studied by many who quoted it.*" The model works as follows: compartments A and B are separated by a copper ferrocyanide membrane (M_1)

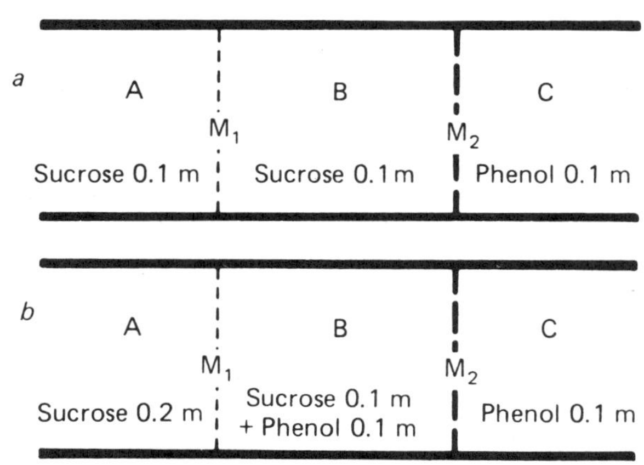

Figure 17. Countercurrent-multiplier model of Kuhn and Ryffel. [Figure based on Kuhn and Ryffel (36).]

permeable to water but not to solute. The solution in both A and B is initially 0.1 M sucrose. Compartment C is separated from compartment B by a rubber membrane permeable to phenol but not to water or sucrose. The solution in C is 0.1 M phenol. Phenol diffuses from compartment C to compartment B until solution B is 0.1 M in both phenol and sucrose; that is, until it has twice its original osmolality. Water now diffuses from A to B, raising the concentration of sucrose in A to 0.2 M.

This model can be transformed into that proposed by Kokko and Rector and by Stephenson as follows: sodium chloride replaces sucrose, and urea replaces phenol. Compartment C represents the collecting duct containing a high urea concentration, compartment B is the medullary interstitium initially containing salt, and compartment A is the lumen of the loop containing salt initially at the same concentration as that in B. Membrane M_2 is permeable to urea and to water but not to salt, and membrane M_1 is permeable first to water but not to salt (descending limb), then to salt but not to water (ascending limb). Urea diffuses from C to B, raising the osmolality of B and drawing water from A, thereby raising the salt concentration in A above that in B. Fluid flows around from descending to ascending limb, M_1 is now permeable to salt instead of to water, and salt diffuses from A to B. Thus salt moves only down concentration gradients, but the ascending limb concentration is lower than that in the descending limb and salt is supplied to the interstitial space.

Thus in principle it is possible to explain the delivery of salt from loop to interstitium without requiring that the transfer of salt depend on an active process in the cells of the loop epithelium. Whether this is, in fact, the correct explanation remains somewhat uncertain. It should be noted that in the Stephenson model active transport by the thin ascending limb is not excluded but, if present, would be made more efficient by the improvement of the concentration difference against (or along) which the salt is moved. The Kokko-Rector model is essentially the extreme case of the Stephenson model.

In favor of the model are the findings of Kokko and Imai (27, 33) that the permeability characteristics of the two thin limbs in rabbits are precisely those required for the postulated mechanism, including the absence of any evidence of active transport of sodium or chloride. Imai (26) has extended these observations with studies in rats and hamsters with similar results. Perhaps even more favorable to the model is its great explanatory value, not only in rendering active transport by the feeble-looking thin ascending limb less or totally unnecessary, but in explaining the "*economy of water . . . referable to urea.*"

On the other hand there are certain data and observations that are hard to accommodate in this model. The sand rat *Psammomys obesus* has been studied extensively by de Rouffignac and his colleagues (e.g., ref. 13). *Psammomys* has the most highly developed thin segments of any animal that has been studied, yet it is able to produce a highly concentrated urine containing very little urea: osmolalities over 2,000 mosmol have been found in urine containing only a little over 100 mmol urea. Furthermore there is evidence that seems to indicate that the rising osmolality in the thin descending limb is the consequence largely of solute entry rather than water loss (13), but perhaps it is *Psammomys* that is out of line rather than the proposed mechanism. *Psammomys* is unusual in other respects.

More disturbing, however, are some of the data from the rat, which we are usually inclined to consider a more typical mammal. The model of a passive process dependent on urea requires that the urea concentration in the interstitium exceed that in the lumen of the loop by at least as much as the salt concentration in the lumen exceeds that in the interstitial fluid, the latter being the driving force for moving sodium from lumen to interstitium. Assuming that urea enters the interstitial fluid from the collecting ducts by diffusion, as is usually assumed to be the case, the concentration of urea in urine provides an upper limit to the concentration in the interstitial fluid. Jamison and his associates (45) have measured the concentration of urea at the bend of the loop and in the urine and have found that the concentration in the loop is lower, but only slightly lower, than in the urine. The difference, although significant, is small enough to cause concern as to whether it is sufficient to account for passive reabsorption of enough sodium chloride; the single effect in the countercurrent multiplier cannot be greater than the difference in urea concentration.

The long interval between the development by Werner Kuhn and his associates of the theory of urinary concentration by countercurrent multiplication in the loop of Henle and its general acceptance is a telling illustration of the resistance to giving credence to totally new ideas. The evidence, now seen to have been incontrovertible and adduced in its favor by the work of Heinrich Wirz, was largely disregarded for several years by most of the nephrological community; I was no exception. Although the general features of the mechanism for concentrating urine seem now to be fairly well established, important details remain to be worked out.

BIBLIOGRAPHY

1. Berliner, R. W. Discussion of paper by Gottschalk in Symposium on Salt and Water Metabolism. *Circulation* 21: 875, 1960.
2. Berliner, R. W., and D. G. Davidson. Production of hypertonic urine in the absence of pituitary antidiuretic hormone. *J. Clin. Invest.* 36: 1416–1427, 1957.
3. Berliner, R. W., N. G. Levinsky, D. G. Davidson, and M. Eden. Dilution and concentration of the urine and the action of antidiuretic hormone. *Am. J. Med.* 24: 730–733, 1958.

4. BRAY, G. A., and A. S. PRESTON. Effect of urea on urine concentration in the rat. *J. Clin. Invest.* 40: 1952–1960, 1961.
5. BRODSKY, W. A., W. S. REHM, W. H. DENNIS, and D. G. MILLER. Thermodynamic analysis of the intracellular osmotic hypothesis of active water transport. *Science Wash. DC* 121: 302–303, 1955.
6. BRUNN, F. Beitrag zur Kenntnis der Wirkung von Hypophysenextract auf den Wasserhaushalt des Forsches. *Z. Gesamte Exp. Med.* 25: 170–175, 1921.
7. BURG, M. B., and N. GREEN. Function of the thick ascending limb of Henle's loop. *Am. J. Physiol.* 224: 659–668, 1973.
8. BURGESS, W. W., A. M. HARVEY, and E. K. MARSHALL, JR. The site of the antidiuretic action of pituitary extract. *J. Pharmacol. Exp. Ther.* 49: 237–249, 1933.
9. CHABARDÈS, D., M. GAGNAN-BRUNETTE, M. IMBERT-TEBOUL, O. GONTCHAREVSKAIA, M. MONTÉGUT, A. CLIQUE, and F. MOREL. Adenylate cyclase responsiveness to hormones in various portions of the human nephron. *J. Clin. Invest.* 65: 439–448, 1980.
10. CRANE, M. M. Observation on the function of the frog's kidney. *Am. J. Physiol.* 81: 232–243, 1927.
11. CRAWFORD, J. D., A. P. DOYLE, and J. H. PROBST. Service of urea in renal water conservation. *Am. J. Physiol.* 196: 545–548, 1959.
12. DEL GRECO, F., and H. E. DE WARDENER. The effect on urine osmolarity of a transient reduction in glomerular filtration rate and solute output during a "water" diuresis. *J. Physiol.* 131: 307–316, 1956.
13. DE ROUFFIGNAC, C., and F. MOREL. Micropuncture study of water, electrolytes, and urea movements along the loops of Henle in *Psammomys. J. Clin. Invest.* 48: 474–486, 1969.
14. FILEHNE, W., and H. BIBERFELD. Beitrage zur Diurese. *Pfluegers Arch. Gesamte Physiol. Menschen Tiere* 91: 569–573, 1902.
15. FRANK, J., and J. E. MAYER. An osmotic diffusion pump. *Arch. Biochem.* 14: 297–313, 1947.
16. GAMBLE, J. L., C. F. MCKHANN, A. M. BUTLER, and E. TUTHILL. An economy of water in renal function referable to urea. *Am. J. Physiol.* 109: 139–154, 1934.
17. GLIMSTEDT, G. Quantitatif histopochemische Untersuchungen über die Nieren. I. Die Verteilung der Chloride. *Z. Mikrosk. Anat. Forsch. Leipz.* 52: 335–358, 1912.
18. GOTTSCHALK, C. W. Micropuncture studies of tubular function in the mammalian kidney. Fifth Bowditch lecture. *Physiologist* 4 (1): 35–55, 1961.
19. GOTTSCHALK, C. W. Renal tubular functions: lessons from micropuncture. In: *The Harvey Lectures.* New York: Academic, 1962, p. 99–124. (Ser. 58.)
20. GOTTSCHALK, C. W., and M. MYLLE. Evidence that the mammalian nephron functions as a countercurrent multiplier system. *Science Wash. DC* 128: 594, 1958.
21. GOTTSCHALK, C. W., and M. MYLLE. Micropuncture study of the mammalian urinary concentrating mechanism: evidence for the countercurrent hypothesis. *Am. J. Physiol.* 196: 927–936, 1959.
22. GREGER, R. Chloride reabsorption in the rabbit cortical thick ascending limb of the loop of Henle. A sodium dependent process. *Pfluegers Arch.* 390: 38–43, 1981.

23. Hargitay, B., and W. Kuhn. Das Multiplikationsprinzip als Grundlage der Harnkonzentrierung in der Niere. *Z. Elektrochem.* 55: 539–558, 1951.
24. Hilger, H. H., J. D. Klumper, and K. J. Ullrich. Wasserruckresorption und Ionentransport durch die Sammelrohzellen der Saugetiernier. *Pfluegers Arch.* 267: 218–237, 1958.
25. Hirokawa, W. Ueber den osmotischen Druck des Nierenparanchyms. *Hofmeisters Beitr. Physiol. Pathol.* 11: 458–478, 1908.
26. Imai, M. Function of the thin ascending limb of Henle of rats and hamsters perfused in vitro. *Am. J. Physiol.* 232 (*Renal Fluid Electrolyte Physiol.* 1): F201–F209, 1977.
27. Imai, M., and J. P. Kokko. Sodium chloride, urea, and water transport in the thin ascending limb of Henle: generation of osmotic gradients by passive diffusion of solutes. *J. Clin. Invest.* 53: 393–402, 1974.
28. Jamison, R. L. Micropuncture study of segments of thin loop of Henle in the rat. *Am. J. Physiol.* 215: 236–242, 1968.
29. Jamison, R. L., C. M. Bennett, and R. W. Berliner. Countercurrent multiplication by the thin loops of Henle. *Am. J. Physiol.* 212: 357–366, 1967.
30. Jamison, R. L., J. Buerkert, and F. Lacy. A micropuncture study of collecting tubule function in rats with hereditary diabetes insipidus. *J. Clin. Invest.* 50: 2444–2452, 1971.
31. Jørgensen, B. C. The amphibian water economy with special regard to the effects of neurohypophyseal extracts. *Acta Physiol. Scand.* 22, Suppl. 78: 1–79, 1950.
32. Kelman, R. B., D. J. Marsh, and H. Howard. Nonmonotonicity of solutions of linear differential equations occurring in the theory of urine formation. *Soc. Ind. Appl. Math. Rev.* 8: 463, 1966.
33. Kokko, J. P. Sodium chloride and water transport in the descending limb of Henle. *J. Clin. Invest.* 49: 1838–1846, 1970.
34. Kokko, J. P., and F. C. Rector, Jr. Countercurrent multiplication system without active transport in inner medulla. *Kidney Int.* 2: 214–223, 1972.
35. Kuhn, W., and A. Ramel. Aktiver Salztransport als möglicher (und wahrscheinlicher) Einzeleffekt bei der Harnkonzentrierung in der Niere. *Helv. Chim. Acta* 42: 628–660, 1959.
36. Kuhn, W., and K. Ryffel. Herstellung konzentrierter Losungen aus Verdunnten durch blosse Membranwirkung. Ein Modellversuch zur Funktion der Niere. *Z. Phys. Chem.* 276: 145–147, 1942.
37. Levinsky, N. G., and R. W. Berliner. The role of urea in the urine concentrating mechanism. *J. Clin. Invest.* 38: 741–748, 1959.
37a. Ljungberg, E. On the reabsorption of chlorides in the kidney of the rabbit. *Acta Med. Scand. Suppl.* 186: 1–189, 1947.
38. Marsh, D. J. Hyposmotic reabsorption due to active salt transport in perfused collecting ducts of the rat renal medulla. *Nature Lond.* 210: 1179–1180, 1966.
39. Marsh, D. J., and S. P. Azen. Mechanism of NaCl reabsorption by hamster thin ascending limbs of Henle's loop. *Am. J. Physiol.* 228: 71–79, 1975.
40. Marsh, D. J., and S. Solomon. Analysis of electrolyte movement in thin Henle's loops of hamster papilla. *Am. J. Physiol.* 208: 1119–1128, 1965.

41. Marshall, E. K., Jr., and M. M. Crane. The secretory function of the renal tubules. *Am. J. Physiol.* 70: 465–488, 1924.
42. Morel, F. Sites of hormone action in the mammalian nephron. *Am. J. Physiol.* 240 (*Renal Fluid Electrolyte Physiol.* 9): F159–F164, 1981.
43. Morgan, T. Permeability of the thin limbs of the loop of Henle. *Proc. 5th Int. Congr. Nephrol.* 2: 105–111, 1972.
44. Morgan, T., and R. W. Berliner. Permeability of the loop of Henle, vasa recta, and collecting duct to water, urea, and sodium. *Am. J. Physiol.* 215: 108–115, 1968.
45. Pennell, J. P., F. B. Lacy, and R. L. Jamison. An in vivo study of the concentrating process in the descending limb of Henle's loop. *Kidney Int.* 5: 337–347, 1974.
46. Peter, K. *Untersuchungen über Bau und Entwicklung der Niere* (monograph). Jena, GDR: Fischer, 1909.
47. Pinter, G. G., and J. L. Shohet. Origin of sodium concentration profile in the renal medulla. *Nature Lond.* 200: 955–958, 1963.
48. Pitts, R. F. Renal excretion of acid. *Federation Proc.* 7: 418–426, 1948.
49. Rocha, A. S., and J. P. Kokko. Sodium chloride and water transport in the medullary thick ascending limb of Henle. *J. Clin. Invest.* 52: 612–623, 1973.
50. Sakai, F., R. L. Jamison, and R. W. Berliner. A method for exposing the rat renal medulla in vivo: micropuncture of the collecting duct. *Am. J. Physiol.* 209: 663–668, 1965.
51. Sawyer, W. H. Increased renal reabsorption of osmotically free water by the toad (*Bufo marinus*) in response to neurohypophysial hormones. *Am. J. Physiol.* 189: 564–568, 1957.
52. Smith, H. W. *The Physiology of the Kidney.* New York: Oxford Univ. Press, 1937.
53. Smith, H. W. *The Kidney: Structure and Function in Health and Disease.* New York: Oxford Univ. Press, 1951.
54. Smith, H. W. *Principles of Renal Physiology.* New York: Oxford Univ. Press, 1956.
55. Smith, H. W. The fate of sodium and water in the renal tubules. *Bull. NY Acad. Med.* 35: 293–316, 1959.
56. Stephenson, J. L. Concentration in renal counterflow systems. *Biophys. J.* 6: 539–551, 1966.
57. Stephenson, J. L. Concentration of urine in a central core model of the renal counterflow system. *Kidney Int.* 2: 85–94, 1972.
58. Tadokoro, M. Active reabsorption of NaCl in the ascending thin limb of loop of Henle in vivo. *Jpn. J. Nephrol.* 19: 275–282, 1977.
59. Ullrich, K. J. Active sodium transport and oxygen consumption in the outer medulla of the kidney in warm-blooded animals. *Pfluegers Arch. Gesamte Physiol. Menschen Tiere* 266: 55–57, 1957.
60. Ullrich, K. J., F. O. Drenckhan, and K. H. Jarausch. Untersuchungen zum Problem der Harnkonzentrierung und Verdunnung. Ueber das osmotische Verhalten von Nierenzellen und die begleitende Elektrolytanhaufung im Nierendewebe bei verschiedenen Diuresezustanden. *Pfluegers Arch. Gesamte Physiol. Menschen Tiere* 261: 62–77, 1955.
61. Walker, A. M., P. A. Bott, J. Oliver, and M. C. MacDowell. The collection and analysis of fluid from single nephrons of the mammalian kidney. *Am. J. Physiol.* 134: 580–595, 1941.
62. Wesson, L. G., Jr., and W. P. Anslow, Jr. Effect of osmotic and mercurial

diuresis on simultaneous water diuresis. *Am. J. Physiol.* 170: 255–269, 1952.

63. WINDHAGER, E. E. Electrophysiological study of renal papilla of golden hamsters. *Am. J. Physiol.* 206: 694–700, 1964.
64. WIRZ, H. Der osmotische Druck des Blutes in der Nierenpapille. *Helv. Physiol. Pharmacol. Acta* 11: 20–29, 1953.
65. WIRZ, H. Der osmotische Druck in den corticalen Tubuli der Rattenniere. *Helv. Physiol. Pharmacol. Acta* 14: 353–362, 1956.
66. WIRZ, H. The location of antidiuretic action in the mammalian kidney. In: *The Neurohypophysis*, edited by H. Heller. New York: Academic, 1957, p. 157–169.
67. WIRZ, H., and R. DIRIX. Urinary concentration and dilution. In: *Handbook of Physiology. Renal Physiology*, edited by J. Orloff and R. W. Berliner. Washington, DC: Am. Physiol. Soc., 1973, sect. 8, chapt. 13, p. 415–430.
68. WIRZ, H., B. HARGITAY, and W. KUHN. Lokalisation des Konzentrierungsporzesses in der Niere durch direkte Kryoskopie. *Helv. Physiol. Pharmacol. Acta* 9: 196–207, 1951.

IX

Control of Vasopressin Release

JAMES T. FITZSIMONS

MECHANISMS that enable organisms to make the most economical use of available water and to replace it efficiently are of the utmost importance for the successful colonization of dry land. Water is conserved according to need through the operation of a homeostatic mechanism of great sensitivity and precision, of which a crucial component is the release of vasopressin from the posterior lobe of the pituitary gland. The development of ideas on this aspect of posterior pituitary function is described in this chapter together with a brief summary of some of the recent developments in our understanding of the physiology of vasopressin.

VASOPRESSIN RELEASE

Pituitary Secretion Affecting Renal Function

The oldest theory concerning the function of the pituitary survives in the name of the gland itself. The secretion of the mucous membrane of the nose, "pituita," was supposed to be derived from the "glandula pituitaria" and consisted of the waste products from the conversion of vital spirits into animal spirits in the brain. The more recent history of pituitary research is described in a fascinating paper, "Breakthroughs in Hypothalamic and Pituitary Research," by Anderson and Haymaker (2), who drew attention to Sir Henry Dale's opening address at the Colston symposium on the neurohypophysis in 1956. At the start of this address, Dale (14) recalled:

> *The 1891 edition of Michael Foster's then justly famous* Textbook of Physiology, *which provided the basis of my own undergraduate studies of the subject when these began, in 1894, was curtly explicit in its account of the knowledge then available concerning the function of the pituitary body. "With regard to the purposes of the organ as a whole," it stated, "we know absolutely nothing"—a statement which, you may imagine, was not without an aspect of reassurance, for a student with an examination in prospect.*

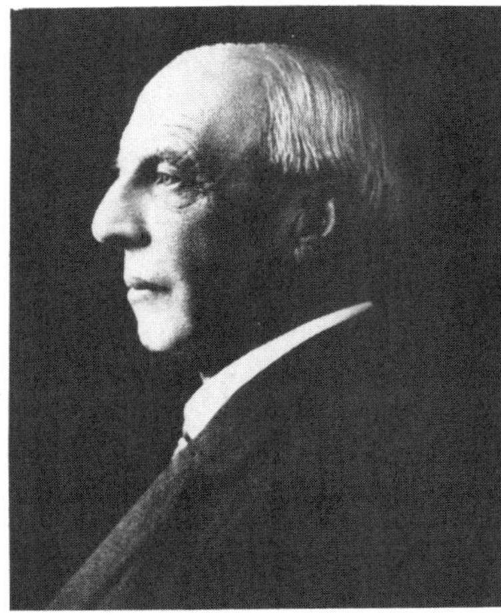

Figure 1. Edward Albert Sharpey-Schafer (1850–1935).

This was soon to change. After demonstrating that suprarenal extracts were pressor, Dr. George Oliver, "the enterprising physician from Harrogate" as Sir Henry Dale described him, and Edward Albert Schäfer (later Sharpey-Schafer) (Fig. 1), professor of physiology at University College, London, turned their attention to the effects of injecting extracts of other glands, including the pituitary. In a short paper presented to the Physiological Society in 1895, they described the striking rise in blood pressure produced by intravenous injection of pituitary extracts (39). In 1898 William Henry Howell (27), professor at Johns Hopkins, reported that the pressor substance was localized to the neurohypophysis and that extracts from other parts of the central nervous system or from the adenohypophysis had no characteristic effects on circulation or respiration. Schäfer and Vincent (46) confirmed this the following year, but they were puzzled as were others at the time by the fact that this potent substance was present in the posterior lobe of the pituitary and not in the obviously glandular anterior lobe. This puzzle was later resolved by the concept of neurosecretion, as described in VASOPRESSIN SINCE 1947, p. 301.

The first indication that the neurohypophysis plays a part in the regulation of urine secretion was in 1901 in a communication to the Physiological Society by Rudolph Magnus, later professor of pharmacology at Utrecht and well known for his work on postural reflexes, and Schäfer, by now professor of physiology at Edinburgh (34). They reported that pituitary extracts caused expansion of the kidney and a marked and often prolonged diuresis. On the basis of these and later experiments with Percy Theodore Herring, who became professor of physiology at St. Andrews University, Schäfer observed that the diuretic action of posterior pituitary extracts seems to be independent of any action on the kidney vessels or blood pressure (45). He concluded that the posterior pituitary, including the pars intermedia, which comes away with the posterior lobe when it is separated from the rest of the pituitary and which was regarded as the source of the active principles (25), produces an internal secretion that has specific actions both on the renal vessels and on the renal epithelium. Schäfer and Herring (45) included several kymographic tracings of the effects of such extracts on circulation and urine flow (Fig. 2). These ideas were developed in the Croonian lecture of 1909 (44) in which Schäfer also referred to an antidiuretic action of posterior pituitary extracts, which can be seen in Figure 2 to precede the increase in urine flow. He suggested (44) that there may be two substances acting on the kidney:

VASOPRESSIN RELEASE

It is further noticeable that in a large proportion of experiments a common phenomenon is a temporary diminution or cessation of urine flow, even although the blood-pressure is raised to a considerable extent and the kidney volume markedly increased; conditions which—on the mechanical or filtration theory of urine secretion—should inevitably produce diuresis. There is, in fact, very often at first an inhibition of secretion (followed in the majority of cases by the characteristic secretory activity), even although the vascular conditions are throughout favourable to the occurrence of free secretion. The extract is therefore liable to cause two effects which are antagonistic to one another. The most reasonable explanation of this is afforded by the supposition that the gland contains not only a substance which stimulates the kidney cells to activity but also another

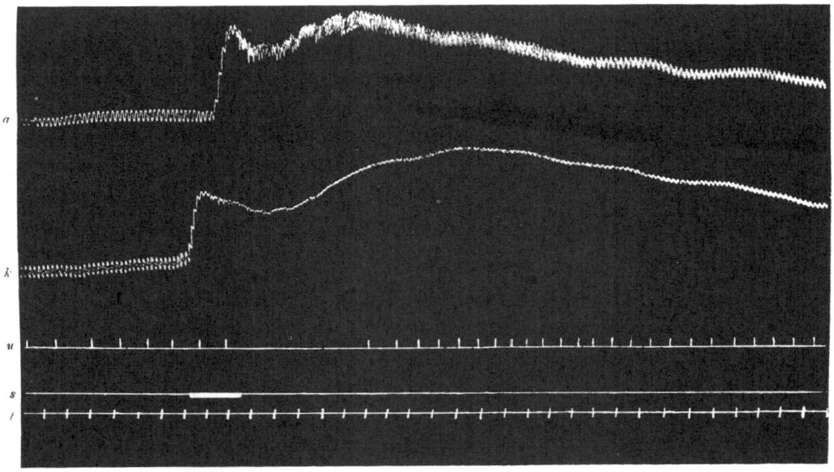

Figure 2. Effect of posterior pituitary extract on blood pressure and urine flow in rabbits. Note initial fall in urine flow before diuresis. a, Carotid blood pressure; k, kidney volume measured in an air oncometer; u, urine flow measured by drop counter; s, injection of 1 ml of a 10% aqueous extract of infundibular pituitary; t, time in 10-s intervals. [From Schäfer and Herring (45).]

substance which depresses their activity, and this to so great an extent in certain cases that the kidney ceases to secrete, although all the vascular conditions for urine excretion are of the most favourable character. Nevertheless, the secretory substance usually ultimately proves the more potent: or it may be that the kidney cells are more susceptible to its influence.

Illustrative of Schäfer's interpretation of the evidence is a section in the Croonian lecture entitled "Stimulation of Pituitary by Injury," in which Schäfer described experiments that produced polyuria by subjecting the pituitaries of three dogs to mechanical injury or "feeble thermocautery."

The bearing of these results upon the polyuria which occurs in injuries and tumours affecting the base of the brain is of considerable clinical interest. . . . The polyuria and glycosuria have generally been set down to injury of a hypothetical centre at the base of the brain. Even when associated, as these symptoms often are in acromegaly, with tumours of the pituitary, they have not been usually ascribed to an increased activity of that gland. . . . Often it (polyuria) does not occur until the disease is more advanced, and may then be due either to the hypertrophy involving the pars intermedia or to this part being stimulated mechanically by the adjacent growth.

There is no doubt that the diuretic effect of posterior pituitary extracts was uppermost in Schäfer's mind and that he interpreted clinical polyuria as caused by excessive secretion of a diuretic hormone owing to irritation or hypertrophy of the pars intermedia. It is interesting to reflect on the fact that as late as 1932, according to Fisher, Ingram, and Ranson (17), Harvey Cushing had stated that it was not known whether diabetes insipidus was an irritative or destructive phenomenon.

In 1912, shortly after Schäfer's Croonian lecture, Erich Frank, who was at the Medical Clinic at Breslau of which Minkowski was director, reviewed the growing body of clinical and pathological evidence on diabetes insipidus in an important paper, "Relationships of the Pituitary to Diabetes Insipidus" (20). He was much influenced by the experiments of Schäfer, to which he refers frequently in his paper, and he therefore assumed that the pituitary secretion was diuretic. His conclusion on the nature of diabetes insipidus (20) was the same as Schäfer's:

It follows from the experimental and clinical facts given, that a gland occupying the pars intermedia of the pituitary affects renal activity through an internal secretion and that true diabetes insipidus of man can be ascribed to a pathological hyperfunction of this gland.

In choosing the pars intermedia as the source of the internal secretion, Frank was following Herring. Herring (25) had suggested that the finely granular epithelial cells in the part of the intermediate lobe that is firmly attached to the posterior lobe were the source of the active principles found in the posterior lobe. He believed that these were contained in hyaline masses of colloid (later called Herring bodies) in the posterior lobe and that this material was carried by lymphatics into the central cavity and then into the third cerebral ventricle. Herring (26) accepted:

The posterior lobe may also furnish secretions into blood-vessels, but its arrangement and histological features suggest a gland which pours its products into the infundibulum, and so into the ventricles of the brain. It may, therefore, be regarded, in part at least, as a special brain gland.

Schäfer and Frank were mistaken in thinking that the main physiological action of posterior pituitary extracts was diuretic, but they deserve credit for focusing attention away from a purely nervous explanation of diabetes insipidus to one involving an internal secretion. The prevailing view had been that the central nervous system played the major role in achieving the constancy of the internal environment, memorably expressed in the celebrated passage in Claude Bernard's *Leçons sur les phénomènes de la vie communs aux animaux et aux végétaux* (8), published in 1878, which begins "*La fixité du milieu intérieur est la condition de la vie libre, indépendante.*" Frank referred to the view, widely held at the time, that Bernard's "piqûre diabète" and the similar puncture polyurias described by other workers provided an explanation of diabetes insipidus; the polyuria of diabetes was regarded as a manifestation of organic brain disease; the lesion caused permanent stimulation of a nervous center for urine flow.

Antidiuretic Effect

Only when pituitary extracts were given to conscious humans instead of to anesthetized animals did the antidiuretic action of such extracts become clear. In 1913 (shortly after Frank's paper appeared) Francesco Farini, assistant physician in the Divisione Medica Ospitale Civile di Venezia, and R. von den Velden, chief physician of the Düsseldorfer Medizinischen Klinik, independently showed that pituitary extracts cause marked reductions in urine flow in humans. In Farini's paper [in the 11 September 1913 issue of the *Gazzetta degli Ospedali e delle Cliniche* (16)] the antidiuretic effect of various posterior pituitary extracts was fully described in one case of diabetes insipidus (Fig. 3) and more briefly in another.

Von den Velden's article (54) (based on a communication made to the Versammlung Deutscher Nuturforscher und Aerzte in Vienna shortly after publication of Farini's article and published on 10 November 1913 in the *Berliner Klinische Wochenschrift*) described the antidiuretic effects of pituitary extracts both in normal subjects and in patients with diabetes insipidus: "*The main result obtained in subjects with healthy kidneys was not an increase but a decrease in urine flow after subcutaneous injections of pituitrin and hypophysin.*

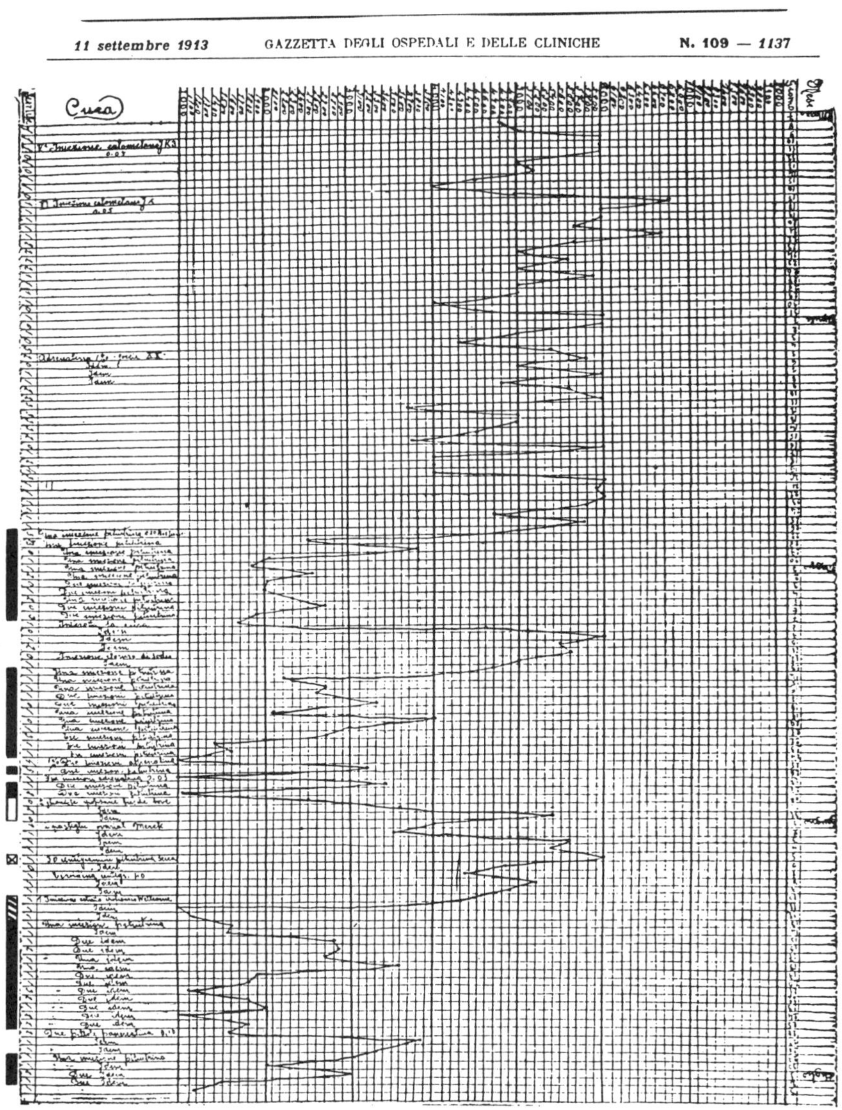

Figure 3. Effects of posterior pituitary extracts and other substances on daily urine volume of patient with diabetes insipidus. Each small division on horizontal axis is 100 ml; total range covered is 1,000–8,000 ml. Each division on vertical axis is 1 day. Patient was given calomel, epinephrine, NaCl, and ovarian, thyroid, and pancreatic extracts, as well as various pituitary preparations. Days on which different pituitary preparations were given are indicated *left* of graph: *solid bars*, Pituitrin (Parke Davis) injections; *open bar*, fresh beef pituitary gland; *cross*, dried whole pituitary gland; *cross hatching*, pituitary extract (Wellcome). [From Farini (16).]

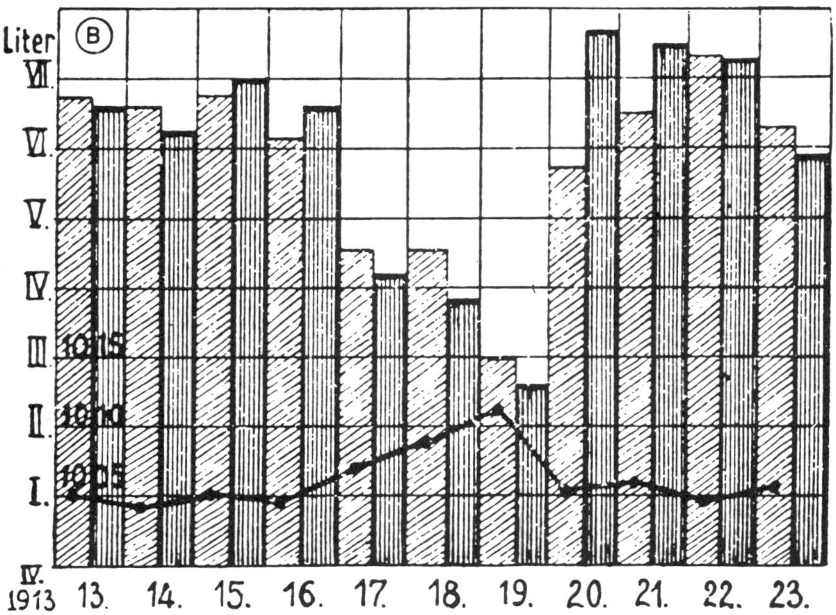

Figure 4. Water intake (*diagonally hatched columns*), urine volume (*vertically hatched columns*), and urine specific gravity (*curve*) of patient with diabetes insipidus after injection of 1 ml Pituitrin each day on April 16 and 17 and 1 ml twice a day on the 2 following days. [From von den Velden (54).]

Water retention, more or less pronounced, was always found and there was parallel retention of NaCl." His case description of patients with diabetes insipidus injected with pituitary extract would be entirely acceptable today:

> *The following curve 2* [Fig. 4] *will demonstrate the effect as a whole; it shows how the amount of urine fell during the injections and the specific gravity rose. The body weight rose, the general health improved strikingly, the feeling of dryness of all the mucous membranes disappeared, and the appetite increased. The patient needed to urinate only once or twice in the night instead of 10 to 12 times; he secretly ate spiced meat and vegetables, which he should not have done, without the secondary intense thirst. The moment therapy was left off, the old state reappeared in unchanged severity; the first 24 hours in fact showed a quite striking excess of diuresis over the supply of liquid of 1 litre.*

Since then numerous observations on humans and unanesthetized animals have confirmed the finding of Farini and von den Velden that the important action of posterior pituitary extracts is to produce antidiuresis. Clear-cut though the results on diabetic patients were, von den Velden was not ready to draw conclusions about normal physiology:

Whether we are dealing here with a "substitution therapy," for which there is little indication, whether the effect is to be explained indirectly by an influence on other internal secretory organs, or whether these changes are brought about only by vascular action in the kidney or by a specific kidney cell stimulation, cannot yet be decided.

Despite this disclaimer the way was now clear for the establishment of an endocrine role of the posterior pituitary based on secretion of an antidiuretic hormone.

Supraopticohypophysial System For Vasopressin Release

Just before World War I, at the very time that the idea was gaining ground that diabetes insipidus was caused by the failure of a diseased or damaged neurohypophysis to secrete some active antidiuretic principle, Jean Camus and Gustave Roussy (11–13), working in the Laboratoires de Physiologie et d'Anatomie Pathologique of the Faculté de Médecine de Paris, introduced a discordant note by claiming that a lesion of the hypothalamus alone was sufficient to cause polyuria (Fig. 5). In a 1914 communication (13) they stated:

The lesion which causes polyuria does not affect the hypophysis in any way. In five cases the experimental puncture did not touch the hypophysis, nevertheless an intense polyuria was produced. This polyuria was neither more nor less intense than when the hypophysis had been affected by the lesion.

Total removal of the hypophysis, performed without lesioning the base of the brain (infundibulum), does not cause polyuria.

In their classic monograph on diabetes insipidus published in 1938 (17), Charles Fisher, Walter R. Ingram, and Stephen Walter Ranson

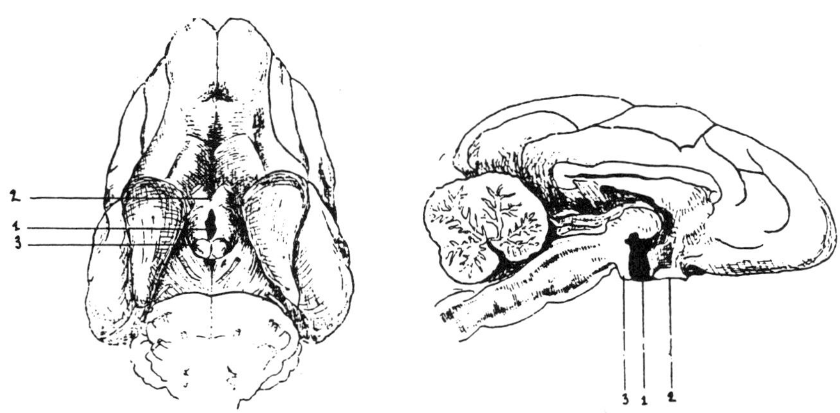

Figure 5. Site of lesion at base of dog brain that resulted in polyuria. *Line 1* points to experimental lesion; *line 2* points to optic chiasma, and *line 3* points to mammillary bodies. [From Camus and Roussy (12).]

(Fig. 6) of the Institute of Neurology at Northwestern University dealt with the early history of diabetes insipidus in comprehensive detail. They pointed out that the experiments of Camus and Roussy brought the pituitary hypothesis into doubt from the very start. They described how there arose two schools of thought on the cause of diabetes insipidus: the "hypophysists" held that the pituitary was all-important, and the "hypothalamists" held that the hypothalamus was paramount. But as they (17) pointed out:

A way out of this impasse was ready at hand but strangely enough appears to have been completely ignored for many years. In 1894 Cajal had shown that the hypothalamus of the rat sends a heavy bundle of unmyelinated fibers into the neural division of the hypophysis by way of the infundibular stem. Here was given a morphological basis for the possibility of a functional interrelation between these two organs.

It was largely as a result of their own extensive experimental work that the two extremes of view were reconciled. Fisher, Ingram, and Ranson produced diabetes insipidus in cats and monkeys by interrupting the supraopticohypophysial tracts, using the Horsley-Clarke stereotaxic instrument that had been introduced at Northwestern University by Ranson (see ref. 2). They found that interruption of the tracts led to polyuria with striking degenerative changes in the neurohypophysis and loss of 95% of its antidiuretic activity. Bilateral lesions in the cat resulted in three separate phases in the onset of

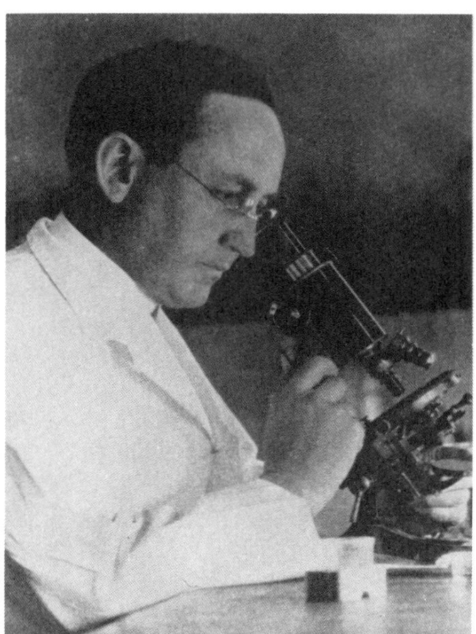

Figure 6. Stephen Walter Ranson (1880–1942).

diabetes insipidus: a phase of transient polyuria from postoperative days one to six; an interphase from days six to ten during which urine flow fell to normal as the denervated posterior pituitary underwent atrophy, releasing hormone into the bloodstream; and finally, a phase of permanent polyuria (Fig. 7). The pattern in the monkey was similar. Conception of the pathological physiology of diabetes insipidus (17) was as follows:

The supraoptico-hypophyseal system regulates the secretion of the antidiuretic hormone by the neural division of the hypophysis. It should be emphasized that the neural division includes the infundibular stem and median eminence. The interruption of the supraoptico-hypophyseal tracts in the hypothalamus causes the neural division to become atrophic and functionally inactive and leads to a deficiency of antidiuretic hormone in the organism. Likewise, section of the stem high enough to cut all of it and the median eminence away from the hypothalamus brings about a similar atrophy and deficiency. Extirpation of the neural division in all its parts leads to the same hormonal deficiency by virtue of the fact that it removes the site of formation of

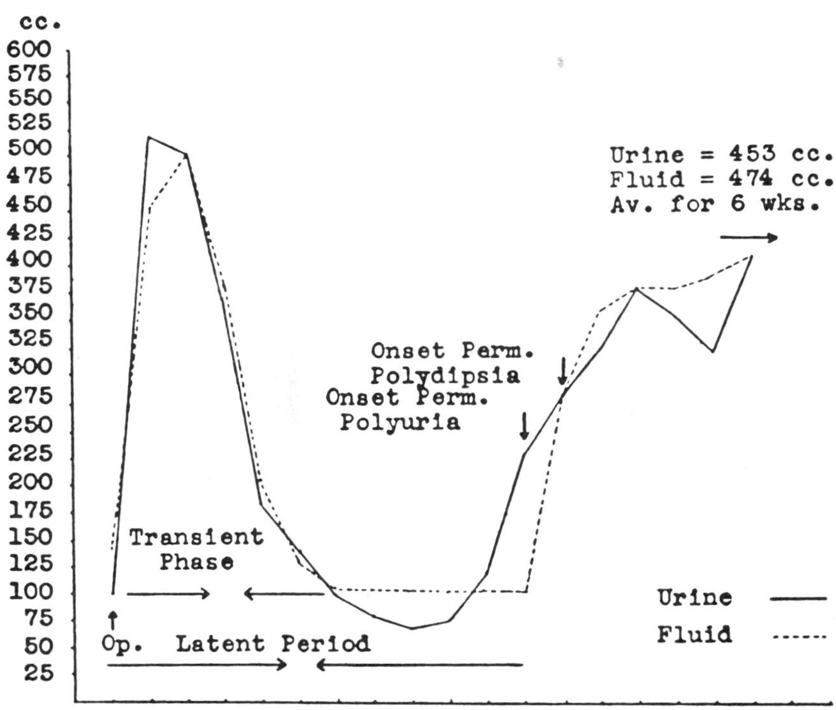

Figure 7. Graph showing course of polyuria and polydipsia of typical case of experimental diabetes insipidus in cats. Note that onset of permanent phase of polyuria occurred 1 day before onset of polydipsia. [From Fisher, Ingram, and Ranson (17).]

the antidiuretic principle. The evidence indicates that the antidiuretic hormone acts mainly on the kidney and prevents the secretion of excessive amounts of urine. The deficiency of this hormone as a result of the types of damage described, brings about a primary polyuria which is followed by a secondary and compensatory polydipsia. The polyuria which develops can be thought of as representing the resultant of diuretic processes in the body unchecked by the antidiuretic mechanism. These diuretic processes are normally under the control of the pars anterior of the hypophysis and the polyuria may, therefore, be thought of as resulting from an uncompensated activity of this gland. In this sense, then, one may speak of diabetes insipidus as being caused by a disturbance of the equilibrium normally obtaining between the neural division and the pars anterior. It should be emphasized that we are speaking of an uncompensated activity of the pars anterior and not a hyperactivity. The pars anterior can be thought of as exerting its diuretic influence through its general control over metabolism and activity, rather than through a specific diuretic hormone. . . . Further, we have been led to conclude that the neural division itself and not the pars intermedia is the site of formation of the antidiuretic principle.

VASOPRESSIN RELEASE

Geoffrey Wingfield Harris, professor of physiology at the Institute of Psychiatry in London, pointed out in his 1955 monograph, *Neural Control of the Pituitary Gland* (24) that if these views are correct, it would be expected that electrical stimulation of the supraopticohypophysial tract would elicit the signs of antidiuretic hormone secretion. An indirect indication of the importance of the nervous connection was provided by the experiments of Ernest Basil Verney, William J. O'Connor, and others, beginning in the early 1930s, on the inhibition of water diuresis by emotional stress (38, 56). Faradic stimulation under the skin, increased in strength until the dog showed signs of resentment, led to inhibition of water diuresis, best seen after removal of the renal and splanchnic nerves. The inhibition could be matched by posterior pituitary extracts and was greatly decreased by removal of the posterior lobe of the pituitary.

Harris referred to experiments in which H. O. Haterius had produced antidiuresis in rabbits anesthetized with intravenous chloralose and urethane undergoing water diuresis by stimulating the pituitary stalk region. Harris improved on this approach by using a remote-control method of stimulation that allowed repeated observations to be made on conscious animals. When the electrode tip was in contact with the supraopticohypophysial tract, stimulation caused a temporary inhibition of water diuresis in hydrated animals. The response could be matched with pituitary extracts. When the electrode was more than 0.5 mm from the supraopticohypophysial tract, no antidiuretic response could be obtained. Antidiuresis was associated with the appearance of an antidiuretic substance in the urine.

The electrical-stimulation experiments of Harris and the lesioning experiments of Fisher, Ingram, and Ranson complemented each other and firmly established the idea that the neurohypophysis depends on its nerve supply to regulate the secretion of antidiuretic hormone.

Is Polyuria Always Primary?

Another controversy in the early history of diabetes insipidus concerned the relationship between polydipsia and polyuria. In 1881, while professor in Jena, Carl Wilhelm Hermann Nothnagel (37) considered the problem of primary polydipsia and asked, "*does the sensation of thirst only depend on stimulation of nerve endings in the parts described* [i.e., the mouth and throat] *through lack of water, or can thirst also be aroused by central stimulation*?" He described (37) what appeared to him to be a case of primary polydipsia in a 35-yr-old man who had been thrown and kicked by a horse. On falling the man had struck the back of his head but had not lost consciousness, although he had vomited.

> *Immediately after the accident— . . . "Half an hour after the fall" is the longest time given—the patient experienced a striking thirst so that in the course of the next 3 hours up to his being brought to the hospital at 11:30 at night he drank a large amount of water and beer, in total quantity about 3 litres of fluid. The first and only time he urinated, up to the time of his admission, was at 11 o'clock, about 2½ hours after the onset of thirst.*

The polydipsia persisted while the patient was under observation; the maximum daily fluid intake reached 18.5 liters. The patient's mouth and throat remained moist, and sucking ice afforded little relief, so that stimulation of nerves in the oropharyngeal region did not appear to be the immediate cause of thirst. Nothnagel suggested that the polydipsia was caused by stimulation of a "durstcentrum" which he thought was in the pons or medulla. The hindbrain was considered to be the most likely site because other vital centers are located there, nerves from the pharynx enter the nervous system in this region, and the patient had pain at the back of the head and neck and showed miosis. However, as Nothnagel himself said, this was all rather inconclusive.

Much later, when the hypothalamus-hypophysis controversy was at its height in 1921, Percival Bailey and Frédéric Bremer (6), working in Harvey Cushing's laboratory at Harvard, published an important paper on experimental diabetes insipidus in the dog, in which they remarked:

> *Polyuria can be preceded by thirst. It is not necessarily preceded by it. The polyuria may appear and persist without any intake of water. But at any rate the polydipsia is not consecutive to the polyuria. The only possible way to reconcile these facts is to suppose that the nervous lesion produces at once thirst and polyuria.*

This work, the first experimental demonstration of primary neurogenic polydipsia (Fig. 8), complemented the clinical observation of Nothnagel, but the question of whether polydipsia is the cause or the consequence of polyuria in diabetes insipidus remained a side issue in the elucidation of the role of the supraopticohypophysial system, and it appeared to be resolved in favor of the latter.

VASOPRESSIN RELEASE

However, because of the work of Bengt Andersson in Stockholm in the early 1950s, there was renewed interest in the central nervous

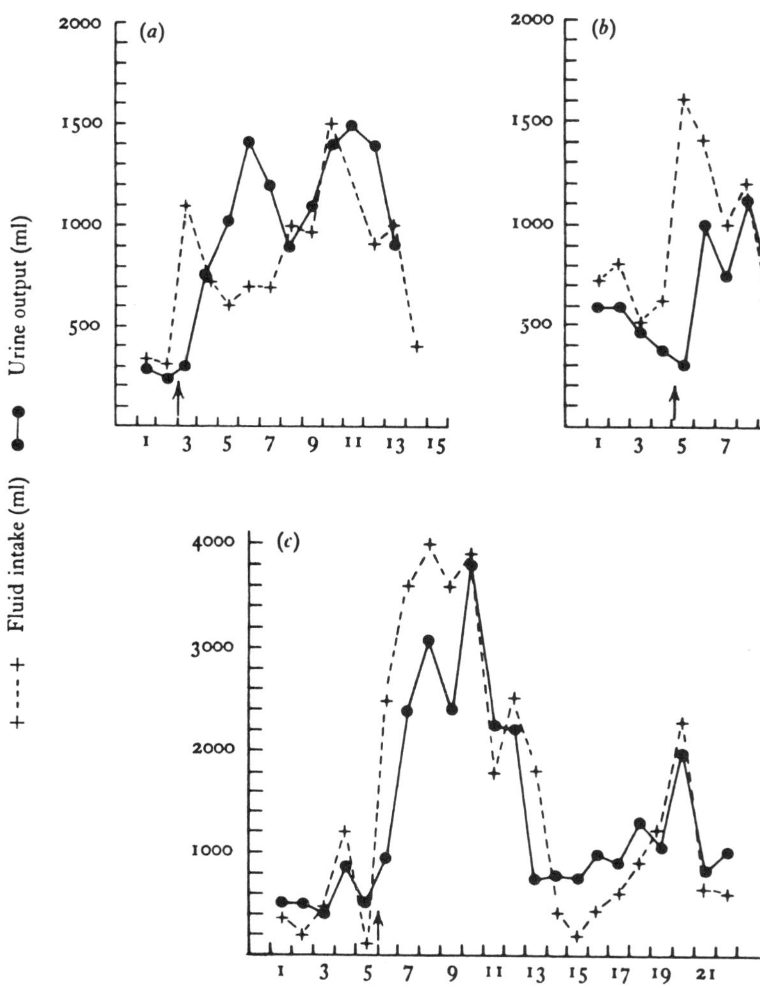

Figure 8. Graphs showing primary neurogenic polydipsia in 3 dogs after lesions in parainfundibular region of hypothalamus; *c*: 2,500-ml intake with 900-ml output on 1st day after operation and 3,600-ml intake with 2,400-ml output on 2nd day. *Arrows*, operation day. [Redrawn from Bailey and Bremer (6).]

structures that control thirst and drinking (see ref. 18). Andersson and McCann (4, 5) used Hess's technique of electrical stimulation of the diencephalon of the conscious animal and showed that stimulation near the anterior columns of the fornix would cause polydipsia in goats. These experiments showed that the hypothalamus controls thirst as well as vasopressin release. As might be expected, the neural organization controlling urine flow and water intake are closely related anatomically.

The debate over whether or not in some cases of diabetes insipidus polydipsia might occur as a consequence of irritation or damage to thirst centers is a reminder that however important is the conservation of water by vasopressin, economy of water without water replenishment is not enough to sustain life for long.

Osmoreceptor Concept

We now turn to a set of key experiments in the analysis of the physiological role of the supraopticohypophysial system. These studies by Ernest Basil Verney (Fig. 9) and his colleagues (56) in Cambridge, UK, led to the elucidation of the factors that determine the release of antidiuretic hormone. Verney had previously introduced the word *osmoreceptor* in the sixth Sharpey-Schäfer memorial lecture (1945), but he presented in the 1947 Croonian lecture (56) a more complete definition:

It becomes justified, therefore, to introduce the term "osmorecep-

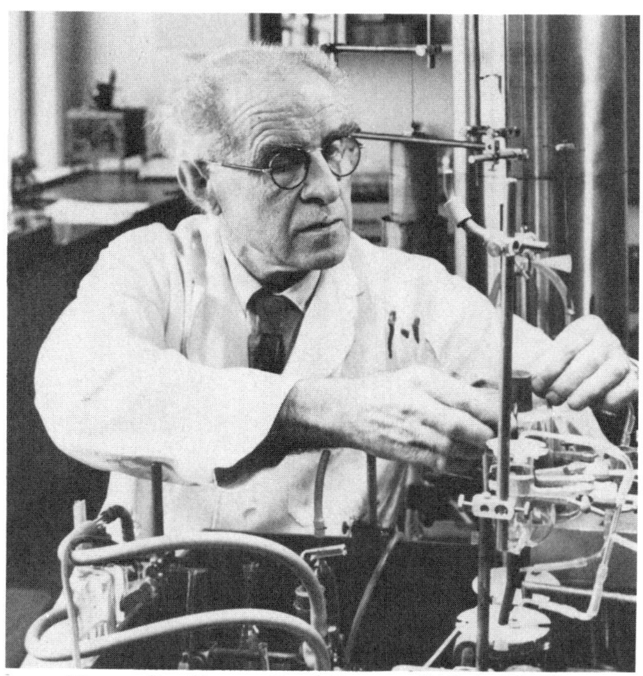

Figure 9. Ernest Basil Verney (1894–1967).

tors" as descriptive of the autonomic receptive elements with which the neurohypophysis is functionally linked, and through whose activation the pituitary antidiuretic substance is released. The term is introduced without prejudice to any specific permeability which they may be shown to exhibit to their ionic and molecular environment; and the facts so far presented show that when they are exposed to short-lived (of the order of 10 sec.) and relatively large (50 to 100%) increases in the osmotic pressure of their environment, their "membrane" is relatively impermeable to sodium chloride, sodium sulphate and sucrose, less impermeable to dextrose, but freely permeable to urea.

Twenty-five years earlier, Verney and Ernest Henry Starling (49, 57) at University College in London had found that the urine produced by an isolated dog kidney perfused by a heart-lung preparation was similar in amount and composition to that produced in diabetes insipidus. The evolutionary significance of this was clearly stated by Starling and Verney (49):

We suggest, therefore, that some substance or substances with an action similar to that of pituitrin are normally present in the intact mammal and serve as the means whereby the kidney is controlled in its important function of regulating the output of water and of chloride. The isolated kidney is divorced from this regulating mechanism—a mechanism which has presumably been produced during phylogenetic development in response to the request for an increasing control over salt-and-water metabolism. It is not surprising, then, that without this aid the kidney functionally reverts to the type of gland characteristic of the fish and amphibian classes of the vertebrate phylum. In these classes, so far as we have been able to find urinary analysis in the literature, the chloride percentage in the urine is always below that in the blood plasma.

The diuresis could be inhibited by adding posterior pituitary extracts to the blood without appreciable diminution of blood flow through the kidney. An even more cogent demonstration of pituitary involvement was provided by Verney in an experiment that allowed a perfused-head preparation to be switched into the circuit of a heart-lung-kidney preparation (55). With the head in circuit, urinary volume and composition became normal again unless the pituitary had been removed previously. These experiments, simple in conception and conclusive in their results, were a technical tour de force. They provided direct evidence that the ability of the kidney to produce concentrated urine depends on the pituitary.

Verney's investigation continued with experiments performed in collaboration with A. Klisiecki, M. Pickford, and P. Rothschild (30, 31) to determine whether or not the diuresis that follows water ingestion has the same explanation as the profuse watery diuresis of isolated perfused kidneys. Was it, too, of pituitary origin? Some of the more reasonable earlier views had supposed that renal nerves were involved in water diuresis or that kidneys were directly responsive to the dilution of blood. That kidneys could be responding directly to the ratio of water molecules to solute molecules (the "diffusion pressure of water," as Haldane and Priestly had believed) was stated by Klisiecki, Pickford, Rothschild, and Verney to be an "*unassailable hypothesis*" for water diuresis, though they covered their position by saying that the hypothesis was "*at present unassailable*" (31). They then promptly laid the foundations for a successful assault on it by pointing out that this hypothesis did not account for the similar polyuria of the heart-lung-kidney preparation, of diabetes insipidus, or after hypophysectomy.

By the 1930s it was becoming clear that alimentary absorption of water occurred well in advance of diuresis and that a pituitary hypothesis fitted the facts better. Verney and his colleagues (30) found that when a large volume of water was given by stomach tube to dogs, there was a 15-min interval between the peak water load in the tissues and the peak diuresis. The diuretic response of a denervated kidney ran parallel with that of an innervated kidney, and it was not accompanied by any change in blood flow through the kidney. They (31) suggested:

> *The secretion of water, over and above that required for the solutes in the urine, is conditioned by and dependent upon a fall in the concentration in blood and kidney of the antidiuretic principle of the pituitary body. The secretion of the antidiuretic principle is itself controlled, through the intermediation of the nervous system, by the concentration of water in blood and tissues.*

This conclusion was contrary to the "unassailable" hypothesis of Haldane and Priestly, which even then had been rendered hardly tenable and which was finally overthrown by the experiments of Verney and his colleagues, culminating in the Croonian lecture of 1947.

Verney's Croonian lecture (56) is a landmark in physiology. In the forty years that have elapsed since its publication, not one of its conclusions has been invalidated. In the experiments described, urine flows were measured in conscious bitches in response to injection or perfusion of various solutions into the carotid arteries that had been exteriorized in skin loops. Verney found that an intracarotid injection of hypertonic NaCl caused a profound inhibition of urine flow in a dog undergoing water diuresis but that a similar injection made into the malleolar vein or an intracarotid injection of isotonic NaCl did not. The failure of intravenous hypertonic NaCl to inhibit urine flow immediately invalidated the Haldane-Priestly hypothesis. The character of the inhibition could be closely matched by intravenous injection of posterior pituitary extracts. Removal of the posterior lobe of the pituitary reduced the inhibitory response to intracarotid hypertonic NaCl to ~10% of what it had been previously.

After establishing that the antidiuretic response to hypertonic NaCl depends on the posterior pituitary, Verney next asked whether NaCl was acting specifically or by virtue of the increase in the osmotic pressure of the plasma it produced. Therefore he compared the antidiuretic responses produced by intracarotid injection of various hyperosmotic solutions, all calculated to cause approximately the same increases in osmotic pressure (mainly ~80%) in the carotid blood. He found that hyperosmotic solutions of NaCl, Na_2SO_4, or sucrose are the most effective at causing similar antidiuretic responses, that glucose is slightly less effective, and that urea is ineffective.

VASOPRESSIN RELEASE

In order to see whether increases in osmotic pressure within the physiological range would release antidiuretic hormone, Verney tried longer-lasting exposures of the osmoreceptors to smaller increases in osmotic pressure, using prolonged intracarotid infusions of hyperosmotic solutions instead of short-period injections. In a 40-min unilateral infusion, a local increase in osmotic pressure of 1.8% brought the urine flow gradually down to 10% of its maximum, which could be matched by posterior pituitary extract given at 1 μU/s (Fig. 10). With these prolonged infusions, sucrose and NaCl gave similar results but glucose was ineffective. Because only half of the osmoreceptors were being exposed in unilateral infusions, it seemed likely that an increase of only 1% of the osmotic pressure in aortic blood is needed to reduce water diuresis to the same extent. Another important finding in the infusion experiments was the gradual recovery of urine flow when the infusion was stopped because this showed that secretion of antidiuretic hormone is inhibited by the local fall in osmotic pressure and consequent depression of osmoreceptor activity.

The importance of these experiments in understanding the phenomenon of water diuresis cannot be overestimated. The conclusions and their significance were clearly stated by Verney (56):

Water diuresis, then, is fitly and accurately described as a condition of physiological diabetes insipidus, and there can be little doubt that the antidiuretic secretion of the neurophypophysis is a hormone in the physiological sense that its liberation is mainly and continually governed by the contemporary concentration of sodium chloride in the carotid arterial plasma. The physiological fitness of this control is emphasized by its quantitative aspects, in that changes within the range and of the order of 1% in the osmotic pressure of the arterial blood lead, through the intermediation of the antidiuretic hormone, to changes in the rate of water excretion within the range and of the order of 1000%: the maintenance of near constancy in the osmotic pressure of the internal environmnent is thereby achieved.

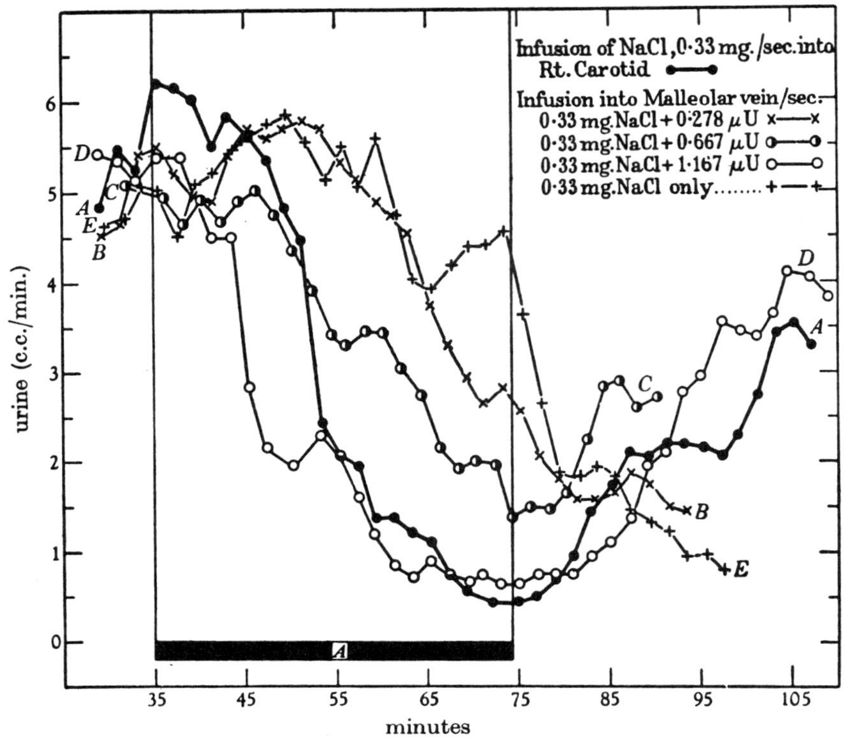

Figure 10. Assay of rate of release of postpituitary antidiuretic substance during prolonged intracarotid infusion (39.5 min, *rectangle* A) of 1.254 M NaCl at 0.2725 ml/min in the bitch "Nicky." Calculated local increase in osmotic pressure is 1.80%. *Curve A*, intracarotid infusion; *curve E*, intravenous infusion of NaCl at same rate; *curves B, C,* and *D* show responses to intravenous infusion with postpituitary extract 0.28, 0.67, and 1.17 μU/s, respectively. *Abscissa*: approximate time after the test dose of water. [From Verney (56).]

Although Verney did not explicitly distinguish between osmosensitivity and osmoreception, he was clearly writing about osmoreception. All cells are osmosensitive in the sense that they are affected by changes in osmotic pressure, but they can only be considered as osmoreceptors if they are particularly responsive in a quantitative manner to changes in osmolality and signal these changes to the central nervous system. The receptors for vasopressin release studied by Verney in dogs clearly meet these criteria and should therefore be regarded as osmoreceptors.

Sodium-Sensitive Receptor?

Is the receptor for vasopressin release exclusively and in all species an osmoreceptor? Andersson, Olsson, and colleagues (see ref. 3), on the basis of experiments in goats, suggested that the receptors for vasopressin release and for thirst are not osmoreceptors but receptors specifically sensitive to the sodium concentration in the cerebrospinal fluid or extracellular fluid. They suggest that the sensitive area is located in the anteroventral walls of the third ventricle where it can be affected by changes in sodium concentration in the cerebrospinal fluid and that it may also be accessible to blood-borne stimuli. Lesions involving the whole anterior wall of the third ventricle caused permanent adipsia and failure to release vasopressin. Antidiuretic responses were obtained in water-loaded goats with intracerebroventricular infusions of sodium-containing hyperosmotic solutions but not with hyperosmotic saccharide solutions that contained no sodium. The antidiuresis was pituitary in origin because it was absent in goats with diabetes insipidus. Decreasing the sodium concentration in the cerebrospinal fluid by intracerebroventricular infusions of saccharide solutions inhibited basal vasopressin secretion in nonhydrated goats and suppressed drinking and antidiuretic responses to intracarotid infusions of hypertonic NaCl.

VASOPRESSIN RELEASE

There are some difficulties with the idea of a specific sodium-sensitive receptor, which means that it must still be regarded as an interesting hypothesis rather than an established mechanism. A stimulus-response relationship has yet to be obtained for vasopressin release and changes in cerebrospinal fluid sodium. Some inconsistencies in the experimental results and the occurrence of other effects, including rises in blood pressure and natriuresis, may mean that the effects of hyperosmotic sodium-containing solutions were caused by nonspecific stimulation of sympathetic centers. The previously made distinction between osmosensitive cells and osmoreceptors is also important when considering the question of a sodium receptor. It is a fundamental property of excitable cells to be sodium sensitive in the sense that the action potential depends on sodium current. We may therefore be dealing with sodium sensitivity rather than sodium reception. The absence of drinking and vasopressin release in response to intracerebroventricular infusions of hyperosmotic solutions of saccharides could be explained by a general depression of nervous activity in the periventricular region, perhaps because of the fall in sodium concentration in the cerebrospinal fluid or because of some toxic effect of the saccharides on neurons (Fig. 11). Similar explanations may account for the inhibition by intracerebroventricular saccharides of drinking and vasopressin release produced by intracarotid infusions of NaCl.

Whatever the position in goats, it is clear that in sheep (36) an osmoreceptor in the sense defined by Verney is additionally required and it may alone be sufficient to account for drinking and vasopressin release. It is equally clear that in dogs (51, 52) an osmoreceptor accounts for the findings. Operationally the distinction between an osmoreceptor and a sodium-sensitive receptor is unimportant because increases in osmolality arising from a lack of water necessarily mean increases in plasma sodium concentration. The evidence at

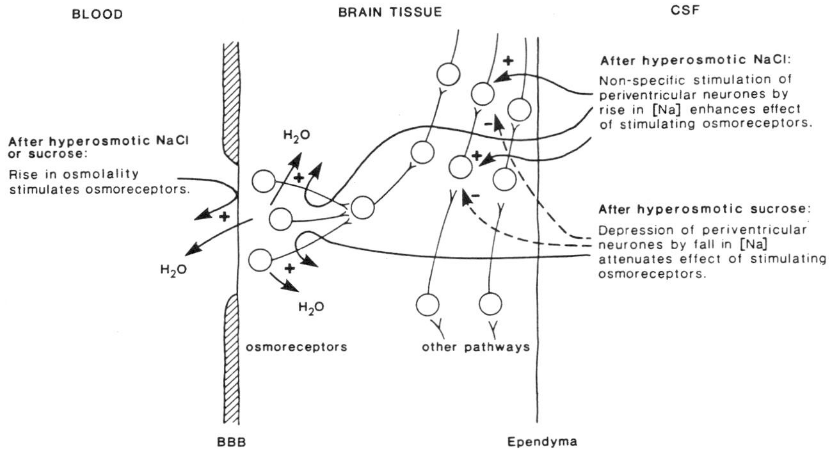

Figure 11. Speculation on how sodium-containing hyperosmotic solutions placed directly into cerebrospinal fluid (CSF) (*right*) could enhance drinking and vasopressin release caused by osmoreceptor stimulation and how hyperosmotic saccharide solutions of the same osmolality could depress such responses. According to this view, nervous conduction in periventricular neurons coming from osmoreceptors and elsewhere is directly affected by solutions placed in cerebrospinal fluid. Osmoreceptors are situated in a part of the diencephalon lacking a blood-brain barrier (BBB), possibly the vascular organ of the lamina terminalis, and are accessible to blood-borne (*left*) increases in osmotic pressure produced by systemic administration of hyperosmotic solutions of osmotically effective solutes.

present still overwhelmingly favors osmoreceptors, though the organization of these may allow the possibility of modulation by sodium concentration at a different anatomical site (see Fig. 12).

Where Are Osmoreceptors?

By selective ligation of intracranial blood vessels, Jewell and Verney (29) narrowed the site of osmoreceptors to the supraoptic region. Verney had previously excluded the carotid sinus and carotid body from consideration by denervation. Subsequently much evidence has been obtained that supports the view that neurons in and around the supraoptic nuclei function as osmoreceptors. However, the effects of blood-borne stimuli on vasopressin release and urine flow indicate that there are osmoreceptors outside the blood-brain barrier. Destruction of the anterior wall of the third ventricle, including the vascular organ of the lamina terminalis that lies outside the blood-brain barrier, disrupts osmoregulation in more than one species.

The central connections and organization of hypothalamic osmoreceptors have been extensively studied since the experiments of Verney. Electrophysiological analysis has shown that supraoptic neurons have many neural inputs, some of which themselves respond to

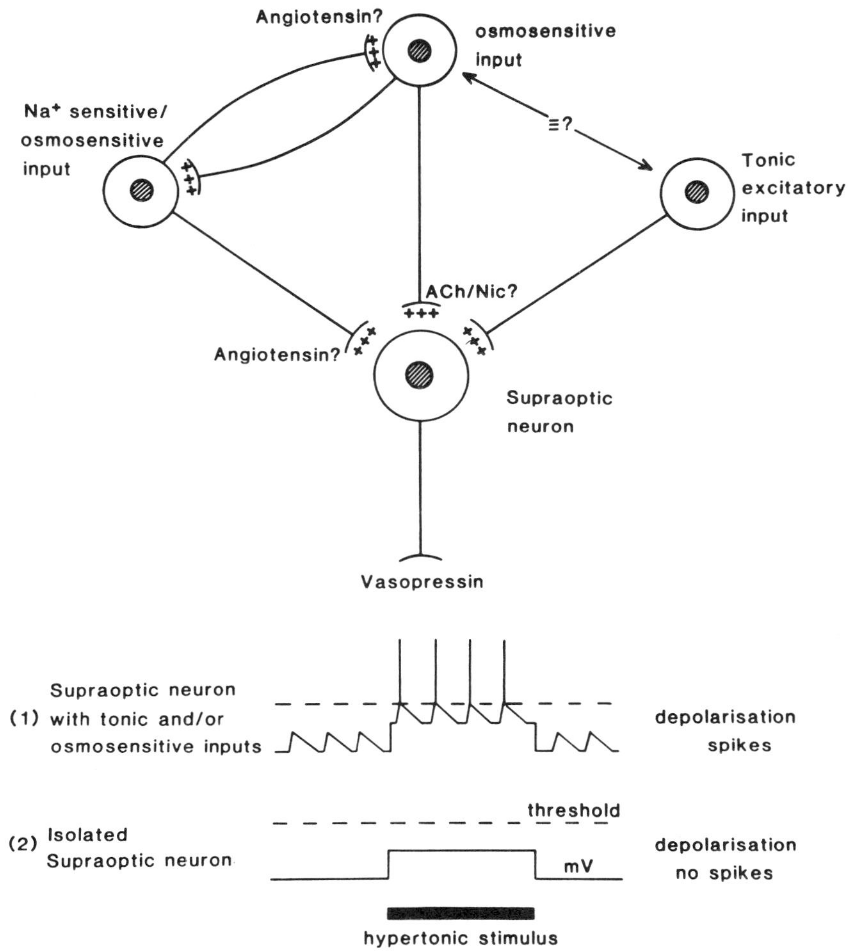

Figure 12. Diagram of proposed hypothalamic osmoreceptor complex. The vasopressin-secreting supraoptic neuron is depolarized by osmotic stimulation, but full expression of osmotic response requires input from other neural elements, some of which are osmosensitive [*above*, *(1) below*]. Thus when communication between neurons is prevented by Co^{2+} or Mg^{2+} and excitatory postsynaptic potentials are abolished, depolarization of supraoptic neurons by osmotic stimulation does not trigger spike generation [(2) *below*]. ACh/Nic, acetylcholine/nicotine [From Leng et al. (32).]

changes in osmolality or sodium concentration (32). The organization of osmoreceptors for vasopressin release is clearly more complex than was first thought (Fig. 12). During release of vasopressin, magnocellular neurons show a phasic pattern of activity, but it is not known whether periodicity is synaptically driven or whether it is a property of the vasopressinergic cells themselves.

The complexity of organization is further illustrated by the long list of putative mediators of vasopressin release that have been described, including catecholamines, acetylcholine, angiotensin II, prostaglandins, endogenous opioids, and calcium (48). Some of these factors may be inhibitory, and of course vasopressin itself may have some negative feedback action on its further release. Since Pickford's pioneering experiments in 1939, the importance of cholinergic pathways to the magnocellular neurons has been recognized. It is also easy to appreciate the significance of angiotensin-induced vasopressin release because this ties in with the role of angiotensin in extracellular fluid volume control. It is difficult at present to imagine how our basic understanding of the physiology of vasopressin release in relation to body fluid homeostasis will be altered by this painstaking analysis, but in view of the other nonrenal roles of vasopressin, it is clearly necessary to understand the nature of the different influences mediating release. Because magnocellular vasopressin-secreting neurons project to many different areas in the brain and presumably have different functions, this may be the significance of the different mediators.

There may even be osmoreceptors outside the central nervous system. For example, F. J. Haberich and his colleagues have suggested that there are hepatic osmoreceptors that participate in the control of water excretion (see ref. 9). They found that infusion of distilled water into the portal vein of a conscious rat caused a significant diuresis that did not occur when a similar infusion was made into the inferior vena cava, whereas a portal infusion of hypertonic NaCl (but not a caval one) caused antidiuresis. There is some electrophysiological evidence to support the idea because afferent activity in hepatic branches of the vagi is increased by moderate changes in osmolality of the fluid perfusing rat or guinea pig livers in vitro.

However, much of the evidence for osmoreceptors outside the central nervous system is inconclusive and in conscious dogs the evidence seems to be against hepatic osmoreceptors. Other sites for osmoreceptors or sodium-sensitive receptors have also been proposed, but the evidence is scanty. The possibility of nonspecific osmosensitivity to large changes in osmolality has not been ruled out, and quantitative stimulus-response data with hormone assays are lacking. In view of the uncertainty of the evidence and the diversity of cardiovascular effects elicited by osmolality changes in blood, with the strong likelihood that these produce changes in sympathetic activity affecting renal hemodynamics, final judgment must await a full physiological analysis, including hormone assays, of any proposed mechanism.

Volume Regulation

In 1935 J. P. Peters (40) wrote, "*It may well be the fulness* [sic] *of the blood stream which provokes the diuretic response on the part of the kidneys.*" Largely through the work of Gauer and Henry (21) and of Guyton et al. (23), it is generally accepted that changes in blood volume without change in concentration affect the kidney, though the mechanisms involved are complicated and not completely understood. It is of course a precondition for successful renal regulation of volume that enough water and electrolyte be ingested. Should the intake of either be insufficient, it is imperative that the body be alerted through the mechanisms of thirst and sodium appetite to the necessity of increasing intake.

VASOPRESSIN RELEASE

Gauer and Henry's view (21) was that blood volume is not fixed but that it is continuously adjusted to the changing size of the vascular bed so that "*at all times an adequate 'fullness of the blood stream' is available to the left ventricle.*" They considered the various mechanisms by which the filling pressure of the heart could be controlled and gave three conditions that must be met for effective monitoring. First, there must be a well-defined compliance relating blood volume and filling pressure of the low-pressure part of the circulation. Second, there must be appropriately located receptor networks capable of recording small changes of tension in the walls of the low-pressure system. Third, these networks must influence the neurohormonal mechanisms that control thirst, excretion of water and sodium, and the distribution of fluid in the extracellular space. With Homer Smith we can agree on the critical importance of sodium as the main determinant of extracellular volume because if osmolality is regulated the volume of the extracellular compartment must reflect the content of its principal cation, though departures from this may occur in some circumstances.

In the context of vasopressin release, one of the suggested mechanisms for extracellular volume control is the left atrial volume–receptor mechanism. An increase in blood volume stimulates stretch receptors in the left atrium and pulmonary veins. Afferent impulses from these receptors travel in myelinated fibers in the vagus nerves and central pathways to reach the supraopticohypophysial system where they inhibit vasopressin secretion leading to increased urine production and therefore a return to normal blood volume. As Folkow (19) pointed out, the most important part of the low-pressure side of circulation is its "functional endpoint," the left ventricle in diastole, hence the particular significance of left atrial pressure because this is the filling pressure of the left ventricle.

The left atrial volume–receptor hypothesis is a simple and logical example of a negative feedback mechanism with an obvious physiological function, but its importance and whether or not vasopressin is involved are matters of some uncertainty. There is considerable discussion about the various factors that could act on the kidneys to alter excretion of water and sodium. Apart from vasopressin these include renal perfusion pressure, renal sympathetic nerves, catecholamines, prostaglandins, kallikrein-kinin system, angiotensin, aldosterone, atrial natriuretic peptides, and an unidentified diuretic factor. According to Linden (33), vasopressin does not seem to be essential. Another authoritative view [by Goetz, Bond, and Bloxham (22)] is that vasopressin secretion is influenced predominantly by osmoreceptors in the hypothalamus and that the left atrial volume–receptor hypothesis adds little to our current understanding of the regulation of extracellular fluid balance.

Although Gauer and Henry were impressed by the particular importance of left atrial pressure, they considered that all chambers of the heart participate in plasma volume control. Because stimulation of atrial receptors is attended by hemodynamic changes throughout the cardiovascular system, it is possible that afferent information from many different receptors is involved. Sensory information carried in the mass of unmyelinated C-fibers arising in the ventricles may be more important in volume control than information from the atria traveling in the myelinated A- and B-fibers. Reflex control of volume may also depend on the arterial baroreceptors.

Up to a point, regulation of osmolality and blood volume are interdependent and some of the effector mechanisms may be shared. There are occasions when volume control overrides the demands of osmoregulation; for example, the hypovolemia of severe sodium depletion leads to increased thirst and fluid retention despite the hyponatremia. In a classic study on experimental sodium deficiency performed on himself and two other subjects, R. A. McCance (35), then at King's College Hospital in London, wrote:

> *It will be noted that at first a removal of sodium was followed* pari passu *by a loss of an equivalent amount of water. So long as this was so, red cell counts may have risen and other signs of anhydraemia appeared, but* no change in the osmotic pressure *of the body fluids had taken place. Further forced removal of sodium was* not *followed by an equivalent loss of water. The volume of the body fluids was relatively well maintained but* only at the expense of the osmotic pressure, *which fell.*

This important finding is shown in Figure 13, in which the scales for sodium and body-weight (i.e., water) loss were so constructed that the curves coincided when sodium and water were lost in the proportions that they are present in extracellular fluid.

The experiments of Robertson et al. (43) have given some quantitative measure of the interaction between osmotic pressure and blood volume on vasopressin release. They have established that there is a highly significant positive correlation between plasma vasopressin and plasma osmolality, thereby providing a system by which small changes in plasma osmolality are rapidly translated into relatively large changes in urine osmolality. However, this system becomes more responsive, with a lower osmotic threshold, when

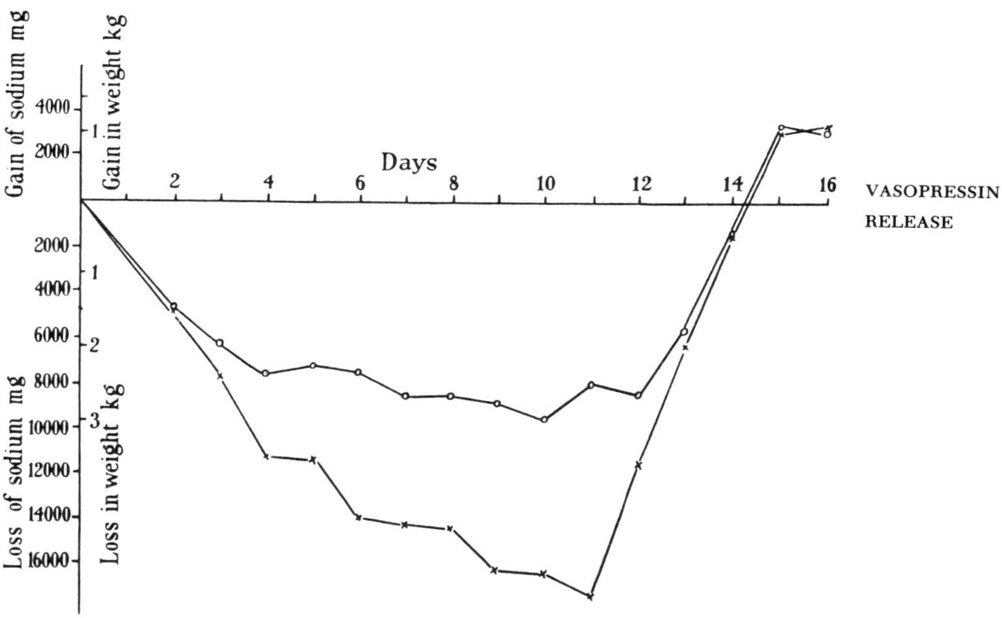

Figure 13. Loss of weight (*circles*) and sodium (*crosses*) during experimental NaCl deficiency in humans. Scales are so constructed that loss of 1 kg water is equal to loss of 3,300 mg (143.5 mmol) sodium, which is the amount of sodium present in 1 liter of extracellular fluid. [From McCance (35).]

blood volume declines by amounts of ~10% or more; it becomes less responsive when blood volume increases.

Vasopressin Since 1947

Conclusive though Verney's analysis of the role of vasopressin in renal osmoregulation was, much experimental effort has been devoted to vasopressin since 1947, some of which has already been mentioned. Some of this work has revealed unsuspected roles for vasopressin (see Physiological Roles of Vasopressin, p. 304), yet to be validated but potentially important. A great body of work has given us an extremely detailed knowledge of the functioning of one hormonal system that has provided valuable insights into how other hormonal systems work. The fields of neuroendocrinology and comparative endocrinology, the concept of prohormones, the physiology of neuroactive peptides and peptidergic transmission, and much else owe a great deal to vasopressin research.

An early stumbling block to acceptance of the idea that the neurohypophysis is an endocrine gland was the lack of any obvious glandular cells in the posterior pituitary. This led Herring to put forward the view that the pars intermedia is the source of pituitary secretion, which he thought is eventually released into the third ventricle via the posterior pituitary. It soon became clear that antidiuretic hormone originates in the neurohypophysis and that it is secreted into the bloodstream. Although as far back as 1924 the hypothalamus was found to contain antidiuretic activity, it was the morphological and experimental work of Berta Scharrer and Ernst Scharrer (47) and then of Wolfgang Bargmann (7) that introduced the idea that the hormones of the posterior pituitary are formed in the nerve cells themselves—the concept of neurosecretion, which eventually resulted in opening up the completely new field of neuroendocrinology. The Herring bodies, already mentioned, are really circumscribed swellings of hypothalamic axons, filled with neurosecretion. The neurons terminating in the posterior pituitary were the first peptidergic neurons to be discovered.

The work of du Vigneaud and his colleagues (see ref. 9) on the structure and synthesis of neurohypophysial hormones has enabled the subsequent development of radioimmunological and immunocytochemical techniques for assaying and identifying vasopressin. These techniques have defined the circumstances in which vasopressin and oxytocin are released separately, a matter on which there had been some disagreement. As recently as 1955, Harris (24) stated that even the evidence for two separate hormones was inconclusive. Physiological evidence and the techniques of molecular biology have established the separate existence and release of two neurohypophysial hormones. The discovery of the rat with hereditary diabetes insipidus, the Brattleboro strain (53), in which there is an inability to synthesize detectable amounts of vasopressin, has provided additional evidence of this.

Neurohypophysial hormones are present in all the vertebrate classes from the fishes upward (1). Each hormone is expressed by one gene that is thought to have arisen from a single ancestral gene 350–450 million years ago, between the emergence of the cyclostomes and the fishes, and that has subsequently evolved by independent mutations. The biological functions of a polypeptide hormone depend on the shape of its molecule and on the shape of the molecule to which it binds because there has to be specific recognition between the reacting molecules. Therefore molecular evolution of hormones by natural selection probably depends on the interaction of at least two molecules, the hormone itself and its receptor, with coordinated changes occurring in the two lines of molecules (1).

Vasopressin and its carrier protein are synthesized as a composite precursor in the magnocellular neurons of the supraoptic and paraventricular nuclei; it is the first hormone shown (by H. Sachs and V. Takabatake in the 1960s) to be formed as part of a common precursor or prohormone molecule. The gene expressing vasopressin (Fig. 14) is 1.85 kilobase pairs long and consists of three exons (42). Exon A encodes vasopressin itself, part of the NH_2-terminal of the neurophysin, an intervening sequence of three amino acids between them,

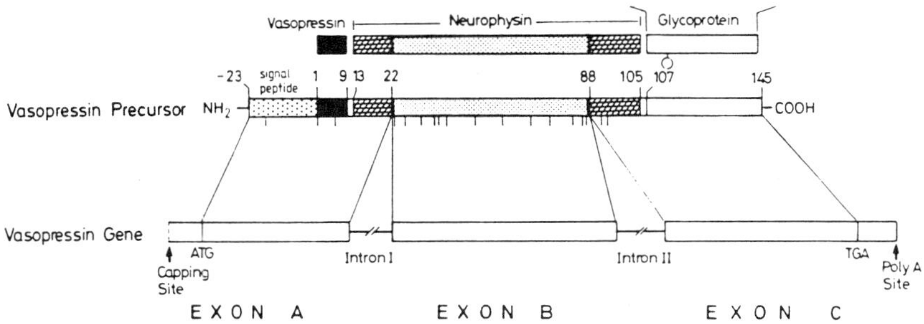

Figure 14. Structural organization of vasopressin gene and hormone precursor. [From Richter (42).]

and a signal peptide. Exon B encodes an internal part of the neurophysin molecule that is constant within and between species. Exon C encodes the COOH terminal of neurophysin, a glycoprotein (not possessed by oxytocin), and one arginine residue between them.

The prohormone travels by rapid axonal transport along the hypothalamohypophysial tracts in neurosecretory granules in which vasopressin, neurophysin, and glycoprotein are cleaved and the COOH-terminal glycine of vasopressin undergoes amidation. Active hormone, neurophysin, and glycoprotein reaching the terminations of the hypothalamohypophysial tracts in the pars nervosa are stored there until released into the general circulation by nervous impulses passing along the same pathways. These impulses depolarize the axon terminals, allowing entry of calcium and release of hormone by the process of exocytosis. The entire contents of the neurosecretory granules are released into the bloodstream, but only vasopressin has been found to have biological activity outside the neuron.

The antidiuretic effect of vasopressin is mediated by cAMP, but in most other sensitive tissues, vasopressin causes an increase in intracellular calcium but does not stimulate adenylate cyclase activity. R. H. Michell, C. J. Kirk, and M. M. Billah suggested in 1979 (see ref. 28) that there are two types of vasopressin receptors: V_2 receptors in the kidney coupled to adenylate cyclase and V_1 receptors in extrarenal tissues coupled to mechanisms that affect calcium; there may be other types. The variety of biological effects of vasopressin has encouraged the search for vasopressin derivatives that could be used as selective agonists or antagonists, experimentally or clinically, and that would be useful in the characterization of vasopressin receptors. Selective antagonists of the pressor and antidiuretic activities of vasopressin are beginning to be available, and some of the problems in their characterization have been recently defined (28).

Deamino-D-arginine vasopressin (DDAVP) was first synthesized by M. Zaoral, J. Kolc, and F. Sorm in 1966 with the aim of producing a more stable molecule with a more prolonged antidiuretic effect (see ref. 41). DDAVP turned out to be a much more potent antidiuretic hormone than arginine vasopressin, and it has very little pressor activity. The cellular action of DDAVP on the kidney is similar to that of vasopressin. An unexpected effect of DDAVP is to enhance plasma levels of factor VIII so that the drug has been used for treating mild hemophilia and for controlling blood clotting in surgery.

Physiological Roles of Vasopressin

Immunocytochemical studies have suggested that vasopressin may be released at sites in the central nervous system other than the neurohypophysis. Since Herring's original suggestion that active pituitary secretion was released into the third ventricle, it has been confirmed on several occasions that there is a vasopressin-like substance in the cerebrospinal fluid. Vasopressin, oxytocin, and neurophysin have been identified in parvicellular as well as magnocellular neurons in many brain regions outside the hypothalamus. Although immunocytochemical findings need to be interpreted cautiously because antibodies typically react with five or fewer amino acids (10), there is tantalizing physiological evidence that, in addition to its peripheral actions, vasopressin acts on the central nervous system.

Among the various functions that have been suggested for centrally released vasopressin are involvement in learning and memory (15), thirst, cardiovascular regulation, temperature regulation, and ACTH release. This does not exhaust the list and at present it is impossible to forsee which, if any, of these effects will prove to be physiologically significant. The sensitizing action on thirst (50), which is found in dogs but not in rats, is the only effect on this list that is in harmony with the antidiuretic effect of vasopressin, because both effects enable the animal to combat dehydration. Because every cell in the body has a full complement of genes, there is no reason why a particular hormone should not be made by any cell, nor is there any reason why it should not have different functions in different parts of the body. There are other examples in evolution of hormones being put to new uses, and vasopressin should not be ruled out in this respect.

Whatever other actions of vasopressin eventually prove to be physiologically significant, there can be little doubt of the importance of its antidiuretic action. The effect of vasopressin on the kidney to produce urine more concentrated than plasma is an adaptation to a terrestrial environment that enables the organism to economize on the use of that enormously valuable commodity water. When too much water is taken, the mechanism is switched off so that the excess water is rapidly and efficiently disposed of without running the risk of water intoxication.

It would be a mistaken view of the role of vasopressin to assume that because it is released in response to increases in effective osmolality, its main function is to enable the body to conserve additional amounts of water in dehydration. It is true that when water supplies fail, further economy of water is possible by releasing more vasopressin. However, urine is normally already fairly concentrated so that the possible reduction in free-water clearance that can be achieved is small, and even with maximal urinary concentration, there is a continued obligatory loss of water through the kidneys, lungs, and skin that has to be replaced. The most appropriate physiological response to dehydration must be an increase in water intake under the control of thirst (18).

In this account of the control of vasopressin release, the renal mechanisms that enable the water-conserving effect of vasopressin to operate have not been considered. The sensitivity and flexibility of the mechanisms that release vasopressin would, of course, be meaningless without the development of a responsive kidney.

BIBLIOGRAPHY

1. Acher, R. Molecular evolution of biologically active polypeptides. *Proc. R. Soc. Lond. B Biol. Sci.* 210: 21–43, 1980.
2. Anderson, E., and W. Haymaker. Breakthroughs in hypothalamic and pituitary research. In: *Progress in Brain Research. Integrative Hypothalamic Activity*, edited by D. F. Swaab and J. P. Schadé, Amsterdam: Elsevier, 1974, vol. 41, p. 1–60.
3. Andersson, B. Sodium versus osmotic sensitivity in cerebral control of water balance. In: *Osmotic and Volume Regulation*, edited by C. B. Jorgensen and E. Skadhauge. Copenhagen: Munksgaard, 1978, p. 84–94.
4. Andersson, B., and S. M. McCann. A further study of polydipsia evoked by hypothalamic stimulation in the goat. *Acta Physiol. Scand.* 33: 333–346, 1955.
5. Anderson, B., and S. M. McCann. Drinking, antidiuresis and milk ejection from electrical stimulation within the hypothalamus of the goat. *Acta Physiol. Scand.* 35: 191–201, 1956.
6. Bailey, P., and F. Bremer. Experimental diabetes insipidus. *Arch. Intern. Med.* 28: 773–803, 1921.
7. Bargmann, W. Über die neuroskretorische Verknüpfung von Hypothalamus und Neurohypophyse. *Z. Zellforsch. Mikrosk. Anat.* 34: 610–634, 1949.
8. Bernard, C. *Leçons sur les phénomènes de la vie communs aux animaux et aux végétaux.* Paris: Baillière, 1878, p. 113 and 115.
9. Bie, P. Osmoreceptors, vasopressin, and control of renal water excretion. *Physiol. Rev.* 60: 961–1048, 1980.
10. Brownstein, M. J. Peptidergic pathways in the central nervous system. *Proc. R. Soc. Lond. B Biol. Sci.* 210: 79–90, 1980.
11. Camus, J., and G. Roussy. Hypophysectomie et polyurie expérimentales. *C. R. Séances Soc. Biol. Fil.* 75: 483–486, 1913.
12. Camus, J., and G. Roussy. Polyurie expérimentale par lésions de la base du cerveau. La polyurie dite hypophysaire. *C. R. Séances Soc. Biol. Fil.* 75: 628–633, 1913.
13. Camus, J., and G. Roussy. Localisation anatomique à la base du cerveau

des lésions qui provoquent la polyurie chez le chien. *C. R. Séances Soc. Biol. Fil.* 76: 877–880, 1914.

14. Dale, H. Evidence concerning the endocrine function of the neurohypophysis and its nervous control. In: *The Neurohypophysis*, edited by H. Heller. London: Butterworths, 1957, p. 1–9.
15. De Wied, D. Behavioural actions of neurohypophysial peptides. *Proc. R. Soc. Lond. B Biol. Sci.* 210: 183–195, 1980.
16. Farini, F. Diabete insipido ed opoterapia ipofisaria. *Gazz. Osp. Clin.* 34: 1135–1139, 1913.
17. Fisher, C., W. R. Ingram, and S. W. Ranson. *Diabetes Insipidus and the Neurohormonal Control of Water Balance: A Contribution to the Structure and Function of the Hypothalamico-Hypophyseal System.* Ann Arbor, MI: Edwards, 1938.
18. Fitzsimons, J. T. *The Physiology of Thirst and Sodium Appetite.* Cambridge, UK: Cambridge Univ. Press, 1979. (Physiol. Soc. Monogr. No. 35.)
19. Folkow, B. Relevance of cardiovascular reflexes. In: *Cardiac Receptors*, edited by R. Hainsworth, C. Kidd, and R. J. Linden. Cambridge, UK: Cambridge Univ. Press, 1979, p. 473–505.
20. Frank, E. Über Beziehungen der Hypophyse zum Diabetes insipidus. *Berl. Klin. Wochenschr.* 49: 393–397, 1912.
21. Gauer, O. H., and J. P. Henry. Neurohormonal control of plasma volume. In: *Cardiovascular Physiology II*, edited by A. C. Guyton and A. W. Cowley. Baltimore, MD: University Park, 1976, vol. 9, p. 145–190. (Int. Rev. Physiol. Ser.)
22. Goetz, K. L., G. C. Bond, and D. D. Bloxham. Atrial receptors and renal function. *Physiol. Rev.* 55: 157–205, 1975.
23. Guyton, A. C., A. E. Taylor, and H. J. Granger. *Circulatory Physiology II: Dynamics and Control of the Body Fluids.* Philadelphia, PA: Saunders, 1975.
24. Harris, G. W. *Neural Control of the Pituitary Gland.* London: Arnold, 1955. (Physiol. Soc. Monogr. No. 3.)
25. Herring, P. T. The histological appearances of the mammalian pituitary body. *Q. J. Exp. Physiol.* 1: 121–159, 1908.
26. Herring, P. T. A contribution to the comparative physiology of the pituitary body. *Q. J. Exp. Physiol.* 1: 261–280, 1908.
27. Howell, W. H. The physiological effects of extracts of the hypophysis cerebri and infundibular body. *J. Exp. Med.* 3: 245–258, 1898.
28. Jard, S. Vasopressin receptors. *Front. Horm. Res.* 13: 89–104, 1985.
29. Jewell, P. A., and E. B. Verney. An experimental attempt to determine the site of the neurohypophysial osmoreceptors in the dog. *Philos. Trans. R. Soc. Lond. B Biol. Sci.* 240: 197–324, 1957.
30. Klisiecki, A., M. Pickford, P. Rothschild, and E. B. Verney. The absorption and excretion of water by the mammal. Part I. The relation between absorption of water and its excretion by the innervated and denervated kidney. *Proc. R. Soc. Lond. B Biol. Sci.* 112: 496–521, 1933.
31. Klisiecki, A., M. Pickford, P. Rothschild, and E. B. Verney. The absorption and excretion of water by the mammal. Part II. Factors influencing the response of the kidney to water-ingestion. *Proc. R. Soc. Lond. B Biol. Sci.* 112: 521–547, 1933.
32. Leng, G., W. T. Mason, and R. G. Dyer. The supraoptic nucleus as an osmoreceptor. *Neuroendocrinology* 34: 75–82, 1982.

33. LINDEN, R. J. Neurocirculatory control of sodium and water excretion. In: *Developments in Cardiovascular Medicine*, edited by C. J. Dickinson and J. Marks. Lancaster, UK: MTP, 1978, p. 191–203.
34. MAGNUS, R., and E. A. SCHÄFER. The action of pituitary extracts on the kidney. *J. Physiol. Lond.* 27: ix–x, 1901.
35. MCCANCE, R. A. Experimental sodium chloride deficiency in man. *Proc. R. Soc. Lond. B Biol. Sci.* 119: 245–268, 1936.
36. MCKINLEY, M. J., D. A. DENTON, L. E. LEKSELL, E. TARJAN, and R. S. WEISINGER. Evidence for cerebral sodium sensors involved in water drinking in sheep. *Physiol. Behav.* 25: 501–504, 1980.
37. NOTHNAGEL, H. Durst und Polydipsie. *Arch. Pathol. Anat.* 86: 435–447, 1881.
38. O'CONNOR, W. J. *Renal Function.* London: Arnold, 1962. (Physiol. Soc. Monogr. No. 10.)
39. OLIVER, G., and E. A. SCHÄFER. On the physiological action of extracts of pituitary body and certain other glandular organs. *J. Physiol. Lond.* 18: 277–279, 1895.
40. PETERS, J. P. *Body Water.* Springfield, IL: Thomas, 1935.
41. PLISKA, V. Pharmacology of Deamino-D-Arginine Vasopressin. *Front. Horm. Res.* 13: 278–291, 1985.
42. RICHTER, D. Vasopressin and oxytocin are expressed as polyproteins. *Trends Biochem. Sci.* 8: 278–281, 1983.
43. ROBERTSON, G. L., R. L. SHELTON, and S. ATHAR. The osmoregulation of vasopressin. *Kidney Int.* 10: 25–37, 1976.
44. SCHÄFER, E. A. The functions of the pituitary body. *Proc. R. Soc. Lond. B Biol. Sci.* 81: 442–468, 1909.
45. SCHÄFER, E. A., and P. T. HERRING. The action of pituitary extracts on the kidney. *Philos. Trans. R. Soc. Lond B Biol. Sci.* 199: 1–29, 1908.
46. SCHÄFER, E. A., and S. VINCENT. The physiological effects of extracts of the pituitary body. *J. Physiol. Lond.* 25: 87–97, 1899.
47. SCHARRER, E., and B. SCHARRER. Über Drusen-Nervenzellen und neurosekretorische Organe bei Wirbeltiere und Wirbellosen. *Biol. Rev.* 12: 185–216, 1937.
48. SKLAR, A. H., and R. W. SCHRIER. Central nervous system mediators of vasopressin release. *Physiol. Rev.* 63: 1243–1280, 1983.
49. STARLING, E. H., and E. B. VERNEY. The secretion of urine as studied on the isolated kidney. *Proc. R. Soc. Lond. B Biol. Sci.* 97: 321–363, 1925.
50. SZCZEPAŃSKA-SADOWSKA, E., J. SOBOCIŃSKA, and B. SADOWSKI. Central dipsogenic effect of vasopressin. *Am. J. Physiol.* 242 (*Regulatory Integrative Comp. Physiol.* 11): R372–R379, 1982.
51. THRASHER, T. N., C. J. BROWN, L. C. KEIL, and D. J. RAMSAY. Thirst and vasopressin release in the dog: an osmoreceptor or sodium receptor mechanism? *Am. J. Physiol.* 238 (*Regulatory Integrative Comp. Physiol.* 7): R333–R339, 1980.
52. THRASHER, T. N., R. G. JONES, L. C. KEIL, C. J. BROWN, and D. J. RAMSAY. Drinking and vasopressin release during ventricular infusions of hypertonic solutions. *Am. J. Physiol.* 238 (*Regulatory Integrative Comp. Physiol.* 7): R340–R345, 1980.
53. VALTIN, H., and H. A. SCHROEDER. Familial hypothalamic diabetes insipidus in rats (Brattleboro strain). *Am. J. Physiol.* 206: 425–430, 1964.
54. VELDEN, R. VON DEN. Die Nierenwirkung von Hypophysenextrakten beim Menschen. *Berl. Klin. Wochenschr.* 50: 2083–2086, 1913.

55. Verney, E. B. The secretion of pituitrin in mammals, as shown by perfusion of the isolated kidney of the dog. *Proc. R. Soc. Lond. B Biol. Sci.* 99: 487–517, 1926.
56. Verney, E. B. The antidiuretic hormone and the factors which determine its release. *Proc. R. Soc. Lond. B Biol. Sci.* 135: 26–106, 1947.
57. Verney, E. B., and E. H. Starling. On secretion by the isolated kidney. *J. Physiol. Lond.* 56: 353–358, 1922.

X

Urea Excretion

BODIL SCHMIDT-NIELSEN

IT is true of the history of science in general that progress is marked by a series of scientific revolutions, and the history of urea excretion is no exception. Paradigms are accepted for a period of time, and only when new facts are found to overwhelmingly conflict with the current ideas are these discarded or modified in favor of new ones (72, 152). Thus it is not possible to write the history of urea excretion without reference to the controversies of the last 150 years between the vitalist beliefs and the beliefs that biological phenomena can be explained by simple physicochemical forces. In 1843 Carl Ludwig (82; author's translation) wrote:

RENAL EXCRETION

We have a vital, chemical and mechanical force, through which the secretion of fluid through membranes, blood vessels and glands takes place. About the first nothing is yet known, and at least it is not sufficiently defined, therefore I shall for the time being bypass it in silence and later as far as the kidney secretion is concerned show its complete uselessness.

The term *active transport*, which is now generally accepted and which describes the movement of many substances through biological membranes, has replaced the old term *vital forces* in our vocabulary. Modern science has unraveled many of the mysteries of active transport, but this does not mean that it is understood to the fullest degree nor that it can be fully duplicated in vitro.

Perhaps to a higher degree than most other excretory products, urea has been the subject of controversy concerning its movements through biological membranes as well as its role in the mammalian kidney, and there are still uncharted areas concerning the tubular handling of urea and its function in the mammalian concentrating mechanism. As recently pointed out by Roch-Ramel and Peters (128), the movement of urea between different body compartments is usually described by three dogmatic statements, each of which is unequivocally based on the totally mechanistic view as expressed by Ludwig or, as discussed subsequently, on the desire to simplify all vital phenomena to the utmost. The dogmas are: *1*) Biological membranes are generally "freely" permeable to urea or, in other words, are practically as permeable to urea as to water. *2*) The main exceptions to this rule are a number of members (including the blood-brain barrier and parts of the renal tubules) that are definitely less permeable to urea than to water. *3*) All movements of urea across biological membranes occur by free diffusion; there are no known membrane carriers for urea. "*Although none of these dogmas can be considered definitely established, a great number of observations support them. There are, however, a number of findings which cannot be reconciled with these dogmatic statements*" (128).

These unresolved issues have had a curious effect on the history of urea excretion and movement through membranes. The knowledge and insights, rather than moving forward along a single path, have taken separate paths that rarely meet. Thus the ambiguities in interpretations make this particular subject rather difficult to approach. The history of urea is not marked by a series of brilliant insights that have increased our understanding but rather by a struggle between opposing views.

Discovery of Urea

The first discovery of urea has been widely attributed to Rouelle le cadet (130) in 1773. However, the discovery was made at least fifty years earlier by Herman Boerhaave (Fig. 1), Professor of Chemistry and Botany at the University of Leyden between 1704 and 1729 (73).

As expressed by V. Robinson (123) in *The Story of Medicine: Boerhaave was a savant, familiar with classic, oriental, and modern tongues, music, poetry, philosophy, history, literature and the bibliography of the sciences. He developed the chemistry of the carbon compounds and the doctrine of affinity. He was not fertile in discovery, not great in original investigations; his role was rather to sum up and interpret the accumulated knowledge of the centuries. Of umblemished character and a great personality, warm-hearted and clear-thinking, he was the medical arbiter of his age.*

In 1727 Boerhaave's students published his lectures under his name. In this book, bitterly resented by Boerhaave, the isolation of urea, which he called "*the native salt of urine*," is first described. In 1732 Boerhaave published the method in his celebrated book *Elementa Chemiae*, with the comment, "*Those experiments which are now contained in this work are what I made in public many years ago, and this I think proper to mention lest anybody should suspect that I borrowed them elsewhere without making mention of the author's name*" (11). Urea was isolated by evaporating the water from fresh

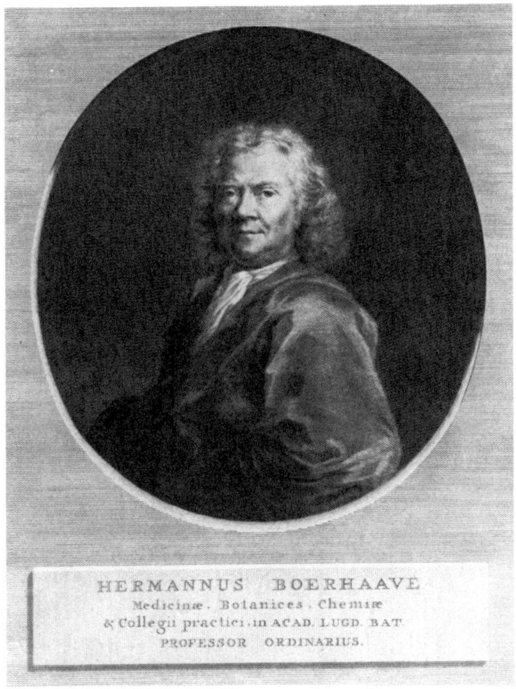
HERMANNUS BOERHAAVE
Medicinæ. Botanices. Chemiæ
& Collegii practici. in ACAD. LUGD. BAT.
PROFESSOR ORDINARIUS.

Figure 1. Herman Boerhaave (1665–1738) occupied most of the chairs at the University of Leyden and was the first to discover urea. (Courtesy of National Library of Medicine, Bethesda, MD.)

urine to a consistency of thick cream that was then left for a year in a tall cylinder covered with paper. By separating the thick black liquid on top from the crystalized salt at the bottom of the vessel, this liquid could be redissolved, and after being cleaned of many of the impurities and evaporated down, "*it will shoot into saline glebes of a particular kind, that are perfectly distinct from every other salt. In their figure and solidity, however, they come pretty near the crystals of sugar. These are not fetid, nor alkaline but very volatile. This is the native Salt of the Urine*" (11). That Boerhaave's method does in fact yield urea was later verified by Backer and De Jonge (see ref. 73).

Boerhaave's discovery of urea was completely overlooked for 200 years, but urea was independently discovered in 1773 by H. M. Rouelle, who in 1768 had succeeded his famous and eccentric older brother G. F. Rouelle as experimental demonstrator of chemistry at the Jardin du Roi in Paris. Rouelle's urea, probably quite impure, was isolated as the alcohol-soluble substance from urine. This saponaceous extract crystalized like a salt and yielded, upon heating, more than half its weight in ammonia. Thus Rouelle (130) was the first to present proof of the high nitrogen content of urea, and he regarded it as the end product from digestion and combustion of the nutritive vegetable matter in the body. The name "urée" was given to this substance in 1799 by Fourcroy and Vanquelin (42), who isolated and analyzed it. A far more accurate analysis of the elements in urea was published in 1817 by Prout (111) (best known for his hypothesis concerning atomic weights).

Synthesis of Urea

The next chapter in the urea story, the synthesis of urea from inorganic compounds by Friedrich Wöhler [Fig. 2; (179)] is of interest for several reasons. On 22 February 1828 (107), Wöhler wrote to his friend and mentor Berzelius in Stockholm:

I can make urea without the necessity of a kidney or even an animal whether man or dog. Ammonium cyanate is urea.... This is an incontrovertible example that two different bodies can contain the same proportions of the same elements, and that only the different kind of combination produces the difference in properties. Can this artificial production of urea be regarded as an example of the formation of an organic substance from inorganic bodies?

At the time of this letter, Wöhler was a teacher in the newly founded *Gewerbeschule* in Berlin. Because a great deal has been written about

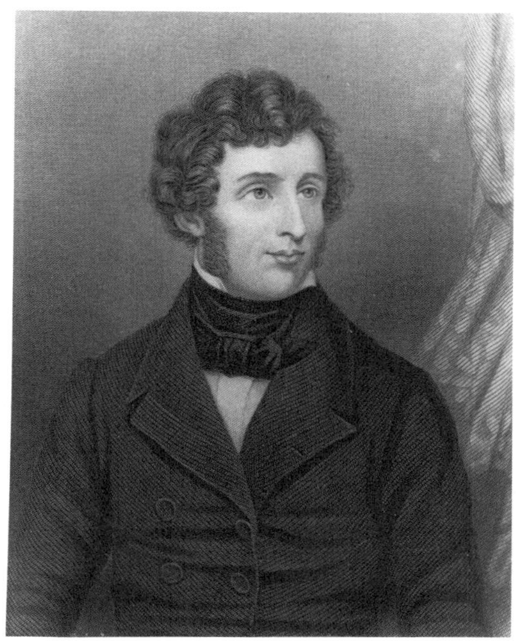

Figure 2. Friedrich Wöhler (1800–1882) was a chemist and teacher at *Gewerbeschule* in Berlin when he synthesized urea in 1828. (Courtesy of National Library of Medicine, Bethesda, MD.)

this outstanding chemist, only a few details are presented here. He was born in 1800, the son of a veterinary surgeon. In 1820 he studied medicine in Marburg, but his real interest was chemistry, which he pursued by carrying out experiments on cyanic acid in his private lodgings. He took his medical degree in 1823, after which he decided to be a chemist and spent a year with Berzelius in Stockholm (107). Wöhler's urea was hailed by many as "*an epoch-making discovery in the real sense of that word*" (16).

Why, we may ask, was so much importance attached to this synthesis? It was not the interesting fact that ammonium cyanate shares the same empirical formula with urea and thus is a clear example of isomerism. As detailed by Brooke (16), the heart of the matter lay in the challenge to the vitalist beliefs. At the forefront of most scientific thinking and experimentation during the nineteenth and a good part of the twentieth century was the question: Is there something peculiar about an organism and is there something peculiar about an organic compound that cannot be duplicated outside the body? Although for some the synthesis of urea spelled an end to vitalist ideas, some chemists and physiologists argued that urea could scarcely be considered organic matter. Even Berzelius argued that urea occupied the milieu between organic and inorganic compounds. Other chemists raised the question that there was something dubious about the synthesis itself because Wöhler used organic compounds as sources for the production of cyanate and ammonia (16). It is also a little peculiar that all these questions were raised about the synthesis of urea because oxalic acid, another organic compound, had been synthesized earlier without raising these arguments. As pointed out by Brooke (16), the synthesis of urea in the laboratory in no way duplicates the synthesis of urea that takes place on the cellular level, and thus in reality it should have very little impact on the vitalist views.

Urea in Organic Fluids

By 1817 the role of urea in metabolism and its elimination in urine was suggested by M. J. E. Berard (6) after analyzing many animal substances: "*Since urea and uric acid are the most azotized substances, the secretion of urine appears to have for its object the separation of the excess azote from the blood.*" This was borne out by repeated observations that the urea content of urine appeared to be directly related to the protein (and hence nitrogen) content of the diet. That urea results from the oxidation of protein was later proved in vitro by M. Bechamp in 1856 (5).

The presence of urea in mammalian blood was demonstrated by J. L. Prevost and J. A. Dumas (110) in 1822. They also found that nephrectomy in cats, dogs, and rabbits increases urea concentration in the blood; they concluded that urea is excreted by the kidneys.

During most of the nineteenth century, it became quite common to measure urea concentration in urine and body fluids of a great variety of animals. In 1827 Cantu demonstrated the presence of urea in the urine of carnivorous birds, although it is absent from the urine of herbivorous birds; in 1831 Hieronymi analyzed the urine of tigers, lions, leopards, and panthers and found concentrations of up to 13% (2.2 M) (73). In 1858 G. Stadeler and F. T. Frerichs discovered that extracts of skate and dogfish muscles contain such colossal quantities of urea that "*the syrup solidified to a solid mass upon the addition of an equal volume of nitric acid*" (160).

Quantitative analysis of urea in urine was carried out by a number of different methods. However, quantitative determination of urea in blood was cumbersome and quite inaccurate. This changed, however, when a young chemist, Eli Kennerly Marshall, Jr., while visiting Aberhalden's laboratory in Germany, became interested in working on urease. [The quotes from Marshall that follow have been cited from Maren (84).] Marshall had received his Ph.D. in Chemistry in the summer of 1912, after which he sailed off to Europe with a letter of introduction to Aberhalden in Halle, Germany. He was accepted but felt quite isolated because of the language barrier, but his time was not wasted: "*I spent time reading in the small department library.... I wanted to study enzyme action, ... ran across literature on urease, and decided to work with it when I returned to Baltimore in the fall.*" That winter (back in Baltimore) Marshall attacked the urease problem with force. He obtained soybeans from the local market at Gay Street and was amazed at the ease and quantitative specificity with which the extracts decomposed urea.

Hudson had used the enzyme invertase to determine cane sugar, and I was suddenly struck with the idea that urease could be used to determine urea and that the procedure could be extremely simple. That evening I left the laboratory with L. G. Rowntree and walked with him across Monument Street to the old Johns Hopkins Club. I asked Rowntree if there were any need for a simple quick method of determining urea in urine, blood and body fluids. He said he was at the time very much interested in determining urea in blood, but the known methods were very difficult, cumbersome and time consuming [Folin's micromethod had just been published and had not come into general use.]. *I told Rowntree I had a very simple method or at least could devise one in a few weeks. He replied that if I did that I could have the chair in Physiological Chemistry in a very few years.... This conversation with Rowntree was a sufficient stimulus to make me go at the matter with great enthusiasm.... In a week or ten days the job was done and my first publication from the medical school was being prepared. I recall that during this exciting week I never left the laboratory until 1:00 to 3:00 a.m.... One of the greatest compliments I ever had was paid me by Otto Folin at our first meeting of the*

Biochemical Society (Christmas 1913). When I was introduced to Folin, he said that when he had read my paper on the determination of urea by using urease he thought it was perfect rot. He continued and said that he had tried my method and it was O.K. and he wanted to congratulate me—this from Folin!—only a few months after my first paper on physiological chemistry had been published.

That same year Marshall refined his techniques and published two more papers on his urease method (85, 87).

In 1914 he published his paper "Urea: Its distribution in and elimination from the body" (93). Between 1914 and 1918, Marshall not only published a series of papers on kidney and liver function, but he also studied medicine. Upon graduation from medical school in 1918, he married and was assigned to Chemical Warfare service in Washington, where he worked until the end of the war. It was then that he met a young enlisted man, Homer W. Smith. The two worked together on mustard gas and published three papers on this subject. When the war was over, Marshall accepted the Chair of Pharmacology at St. Louis, but in less than two years he returned to Baltimore when he was offered the chair at Johns Hopkins (84).

Renal Excretion Studied Prior to the Introduction of Measurements of Glomerular Filtration Rate

Filtration Versus Secretion Hypothesis

The introduction of Marshall's enzyme method had a profound influence on the progress of understanding urea excretion due to the ease of determination of this compound, even in the low concentrations found in mammalian blood. The study of how the kidney excretes urea became the object of several investigations, which more or less followed the lines drawn by the two rival hypotheses for urine formation. One was Carl Ludwig's purely mechanistic theory of glomerular filtration and reabsorption by endosmosis (82); the other was Rudolph Heidenhain's secretory hypothesis, also known as the Bowman-Heidenhain hypothesis (53). In 1917 both were largely replaced by Arthur Cushny's so-called "modern theory" presented in his famous monograph *The Secretion of Urine* (26). Because these theories are described elsewhere (34), I only point out the differences in thinking that so profoundly affected the interpretation of data obtained by various investigators. Ludwig "*carefully avoided attributing any steps in urine formation to 'vital activity' on the part of the glomeruli or tubules.*" As he later said, it was an audacious hypothesis and justified the closing sentence of his second paper: "*Thus we see in these relationships* [between glomeruli and tubules] *a simplicity, a harmony which stands second to no natural process in beauty*" (34). On the other hand, Heidenhain (53) based his hypothesis on his knowledge of secretory glands and on his findings in experiments on rabbit kidneys. When the dye indigo carmine (blue dye sodium sulfindigotate) was injected intravenously in animals in which urine flow had been arrested by section of the cervical cord or by hemorrhage (each of which lowers blood pressure below the pressure necessary for filtration), it accumulated in the cells and lumina of the renal tubules and no color could be discerned in the Bowman's capsules. He argued that the dye is secreted directly from the blood into the tubules independently of any glomerular activity (34, 53). The arguments against Heidenhain's hypothesis then and later were: "*The presence of indigo carmine or any other dye in the tubular lumen at a time when it is not 'visible' in Bowman's capsule does not exclude the possibility of filtration in dilute (not visible) solution and subsequent concentration in the tubular urine by the reabsorption of water*" (26, 34).

To clarify this point and to avoid the ambiguity ascribed to Heidenhain's experiment, Moritz Nussbaum (102, 103) took advantage of the anatomical fact that the amphibian kidney has a separate arterial blood supply to the glomeruli, whereas the tubules are also supplied with blood by a capillary net originating from the renal portal vein. Because Nussbaum's 1878 experiment has special bearing on urea excretion, I present it in some detail. In carefully controlled experiments, he ligated the renal arteries of *Rana esculenta* to cut off the blood supply to the glomeruli while leaving the renal portal circulation intact. He then introduced into the vena abdominalis anterior 2 ml of a saturated solution of indigo carmine. He observed that shortly after the injection the dye was present in the tubuli on the dorsal side of the kidney where the proximal tubules are located. All other parts of the nephron (including the glomeruli) were free of the dye, and no urine was formed, as evidenced by the empty bladder. When he then injected 1–1.5 ml of a 10% urea solution into the vena abdominalis, urine production resumed and the previously empty bladder became full after two to three hours. At the end of the experiment, he injected dye into the aorta and found that no dye entered the glomerular capillaries. Nussbaum (102; author's translation) concluded: "*1. Urea is secreted through the cells of the tubuli. With the help of the sodium sulphindigotate it is even possible to see the secretory cells clearly outlined. 2. The water excretion of the kidneys is not solely dependent on blood pressure but also on the nature of the substances present in the blood.*"

Nussbaum's experiments drew wide attention, and similar perfusion experiments were repeated later by several other investigators, with the same result. Among these were Rowntree and Geraghty, who found in 1912 that phenolsulfonphthalein (phenol red) added to the fluid did not cause secretion of urine, but when urea was added the urine contained the pigment (26). (This explains why Rowntree welcomed with open arms the proposal by Marshall to develop the urease method for urea determination.)

At the time Cushny published his monograph (26), Ludwig's theory had become untenable, partly because a better understanding of osmotic forces had been reached. Cushny (26) dismissed both the Ludwig and the Bowman-Heidenhain hypotheses and proposed instead his modern view:

[It] *accepts the general scheme of filtration and reabsorption of Ludwig, but, appreciating the inadequacy of the known physical forces, supplements them as far as necessary by the 'vital activity' postulated by Heidenhain.... The formation of the glomerular filtrate is due to a blind force. The absorption in the tubules is equally independent of any discrimination, for the fluid absorbed is always the same, whatever the need of the organism at the moment.*

He further proposed that the colloids are filtered out in the glomeruli and that substances can be divided into threshold and no-threshold substances (26). Cushny (26), like Ludwig, saw beauty in the greatest simplicity and wrote, "*It reduces the kidney to a machine instead of postulating for it the capacity of a highly trained chemist.*" Smith (34) remarked: "*If Cushny's position concerning 'vital activity' seems inconsistent; it is inconsistent; the difficulty lies in the paradox that though we name the things we know, we do not necessarily know them because we name them.*"

Cushny (26) described Nussbaum's experiments in great detail, pointing out what he considered possible discrepancies and sources of error, and then added:

I have no desire to belittle the importance of this experiment in determining the theory of renal secretion, but the usual interpretation runs counter to the evidence regarding the excretion of urea and dyes in mammals.... The final determination of secretion of urea in the frog would of course weigh the scales heavily in favour of a similar point of excretion in mammals.... But it is obvious that while the results of perfusion in the frog may lend support to the modern view of renal secretion, it cannot be said to have yielded any decisive argument in its favour. On the other hand, far from supporting the view of vital secretion, it renews doubt as to the cogency of Nussbaum's experiment.

After World War I, Marshall returned to his interest in urea and studied the influences of diuresis on the elimination of urea, creatinine, and chloride. At the time, Marshall (88) did not attempt to measure the rate of glomerular filtration, and his findings in 1920 were rather inconclusive. However, he became increasingly convinced that the hypothesis proposed by Cushny was insufficient because it did not include tubular secretion. In 1966 Marshall (91) wrote:

I had started some work back in 1916 during World War I which I took up again after the war was over.... The results could not be explained, I believed, by filtration and reabsorption alone. However, I had no real conclusive proof and started in again in an attempt to find out whether one could obtain conclusive evidence of secretion of any substance by the renal tubule. During this early period of my work (in the early 1920's) both Cushny (who died in 1926) and Newton Richards, were violently opposed to secretion and would scarcely listen to any argument in favor of it.

Marshall's experiments with secretion of phenol red in dogs were based on the same argument as that used by Nussbaum, namely, that cellular (and in Nussbaum's case intratubular) accumulation could occur even when the glomeruli were not perfused (95). Marshall, together with Crane, then compared the elimination of phenol red and urea by amphibian and mammalian kidneys. Part of their proof was the cellular accumulation of urea as an indication of secretion by the tubules. The other part was the rate of excretion as it is affected by plasma concentrations. In a paper published in 1924 (92) they wrote:

The observations by Marshall and Vickers for secretion of phenol red by the mammal have been extended and found to hold for the frog's kidney. Phenol red is concentrated in the cells of both the amphibian and mammalian kidneys. The efficiency of the kidneys of both classes of animals is much lower for this body [substance] *when plasma concentrations are high than at lower ones. This is taken to mean a saturation of the secreting cells. Urea is concentrated in the frog's kidneys in a similar way to phenol red, but no evidence of such concentration in the cells can be obtained for the mammalian kidney. Also the efficiency of elimination of urea is practically the same at all plasma levels in the mammal, while in the frog its behavior is different and similar to that of phenol red. It is concluded from these observations that phenol red is secreted by both amphibian and mammalian kidney, while urea is secreted by the former.*

This conclusion concerning urea secretion in the frog, which was essentially correct, had to wait for almost thirty years before it was validated by modern clearance techniques and fully accepted.

Urea Clearance and Glomerular Filtration Rate

Mammals

Cushny's simplified view of the kidney soon came under attack from other sides; this time it concerned the meaning of 'threshold' substances. Poul Brandt Rehberg (Fig. 3) was born in Denmark in 1895 and studied at the University of Copenhagen where he received the degree of Cand. Mag. in zoology in 1921. He then obtained a position in August Krogh's laboratory of zoophysiology, where in-

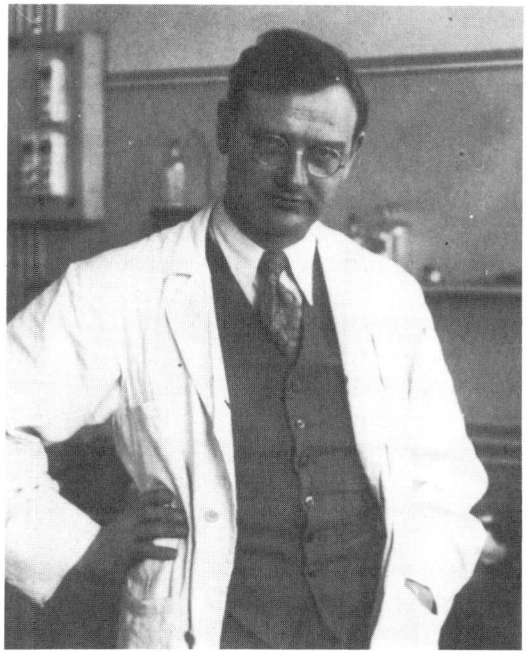

Figure 3. Poul Brandt Rehberg (b. 1895) shown in Zoophysiological Laboratory at Rockefeller Institute in Copenhagen around 1939.

tense research on capillary function was under way. Rehberg became involved in many aspects of this research. At that time Krogh and G. A. Harrop were very interested in the causes of edema, especially as it pertained to capillary function and the colloid osmotic substances of the blood. Rehberg's interest in the kidney was kindled by a study of edema caused by nephritis in humans.

During Marshall's visit to Krogh's laboratory in 1923, he and Rehberg daily discussed the kidney. Marshall (91) later remarked on the curious way in which Rehberg went about his studies. "*He read for a year and evolved a theory and then set out perfectly fairly, I think, to test it out.*" Rehberg (119) wished to test experimentally Cushny's modern theory. He wrote:

In recent years a number of investigations have resulted in that more and more substances have been transferred to the group of threshold substances and at the same time doubt has been cast on the constant composition of the reabsorbed fluid. This has resulted in that the theory has become very complicated and no longer has the same advantages it previously had. The reason, I believe, is that the definition of 'threshold substances' in the reabsorbed fluid does not distinguish between substances that are actively reabsorbed or substances that simply diffuse back due to a concentration difference between the urine in the tubuli and the blood in the surrounding capillaries.

About several more recent contributions he wrote, "*The results of these experiments completely rob the 'modern theory' of its simplicity which was one of its main advantages. In reality the theory is now left in a state where one may turn against it the objection raised by Cushny against the secretion theory 'that it endows the renal cells with powers of discrimination of a very high order.'*"

However, the beauty of a clearly stated hypothesis is that it can be tested, and this is what Rehberg set out to do. For the quantitative calculations of the composition of the reabsorbed fluid, he needed to be able to measure the glomerular filtration rate (GFR); he decided to use creatinine on purely theoretical grounds. His kidney studies culminated in two superb short papers on kidney function published in 1926. "*This amount* [GFR]," he wrote (119), "*can be calculated if one has determinations in blood and urine of a substance that is a 'non-threshold' substance according to Cushny's definition, i.e., a substance that neither diffuses nor is reabsorbed during the movement of the glomerular filtrate through the tubules. This property, I think I can assign to creatinine.*" He chose creatinine because its concentration ratio had been found to be the highest of any natural substance that had been measured in the urine.

Using himself as the experimental subject, Rehberg investigated the renal handling of chloride and urea. Earlier E. B. Mayrs had proposed that urea was a threshold substance because it is of value to the body, but Rehberg's very careful analysis of the effect of blood concentrations and urine flow on the fraction excreted and the concentration of the reabsorbed fluid made him conclude, "*Urea is a no-threshold substance which is never actively reabsorbed. Its presence in the reabsorbed fluid is supposed to be due to mere diffusion.*" This conclusion was based on his finding that the concentration of urea in the reabsorbed fluid increased with increasing concentration index [creatinine urine-plasma ratio (U/P)], whereas the fraction of filtered urea excreted decreased with increasing concentration index. He further concluded that chloride is a threshold substance that is actively reabsorbed but not in the simple manner proposed by Cushny (120).

Similar conclusions concerning urea excretion in mammals were later reached by Homer W. Smith and his many co-workers, notably James Shannon. When Marshall became interested in working on the aglomerular fish to find definite proof of renal tubular secretion, he chose to do the work at Mount Desert Island Biological Laboratory (MDIBL) in Maine. This decision had profound effects on future developments in renal physiology. Not only did Marshall find the proof for renal tubular secretion of fluid and a number of solutes, but he also became reassociated with Smith. Marshall and his students and co-workers abruptly changed the emphasis of research at the laboratory, and this in turn shifted Smith's interest toward renal function. During the summer of 1926, when Marshall came to the summer laboratory in Salisbury Cove, Smith was working on the influence of hydrogen ions on cell division in sand dollar eggs. Smith had in the meantime earned his doctoral degree (D.Sc.) and was now chairman of the Department of Physiology of the University at Virginia School of Medicine. When World War I ended, Marshall had arranged for Smith to undertake graduate studies under William H. Howell of Johns Hopkins School of Medicine from which institution Smith had earned his D.Sc. degree in 1921 (84). Smith's interests, as witnessed by his publications, were concerned with physiological chemistry and the effect of toxins on living organisms. During the following years, Smith increasingly concerned himself with the role of urea in the body fluids of fishes and its excretion through gills and kidneys.

Effect of Urine Flow and GFR on Urea Clearance

By 1903 the determination of blood urea concentration had been introduced into clinical medicine as a diagnostic test for kidney function (20). In the following years several attempts were made to evaluate kidney function in patients with renal disease by measuring urine urea concentration, urea excretion rate, and blood urea concentration. However, the equations used lacked any physiological meaning. It was not until Marshall and D. M. Davis (93) in dogs and Thomas Addis (1) in rabbits found that the rate of urea excretion is directly proportional to the blood urea concentration that the equations began to have some physiological meaning. Addis (1) was the first to show that the ratio (UV/B) between the urea concentration in urine (U) times the urine flow rate (V) and the blood urea concentration (B) is relatively constant at high urine flow rates, but the understanding of the mechanism was still far from clear. As Addis said, "*All we know for certain about the kidney is that it makes urine*" (20). In 1921, Austin, Stillman, and van Slyke (4) showed that the excretion efficiency of dog kidneys can be expressed as UV/B, which in any dog is constant at high urine flow rates, whereas at low flow rates $U\sqrt{V}/B$ is constant.

According to Smith (20) the expression *urea clearance* was born of necessity:

In 1926 van Slyke had been on his way to Baltimore to give an address on kidney function, and on the train his courage failed him when he thought of facing an audience again with a mathematical formula.... Seeking a solution of how to dispense with mathematics for the benefit of the medical profession, it occurred to him that all that the equation for high urine flow said was that in effect some constant volume of blood was being cleared of urea in each minute's time.... In my opinion this word has been more useful to renal physiology than all the equations ever written.

In the next several years when it became possible to measure GFR, the word *clearance* took on a much wider meaning, covering not just urea but any substance cleared from the blood by the kidneys.

In 1928 Smith was consulted by William Goldring concerning urea clearance data from patients with acute infection (20). The data showed marked deviations from the normal despite standard conditions and no apparent renal pathology. It became clear to Smith that without more functional data, including measurements of GFR, the data could not be interpreted. In collaboration with Jolliffe (62, 63), he undertook studies in dogs comparing the urea and creatinine clearances. Smith was careful not to call the creatinine clearance the GFR because Marshall and Grafflin (94) had found that in the aglomerular goosefish, creatinine is secreted by the renal tubules but glucose is not. These facts suggested to Smith (25) that "*nonmetabolized sugars might be used to evaluate the quantity of glomerular filtrate in fishes and higher animals.*" In 1932 Jolliffe, Shannon, and Smith (61) compared urea clearance with the clearance of the pentose xylose, calling the xylose clearance the glomerular clearance.

Searching for a larger molecule less likely to be reabsorbed by the renal tubules than xylose, Smith and A. Newton Richards et al. (20, 122) simultaneously and independently began using inulin to measure glomerular filtration. Shannon, Smith, Herbert Chasis and others now compared urea clearance with filtration rate (inulin clearance in humans and creatinine clearance in dogs) under a variety of physiological and pathological conditions. The results of these experiments became the foundation for the concept of urea excretion by filtration and reabsorption by simple backdiffusion (21, 22, 146, 148, 149, 157).

Many of the conclusions reached were based on the carefully executed experiments by Shannon. James A. Shannon (Fig. 4) was born in 1904 in Hollis, New York, and was studying medicine at New York University when Smith became Professor of Physiology and Director of the Physiological Laboratories there in 1928. In 1931 Shannon joined Jolliffe and Smith (61), who were using xylose to measure GFR; in the summer of 1932 he worked at MDIBL on the excretion of sugars and creatinine in dogfish. His association with Homer Smith continued at both New York University and MDIBL until 1940 when he moved to the Department of Medicine at New York University.

In 1938 Shannon showed that the fraction of filtered urea excreted (FE_{urea}) in dogs depends on the concentration index (creatinine U/P) in a specific manner. At urine flows ranging from extreme water diuresis (creatinine U/P = 10) to low urine flows (creatinine U/P = 400), FE_{urea} decreased only slightly. However, at lower urine flows (higher concentration indexes), FE_{urea} decreased more abruptly, indicating a greater backdiffusion when the urine became more

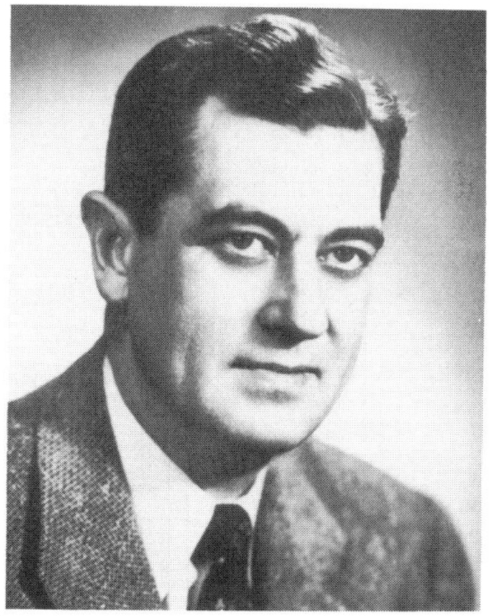

Figure 4. James A. Shannon (b. 1904) was an instructor and Assistant Professor of Medicine at New York University from 1931 to 1940, where he published a series of important papers on urea clearance in dogs, and later became director of the National Institutes of Health.

concentrated (22). Creatinine U/P ratios below those measured at extreme water diuresis are unphysiological and can only be achieved during osmotic diuresis. At such high urine flows, FE_{urea} approached unity. Shannon (148) interpreted his results (Fig. 5) as follows:

The reabsorption of urea is interpreted under the hypothesis that water reabsorption takes place at two sites in the nephron. The diffusion gradient created by the reabsorption of water in the proximal tubule accounts for the deficit in the urea clearance at the highest urine flow during water diuresis. The further deficit associated with low urine flows is attributed to the diffusion in the distal portions of the nephron.

This interpretation, which was reached by the use of a noninvasive technique in conscious dogs that essentially treated the kidney as a black box, was later confirmed, at least in principle, by micropuncture studies, although the overall picture is a great deal more complex.

Similar results were obtained in humans by Chasis and Smith (21) under both normal and pathological conditions. As seen in Figure 6, FE_{urea} was entirely independent of GFR. In his monograph Smith (157) wrote:

The urea clearance ranges from 30–60 percent of the inulin clearance, depending on the urine flow. Urea is completely filterable, and there is as yet no evidence that it is destroyed in the tubular urine so we must interpret the deficit in the urea clearance below the filtration rate as indicating that a considerable fraction of the filtered urea

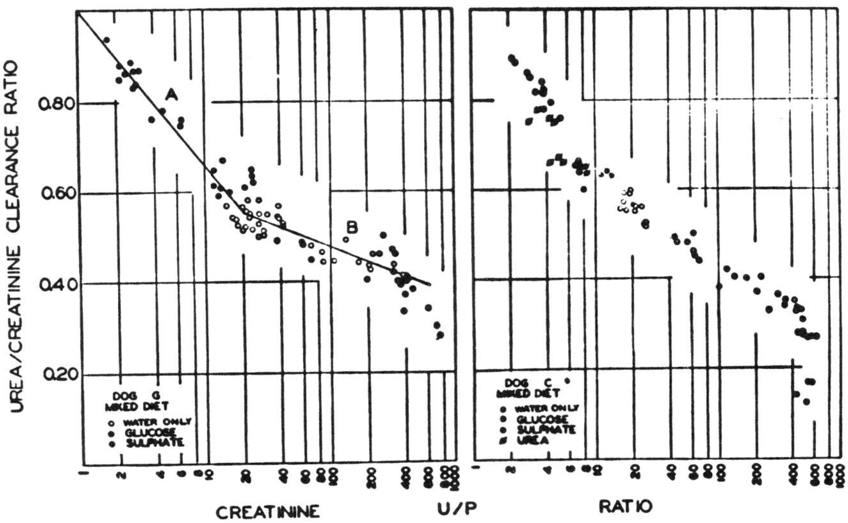

Figure 5. Urea–creatinine clearance ratios in dogs plotted against the concentration index [creatinine urine-plasma ratio (U/P)]. [From Shannon (148).]

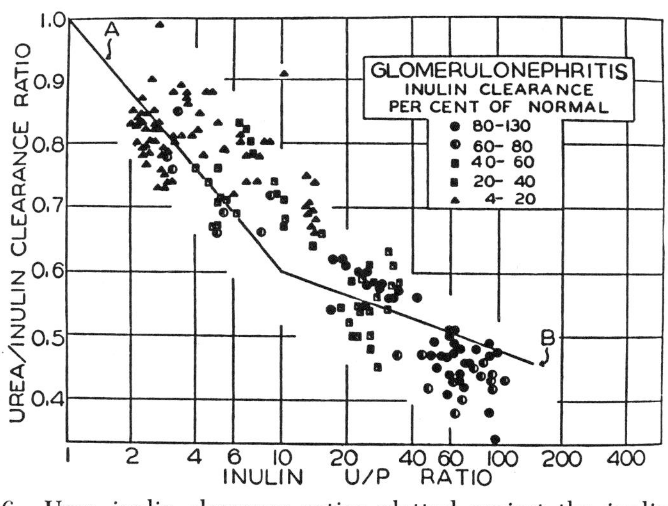

Figure 6. Urea–inulin clearance ratios plotted against the inulin urine-plasma ratios (U/P) of patients with glomerulonephritis and reduced glomerular filtration rates. [From Smith (157).]

diffuses back through the tubules. This back diffusion is readily understood in light of the fact that urea is one of the most diffusible compounds known (as it would have to be to escape the tissues from which it is formed by metabolism) and that when it is administered it is distributed, as first shown by Marshall, throughout the body water.

This conclusion was based also on the mathematical treatment by Dole (32) of the diffusion of urea from the renal tubule to the surrounding blood. Dole's formulation was based on the assumption that the decrease in urea clearance with an increase in urine volume is caused by tubular reabsorption of urea in accordance with quantitative laws of diffusion. It was also based on the assumption that all parts of the renal tubule were surrounded by tissue and capillaries with the same osmolality and urea concentration as that of the systemic plasma. It must be recalled that at the time the countercurrent hypothesis for the urinary concentrating mechanism had not yet been proposed and would not be accepted for several years after it was proposed. Thus the true environment of the nephrons was not known. For practical reasons Smith (157) depicted the renal tubule as straight and wrote, "*The writer sees no reason at the moment to give this hairpin pattern* [of the nephrons] *any special functional significance.*"

Effect of Nitrogen Intake on GFR

Smith's first published work on excretion appeared in 1928. He had read a paper by B. E. Read, who reported that he had found practically no urea in camel urine. This startling finding excited Smith, and the next time a circus came to town, he followed the camels through town carrying a pail in which he collected their urine. When he found normal amounts of urea in the camel urine he concluded that Read's observation was erroneous due to faulty methodology (159). As described subsequently, the analyses by both Read and Smith were correct, the discrepancy in results being due to a difference in nitrogen intake and renal handling of urea in camels on a low-protein diet. That is, urea is conserved by the kidneys when the need for nitrogen conservation arises.

Urea, being the major nitrogenous end product of protein catabolism in mammals, has by many been considered mainly a waste product that the kidneys had to eliminate. This notion was based on the fact that vertebrate tissues do not produce urease, and therefore, once formed, urea seemed unavailable for protein synthesis. It has long been known, however, that this is incorrect; it is well documented that urea in blood may enter the gastrointestinal tract, where it is broken down by urease-producing bacteria (the ammonia formed is utilized by microorganisms in amino acid and protein synthesis) (19, 55–57, 129, 162, 175). In an investigation using Pavlov-type pouches in sheep and goats, Houpt and Houpt (57) found that in these ruminants urea diffuses across the wall of the rumen, where it is hydrolyzed by bacterial urease activity in the ruminal epithelium. The microflora present in the rumen synthesize amino acids and protein that then enter the stomach, where they are digested. Houpt and Houpt (57) concluded that "*the transfer of nitrogen into the rumen is most important when the animal is on a low-protein ration. Under these nutritional conditions, rumen ammonia is extensively utilized in microbial protein synthesis and rumen ammonia concentration is comparatively low.*" A similar utilization of urea takes place in rabbits and other rodents in which urea enters the cecum from the blood. When the fecal pellets are reingested (coprophagy), the protein formed by the microorganisms is digested (56). In humans on a very low-protein diet (such as the Papua and New Guinea Highlanders, who live on a diet mainly composed of sweet potatoes), incorporation of orally ingested urea nitrogen into essential amino acids was observed (162). Because of the recycling of urea nitrogen into amino acids and protein, it is advantageous to a mammal maintained on a low-protein diet to conserve urea formed by protein catabolism. This is particularly important to the growing animal (56, 143, 162), and it serves to maintain plasma urea concentrations at or near normal levels (134).

Urea can be conserved by the kidneys by lowering the urea clearance. When Jolliffe and Smith (62, 63) started their comprehensive studies of urea-excretion patterns in dogs, they were not only interested in the effect of urine flow but also in the effect that changes in protein intake might have on urea clearance. They studied dogs on pure beef (high-protein), maintenance (medium-protein), and cracker-meal (low-protein) diets and found the creatinine clearance to be 30%–50% higher on a mixed diet than on a protein-poor diet and 100% higher on a pure meat diet. However, they found no effect of diet on the urea–creatinine clearance ratio, indicating that both clearances changed in parallel (63). [Far more pronounced effects of diet and feeding were later found by Shannon, Jolliffe, and Smith (149) using xylose to estimate GFR; however, these results were probably inaccurate because it was demonstrated later that xylose is reabsorbed in the renal tubules (147).] The effects of protein feeding on GFR were confirmed repeatedly in dogs and other species including humans (2, 7, 15, 54, 104, 105). There is a rise in GFR starting about 100 minutes after a high-protein feeding; the increase lasts from 2 to 8 hours, depending on the amount of protein ingested. In fasting animals the GFR returned to the level seen in animals maintained on low-protein diets (63). The signal that causes GFR to change with protein intake is still obscure, but it is believed to be related to deamination of amino acids because the increase in GFR could be reproduced by infusion of various amino acids but not by glucose, lactic acid, or pyruvic acid, nor could it be reproduced by acute infusion of urea (157).

In the 1930s several investigators observed that uremic symptoms were provoked by high-protein intake, which shortened the survival of animals with experimental renal failure; a low-protein diet was then proposed for conservative treatment of acute and chronic uremia (7). Recently this treatment has received renewed attention, and it has been suggested that the high filtration rate resulting from high-protein intake aggravates the damage to the glomeruli (15).

Effect of Nitrogen Intake on Tubular Handling of Urea.

Smith (157) became convinced that the only effect of a low-protein intake on renal function was on GFR and renal plasma flow and thus that the basic pattern of filtration–passive tubular backdiffusion did not change with changes in nitrogen intake. Therefore when A. L. Nielsen and H. O. Bang (100, 101), in their experiments on fasting humans on normal- and low-protein intake, found only a 7% decrease in GFR on the low-protein diet but a 33% decrease in urea clearance (measured at the same inulin U/P), Smith (157) dismissed the finding with, "*The reason for the drop in urea/inulin clearance is obscure.*"

Much of my own interest in urea excretion stems from my early observation of an effect of protein intake on the fraction of filtered urea excreted in kangaroo rats and in camels (134, 143). During the summer of 1947, Knut Schmidt-Nielsen and I (142), together with two students, studied the water metabolism of kangaroo rats (*Dipodomys merriami*) in the Arizona desert. One of the adaptations of these animals for water conservation is the ability to excrete an extremely concentrated urine. The highest osmotic concentration of urine in kangaroo rats (estimated to be 6,000 mosmol) was found when the animals were fed dry soybeans; the highest urea concentration exceeded 3,500 mM (134). Another peculiarity of these desert rodents was the very long papilla renis. I decided to learn more about renal function and studied Homer Smith's book *The Physiology of the Kidney* (156) in great detail. Impressed with the power of the clearance technique to determine if a substance is reabsorbed or secreted by the renal tubules, I attempted to measure simultaneous inulin and urea clearances in conscious kangaroo rats. The results (which cannot be considered conclusive due to the impossibility of obtaining plasma samples from these small animals during the clearance periods) indicated tubular secretion of urea in kangaroo rats on a high-protein diet at inulin U/P ratios below 50 and showed that kangaroo rats maintained on a high-protein (40%) diet showed higher urea–inulin clearance ratios than animals on a low-protein (6%) diet at the same concentration index (134).

Shortly after completing these studies, we went to the Sahara desert in Algeria to study the water metabolism of camels. Camels in the Sahara are usually permitted to graze in the sand dunes, but when maintained at our desert laboratory in the Beni Abbes oasis, they were fed a low-protein diet of dates and hay, which is the usual diet given camels when they are not grazing. Urine and blood samples taken daily from our young growing camel revealed a gradual decrease in urine urea concentration, which at times was as low as 5–6 mM. The urea U/P ratio remained around 5 even when the plasma urea concentration gradually rose during dehydration from 1 to 7 mM. Measurement of GFR and urea clearance showed that the fraction of filtered urea excreted decreased in the camel on the low-protein diet to values as low as 0.01–0.05, whereas in the grazing camel it was 0.24. The filtration rate in the camel varied with the salt intake, but the urea clearance decreased independently of the filtration rate. The urea clearance was also independent of plasma urea concentration because dehydration as well as urea injection increased the plasma urea concentration but did not change the fractional excretion of urea (143).

During the following years, my colleagues and I studied the effect of low-protein diet in ruminants and monogastric animals and found clear evidence of renal tubular regulation of urea excretion in sheep (139), dogs (134, 140), humans (99), and rats (163) and no significant decrease in GFR in sheep, humans, and rats. In ruminants the effect of a low-protein diet on tubular handling of urea was particularly pronounced, and the urea U/P ratio decreased with low-protein intake to the same ratio as the osmolar U/P (about 5) (139). The results clearly showed that tubular regulation is independent of blood urea concentration and GFR. Also, humans, dogs, and rats showed a highly significant decrease in the fractions of filtered urea excreted. In these experiments, it became clear that the nutritional value of the diet and the salt intake are both important factors in determining GFR. In my own experiment I observed that a nutritionally incomplete diet lowers the filtration rate; we therefore used a well-balanced low-protein diet. Furthermore salt was added to the low-protein diets in an amount calculated to give the same osmotic clearance as the normal-protein diet. Finally, to ensure that nitrogenous waste was excreted in the form of urea and not ammonia, sodium bicarbonate was added to the drinking water to make the urine alkaline. Differences in diet may explain why the human subjects investigated by Nielsen and Bang (100, 101) showed only a 7% decrease in filtration rate on the low-protein diet, whereas those investigated by Smith and his colleagues showed a greater decrease in GFR. Similarly, both GFR and fractional excretion of urea may decrease, depending on diet (28, 79, 83, 140, 151).

Thus the evidence of tubular regulation of urea excretion in no way contradicted or conflicted with the findings by Jolliffe and Smith (62, 63) that the GFR may be affected by protein intake. A decrease in urea clearance can occur parallel to a decrease in filtration rate, but if the filtration rate remains constant, the urea clearance decreases on the low-protein diet independently of the filtration rate. However, the tubular effect on urea excretion introduced the element of regulation into the simpler model of filtration and passive backdiffusion of urea, but there was no understanding of the factors governing the regulation of GFR and urea clearance, nor was there any understanding of how and in what part of the nephron tubular regulation takes place.

In addition to the effect of the low-protein diet, there were other unexplained phenomena such as the effect of anesthesia and excitement on the fraction of filtered urea excreted (76, 134), the exaltation first noted by Shannon in urea clearance during rising urine flow, and the abrupt decrease in urea clearance at very low urine flow rates (148).

Lower Vertebrates

Among the vertebrates three groups excrete urea as the primary nitrogenous end product of protein metabolism: *1)* some of the fishes inhabiting a marine environment (this group encompasses sharks and rays, the rat fish, and the only living coelacanth *Latimeria*); *2)* freshwater forms adapted to tolerate not only their freshwater environment but also terrestrial conditions and, for a few, a saltwater environment (this group includes the African lungfish, most amphibians, and some reptiles); and *3)* all mammals, regardless of habitat (38, 39, 137).

In the first group, urea serves to maintain the osmolality of the body fluids equal to or higher than the seawater. This prevents water loss to the saltwater environment (155, 158). In this group the kidneys conserve urea by maintaining a high plasma urea concentration (about 350 mM). In the second group, detoxification of ammonia is important because an animal leaving its aquatic environment can no longer excrete ammonia through its integument. Therefore, semiaquatic forms must synthesize urea (38). However, urea also serves in osmotic water retention in amphibians such as frogs in saltwater (144) and toads that burrow (131, 150). Thus urea excretion is regulated to maintain a low plasma urea concentration when the frog or toad is in freshwater and to increase the plasma concentration when desiccation is a problem. Most reptiles are predominantly terrestrial, but some are more water loving than others, and these generally excrete part of their nitrogenous waste as urea (ureotelic) and the rest as uric acid (141). In mammals the fact that urea and not uric acid is the major nitrogenous end product has resulted in the development of a kidney that can concentrate urine to a higher degree than that of any other vertebrate and that is also capable of great flexibility in its excretory function. The role that urea plays in the concentrating mechanism is discussed in the next section.

With the varied roles urea plays in vertebrates, renal mechanisms have developed for retention as well as secretion of urea. The means by which the kidneys regulate plasma urea concentration are changes in GFR, tubular secretion of urea, reabsorption of filtered urea by backdiffusion, and active reabsorption (137).

Fishes

Homer Smith's first interest in the kidney concerned excretion in fishes (153–155). From the literature and from his own studies, he found that elasmobranchs and chimaeroids normally maintain a plasma urea concentration of about 350 mM, and he confirmed that the osmolality of their plasma is slightly higher than that of the surrounding seawater, which permits these fishes to absorb water by osmosis via the gills. He clearly saw the role that urea plays in the osmotic regulation of the elasmobranch and wrote, "*Frédéricq (1903) approached what we believe to be the crux of the problem when he emphasized osmotic pressure and pointed out that because urea freely permeates the tissues it is osmotically indifferent to them; but because it does not freely permeate the gills and integuments it is osmotically active toward the milieu exterieur*" (153). Smith (155) found that the urine of elasmobranchs has a substantially lower urea concentration than the blood and concluded:

> *Accepting the highly probable supposition* [that urea is filtered in the glomeruli], *it follows from the relatively lower concentration in the urine that the urea must be reabsorbed by the tubules. Since the reabsorption involves the movement of urea from a low concentration in the urine this reabsorption must be an active one in the same sense in which glucose is actively reabsorbed from the urine by the tubules of all glomerular vertebrates.*

That this reabsorption is indeed active was later questioned, and it has been suggested that the spatial arrangements of the tubules may be responsible for creating an environment around the distal tubule with a lower urea concentration than the blood; regulation of the reabsorption was found by Roy Forster et al. (40).

Prior to Smith's study of elasmobranchs, he studied the African lungfish and found that during estivation, while kidney function is completely suspended, urea accumulates in the tissues up to 3%–4% of the total body weight (158). This corresponds to a urea concentration of about 1 M. Smith did not suggest that the high accumulation of urea in the tissues might serve an osmotic function in protecting this fish against dehydration because the fish is sealed in a tight cocoon [Fig. 7; (158)]. It was later found that the coelacanth also retains urea in its tissues and thereby maintains an osmotic pressure as high as the milieu exterieur (45).

Amphibians, Reptiles, and Birds

As discussed previously, the disputed Nussbaum experiment had strongly suggested that the renal tubules of frogs secrete urea (102, 103). When the conclusions of Marshall and Crane, that urea is secreted by the frog tubules (89, 92), were challenged by Rehberg and Blem and by Walker, Marshall compared the urea excretion in frogs with the xylose clearance and found urea clearance to be as much as twenty times greater than xylose clearance (90). Twenty years later, Roy P. Forster (Fig. 8) from Dartmouth College reinvestigated urea secretion in bullfrogs, using exogenous creatinine clear-

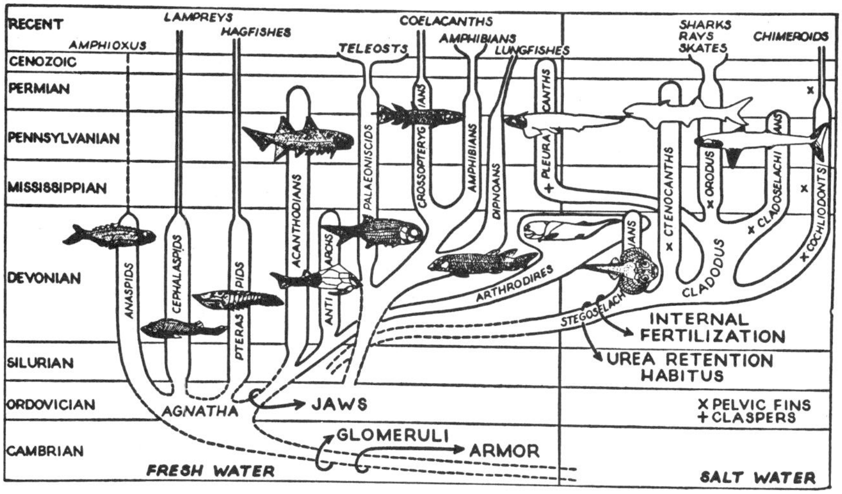

Figure 7. Urea retention in fishes. [From Smith (158).]

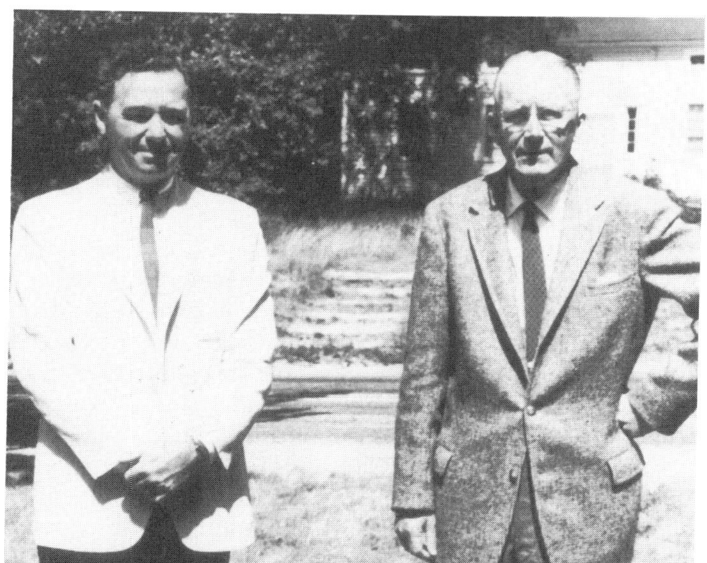

Figure 8. Roy P. Forster (b. 1907) (*left*) and Eli Kennerly Marshall, Jr., (1889–1966) (*right*) at Mount Desert Island Biological Laboratory. (Courtesy of Mount Desert Island Biological Laboratory.)

ance to measure the filtration rate. In 1952 Forster, who had been a regular summer investigator at MDIBL since 1937 and who had worked extensively with secretion of organic compounds in the aglomerular goosefish (36), took up the problem of urea secretion in frogs. Forster (37, 38) then carried out a classic clearance study (Fig. 9) demonstrating that "*the urea secretory process in the bullfrog*

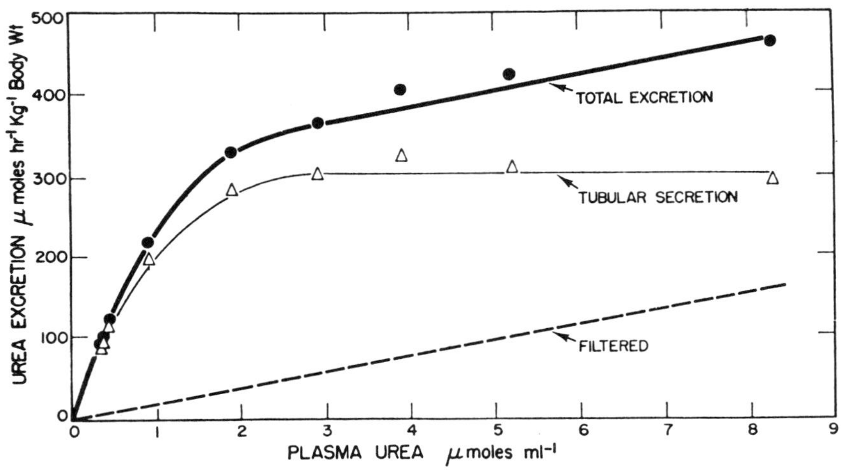

Figure 9. Urea excretion rates in frogs plotted against plasma urea concentrations, showing saturation of tubular secretion. [From Forster (37).]

exhibits characteristics shared with the well-known organic acid transfer system, namely a sharply defined tubular transport maximum, dependence upon aerobic phosphorylation as an energy source, and competitive inhibition." This important study showed that the urea secretory mechanism was fully saturated at a plasma urea concentration of 2–3 mM and that maximal secretory rates were 260 μmol·kg body $wt^{-1} \cdot h^{-1}$.

The earlier findings by Marshall and Crane (92) indicated that a cellular accumulation of urea is a part of the secretory process and therefore that urea secretion takes place in two steps: an active transport step across the basolateral membrane and a passive diffusion step across the apical membrane. This was confirmed in further studies that showed that urea, labeled or unlabeled, is concentrated in the renal tissue to an average of eight times the plasma concentration and is secreted by the tubules (136). (Thus urea secretion cannot be attributed to de novo urea formation in the kidneys of frogs.) Thiourea was found to be secreted by frog tubules, whereas methylurea and acetamide were not (136).

A bidirectional movement of urea was suggested by the reversal of net flux that resulted from the administration of metabolic and competitive inhibitors (36–38, 136). The bidirectional movement of urea was further demonstrated in the doubly perfused frog kidney by Love and Lifson (81), who measured a urea influx rate to the lumen that was greater than the efflux rate. Later, tubular secretion was also proven in micropuncture studies to be present in both proximal and distal convolutions of the frog kidney (80).

When Marshall first described urea secretion in frogs, it had not been found in other animals, although Marshall and Grafflin (94) suggested that it may occur in aglomerular fish. Since that time, however, urea secretion has been demonstrated in various frogs and toads (18, 134, 144), in some reptiles (141), and even in birds (161). The reason for the elusiveness of the secretion is that in these animals urea may be both secreted and reabsorbed, and thus the urea clearance is found to exceed GFR only at high urine-flow rates (low concentration index). Retention of urea is caused by a decrease in GFR and an increase in urea permeability of distal segments of the nephron and bladder with the release of antidiuretic hormone. In the more aquatic frog which estivates under water, the nephron and bladder do not become permeable to urea with antidiuretic hormone (137, 144).

The ability to secrete urea via the renal tubules is found in fully aquatic amphibians such as *Necturus* (121) and is not present in the tadpole (41). Metamorphosing tadpoles begin active urea secretion at exactly the time when they become ready for life on land (41). Urea synthesis increases abruptly in estivating toads as the soil dries out, but there has been no evidence of active reabsorption from the tubules as in the elasmobranchs (131, 150).

Diffusion and Carrier-Mediated or Active Reabsorption of Urea

These processes have not been as well defined as the secretory process. In contrast to urea secretion (serosal to mucosal), saturation of the reabsorptive mechanism (mucosal to serosal) has not been shown in any membrane. This is true of urea reabsorption in elasmobranch tubules, in toad bladder, and in mammalian collecting ducts (38, 136) (discussed subsequently). Also in contrast to the urea-secretion mechanism, each of these membranes exhibits a transport specificity for urea that is shared with other amides such as acetamide and methylurea but not thiourea (27, 114, 136, 163). The reabsorptive mechanism has been studied in toad bladder and in elasmobranchs. In toad bladder the permeability to urea increases tenfold after the serosal application of vasopressin, but it does not differ in either direction, which indicates that urea moves passively across the epithelium (33, 51, 52, 77). Various questions have been raised concerning this movement: Is the vasopressin-induced increase in urea and water permeability simply due to an opening of aqueous pores that permits both water and urea to move more freely through the membrane? Are the effects on urea and water independent, and if so, is urea movement subject to carrier-mediated diffusion?

Alexander Leaf and his colleagues at Massachusetts General Hospital tested the permeability of a number of inorganic and organic ions as well as organic molecules of various sizes and found that amides penetrate the membrane most rapidly after vasopressin and that the greatest effect is on urea, methylurea, and acetamide. In contrast, no effect was found on the penetration of thiourea. Leaf (77), commenting on the striking ability of the tissue to discriminate between urea and thiourea, wrote:

It seems that molecular size alone cannot be the distinguishing feature as the dimensions of compounds in the 'amide' group must overlap in the group unaffected by hormone. Since recognition in molecular terms must mean interaction, some more specific steric fit by the amide group to the accessible channel is required or some specific binding to a membrane constituent must occur.

In Leaf's studies saturation of a carrier was not shown, even when the medium urea concentration was raised to 100 mM. Leaf (77) wrote, "*Although we have been unable to demonstrate self-depression or competition for possible binding sites, interaction with the membrane by hydrogen bonding is not excluded by these observations. Urea and the 'amide group'... all share ability to hydrogen bond.*" Later, Eggena (33) found that at a concentration of 100 mM thiourea inhibits urea transport in toad bladder.

The urea transport system in elasmobranch tubules shares the same specificity for urea analogues as does toad bladder. The amides methylurea and acetamide are reabsorbed from the tubular fluid against a concentration gradient (as urea), whereas thiourea is not (136).

The conclusion from the studies of lower vertebrates is that urea production and excretion are regulated according to the need for maintaining either a low or a high plasma urea concentration. The kidneys regulate the plasma urea concentration by changes in GFR, tubular secretion of urea, and reabsorption of filtered urea (137). Forster (38) stated:

Studies of the kinetics of urea transport in various biological membranes demonstrate that the carrier for secretion into the lumen has a low saturation level and an affinity for thiourea but not for urea analogues that have an amide group. The carrier for reabsorption is similar in all systems involving active and facilitated urea transport in this direction and is characterized by a high saturation level.... The reabsorptive carrier has an affinity for urea analogues with an amide-like group, but not for thiourea.

Urea in Renal Countercurrent System

The introduction of the countercurrent hypothesis in renal physiology had an enormous impact on the concepts of urine concentration and tubular function. It renewed interest in renal function and left the field open for further experimentation. The fact that the tubules are not surrounded by a fluid with the same composition and osmolality as those of blood changed ideas concerning movement between both passive and active compartments. Although in the past the clearance techniques and the micropuncture studies of cortical nephrons dominated the field, other methods were developed, such as tissue analysis, micropuncture of both cortical and papillary tubules and collecting ducts, microperfusion of tubules in situ and in vitro, microcatheterization of collecting ducts, recirculation studies after microinjections, and so forth. More detailed anatomical studies also became of the utmost importance as the need to understand spatial arrangements between tubular segments, capillaries, collecting tubules, and papillary ducts arose.

Interest in the countercurrent hypothesis started to mount after three important publications (50, 176, 178). B. Hargitay and Werner Kuhn (50) proposed on theoretical grounds that the mammalian kidney may function as a countercurrent multiplier. Heinrich Wirz, Hargitay, and Kuhn (178) demonstrated that in a kidney producing hypertonic urine the osmotic pressure in the water phase of the kidney increases in a regular manner from the cortex to the tip of the papilla. Wirz (176) also showed that blood from a capillary at the tip of the papilla has practically the same osmotic pressure as that of urine from the collecting ducts. These results fascinated and inspired a young German, Karl J. Ullrich (Fig. 10), who after graduating from medical school in 1951, worked with Kurt Kramer at the Physiological Institute in Marburg, West Germany.

In 1951 Ullrich turned his attention to the renal countercurrent system and determined osmotic and Na^+ gradients in dog kidneys (169). Together with K. H. Jarausch, he determined the distribution from cortex to medulla of six electrolytes, as well as urea, amino

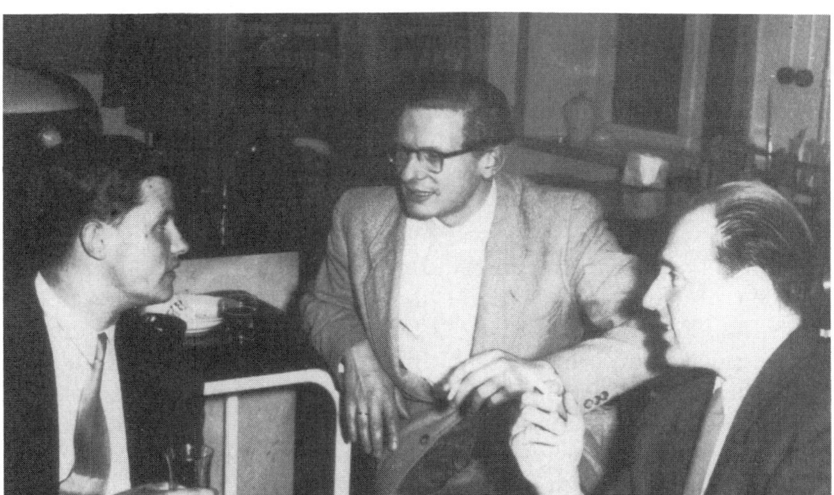

Figure 10. Karl J. Ullrich (b. 1925) (*center*) in his laboratory in Göttingen, West Germany in 1958 with his collaborators J. D. Klümper (*left*) and H. H. Hilger (*right*). (Courtesy of K. J. Ullrich.)

acids, and exogenous creatinine during diuresis and antidiuresis (170). This comprehensive study firmly established the major role played by Na^+, Cl^-, and urea in the renal concentrating mechanism. It is interesting to note that Cushny had already determined urea concentration in the inner medulla, but without the countercurrent hypothesis the high tissue urea concentration was assumed to be caused by a high concentration in the collecting ducts. Ullrich proceeded to develop his own techniques for micropuncture and for a series of ultramicroanalysis techniques. Together with Jarausch, he developed a technique for microcatheterization of hamster collecting ducts, taking samples at different distances from the papilla tip.

In the meantime (1957) an article by P. F. Sholander was published in *Scientific American* in which he compared the rete mirabile in fish swim bladder with the countercurrent system in kidney. An illustration showed a cross-section of kidney in which the increasing urea concentration toward the papilla was shown by increasing color intensity. Although I had read the Wirz (176, 178) papers before, this illustration actually started my own interest in the countercurrent mechanism and prompted my first studies on solute distribution in the kidney.

It became firmly established that urea accumulates in the renal medulla of mammals during antidiuresis. On a normal-protein diet, the mean urea concentration in tissue water rises in the outer medulla (particularly in the inner stripe) and then rises more steeply throughout the inner medulla, in which the highest urea concentration is reached in dogs and rats at the tip of the papilla (126, 132, 133, 138, 140, 163, 170, 173). In dogs and rats the concentration of urea in the kidneys may account for approximately half of the osmotic concentration of the inner medulla and rises to 1000–1200 mM in tissue water at the tip of the papilla. In diuretic animals the urea concentrations in the outer and inner medulla are greatly decreased (20–39 mM). In desert rodents with a higher osmotic concentration of urine, urea accumulation in the papilla is less pronounced and urea concentration in the inner medulla levels off at 500–700 mM in tissue water and does not rise in the tip of the papilla (135).

In 1958 I proposed that urea is concentrated in the inner medulla through active urea transport and countercurrent multiplication in the loop of Henle (134). Later in the same year, Berliner et al. published a paper (10) that had a major impact on current thinking with respect to urea movements in the renal medulla. Although in this paper Berliner et al. rejected countercurrent multiplication for Na^+ in the loop of Henle, a suggestion that proved to be wrong (49), the authors in other ways anticipated facts not yet gathered. They proposed that the high concentration of urea found in the inner medulla of the kidney is caused by diffusion of urea out of the collecting ducts (10). They wrote:

Now if it is assumed that in the presence of ADH [antidiuretic hormone] *the collecting ducts are permeable to urea as well as water, circumstances are suitable for the collecting ducts to feed urea continuously to the medullary interstitial space, the concentration of urea in this area rises to considerable levels because, as in the case with the sodium salts contributed by the loop, 1) the blood flow is low or 2) the countercurrent flow of blood keeps low the effective blood flow with respect to urea, a highly diffusible substance.*

The proposal was supported by the finding that the urea concentration in urine is usually higher than that in the tissue water of the inner medulla (10). That same year, Klümper et al. (68), investigating urea movements in the collecting ducts with the technique developed by Ullrich and his colleagues (60), concluded, "*Urea in the urine while passing through the collecting duct is concentrated due to water reabsorption and ... urea leaves the collecting duct together with water.*" Furthermore, the permeability of the collecting duct epithelium to urea was later found to be low in the outer medullary collecting tubules and unaffected by antidiuretic hormone, whereas the inner medullary collecting ducts were found to have a higher urea permeability that increases in the presence of antidiuretic hormone (9, 12).

In 1959 I invited Ullrich to come to Duke University for collaboration. Following discussions with Carl. W. Gottschalk at the nearby University of North Carolina, it was decided that we join forces in micropuncture studies with Gottschalk and his associates William E. Lassiter and Margaret Mylle (47, 172). These studies and an earlier micropuncture study from Gottschalk's laboratory on cortical nephrons and long loops of Henle in hamsters and rats (74) showed (as suggested by Shannon from clearance studies) that about 50% of the filtered urea leaves the proximal tubules as NaCl and water are reabsorbed from the tubule (74–76, 172). Urea is added to the short loops of Henle, as shown by micropuncture of the early distal convolutions of these nephrons (which are present on the cortical surface of the kidney), and the amount present at this site exceeds the amount of urea filtered by the glomeruli [in some rodents the amount is four times the amount filtered (29, 30, 47, 74, 127, 172, 174)]. In rats maintained on a low-protein diet, the relative amount of urea added to the short loops is greater than that in rats maintained on normal-protein diets (28). Urea is also added to the descending limb of the long loops of Henle (which in intact kidneys are accessible for micropuncture only at and near the tip of the papilla), in which it is present in greater amounts than that filtered (47, 74). The concentration increases toward the bend of the loop, and the amount of urea present may be as much as nine times the amount filtered (109).

In comprehensive and carefully executed experiments, Ullrich and his colleagues evaluated active transport of urea and determined the permeability coefficient and reflection coefficient in mammalian proximal and distal convoluted tubules and in collecting ducts in vivo (17, 165–168). They used the standing-drop method and micro-perfusion techniques. The measurements confirmed that urea moves by simple passive diffusion through the epithelium of proximal and distal convolutions and papillary collecting duct in rats on a normal-protein diet. However, in rats on a low-protein diet, active transport out of the collecting ducts was indicated (Fig. 11). As expected, the permeability of the proximal tubules was higher than that of the distal tubules. Permeability of the loops of Henle was measured during microperfusion of isolated rabbit tubules in vitro by Kokko and his collaborators (58, 69, 70, 124), and in rat papillae by Morgan et al. (97).

Urea-Recycling Theory

The theory for urea recycling, which came to be widely accepted as explaining most of the facts that emerged, is depicted in Figure 12 (8–10, 71, 96, 177). Mudge et al. (98) stated, "*Urea is recirculated by the mammalian nephron during antidiuresis. It is reabsorbed from the distal tubules and collecting ducts and secreted into the loops of Henle.*"

The recirculation hypothesis is supported by data obtained by injecting labeled inulin and urea together either into the renal artery (23) or into a late distal tubule (48, 64); urine is then collected at or near the papillary tip every minute. In both of these types of experiments, the recovery of urea is delayed relative to the recovery of inulin (which does not leave the tubules) (48). At the lowest urine flow rates, about 80% of the injected urea was found to be delayed

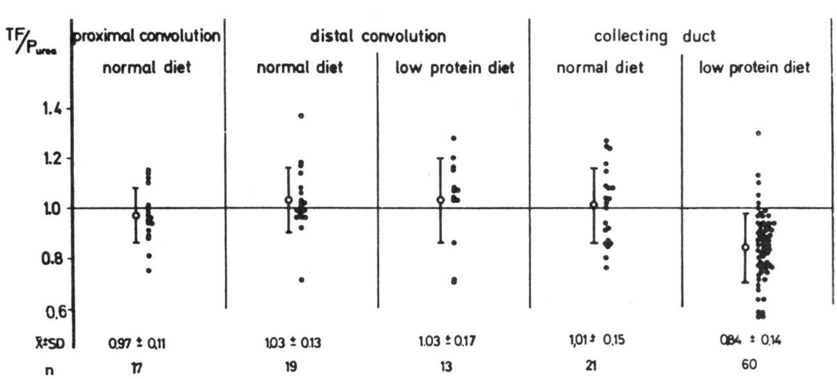

Figure 11. Comparison of the ^{14}C or chemical urea concentration in an equilibrium solution of a "standing droplet" in the renal tubules of rats maintained on normal- and low-protein diets. TF/P, tubule fluid-plasma ratio. [From Ullrich (166).]

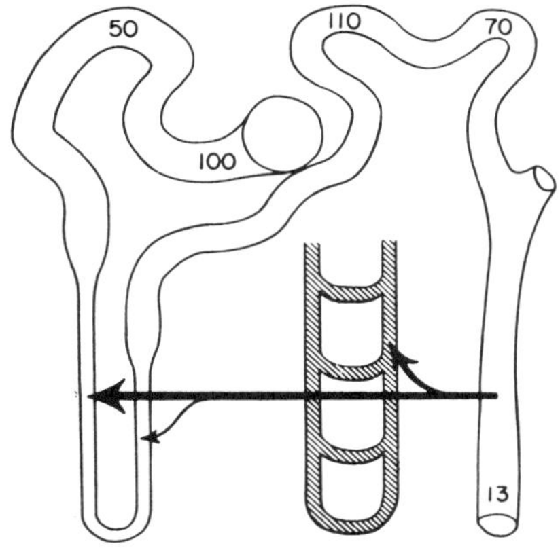

Figure 12. Recirculation of urea in the countercurrent system. [Adapted from Ullrich et al. (164a), incorporating data of Lassiter et al. (74).]

(recirculated) relative to the inulin, whereas at higher urine flows, only 20% was delayed (27, 28, 164). In rats maintained on low-protein diets, a substantially greater fraction of urea leaves the collecting ducts and only 2% of the injected urea is excreted with the inulin, compared to 20% in rats maintained on normal-protein diets (27, 28, 164). That in fact recirculation takes place was supported by the finding that the injected urea was recovered in a series of peaks with a regular interval of 1.5–2 min (28).

Anatomical investigations have shown that the spatial arrangement of loops of Henle and vasa recta bundles in the outer medulla favors an exchange of solutes and water between vasa recta and thin loops of Henle from the short-looped nephrons. In various rodents the thin segments of short-looped nephrons are either partially or totally imbedded in the vascular bundles in the inner stripe of the outer medulla (65, 66) and thus are adjacent to ascending vasa recta, carrying blood with a higher osmotic and urea concentration from the inner medulla.

One of the questions that has occupied several investigators in recent years is whether active sodium transport is required in the inner medullary thin limbs of the loops of Henle to explain the solute gradient (3, 30, 59, 71, 108, 109, 128). Independently and almost simultaneously, J. L. Stephenson (160a) and Juha Kokko and Floyd Rector (71) proposed similar passive models for the operation of the countercurrent multiplier in the inner medulla. The passive model proposed by Kokko and Rector (71) was based on their permeability measurements in long loops of Henle from rabbits. They suggested that "*papillary interstitial urea abstracts water out of the descending limbs generating high intraluminal NaCl concentrations which allows the entire system to operate by passive diffusion of NaCl out of the thin ascending loop of Henle.*" The hypothesis has not been validated because several studies have shown a substantial addition of urea to the descending limb in rats and other rodents (30, 74, 106, 108, 109). Other studies have suggested differences in the function of the countercurrent mechanism among mammalian species.

Another question that has received wide attention since it was first proposed by Gamble et al. (43) is the enhancement of the concentrating mechanism caused by urea. They found that the ability of the rat to concentrate urine is highest when the amount of urea in the urine constitutes 65% of the solute excreted. This phenomenon has been confirmed repeatedly, and it has been shown that not only is the osmotic concentration of urine enhanced by the urea in urine but other solutes are excreted in a smaller volume of water (78). As shown by Rabinowitz and his colleagues (115, 116, 118), this mechanism is not present in all mammals. However, the enhancement is not confined to urea but can also be produced by the infusion of urea analogues of the amide group such as methylurea and acetamide (112, 113).

Urea Movement Through Membranes in Mammalian Kidney

As stated by Wirz and Dirix (177), "*The role of urea in the countercurrent system is very involved and still incompletely understood.*" Although recirculation has been generally accepted, the manner of urea transport across the tubular epithelium has not been generally agreed upon. As in the past, controversies center around the questions of passive diffusion, carrier-mediated diffusion, and active transport of urea. Many proponents of simple diffusion have stated that all movements of urea in the countercurrent system can be explained by simple diffusion, whereas others point to experimental findings that are at odds with this hypothesis. The complex anatomical features of the mammalian kidney and the differences in urea concentration of blood and tissue fluid in different regions of the kidney have contributed to this confusion and have left some studies open to criticism and alternative interpretations.

Several attempts have been made to determine if the amount of urea added to the proximal tubules can be adequately accounted for by urea reabsorption from the collecting ducts. Although in most cases the amount calculated to leave the collecting ducts approximately equals the amount added to the loops of Henle (98), there are other physiological conditions in which this is not the case. Françoise Roch-Ramel et al. (126, 128) found that when large loads of urea were given to rats, no urea was reabsorbed from the collecting ducts (to the contrary, urea was added to collecting duct fluid), but an amount corresponding to 25% of the filtered load was added to the short loops of Henle between late proximal and early distal tubules (31). Urea was also found to be added to the short loops of Henle in saline diuresis under conditions for which it could not be accounted by the amount leaving the collecting ducts (125). This was found in a specific strain (Kraus) of Wistar rats but not in two other Wistar rat strains (125). These findings, which suggest active secretion of urea into the proximal tubule, were supported by the findings by Kawamura and Kokko (67), who demonstrated active secretion of urea in the isolated straight proximal tubules of both cortical and juxtamedullary nephrons in rabbits. The secretion occurred when both sides of the tubular epithelium were bathed with a 1 mM urea solution and was reversibly inhibited by cyanide and phloretin. This study is in good agreement with the secretion-mechanism seen in frogs that also shows a low tubular maximum (35).

The regulation of urea excretion found in animals maintained on a low-protein diet has not been explained by the passive-diffusion mechanism. In animals regulating urea excretion on a low-protein diet, urea concentration does not rise to the tip of the papilla but the highest concentration is seen in the inner stripe of the outer medulla in ruminants and in the outer part of the inner medulla in rats. Not in agreement with the diffusion hypothesis was the finding that, whereas in animals on a normal-protein diet the urine urea concentration is higher than that of the inner medulla and therefore favors inward diffusion from the collecting ducts to the tissue, this gradient is reversed in the animals on a low-protein diet, which show a significantly lower urine urea concentration than that in any of the inner medullary zones (139, 140, 163). Experiments performed by several investigators on rats on low- and normal-protein diets all showed a greatly increased urea reabsorption from the collecting ducts of rats on low-protein diets compared to those on normal- or high-protein diets when measurements were made under free-flow conditions (13, 14, 24, 28, 44, 76, 171) as well as steady-state (zero net flux) conditions (171). That this reabsorption occurred against a concentration gradient was indicated by urea-concentration measurements in tissue water (24) or vasa recta blood (76, 171) (see Fig. 11).

In animals maintained on a normal-protein diet, the urea gradient from collecting duct to tissue water, during steady-state antidiuresis, favors passive diffusion. However, Martin Goldberg et al. (44) examined the question of whether urea delivery to the renal medulla is dependent on the Na^+ gradient in the kidney. They found that when the Na^+ gradient was abolished in anesthetized dogs by ethacrynic acid, urea still accumulated in the inner medulla, showing an uphill gradient toward the papilla tip. The gradient was markedly reduced by inhibitors of anaerobic glycolysis and by acetamide. The results of George Bray and Agnes Preston (13, 14) also suggest active urea reabsorption in the collecting ducts of rats on normal diets during extreme diuresis.

Conclusion and Afterthoughts

The understanding of how urea is handled by the kidney has come a long way since Thomas Addis remarked that "*all we know about the kidney is that it makes urine.*" Facts have been gathered by many investigators from lower vertebrates as well as from mammalian kidneys, but what I find striking in my survey of the literature is that these facts have not really been integrated. The mammalian kidney has evolved from the kidney of lower vertebrates, more specifically from that of primitive amphibians. In many lower vertebrates urea functions in osmotic water retention in much the same way that high urea concentration in the mammalian renal medulla functions in abstracting water from the collecting ducts. Mechanisms have evolved in lower vertebrates to regulate urea excretion; these include diffusion, tubular secretion and reabsorption. Obviously, if these mechanisms are possible in lower vertebrates, they should also be possible in mammals and have indeed been shown to be present in the straight proximal tubules and in the collecting ducts. Yet efforts have consistently been made to explain what happens in the mammalian kidney on the basis of simple diffusion alone. This tendency is based on the desire, which has dominated our thinking for 100 years, to explain biological phenomena in the simplest possible mechanistic terms. In the meantime, however, what has been revealed by biological research is a far greater complexity of cellular function than could ever have been imagined.

In the renal countercurrent mechanism, active Na^+ transport has been the only force seriously considered responsible for creating the osmotic gradient from the cortex to the tip of the papilla, whereas no attempts have been made to include active transport of urea in the countercurrent models despite the evidence of active urea secretion in straight proximal tubules and active reabsorption in the collecting ducts presented by many investigators. Inclusion of these facts in a more comprehensive countercurrent model might serve to clarify some of the points that are difficult to explain by the current models.

BIBLIOGRAPHY

1. Addis, T. The ratio between the urea content of the urine and of the blood after the administration of large quantities of urea. *J. Urol.* 1: 263–287, 1917.
2. Addis, T., E. Barrett, L. J. Poo, H. J. Wreen, and R. W. Lippman. The relation between protein consumption and diurnal variations of the endogenous creatinine clearance in normal individuals. *J. Clin. Invest.* 30:206–209, 1951.
3. Andreoli, T. E., R. W. Berliner, J. P. Kokko, and D. J. Marsh. Questions and replies: renal mechanisms for urinary concentrating and diluting processes. *Am. J. Physiol.* 235 (*Renal Fluid Electrolyte Physiol.* 4): F1–F11, 1978.
4. Austin, H. J., E. Stillman, and D. D. van Slyke. Factors governing the excretion rate of urea. *J. Biol. Chem.* 46: 91–112, 1921.
5. Bechamp, M. Extrait d'une thèse sur les substances albuminoïdes et sur leur transformation en urée. *Ann. Chim. Phys.* 48: 348–355, 1856.

6. Berard, M. J. E. Essay sur l'analyse de substance animales. *Ann. Chim. Phys.* 5: 290–298, 1817.
7. Bergström, J. Discovery and rediscovery of low protein diet. *Clin. Nephrol.* 21: 29–35, 1984.
8. Berliner, R. W. The concentrating mechanism in the renal medulla. *Kidney Int.* 9: 214–222, 1976.
9. Berliner, R. W., and C. M. Bennett. Concentration of urine in the mammalian kidney. *Am. J. Med.* 42: 777–789, 1967.
10. Berliner, R. W., N. G. Levinsky, D. G. Davidson, and M. Eden. Dilution and concentration of the urine and the action of antidiuretic hormone. *Am. J. Med.* 24: 730–744, 1958.
11. Boerhaave, H. *Elements of Chemistry: Being the Annual Lectures of Herman Boerhaave,* translated by T. Dallowe. London: Pemberton, 1735, vol. 1.
12. Bowman, F. J., and E. C. Foulkes. Antidiuretic hormone and urea permeability of collecting ducts. *Am. J. Physiol.* 218: 231–233, 1970.
13. Bray, G. A., and A. Preston. Effect of urea on urine concentration in the rat. *J. Clin. Invest.* 40: 1952–1960, 1961.
14. Bray, G. A., and A. S. Preston. The role of urea in the concentration of non-urea solutes by the kidney. In: *Urea and the Kidney,* edited by B. Schmidt-Nielsen. Amsterdam: Excerpta Med., 1970, p. 284–292.
15. Brenner, B. M., T. W. Meyer, and T. H. Hostetter. Dietary protein intake and the progressive nature of kidney disease: the role of hemodynamically mediated glomerular injury in the pathogenesis of progressive glomerular sclerosis in aging. *N. Engl. J. Med.* 307: 652–659, 1982.
16. Brooke, J. H. Wöhler's urea and its vital force?—A verdict from the chemists. *Ambix* 15: 84–114, 1968.
17. Capek, K., G. Fuchs, G. Rumrich, and K. J. Ullrich. Harnstoffpermeabilität der corticalen Tubulusabschnitte von Ratten in Antidiurese und Wasserdiurese. *Pfluegers Arch. Gesamte Physiol. Menschen Tiere* 290: 237–249, 1966.
18. Carlisky, N. J. Urea excretion and arginase in the anuran kidney. In: *Urea and the Kidney,* edited by B. Schmidt-Nielsen. Amsterdam: Excerpta Med., 1970, p. 263–271.
19. Chalmers, M. I., and R. L. M. Synge. The digestion of protein and nitrogenous compounds in ruminants. *Adv. Protein Chem.* 9: 93–120, 1954.
20. Chasis, H., and W. Goldring (editors). *Homer William Smith, Sc. D.: His Scientific and Literary Achievements.* New York: New York Univ. Press, 1965.
21. Chasis, H., and H. W. Smith. The excretion of urea in normal man and in subjects with glomerulonephritis. *J. Clin. Invest.* 17: 347–359, 1938.
22. Chelsley, L. C. Urea excretion at low urine volumes. The calculation of "minimal" urea clearance. *J. Clin. Invest.* 17: 119–123, 1937.
23. Chinard, F. P., and T. Enns. Relative renal excretion patterns of sodium ion, chloride ion, urea, water and glomerular substances. *Am. J. Physiol.* 182: 247–250, 1955.
24. Clapp, J. R. Renal tubular reabsorption of urea in normal and protein-depleted rats. *Am. J. Physiol.* 210: 1304–1308, 1966.

25. CLARKE, R. W., and H. W. SMITH. Absorption and excretion of water and salts by the elasmobranch fishes. III. The use of xylose as a measure of the glomerular filtrate in *Squalus acanthias*. *J. Cell. Comp. Physiol.* 1: 131–143, 1932.
26. CUSHNY, A. R. *The Secretion of Urine*. London: Longmans, Green, 1917.
27. DANIELSON, R. A., and B. SCHMIDT-NIELSEN. Recirculation of urea analogs from renal collecting ducts of high- and low-protein-fed rats. *Am. J. Physiol.* 223: 130–137, 1972.
28. DANIELSON, R. A., B. SCHMIDT-NIELSEN, and C. HOHBERGER. Micropuncture study of the regulation of urea excretion by the collecting ducts in rats on high and low protein diets. In: *Urea and the Kidney*, edited by B. Schmidt-Nielsen. Amsterdam: Excerpta Med., 1970, p. 375–384.
29. DE ROUFFIGNAC, C. Physiological role of the loop of Henle in urinary concentration. *Kidney Int.* 2: 297–303, 1972.
30. DE ROUFFIGNAC, C., and F. MOREL. Micropuncture study of water, electrolytes, and urea movements along the loops of Henle in *Psammomys*. *J. Clin. Invest.* 48: 474–486, 1969.
31. DIEZI, J. The adaptation of renal urea excretion after unilateral nephrectomy and after overloading with urea. *Pfluegers Arch.* 344: 287–298, 1973.
32. DOLE, V. P. Back-diffusion of urea in the mammalian kidney. *Am. J. Physiol.* 139: 504–513, 1943.
33. EGGENA, P. Inhibition of vasopressin-stimulated urea transport across the toad urinary bladder. *J. Clin. Invest.* 52: 2963–2970, 1973.
34. FISHMAN, A. P., and D. W. RICHARDS (editors). *Circulation of the Blood: Men and Ideas*. Bethesda, MD: Am. Physiol. Soc., 1982.
35. FORSTER, R. P. Active cellular transport of urea by frog renal tubules. *Am. J. Physiol.* 179: 372–377, 1954.
36. FORSTER, R. P. Renal transport mechanisms. *Federation Proc.* 26: 1008–1019, 1967.
37. FORSTER, R. P. Active tubular transport of urea and its role in environmental physiology. In: *Urea and the Kidney*, edited by B. Schmidt-Nielsen. Amsterdam: Excerpta Med., 1970, p. 229–237.
38. FORSTER, R. P. Comparative vertebrate physiology and renal concepts. In: *Handbook of Physiology. Renal Physiology*, edited by J. Orloff and R. W. Berliner. Washington, DC: Am. Physiol. Soc., 1973, sect. 8, chapt. 8, p. 161–184.
39. FORSTER, R. P., and L. GOLDSTEIN. Formation of excretory products. In: *Fish Physiology*, edited by W. S. Hoar and D. J. Randall. New York: Academic, 1969, vol. 1, p. 313–350.
40. FORSTER, R. P., L. GOLDSTEIN, and J. K. ROSEN. Intrarenal control of urea reabsorption by renal tubules of the marine elasmobranch, *Squalus acanthias*. *Comp. Biochem. Physiol. A Comp. Physiol.* 42: 3–12, 1972.
41. FORSTER, R. P., B. SCHMIDT-NIELSEN, and L. GOLDSTEIN. Relation of renal tubular transport of urea to its biosynthesis in metamorphosing tadpoles. *J. Cell. Comp. Physiol.* 61: 239–244, 1963.
42. FOURCROY, A.-F., and L.-N. VANQUELIN. Memoire, Pour servir a l'histoire naturellc chimique et medicale de l'urine humaine, dans lequel on s'occupé spécialement des propríetés de la matière particulière qui

la caractérise. *Ann. Chim. Paris* 80–162, 1799.

43. GAMBLE, J. L., C. F. MCKHANN, A. M. BUTLER, and E. TUTHILL. An economy of water in renal function referable to urea. *Am. J. Physiol.* 109: 139–154, 1934.
44. GOLDBERG, M., A. M. WOJTZAK, and M. A. RAMIREZ. Uphill transport gradient for urea in the renal medulla. In: *Urea and the Kidney,* edited by B. Schmidt-Nielsen. Amsterdam: Excerpta Med., 1970, p. 293–304.
45. GOLDSTEIN, L., S. HARLEY-DEWITT, and R. P. FORSTER. Activities of ornithine-urea cycle enzymes and of trimethylamine oxidase in the coelacanth, *Latimeria chalumnae. Comp. Biochem. Physiol. B Comp. Biochem.* 44: 357–362, 1973.
46. GORDON, M. S., K. SCHMIDT-NIELSEN, and H. M. KELLY. Osmotic regulation in the crab-eating frog (*Rana cancrivora*). *J. Exp. Biol.* 38: 659–678, 1961.
47. GOTTSCHALK, C. W., W. E. LASSITER, M. MYLLE, K. J. ULLRICH, B. SCHMIDT-NIELSEN, R. O'DELL, and G. PEHLING. Micropuncture study of composition of loop of Henle fluid in desert rodents. *Am. J. Physiol.* 204: 532–535, 1963.
48. GOTTSCHALK, C. W., F. MOREL, and M. MYLLE. Tracer microinjection studies of renal tubular permeability. *Am. J. Physiol.* 209: 173–178, 1965.
49. GOTTSCHALK, C. W., and M. MYLLE. Micropuncture study of the mammalian urinary concentrating mechanism: evidence for the countercurrent hypothesis. *Am. J. Physiol.* 196: 927–936, 1959.
50. HARGITAY, B., and W. KUHN. Das Multipoikationsprinzip als Grundlage der Harnkonzentrierung in der Niere. *Z. Elektrochem.* 55: 539–558, 1951.
51. HAYS, R. M. Antidiuretic hormone. *N. Engl. J. Med.* 295: 659–665, 1976.
52. HAYS, R. M., S. H. HARKNESS, and N. FRANKI. The movement of urea and other small molecules across the toad bladder. In: *Urea and the Kidney,* edited by B. Schmidt-Nielsen. Amsterdam: Excerpta Med., 1970, p. 149–158.
53. HEIDENHAIN, R. Versuche über den Vorgang der Harnabsonderung. *Pfluegers Arch. Gesamte Physiol. Menschen Tiere* 9: 1–27, 1874.
54. HERRIN, R. C., A. RABIN, and R. N. FEINSTEIN. The influence of diet upon urea clearance in dogs. *Am. J. Physiol.* 119: 87–92, 1937.
55. HOUPT, T. R. Utilization of blood urea in ruminants. *Am. J. Physiol.* 197: 115–120, 1959.
56. HOUPT, T. R. Urea utilization by rabbits fed a low-protein ration. *Am. J. Physiol.* 205: 1144–1150, 1963.
57. HOUPT, T. R., and K. A. HOUPT. Transfer of urea nitrogen across the rumen wall. *Am. J. Physiol.* 214: 1296–1303, 1968.
58. IMAI, M., and J. P. KOKKO. Sodium chloride, urea and water transport in the thin ascending limb of Henle. *J. Clin. Invest.* 53: 393–402, 1974.
59. IMBERT, M., and C. DE ROUFFIGNAC. Role of sodium and urea in the renal concentrating mechanisms in *Psammomys obesus. Pfluegers Arch.* 361: 107–114, 1976.
60. JARAUSCH, K. H., and K. J. ULLRICH. Zur Technik der Entnahme von

Harnproben aus Einzelnen Sammelrohren der Saugetierriere mittels Polyathylen-Capillaren. *Pfluegers Arch. Gesamte Physiol. Menschen Tiere* 264: 88–94, 1957.

61. JOLLIFFE, N., J. A. SHANNON, and H. W. SMITH. The excretion of urine in the dog. III. The use of non-metabolized sugars in the measurement of the glomerular filtrate. *Am. J. Physiol.* 100: 301–312, 1932.
62. JOLLIFFE, N., and H. W. SMITH. The excretion of urine in the dog. I. The urea and creatinine clearances on a mixed diet. *Am. J. Physiol.* 98: 572–577, 1931.
63. JOLLIFFE, N., and H. W. SMITH. The excretion of urine in the dog. II. The urea and creatinine clearance on cracker meal diet. *Am. J. Physiol.* 99: 101–107, 1931.
64. JONES, N. F., M. MYLLE, and C. W. GOTTSCHALK. Renal tubular microinjection studies in normal and potassium-depleted rats. *Clin. Sci.* 29: 261–275, 1965.
65. KAISSLING, B., C. DE ROUFFIGNAC, J. M. BARRETT, and W. KRIZ. The structural organization of the kidney of the desert rodent *Psammomys obesus. Anat. Embryol.* 148: 121–143, 1975.
66. KAISSLING, B., W. KRIZ, and J. M. BARRETT. Structural analysis of the rabbit kidney: thin limb ultrastructure. *Adv. Anat. Embryol. Cell Biol.* 56: 51–63, 1979.
67. KAWAMURA, S., and J. P. KOKKO. Urea secretion by the straight segment of the proximal tubule. *J. Clin. Invest.* 58: 604–612, 1976.
68. KLÜMPER, J. D., K. J. ULLRICH, and H. H. HILGER. Das Verhalten des Harnstoffs in den sammelrohren der Saugetierniere. *Pfluegers Arch. Gesamte Physiol. Menschen Tiere* 267: 238–243, 1958.
69. KOKKO, J. P. Sodium chloride and water transport in the descending limb of Henle. *J. Clin. Invest.* 49: 1838–1846, 1970.
70. KOKKO, J. P. Urea transport in the proximal tubule and the descending thin limb of Henle. *J. Clin. Invest.* 51: 1999–2008, 1972.
71. KOKKO, J. P., and F. C. RECTOR, JR. Countercurrent multiplication system without active transport in inner medulla. *Kidney Int.* 2: 214–233, 1972.
72. KUHN, T. S. *The Structure of Scientific Revolutions* (2nd ed.). Chicago, IL: Univ. of Chicago Press, 1970.
73. KURZER, F., and P. M. SANDERSON. Urea in the history of organic chemistry. *J. Chem. Educ.* 33: 452–459, 1956.
74. LASSITER, W. E., C. W. GOTTSCHALK, and M. MYLLE. Micropuncture study of net transtubular movement of water and urea in nondiuretic mammalian kidney. *Am. J. Physiol.* 200: 1139–1147, 1961.
75. LASSITER, W. E., M. MYLLE, and C. W. GOTTSCHALK. Net transtubular movement of water and urea in saline diuresis. *Am. J. Physiol.* 206: 669–673, 1964.
76. LASSITER, W. E., M. MYLLE, and C. W. GOTTSCHALK. Micropuncture study of urea transport in rat renal medulla. *Am. J. Physiol.* 210: 965–970, 1966.
77. LEAF, A. Transport of urea across a living membrane. In: *Urea and the Kidney,* edited by B. Schmidt-Nielsen. Amsterdam: Excerpta Med., 1970, p. 83–88.
78. LEVINSKY, N. G., and R. W. BERLINER. The role of urea in the urine concentrating mechanism. *J. Clin. Invest.* 38: 741–748, 1959.

79. Lintern, S. M., and S. Barker. Renal retention of urea in the Kangaroo Island wallaby, *Protemnodon eugenii* (Desmarest). *Aust. J. Exp. Biol. Med. Sci.* 47: 243–250, 1969.
80. Long, W. S. Renal secretion of urea in *Rana catesbeiana*. In: *Urea and the Kidney*, edited by B. Schmidt-Nielsen. Amsterdam: Excerpta Med., 1970, p. 216–222.
81. Love, J. K., and N. Lifson. Transtubular movements of urea in the doubly perfused bullfrog kidney. *Am. J. Physiol.* 193: 662–668, 1958.
82. Ludwig, C. F. W. *Beitrage für Lehre vom Mechanismus der Harn Secretion.* Marburg, Germany: Elwert, 1843.
83. Maltz, E., N. Silanikova, and A. Shkolnik. Renal performance in relation to water and nitrogen metabolism in Bedouin goats during lactation. *Comp. Biochem. Physiol. A Comp. Physiol.* 70: 145–147, 1981.
84. Maren, T. H. Eli Kennerly Marshall, Jr. *Biogr. Mem. Natl. Acad. Sci.* 56: 313–352, 1986.
85. Marshall, E. K., Jr. A rapid clinical method for the estimation of urea in urine. *J. Biol. Chem.* 14: 283–290, 1913.
86. Marshall, E. K., Jr. A new method for the determination of urea in the blood. *J. Biol. Chem.* 15: 487–494, 1913.
87. Marshall, E. K., Jr. The determination of urea in urine. *J. Biol. Chem.* 15: 495–496, 1913.
88. Marshall, E. K., Jr. The influence of diuresis on the elimination of urea, creatinine and chlorides. *J. Pharmacol. Exp. Ther.* 16: 141–154, 1920.
89. Marshall, E. K., Jr. The secretion of urine. *Physiol. Rev.* 6: 440–473, 1926.
90. Marshall, E. K., Jr. The secretion of urea in the frog. *J. Cell. Comp. Physiol.* 2: 349–353, 1932.
91. Marshall, E. K., Jr. Two lectures on renal physiology. *Physiologist* 9: 367–384, 1966.
92. Marshall, E. K., Jr., and M. M. Crane. The secretory function of the renal tubules. *Am. J. Physiol.* 70: 465–488, 1924.
93. Marshall, E. K., Jr., and D. M. Davis. Urea: Its distribution in and elimination from the body. *J. Biol. Chem.* 18: 53–80, 1914.
94. Marshall, E. K., Jr., and A. L. Grafflin. The structure and function of the kidney of *Lophius piscatorius*. *Bull. Johns Hopkins Hosp.* 43: 205–235, 1928.
95. Marshall, E. K., Jr., and V. L. Vickers. The mechanism of the elimination of phenolsulphonephthalein by the kidney—a proof of secretion by the convoluted tubules. *Bull. Johns Hopkins Hosp.* 34: 1–7, 1923.
96. Morel, F., and C. de Rouffignac. Micropuncture study of urea medullary recycling in desert rodents. In: *Urea and the Kidney*, edited by B. Schmidt-Nielsen. Amsterdam: Excerpta Med., 1970, p. 401–413.
97. Morgan, T., F. Sakai, and R. W. Berliner. In vitro permeability of medullary collecting ducts to water and urea. *Am. J. Physiol.* 214: 574–581, 1968.
98. Mudge, G. H., W. O. Berndt, and H. Valtin. Tubular transport of urea, glucose, phosphate, uric acid, sulfate, and thiosulfate. In: *Handbook of Physiology. Renal Physiology*, edited by J. Orloff and R. W.

Berliner. Washington, DC: Am. Physiol. Soc., 1973, sect. 8, chapt. 19, p. 587–652.

99. Murdaugh, H. V., Jr., B. Schmidt-Nielsen, E. M. Doyle, and R. O'Dell. Renal tubular regulation of urea excretion in man. *J. Appl. Physiol.* 13: 263–268, 1958.

100. Nielsen, A. L., and H. O. Bang. The influence of diet on renal function in healthy persons. *Acta Med. Scand.* 130: 382–388, 1948.

101. Nielsen, A. L., and H. O. Bang. The protein content of the diet and the function of the kidneys in human beings. *Scand. J. Clin. Lab. Invest.* 1: 295–297, 1949.

102. Nussbaum, M. Ueber die Secretion der Niere. *Pfluegers Arch. Gesamte Physiol. Menschen Tiere* 16: 189–148, 1878.

103. Nussbaum, M. Fortgesetzte Untersuchungen über die Secretion der Niere. *Pfluegers Arch. Gesamte Physiol. Menschen Tiere* 17: 580–593, 1878.

104. O'Connor, W. J., and R. A. Summerill. The effect of a meal of meat on glomerular filtration rate in dogs at normal urine flows. *J. Physiol. Lond.* 256: 81–91, 1976.

105. O'Connor, W. J., and R. A. Summerill. The excretion of urea by dogs following a meat meal. *J. Physiol. Lond.* 256: 93–102, 1976.

106. Oliver, R. E., D. R. Roy, and R. L. Jamison. Urinary concentration in the papillary collecting duct of the rat. *J. Clin. Invest.* 69: 157–164, 1982.

107. Partington, J. R. *History of Chemistry.* London: Macmillan, 1964, vol. 4, p. 321–335.

108. Pennell, J. P., F. B. Lacy, and R. L. Jamison. An in vivo study of concentrating process in the descending limb of Henle's loop. *Kidney Int.* 5: 337–347, 1974.

109. Pennell, J. P., V. Sanjana, N. R. Frey, and R. L. Jamison. The effect of urea infusion on the urinary concentrating mechanisms in protein-depleted rats. *J. Clin. Invest.* 55: 399–409, 1975.

110. Prevost, J. L., and J. A. Dumas. Examen du sang et de son action dans les divers phénomènes de la vie. *Ann. Chim. Phys.* 23: 90–104, 1823.

111. Prout, W. Observations on the nature of some of the proximate principles of the urine. *Med. Chir. Trans.* 7: 520–544, 1817.

112. Rabinowitz, L. Enhancement of renal concentrating ability in the rat by acetamide and methylurea. *Am. J. Physiol.* 214: 737–744, 1968.

113. Rabinowitz, L. Accumulation of organic nonelectrolytes in the renal medulla: mechanism and consequences. In: *Urea and the Kidney,* edited by B. Schmidt-Nielsen. Amsterdam: Excerpta Med., 1970, p. 323–332.

114. Rabinowitz, L., and A. D. Baines. Microinjection studies of renal tubular permeability to methylurea and acetamide in the rat. *Am. J. Physiol.* 214: 745–748, 1968.

115. Rabinowitz, L., and R. A. Gunther. Renal concentrating ability in sheep during urea, mannitol, and methylurea diuresis. *Am. J. Physiol.* 222: 801–806, 1972.

116. Rabinowitz, L., and R. A. Gunther. Excretion of urea in sheep during urea, mannitol, and methylurea osmotic diuresis. *Am. J. Physiol.* 222: 807–809, 1972.

117. Rabinowitz, L., and R. H. Kellogg. Enhancement of renal concentrat-

ing ability in the dog by urea and related compounds. *Am. J. Physiol.* 205: 112–116, 1963.
118. Rabinowitz, L., A. B. Thompson, and R. B. Wagman. Effect of acute urea administration on urinary nonurea solute concentration. *Am. J. Physiol.* 221: 242–245, 1971.
119. Rehberg, P. B. Studies on kidney function. I. The rate of filtration and reabsorption in the human kidney. *Biochem. J.* 20: 447–460, 1926.
120. Rehberg, P. B. Studies on kidney function. II. The excretion of urea and chlorine analyzed according to a modified filtration-reabsorption theory. *Biochem. J.* 20: 461–482, 1926.
121. Richards, A. N., and A. M. Walker. Urine formation in the amphibian kidney. *Am. J. Med. Sci.* 190: 727–746, 1935.
122. Richards, A. N., B. B. Westfall, and P. A. Bott. Renal excretion of inulin, creatinine and xylose in normal dogs. *Proc. Soc. Exp. Biol. Med.* 32: 73–75, 1934.
123. Robinson, V. *The Story of Medicine.* New York: Tudor, 1935.
124. Rocha, A. S., and J. P. Kokko. Permeability of medullary nephron segments to urea and water: effect of vasopressin. *Kidney Int.* 6: 379–387, 1974.
125. Roch-Ramel, F., M. Churchill-Borloz, D. Carmignac, P. Michoud, and G. Peters. Excretion of urea by the rat kidney in isotonic saline diuresis: a micropuncture study. *Am. J. Physiol.* 222: 489–494, 1972.
126. Roch-Ramel, F., J. Diezi, F. Chomety, P. Michoud, and G. Peters. Urea concentrations in tubular fluid and in renal tissue of rats overloaded with urea or with saline solutions. In: *Urea and the Kidney,* edited by B. Schmidt-Nielsen. Amsterdam: Excerpta Med., 1970, p. 333–341.
127. Roch-Ramel, F., and G. Peters. Intrarenal urea and electrolyte concentrations as influenced by water diuresis and by hydrochlorothiazide. *Eur. J. Pharmacol.* 1: 124–139, 1967.
128. Roch-Ramel, F., and G. Peters. Renal transport of urea. In: *Renal Transport of Organic Substances,* edited by R. Gregor, F. Lan, and S. Silbernagi. New York: Springer-Verlag, 1981, p. 134–153.
129. Rose, W. C., L. C. Smith, M. Womack, and M. Shane. The utilization of the nitrogen of ammonium salts, urea, and certain other compounds in the synthesis of non-essential amino acids in vivo. *J. Biol. Chem.* 181: 307–316, 1949.
130. Rouelle, H. M. Observation sur l'urine humaine, et sur celles de vache et cheval, comparées ensemble. *J. Med. Chir. Pharm.* 40: 451–468, 1773.
131. Ruibald, R., W. Trevis, and V. Roig. The terrestrial ecology of the spadefoot toad *Scapiopus hammondii. Copeia* 3: 571–584, 1969.
132. Ruiz-Guiñazú, A. The contribution of urea to the renal osmotic gradient in normal and diseased kidneys. In: *Urea and the Kidney,* edited by B. Schmidt-Nielsen. Amsterdam: Excerpta Med., 1970, p. 305–313.
133. Ruiz-Guiñazú, A., E. E. Arrizurieta, and L. Yelinek. Electrolyte, water, and urea content in dog kidneys in different states of diuresis. *Am. J. Physiol.* 206: 725–730, 1964.
134. Schmidt-Nielsen, B. Urea excretion in mammals. *Physiol. Rev.* 38: 139–168, 1958.
135. Schmidt-Nielsen, B. Comparative physiology of urea excretion. In:

Progress in Nephrology, edited by G. Peters and F. Roch-Ramel. Heidelberg, FRG: Springer-Verlag, 1969, p. 1–12.

136. SCHMIDT-NIELSEN, B. Urea analogues and tubular transport competition. In: *Urea and the Kidney,* edited by B. Schmidt-Nielsen. Amsterdam: Excerpta Med., 1970, p. 252–262.
137. SCHMIDT-NIELSEN, B. Mechanisms of urea excretion by the vertebrate kidney. In: *Nitrogen Metabolism and the Environment,* edited by J. W. Campbell and L. Goldstein. New York: Academic, 1972, p. 79–103.
138. SCHMIDT-NIELSEN, B., and R. O'DELL. Effect of diet on distribution of urea and electrolytes in kidneys of sheep. *Am. J. Physiol.* 197: 856–860, 1959.
139. SCHMIDT-NIELSEN, B., H. OSAKI, H. V. MURDAUGH, JR., and R. O'DELL. Renal regulation of urea excretion in sheep. *Am. J. Physiol.* 194: 221–228, 1958.
140. SCHMIDT-NIELSEN, B., and R. R. ROBINSON. Contribution of urea to urinary concentrating ability in the dog. *Am. J. Physiol.* 218: 1363–1369, 1970.
141. SCHMIDT-NIELSEN, B., and D. SCHMIDT. Renal function of *Shenodon punctatum. Comp. Biochem. Physiol. A Comp. Physiol.* 44: 121–129, 1973.
142. SCHMIDT-NIELSEN, B., K. SCHMIDT-NIELSEN, A. BROKAW, and H. SCHNEIDERMAN. Water conservation in desert rodents. *J. Cell. Comp. Physiol.* 32: 331–360, 1948.
143. SCHMIDT-NIELSEN, B., K. SCHMIDT-NIELSEN, T. R. HOUPT, and S. A. JARNUM. Urea excretion in the camel. *Am. J. Physiol.* 188: 477–484, 1957.
144. SCHMIDT-NIELSEN, K., and P. LEE. Kidney function in the crab-eating frog (*Rana cancrivora*). *J. Exp. Biol.* 39: 167–177, 1962.
145. SCHOLANDER, P. E. The wonderful net. *Sci. Am.* 196: 96–107, 1957.
146. SHANNON, J. A. Glomerular filtration and urea excretion in relation to urine flow in the dog. *Am. J. Physiol.* 117: 206–225, 1936.
147. SHANNON, J. A. The tubular reabsorption of xylose in the normal dog. *Am. J. Physiol.* 122: 775–781, 1938.
148. SHANNON, J. A. Urea excretion in normal dog during forced diuresis. *Am. J. Physiol.* 122: 782–787, 1938.
149. SHANNON, J. A., N. JOLLIFFE, and H. W. SMITH. The excretion of urine in the dog. IV. The effect of maintenance diet feeding, etc., upon quantity of glomerular filtration. *Am. J. Physiol.* 101: 625–638, 1932.
150. SHOEMAKER, V. H., L. MCCLANAHAN, and R. RUIBALD. Seasonal changes in body fluids in field populations of spadefoot toads. *Copeia* 3: 585–591, 1969.
151. SILANIKOVE, N., H. TAGARI, and A. SHKOLNIK. Gross energy digestion and urea recycling in the desert black Bedouin goat. *Comp. Biochem. Physiol. A Comp. Physiol.* 67: 215–218, 1980.
152. SINGER, C. *A Short History of Scientific Ideas to 1900.* Oxford, UK: Oxford Univ. Press, 1959.
153. SMITH, H. W. The absorption and excretion of water and salts by the elasmobranch fishes. I. Fresh water elasmobranchs. *Am. J. Physiol.* 98: 279–295, 1931.
154. SMITH, H. W. The absorption and excretion of water and salts by the elasmobranch fishes. II. Marine elasmobranchs. *Am. J. Physiol.* 98:

296–310, 1931.
155. SMITH, H. W. The retention and physiological role of urea in the elasmobranchii. *Biol. Rev. Camb. Philos. Soc.* 11: 49–82, 1936.
156. SMITH, H. W. *The Physiology of the Kidney.* Oxford, UK: Oxford Univ. Press, 1937.
157. SMITH, H. W. *The Kidney: Structure and Function in Health and Disease.* Oxford, UK: Oxford Univ. Press, 1951.
158. SMITH, H. W. *From Fish to Philosopher* (lst ed.). Boston, MA: Little, Brown, 1953.
159. SMITH, H. W., and H. SILVETTE. Note on the nitrogen excretion of camels. *J. Biol. Chem.* 82: 409–411, 1928.
160. STADELER, G., and F. T. FRERICHS. Über das Vorkommen von Harnstoff, Taurin and Scyllit in den Organen der Plagiostomen. *J. Pract. Chem.* 73: 48–55, 1858.
160a. STEPHENSON, J. L. Concentration of urine in a central core model of the renal counterflow system. *Kidney Int.* 2: 85–94, 1972.
161. STEWART, D. J., W. N. HOLMES, and G. FLETCHER. The renal excretion of nitrogenous compounds by the duck (*Anas platyrhynchos*) maintained on freshwater and on hypertonic saline. *J. Exp. Biol.* 50: 527–539, 1969.
162. TANAKA, N., K. KUBO, K. SHIRAKI, H. KOISHI, and H. YOSHIMURA. A pilot study on protein metabolism in the Papua New Guinea highlanders. *J. Nutr. Sci. Vitaminol.* 26: 247–259, 1980.
163. TRUNIGER, B., and B. SCHMIDT-NIELSEN. Intrarenal distribution of urea and related compounds: effects of nitrogen intake. *Am. J. Physiol.* 207: 971–978, 1964.
164. TRUNIGER, B., and B. SCHMIDT-NIELSEN. Transtubular movements of urea and related compounds. In: *Progress in Nephrology,* edited by G. Peters and F. Roch-Ramel. Heidelberg, FRG: Springer-Verlag, 1969, p. 26–31.
164a. ULLRICH, K. J. Introduction to the session on urea movement across the renal tubules. In: *Urea and the Kidney,* edited by B. Schmidt-Nielsen. Amsterdam: Excerpta Med., 1970, p. 171–174.
165. ULLRICH, K. J. *Physiologie der Harnkonzentrierung und Verdünnung.* Heidelberg, FRG: Springer-Verlag, 1959.
166. ULLRICH, K. J. Die Nierenphysiologie auf dem Weg zur molecularen Betrachtungsweise. *Max-Planck-Ges. Jahrb.* 153–174, 1969.
167. ULLRICH, K. J. "Anatomie" eines Epithels, Analyse des Stofftransportes durch den proximalen Nierebtubulus. *Naturwissenschaften* 60: 290–297, 1973.
168. ULLRICH, K. J. Permeability characteristics of the mammalian nephron. In: *Handbook of Physiology. Renal Physiology,* edited by J. Orloff and R. W. Berliner. Washington, DC: Am. Physiol. Soc., 1973, sect. 8, chapt. 12, p. 377–398.
169. ULLRICH, K. J., F. O. DRENCKHAHN, and K. H. JARAUSCH. Untersuchungen zum Problem der Harnkonzentrierung und Verdünnung. *Pfluegers Arch. Gesamte Physiol. Menschen Tiere* 261: 62–77, 1955.
170. ULLRICH, K. J., and K. H. JARAUSCH. Untersuchungen zum Problem der Harnkonzentrierung und Harnverdünnung. *Pfluegers Arch. Gesamte Physiol. Menschen Tiere* 262: 537–550, 1956.
171. ULLRICH, K. J., G. RUMRICH, and B. SCHMIDT-NIELSEN. Urea transport in

the collecting duct of rats on normal and low protein diets. *Pfluegers Arch. Gesamte Physiol. Menschen Tiere* 295: 147–156, 1967.

172. Ullrich, K. J., B. Schmidt-Nielsen, R. O'Dell, G. Pehling, C. W. Gottschalk, W. E. Lassiter, and M. Mylle. Micropuncture study of composition of proximal and distal tubular fluid in rat kidney. *Am. J. Physiol.* 204: 527–531, 1963.
173. Valtin, H. Sequestration of urea and nonurea solutes in renal tissues of rats with hereditary hypothalamic diabetes insipidus: effect of vasopressin and dehydration on countercurrent mechanism. *J. Clin. Invest.* 45: 337–345, 1966.
174. Valtin, H. Structural and functional heterogeneity of mammalian nephrons. *Am. J. Physiol.* 233: (*Renal Fluid Electrolyte Physiol.* 2): F491–F501, 1977.
175. Walser, M. Use of isotopic urea to study the distribution and degradation of urea in man. In: *Urea and the Kidney*, edited by B. Schmidt-Nielsen. Amsterdam: Excerpta Med., 1970, p. 421–429.
176. Wirz, H. Der osmotische Druck des Blutes in der Nierenpapille. *Helv. Physiol. Pharmacol. Acta* 11: 20–29, 1953.
177. Wirz, H., and R. Dirix. Urinary concentration and dilution. In: *Handbook of Physiology. Renal Physiology*, edited by J. Orloff and R. W. Berliner. Washington, DC: Am. Physiol. Soc., 1973, sect. 8, chapt. 13, p. 415–430.
178. Wirz, H., B. Hargitay, and W. Kuhn. Lokalisation des Konzentrierungsprozesses in der Niere durch direkte Kryoskopie. *Helvet. Physiol. Pharmacol. Acta* 9: 196–207, 1951.
179. Wöhler, F. Ueber kunstiliche Bildung des Harnstoffs. *Ann. Phys. Chem.* 12: 253–256, 1828.

XI

Acidification of Urine

FLOYD C. RECTOR, JR.

THE properties of acids and bases have intrigued chemists and physicians since antiquity. The ancients learned to distinguish them by the difference in color of certain vegetable dyes in acid and alkaline solutions. The Greek physician Galen (A.D. 129–199) in fact was aware of the acidic nature of certain body fluids, including urine. In his work *On the Natural Faculties* (17), he wrote: "*The urinary bladder continues to collect urine up to the time that it becomes uncomfortable through the increasing quantity of urine or the irritation caused by its acidity.*" Strong acids were first produced in India, and their use spread to China and the Arab world in the eighth and ninth centuries. Knowledge of acids was brought to Europe in the thirteenth and fourteenth centuries by Arab alchemists. The dramatic ability of strong acids to dissolve metals and other hard substances had great appeal to the alchemists of this age, who were engrossed in efforts to produce the "philosopher's stone," a mystical substance thought to be able to dissolve all other substances, convert base metals to gold, cure all ills, and sustain life eternal. The first step in the process was to produce a strong acid, usually nitric acid formed from niter or "Chinese salt." Strong bases were also first produced in India, either by heating lime or by burning wood, the ash of which contained potash plus potassium carbonate. The term *alkali* is derived from the Arabic word for ash, *al qali*. Although the strong bases did not have the dramatic qualities of the acids, they were used extensively in medicine. In India alkalies were used to cauterize skin lesions and were given as dilute solutions for ascites, tumors, calculi, and other ailments (2).

URINE ACIDIFICATION

In the early sixteenth century the Swiss alchemist and physician Theophrastus Bombastus von Hohenheim, better known as Paracelsus (1493–1541), moved medicine away from the strict mechanical-anatomical concept of the Italian school and introduced the concept that chemical reactions were responsible for many physiological phenomena (16). This prompted chemists and physicians to master the skills of making acids, bases, and salts and to experiment with their use in many ills. The Belgian physician Jan Baptist van Helmont(1580–1644), while studying the effervescence that occurs when acids and alkalies react, discovered CO_2 and proposed that many of the reactions occurring in the digestive tract and in blood were fermentation processes similar to the effervescent reaction. The chemist Johann Rudolf Glauber (1604–1668) improved the method for making hydrochloric acid, prepared sodium sulfate [(*sal mirabile dictu*), also known as Glauber's salt], and fostered the idea that salts result from a union of acids and bases. This idea was supported by the Westphalian physician Otto Tachenius (ca. 1620–1690), who considered acids and bases as the primary substances of nature, present in all animate and inanimate objects. These concepts were extended by a pupil of Glauber, François de le Boë, better known by his latin name Franciscus Sylvius (1614–1672). Sylvius, while Professor of Medicine at the University of Leiden, founded the iatrochemical school of medicine on the precept that all disorders were due to disturbances in the balance between acids and bases in the organism and its secretions because of abnormal fermentations. Disorders due to excess acid fermentation required therapy with alkalinizing regimens, and vice versa. There was also recognition at this time that blood is alkaline, whereas urine is acid (16). The implications of this phenomenon, however, were not appreciated for another two hundred years.

During the eighteenth and nineteenth centuries there was little important work on the role of acids and bases in medicine and physiology. Rather, this was the period in which the chemists and physical chemists were defining the nature of acids and bases (2). Robert Boyle and his contemporaries at Oxford made a systematic study of indicators and found that only acids turned vegetable matter red, whereas only alkalies turned them green. Boyle was the first to characterize alkalies as fixed or volatile. Fixed alkalies were the carbonate salts of alkali metals (sodium, potassium), whereas a volatile alkali was ammonium carbonate. He also found that only acids were able to generate an inflammable gas when poured on iron. The early concepts of acids were strongly influenced by the phlogiston theory of chemistry created by Johann Becher and Georg Stahl, who believed that just as all inflammable materials contained phlogiston, all acids contained a substance *acidum universalis*. Much debate and controversy occurred over the identity of this universal substance. The Parisian physician and chemist Nicholas Lémery (1678–1721) believed that atmospheric air contained an acid that penetrated into metals and increased their weight when heated and that the same substance existed in niter. (It was this substance that Lavoisier eventually discovered to be oxygen.) Others such as Claude-Louis Berthollet (1749–1822) in Paris and Joseph Priestley (1733–1804) in England believed that the universally occurring substance must be "fixed air," carbon dioxide, or carbonic acid. In 1766 the English chemist Henry Cavendish turned his attention to an earlier discovery of Boyle's and observed that a given quantity of sulfuric acid always produced the same amount of inflammable gas. He was convinced that the gas was pure phlogiston derived from the metal. Ten years later in 1776, Antoine-Laurent Lavoisier in Paris determined that the gas was derived from the acid, not the metal. He named this newly discovered gas *oxygen*, meaning derived from acid, and believed that it occurred in all acids and was responsible for their acidic properties. By the early 1800s, however, the discovery of the halogenous acids (HCl, HBr, HI) made it apparent that oxygen was not a constituent of all acids, thus necessitating a broader definition. In 1838 Justus von Liebig, while Professor of Chemistry in Giessen, defined acids as substances, the hydrogen content of which could be replaced by a metal. Liebig's theory was widely accepted for many years but ultimately was displaced in 1887 when the great Swedish chemist and physicist Svante August Arrhenius (1859–1927) introduced his theory of electrolytic dissociation. For this contribution Arrhenius received the Nobel prize in 1903. According to this theory, acids and alkalies in aqueous solutions dissociate, releasing H^+ and OH^-, respectively. The quantity of the released H^+ or OH^- could be used to quantify the strength of the acid or alkali. In 1909–1912 Sören Peter Lauritz Sorensen (Fig. 1, *left*), working at the Carlsberg laboratory in Copenhagen, introduced a refined electrometric method for measuring H^+ concentration, the pH scale for expressing H^+ concentration, and the use of buffers for controlling pH in enzymatic reactions (39). At about the same time, Lawrence Joseph Henderson (Fig. 1, *right*) at Harvard University began his

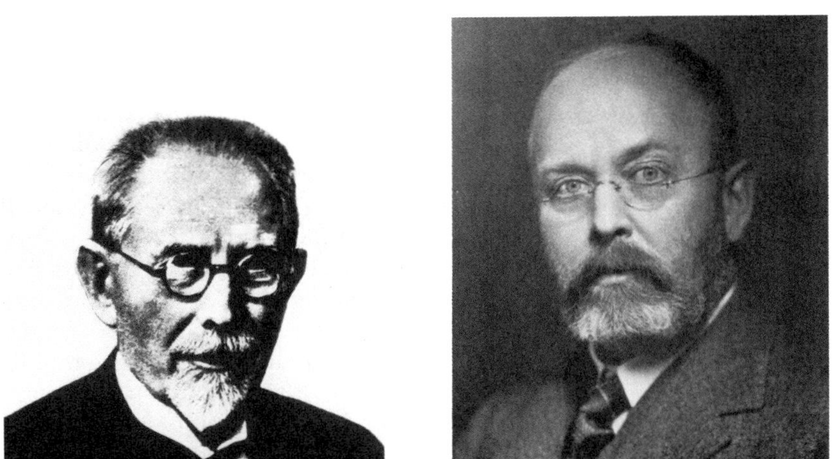

Figure 1. *Left*: Soren Peter Lauritz Sorensen (1868–1939). (Courtesy of National Library of Medicine.) *Right*: Lawrence Joseph Henderson (1878–1942). (Courtesy of National Academy of Sciences.)

studies on the buffering properties of blood and introduced the Henderson equation for evaluating the buffering properties of weak acids and bases from their dissociation constants (21). The logarithmic transformation of this equation by the Danish chemist Karl A. Hasselbalch yielded the familiar Henderson-Hasselbalch equation.

Against this background of the evolving concepts of the physicochemical nature of acids and bases, a renewed interest in acid-base physiology emerged in the mid-nineteenth century. In 1871 Frederich Hoffman (22), while working in the Physiological Institute in Munich, observed that the urine of an animal tested with acid-base indicators gave an acidic reaction, whereas the blood gave an alkaline reaction. This led to the conclusion that the body must be producing acids and that the kidney, by excreting the acids into the urine, maintained the normal alkalinity of the blood. The first physiological studies on the ability of the kidneys to regulate acid excretion were performed by Fredrich Walter in Strassburg, Germany, in 1877. Walter (48) found that when dogs were given hydrochloric, phosphoric, or salicylic acid for several days, there was a reduction in the concentration of HCO_3^- in the blood and an increased excretion of acid and ammonium in the urine. Walter also observed that, in comparison with dogs, rabbits succumbed when given small amounts of acid, a fact he attributed to their inability to excrete urinary ammonia. At that time the concept arose that acids ingested in the diet or produced by the body were in part neutralized by reaction with basic ammonia, which was also produced in the body, and were then excreted into the urine as the neutral ammonium salts of the acids. The metabolic acids were also excreted in part as free acids, but the rather crude and technically inaccurate methods for estimating the quantity of acid excreted in the urine limited these early studies. However, in 1903 the superb analytic chemist Otto Folin (Fig. 2, *left*), working in the Clinical Laboratory at McLean Hospital for the Insane in Waverly, Massachussetts, showed by careful analysis that the excess of anions over cations in the urine was equal to the quantity of H^+ excreted bound to nonammonia buffers; in addition, if precautions were taken to prevent precipitation of calcium salts, this quantity could be accurately assessed by the amount of alkali required to titrate urine to the alkalinity of blood, estimated colorimetrically (14). In 1911 Henderson was the first to recognize that the excretion of titratable acid and ammonium into the urine would restore an equivalent quantity of alkali back to blood, reversing the process in which blood alkali had initially neutralized the metabolic acids (21).

From the time of Walter it was thought that ammonia, produced in various parts of the body, reacted with metabolically produced acids to form neutral ammonium salts, which were subsequently extracted by the kidney and excreted into the urine. In 1921, however, T. Nash and Stanley Benedict (29) found that renal venous

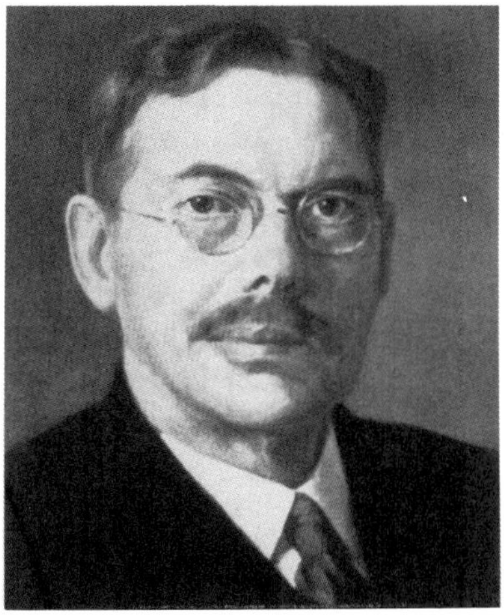
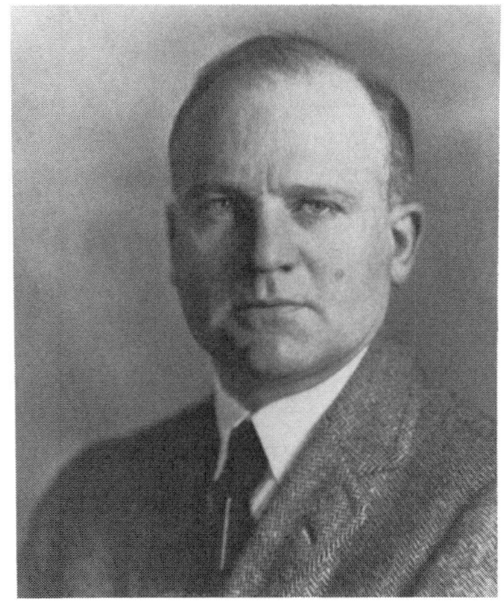

Figure 2. *Left*: Otto Folin (1861–1931). (Courtesy of National Library of Medicine.) *Right*: Donald Dexter Van Slyke (1883–1971). (Courtesy of National Academy of Sciences.)

ammonium was higher than arterial ammonium, indicating that the kidney was not extracting ammonium salts from the arterial blood but rather was actually synthesizing ammonium for secretion into urine. They also observed in acidotic dogs that the increase in the excretion of ammonium nitrogen was associated with a parallel decrease in the excretion of urea nitrogen, suggesting that urea was serving as the substrate for the synthesis of urinary ammonium. This view was subsequently disproved in 1941 by Donald D. Van Slyke (Fig. 2, *right*) and his co-workers at the Rockefeller Institute when they demonstrated that in an acidotic dog the ammonium excreted into the urine could be quantitatively accounted for by the extraction of glutamine by the kidney, whereas all of the urea extracted by the kidney was excreted into the urine as urea (44). In alkalotic dogs there was neither excretion of ammonia nor extraction of glutamine by the kidney. The reciprocal relationship between ammonium and urea excretion was thought to reflect prerenal regulation, probably hepatic, of the distribution of nitrogen between urea and the major precursor of urinary ammonium, glutamine. Subsequent studies have confirmed that glutamine is the major precursor of urinary ammonia, but there are small contributions from glycine and alanine (36).

The mechanism by which an acidic urine was produced by the kidney was poorly understood, and this question was part of the larger controversy concerning the formation of urine. William Bowman (in 1844) and later Rudolph Heidenhain (in 1874) believed that the tubules secreted solid waste that was flushed out of the tubules by water that was either secreted or filtered by the glomeruli. According to this view, the volume of urine was equal to the quantity of fluid formed by the glomerulus. In 1844 the great German physiologist Carl Ludwig proposed the alternative view that a large volume of fluid, containing the dissolved constituents of blood, was formed through passive filtration by the glomerulus and that most of this fluid was reabsorbed passively by the tubules. The force for this passive reabsorption was thought to be primarily the hydraulic pressure differences across the tubules, but there was also a hint that the "sucking" force of plasma proteins might play a role (thus anticipating the later discovery of colloid osmotic forces by Ernest Henry Starling). In order to account for the compositional differences between urine and blood, Ludwig modified his view over the years to make the tubules permselective, thus permitting selective reabsorption of filtered solutes. Against this background the question concerning the origin of acid in the urine was whether the tubules secreted acid or whether both acids and alkalies in blood were filtered by the glomeruli, with the alkali being preferentially reabsorbed by the tubules.

This latter possibility was most clearly delineated by Henderson (21) in 1911. In his characterization of the buffer systems in blood and urine, Henderson noted that the principal acid in urine was NaH_2PO_4 and suggested that, rather than being secreted by tubules, both the alkaline and acid forms of phosphate were filtered but that only the alkaline form was reabsorbed by the tubule, leaving behind the acid form. In 1924 Joseph T. Wearn and A. Newton Richards (49), at the University of Pennsylvania, confirmed that the glomerular filtrate is alkaline, as is blood, whereas urine drawn from the bladder at the same time is acidic. The line of reasoning proposed by Henderson was extended by Arthur R. Cushny (12) in his monograph *The Secretion of Urine*, first published in 1917. Cushny, who at various times was at the University of Michigan, the University of London, and the University of Edinburgh, proposed that the filtrate contained both alkaline and acidic forms of phosphate, bicarbonate, and carbonic acid, and that the tubules, by reabsorbing all of the filtered bicarbonate plus the bicarbonate associated with the carbonic acid, would liberate H^+ that could then titrate alkaline phosphate to the acidic form (Fig. 3). This extension does not require that alkaline phosphate necessarily be reabsorbed. In 1934 Sendroy, Seelig, and Van Slyke (35) found that in acidotic patients the amount of acid excreted in the urine could be quantitatively explained by this theory. In addition they confirmed the earlier observation of James Gamble (18), at Harvard University, that if the urine was promptly removed from the bladder with precaution against loss of CO_2, the CO_2 tension could be several times as great as in venous blood. To explain this observation, Van Slyke and co-workers (35) proposed that the acidity of the urine was the consequence of specific tubular reabsorption of bicarbonate, and that because bicarbonate and water were reabsorbed more rapidly than H_2CO_3, the CO_2

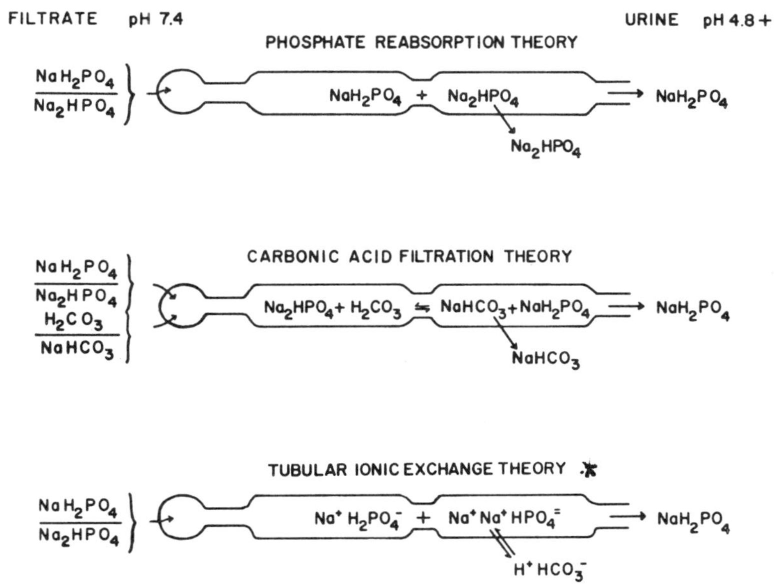

Figure 3. Theories to account for acidification of urine. [From Pitts and Alexander (32).]

tension of urine was higher than that of venous blood. Cushny (12) summarized the two opposing views as follows:

> *Thus the followers of Bowman and Heidenhain hold that the tubular epithelium, taking up neutral phosphate from the blood, throws it in a more acid form into the tubules and returns the alkali to the blood again; the modern theory, on the other hand, states that glomerular filtrate corresponds to the plasma in its phosphate content, and that the epithelium absorbs the sodium and hydroxyl ions in the form of bicarbonate, while the phosphate ion is rejected by it for the most part and passes into the ureter enriched in hydrogen. The one school asserts that acid is actively excreted, the other that alkali is actively reabsorbed.*

In 1937 Hugh Montgomery and J. A. Pierce (27), working at the University of Pennsylvania in Richards's laboratory, found in micropuncture studies on frogs and *Necturi* that glomerular filtrate and proximal tubule fluid are isohydric to plasma and that acidification occurs in the distal tubule (Fig. 4). In addition they found that when a solution of 0.33 M Na_2PO_4 at pH 7.4 and containing phenol red was instilled into the lumen of the distal tubule of the frog, the fluid became yellow (pH < 6.8) in 60 sec. Because the fluid was free of bicarbonate and carbonic acid, it was reasoned that bicarbonate reabsorption was excluded as the mechanism of acidification. The pH change could have been caused by selective reabsorption of the basic Na_2HPO_4 or by secreting H^+ in exchange for the Na^+. In his

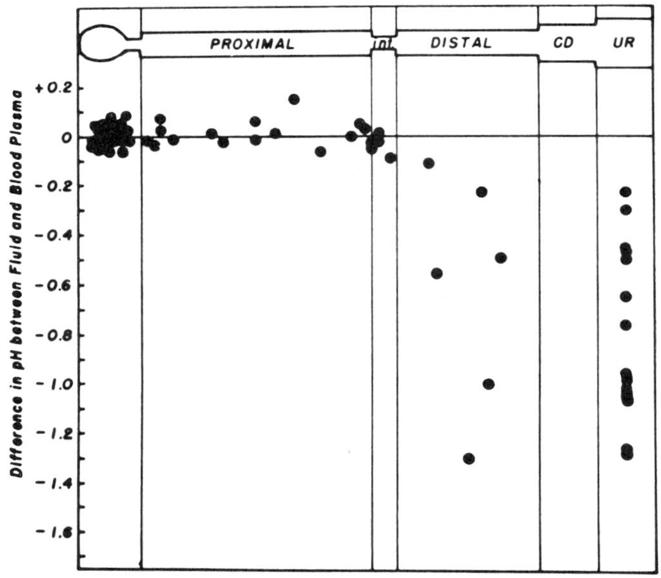

Figure 4. Site of acidification of urine in amphibian kidneys. CD, collecting duct; UR, ureter; int., intermediate tubule. [Adapted from Montgomery and Pierce (27).]

monograph *The Physiology of the Kidney*, published in 1936 (38), Homer W. Smith (Fig. 5), in the Department of Physiology at New York University, argued that inasmuch as the frog distal tubule has very little capacity to reabsorb phosphate, the acidification of the fluid in the tubule must be due to reabsorption of Na^+ in exchange for secreted H^+. Thus Smith was the first to propose Na^+-H^+ exchange as the mechanism of urine acidification. Smith also addressed the question of the origin of the high urine CO_2 tension observed by Gamble (18) and by Van Slyke and co-workers (35). Smith argued that because of the high diffusivity of CO_2 in tissues, it was unlikely that CO_2 would remain behind in the tubule lumina as fluid was reabsorbed and thus it was unlikely that this was the explanation for the high urine CO_2 tension. As an alternative explanation, he suggested that the secretion of H^+ into bicarbonate-containing distal tubule fluid produced carbonic acid that was swept into the ureters where it evolved into CO_2.

In 1948, in an elegant series of experiments, Robert F. Pitts (Fig. 5) and his associate Robert Alexander (32), in the Department of Physiology at Cornell University School of Medicine in New York, reported that infusion of weak buffer salts, either phosphate or creatine, into acidotic dogs increased the excretion of titratable acid to a level far in excess of the total carbonic acid and acid phosphate present in the glomerular filtrate. They reasoned that the quantity of acid in urine could not be explained by reabsorption of the filtered

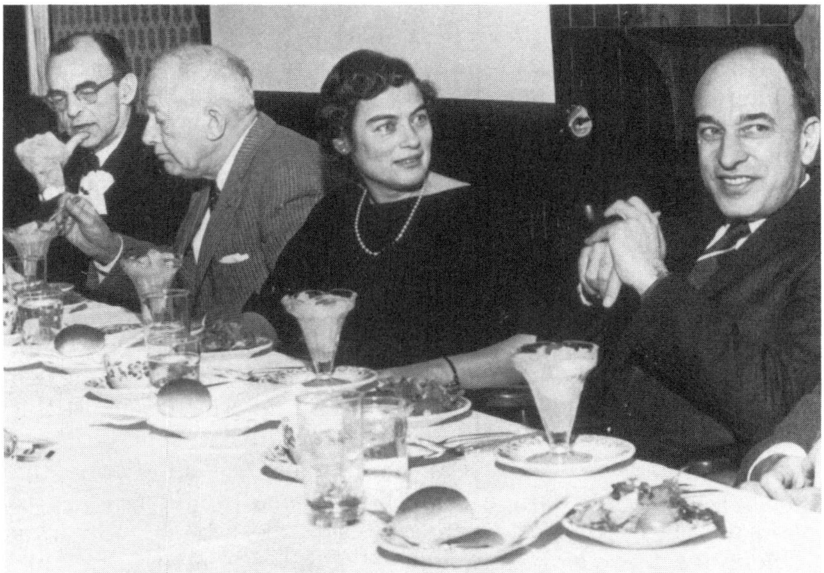

Figure 5. Photograph taken at dinner honoring Homer Smith in 1962. *Left* to *right*: Robert Pitts, Homer Smith, Lea Berliner, Robert Berliner. (Courtesy of R. W. Berliner.)

alkaline salts (bicarbonate, dibasic phosphate) and that H^+ must be secreted by the renal tubules. Because the quantity of acid excreted exceeded that of nonbuffer anions, they concluded that the H^+ could not have been accompanied by secreted anions (e.g., HCl) and therefore must have been secreted in exchange for some filtered cation, presumably Na^+. To explore the possible source of the secreted H^+, Pitts and Alexander (32) examined the effects of sulfanilamide, which had been discovered earlier by Keilin and Mann to be an inhibitor of carbonic anhydrase. The marked reduction of acid excretion resulting from sulfanilamide administration led them to propose that hydration of CO_2 to H_2CO_3, catalyzed by carbonic anhydrase within renal tubule cells, was the source for the secreted H^+.

Two lines of argument, however, questioned the validity of these conclusions. First, Walter Menaker, at Yale University, pointed out that reabsorption of either CO_3^{2-} or OH^- could liberate H^+ from HCO_3^- and H_2O, respectively, which in turn could titrate dibasic phosphate to acidic monobasic phosphate (26). This possibility was considered very unlikely, however, because of the very low concentration of these ions in acidic urine. William Brodsky (9), then at the University of Louisville, raised a more likely objection. If the tubule epithelium were freely permeable to CO_2, then hydration of CO_2 in the tubule lumina could provide a continuous supply of H_2CO_3, which, when HCO_3^- was reabsorbed, would liberate H^+ that could then titrate nonbicarbonate buffers. The rebuttal of this latter possibility depended on a theoretical analysis of the possible rate of CO_2 hydration in the tubule lumina and was undertaken primarily by Robert W. Berliner (Fig. 5) at the National Institutes of Health in Bethesda, MD. This approach was only possible because of the elegant studies performed in the 1930s and 1940s by the English physical chemist F. J. W. Roughton, defining the rate constants of the CO_2-H_2CO_3 hydration and dehydration reactions. The analysis by Berliner revealed that the uncatalyzed hydration of CO_2 in tubule lumina could not account for the maximum rates of titratable acid formation in acidotic dogs and in addition would drive the urine CO_2 tension far below that of plasma. Berliner realized that this constraint could be overcome by the presence of carbonic anhydrase in the cell membranes lining tubule lumina. However, he argued against this possibility on the basis of the findings of Bruno K. Ochwadt and Pitts. They found that, during the excretion of an alkaline urine, the very high urine CO_2 tension could be reduced to a level equal to that in plasma by the intravenous infusion of carbonic anhydrase sufficient to achieve a measurable level of the enzyme in urine (30). As Berliner pointed out, this finding was not consistent with the existence of carbonic anhydrase in the luminal membrane of distal tubular cells and therefore the hypothesis proposed by Brodsky was not kinetically feasible. Subsequent histochemical studies on the cellular localization of carbonic anhydrase confirmed that the enzyme was not present in the luminal cell membrane in the distal nephron. Thus the conclusion that the formation of titratable acid was the consequence of H^+ excretion in the distal position of the nephron appeared inescapable.

The thrust of these studies and controversies concerned the mechanism by which urinary buffers were excreted in the acidic form to accomplish elimination of acid from the body. Equally important, however, is the mechanism by which filtered bicarbonate is reclaimed by the renal tubule. In the early micropuncture studies in amphibians (frog and *Necturus*), Montgomery and Pierce (27) found that the pH of proximal tubule fluid measured with a quinhydrone microelectrode was isohydric to both plasma and glomerular filtrate (see Fig. 4). Because the total volume of tubular fluid was reduced during passage through the proximal tubule, it was generally thought that bicarbonate must have been reabsorbed in the proximal tubule, but by a process that did not result in acidification of the tubular fluid and therefore was probably different from the process occurring in the more distal parts of the nephron. In 1961, however, Carl Gottschalk, William Lassiter, and Margaret Mylle (20), at the University of North Carolina, observed that proximal tubule fluid in a mammalian species (rat) was acidified to approximately 6.8 (Fig. 6). In order for the tubule fluid to fall to this pH, it was necessary that 85%–90% of the filtered bicarbonate be reabsorbed by the proximal

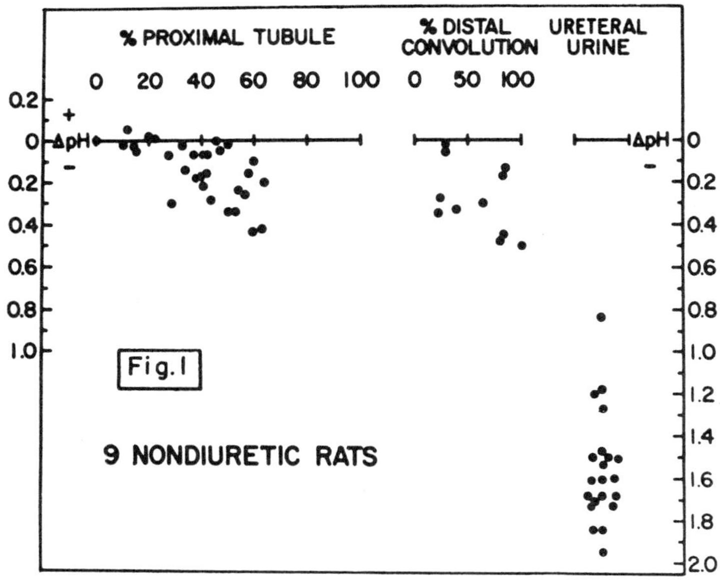

Figure 6. Difference in pH of tubular fluid and ureteral urine from that of arterial blood in 9 nondiuretic rats. Negative △ pH values represent acidification relative to arterial pH. [From Gottschalk et al. (20).]

tubule. Although this study did not identify the mechanism by which bicarbonate was reabsorbed, an earlier study by Berliner (3) showed that large doses of the potent carbonic anhydrase inhibitor acetazolamide caused the excretion of at least 40% of the filtered HCO_3^-. Because this quantity exceeded the amount that could be reasonably ascribed to the distal nephron, he concluded that acetazolamide was inhibiting a carbonic anhydrase–dependent process in the proximal tubule. Berliner proposed that bicarbonate was reabsorbed in the proximal tubule by a mechanism similar to that proposed for the distal nephron, namely that H^+ was secreted into the tubule lumen in exchange for Na^+ and that the H^+ was produced in the cell by the hydration of CO_2 under the catalytic action of carbonic anhydrase. In the lumen the secreted H^+ reacted with filtered bicarbonate to form carbonic acid which subsequently broke down to CO_2, thus completing the reabsorptive process.

In 1960 Mackenzie Walser and Gilbert Mudge (47), at Johns Hopkins School of Medicine, pointed out an important consequence of the above mechanism for the reabsorption of bicarbonate. For this mechanism to operate in the steady state, the rate at which carbonic acid is formed and subsequently broken down in the tubule lumen must equal the rate of bicarbonate removal. From Roughton's rate constant for the uncatalyzed dehydration of carbonic acid, they calculated that, in order for the breakdown of carbonic acid to be driven at a rate equal to the rate of bicarbonate reabsorption, the concentration of carbonic acid would have to rise to a level approximately ten times higher than the equilibrium value in an unperturbed system in which H^+ were not being secreted. Consequently the actual intratubular pH in situ would be approximately 1.0 pH unit below the predicted value, if the latter is predicted on the assumption of equilibrium between carbonic acid and CO_2. This analysis by Walser and Mudge provided the basis for an experimental assessment of the mechanism of bicarbonate reabsorption in the proximal tubule. In the early 1960s, Norman W. Carter in Dallas was developing pH-sensitive glass microelectrodes for the measurement of intracellular pH (Fig. 7). It was obvious that these microelectrodes could provide the means for testing the hypothesis proposed by Walser and Mudge. In 1965 Floyd Rector along with Carter (Fig. 8, *left*) and Donald Seldin (Fig. 8, *right*) reported that the pH of proximal tubule fluid measured in situ with these microelectrodes is equal to the predicted equilibrium pH, calculated from the measured bicarbonate concentration and plasma CO_2 tension, using the Henderson-Hasselbalch equation (33). This result was not consistent with the proposed mechanism of H^+ secretion unless the tubule fluid was in functional contact with carbonic anhydrase. To test this latter possibility these investigators inhibited carbonic an-

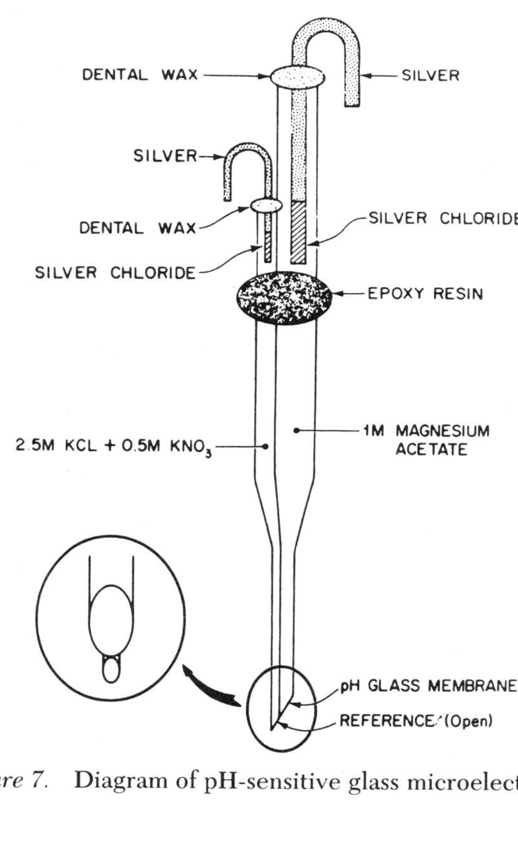

Figure 7. Diagram of pH-sensitive glass microelectrode.

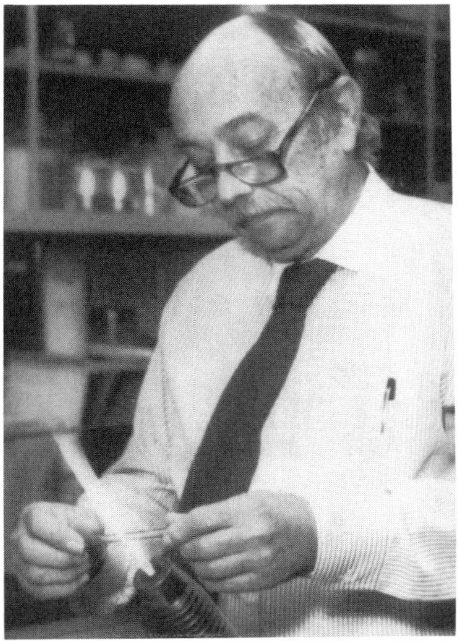

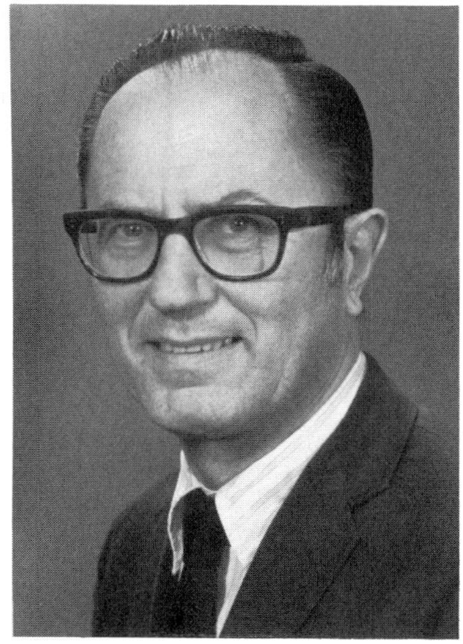

Figure 8. Left: Norman W. Carter (b. 1925). *Right*: Donald W. Seldin (b. 1920). (Courtesy of N. W. Carter and D. W. Seldin.)

hydrase and found that, although bicarbonate reabsorption was partially inhibited, tubule pH became about 0.8 pH unit more acid than the predicted equilibrium pH (Fig. 9). These findings were confirmed in 1968 by Frederico L. Vieira and Gerhard Malnic (45) in Brazil. In the studies by both Rector et al. (33) and Vieira and Malnic (45), the tubule carbon dioxide tension used to calculate the equilibrium pH was assumed to be equal to that in arterial blood. Micropuncture studies by Thomas DuBose and co-workers (13) in Dallas, in which in situ pH and carbon dioxide tension as well as bicarbonate concentration were all measured directly, have confirmed that there is indeed an acid disequilibrium pH in the proximal tubule after inhibition of carbonic anhydrase. These results established that bicarbonate reabsorption is mediated by H^+ secretion and that the enzyme carbonic anhydrase must be present in the luminal cell membrane of the proximal tubule and, by its functional contact with the tubule fluid, prevents accumulation of excess carbonic acid that would otherwise retard the rate of H^+ secretion.

The evidence is convincing that both proximal and distal portions of the nephron secrete H^+ and thereby affect the conservation of filtered bicarbonate, the titration of filtered nonbicarbonate buffers to form urinary titratable acid, and the excretion of NH_4^+. Since two-thirds of the H^+ excreted into the urine is bound to ammonia, the formation and excretion of ammonia plays a key role in acid-base homeostasis. In 1948 Pitts (31) examined the relationship between urinary ammonia excretion and urine pH in normal and chronically

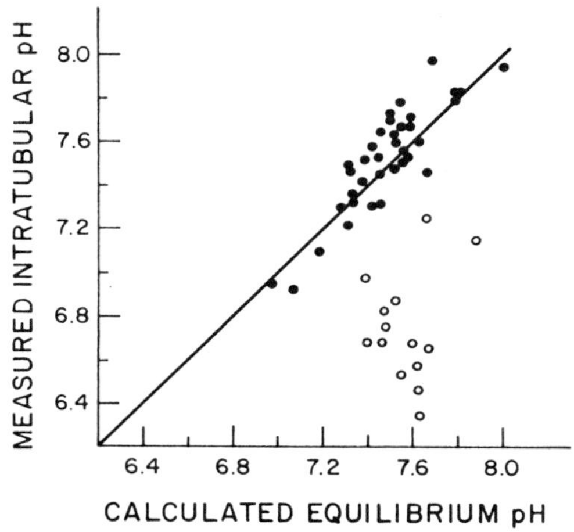

Figure 9. Comparison of measured intratubular pH with equilibrium pH, calculated from arterial P_{CO_2} and tubule fluid bicarbonate concentration using the Henderson-Hasselbalch equation. ●, Rats infused with $NaHCO_3$; ○, rats infused with $NaHCO_3$ after inhibition of carbonic anhydrase with benzolamide. After inhibition of carbonic anhydrase, tubule fluid was significantly more acid (acid disequilibrium pH) than the calculated equilibrium value. [From Rector et al. (33), by copyright permission of The American Society for Clinical Investigation.]

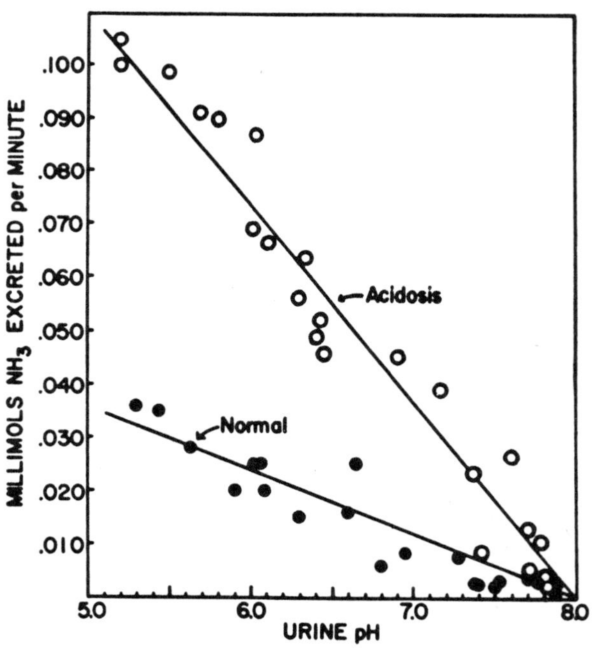

Figure 10. Rate of excretion of ammonia by a single dog under two conditions of acid-base balance. In both conditions sodium bicarbonate was infused to increase urine pH. [From Pitts (31).]

acidotic dogs. In both groups, when urine was acutely alkalinized by an infusion of sodium bicarbonate, ammonia excretion decreased: urinary ammonia excretion fell in a linear fashion as urine pH increased (Fig. 10). For any given urine pH, urinary ammonia was higher in the acidotic than in the normal dogs. Pitts proposed that ammonia was excreted by a process of nonionic diffusion in which nonionic ammonia, produced in renal tubule cells from glutamine, diffused into the tubule lumen where it reacted with secreted H^+ and was trapped as nondiffusible NH_4^+ (Fig. 11). The more acid the urine, the greater the amount of ammonia trapped in the tubule urine as NH_4^+. Thus urine pH, determined by H^+ secretion, is an important determinant of ammonia excretion. This concept, proposed in 1948 with some modifications concerning the diffusion of ammonia from the loop of Henle to the collecting duct, is still the accepted view of the mechanism of ammonia excretion. Pitts also concluded that the rate of ammonia production from glutamine can regulate ammonia excretion. Chronic metabolic acidosis produces an adaptive increase in ammonia production so that the cellular concentration of ammonia, the amount diffusing from cell to tubule lumen, and the amount trapped as NH_4^+ at any given tubule pH are all increased. Since these early studies, a large body of research has been directed toward an elucidation of the details of this adaptive increase in ammonia production, but a review of this area is outside the scope of this chapter.

By 1965 the evidence was reasonably persuasive that the secretion of H^+ occurs in both the proximal and distal parts of the nephron and is the process responsible for the formation of an acidic urine. In the succeeding twenty years research has been directed toward

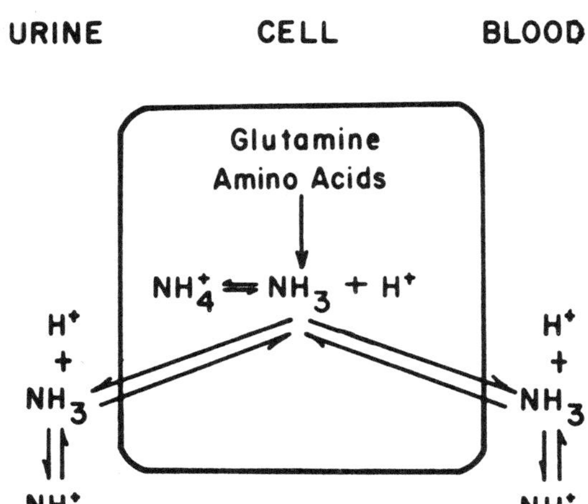

Figure 11. Passive secretion of free ammonia by nonionic diffusion. The major fraction is trapped in acid urine as relatively nondiffusible ammonium ion.

elucidation of the cellular and molecular mechanisms of the acidification process in the various parts of the nephron. The development of the technique of in vitro microperfusion of isolated tubule segments by Maurice Burg, Jared Grantham, and Jack Orloff (10) at the National Institutes of Health in Bethesda, the development of the microcalorimetric method for measuring the concentration of total carbon dioxide content of tubule fluid by Gerald Vurek (46) (also at the National Institutes of Health), the development of the technique of preparing isolated cell membrane vesicles from mammalian epithelial tissue for the study of ion transport in the laboratory of Kurt Isselbacher (15) at Harvard Medical School, the application of the turtle bladder to the study of the mechanism of urinary acidification by Theodore Schilb and William Brodsky (34) at Mount Sinai School of Medicine, and the development of microelectrode and fluorescent-probe techniques for the measurement of intracellular pH in renal tubular cells have all played important roles in this more detailed segmental analysis of the acidification process.

Studies utilizing the isolated tubule, performed primarily in Burg's laboratory, demonstrated that the proximal convoluted tubule, proximal straight tubule, and the thick ascending limb reabsorb bicarbonate and acidify the tubule fluid. Burg and co-workers (11, 19, 24) demonstrated that the reabsorption of bicarbonate in these three areas of the nephron is coupled to sodium transport and is dependent on the presence of sodium, findings consistent with the view that the process of H^+ secretion was mediated by Na^+-H^+ exchange. A more direct demonstration of Na^+-H^+ exchange came from studies on isolated kidney cell membranes. Heine Murer, Ullrich Hopfer, and Rolf Kinne, at the Max Planck Institute in Frankfurt, prepared brush-border membrane vesicles from kidney cortex, presumably primarily luminal membranes from proximal convoluted tubules. With these vesicles they found that sodium-free vesicles, when placed in media containing sodium, extruded H^+. This process occurred when the vesicles were voltage clamped with equal concentrations of potassium inside and out, plus valinomycin. Thus the coupling between Na^+ and H^+ transport was not dependent on electrical forces but was direct coupled exchange. Subsequent studies by James Kinsella and Peter Aronson (23), then at the National Institutes of Health in Baltimore, showed that pH gradients could drive sodium uptake, that the coupling between H^+ and Na^+ transport was 1:1 and electroneutral, and that the exchanger could be inhibited by relatively high concentrations of amiloride.

The secretion of H^+ in exchange for Na^+ by the proximal nephron generates a HCO_3^- inside the cell that must cross the basolateral cell membrane in order to return to the blood. The mechanism for this process was elucidated in the proximal tubule of the salamander kidney by Walter Boron and Emile Boulpaep. As a graduate student, Boron had worked in the laboratory of Albert Roos at Washington

University School of Medicine studying the regulation of cell pH in barnacular muscle and squid axon. The work of Boron and Roos, as well as others, demonstrated that, in the maintenance of cell pH in invertebrates, H^+ was extruded from and HCO_3^- transported into the cells by Na^+-coupled processes (8). It was against this conceptual framework that Boron began his studies on the regulation of renal tubule cell pH at Yale University. In 1983 Boron and Boulpaep (6) reported the existence of amiloride-sensitive Na^+-H^+ exchangers in both the apical and basolateral cell membranes of the proximal tubule of the salamander kidney. These two exchangers both functioned to extrude H^+ from the cell and consequently could not account for vectorial transport of bicarbonate from cell to blood. In addition they found that bicarbonate is transported across the basolateral cell membrane directly coupled to Na^+ by a stilbene-inhibitable cotransport system (7). The coupling ratio between HCO_3^- and Na^+ was at least two HCO_3^- for one Na^+. Consequently the transport system was electrogenic and influenced by the basolateral membrane potential difference, in addition to the intracellular concentrations of HCO_3^- and Na^+. Initially these findings were met with skepticism by most renal physiologists, who felt that this coupled system was too cumbersome to account for the very high rates of vectorial transport of bicarbonate that occurs in the mammalian proximal tubule and that this transport system was probably unique to the invertebrate kidney. However, in the past three years a similar cotransport system has been identified in the mammalian kidney by Robert Alpern (1) in San Francisco, by Bruce Biagi (5) at the University of Ohio School of Medicine, and by K. Yoshitoma et al. (50) working in Eberhard Fromter's laboratory in Frankfurt. This cotransport system has also been characterized in basolateral membrane vesicles prepared from mammalian kidneys. Currently this cotransport system appears to have a coupling ratio of three HCO_3^- to one Na^+. At this point it is clear that the Na^+-HCO_3^- cotransport system has several advantages over simple uncoupled bicarbonate conductance: it is energetically more efficient, it provides free transport of some Na^+ out of the cell independent of the Na^+-K^+-ATPase system, and it provides a means of regulating the rate of bicarbonate transport with only minimal changes in cell pH.

The technique of in vitro microperfusion of isolated nephron segments has also been applied to the study of the acidification process in the collecting duct system. As expected, Dwight McKinney and Burg (25) found that collecting tubules reabsorb bicarbonate and acidify tubule fluid. These studies, however, yielded an unexpected surprise. They found that cortical collecting tubules isolated from animals pretreated with acid reabsorbed bicarbonate, whereas tubules isolated from animals pretreated with alkali secreted bicarbonate. This finding was completely unexpected and could not have been predicted from previous clearance or micropuncture studies. In contrast to the more proximal portions of the nephron, the acidification process in the collecting tubule was found to be independent of sodium transport, and in fact Dennis Stone and co-workers (43) in Dallas have shown electrogenic hydrogen secretion in the inner stripe of the outer medulla, a region of the nephron in which no sodium transport occurs. The acidification process in the collecting duct system, therefore, does not fulfill the criteria for Na^+-H^+ exchange as originally proposed by Smith and instead is an independent, electrogenic process similar to that found in the turtle bladder.

In 1929 Smith (37) found that the coelomic fluid surrounding the distended urinary bladder of the turtle was very alkaline, containing high concentrations of bicarbonate. Eugene Robin and co-workers, working at the Mt. Desert Island Biological Laboratory provided evidence that this coelomic fluid served to buffer the acidosis that developed during the anaerobic period of diving. The origin of this alkaline coelomic fluid was not known, although it was suspected that the urinary bladder might be involved. In 1966 Theodore Schilb and William Brodsky (34) observed that sacs of turtle bladder acidify the fluid in contact with the mucosal surface of the bladder. Shortly thereafter Philip Steinmetz (40), then at Harvard Medical School, demonstrated that this acidification of the mucosal fluid was associated with an equivalent addition of bicarbonate to the serosal fluid. Based on these observations, the turtle has been used primarily by Steinmetz and his many co-workers as a model system to study the mechanism of distal urinary acidification. Embryologically the amphibian urinary bladder is phylogenetically related to the collecting duct system of the mammalian kidney. Both are derived from the persistent ureteric bud that arises from the primitive mesonephric kidney. The kidney of the turtle is a poorly developed remnant of the mesonephric kidney, whereas in the mammalian kidney the portions of the nephron proximal to the collecting duct arise from the metanephric blastema. The functional similarities between the amphibian bladder and the collecting duct system of the mammalian kidney are also quite striking. Both have electrogenic aldosterone-sensitive sodium transport and vasopressin-sensitive water permeability, and both secrete H^+ and HCO_3^- when appropriately stimulated. In 1967 Steinmetz (42) reported that the hydrogen secretory process was independent of sodium and sodium transport and was electrogenic, generating a mucosal positive potential difference. Moreover the short-circuit current generated in bladders in which sodium transport was inhibited was in the direction of positive charge transfer into the mucosal fluid and was quantitatively equal to the rate of H^+ transport. This transport process, which is probably energized by ATP, can secrete H^+ against very steep electrochemical gradients and alters its rate of secretion inversely to the electrochemical gradient against which H^+ is secreted. The cell populations in both the bladder and collecting duct are heterogeneous. There is now strong evidence that the mitochondrial-rich cells that stain densely for carbonic anhydrase (intercalated cells) are responsible for hydrogen secretion, whereas the remaining cells (principal cells) are responsible for electrogenic sodium transport (41). The mechanism by which the base generated by H^+ secretion exits the cell in the turtle and the collecting duct is different from that in the proximal tubule. Bases, either as OH^- or HCO_3^- leave the cell by electroneutral exchange with Cl^- in the serosal fluid (41, 43).

This long thread of research, stretching from the mid-nineteenth century to the present, has led to the current view that most portions of the nephron, with the exception of the thin limbs of Henle's loop, participate in the process of urinary acidification by secreting H^+. However, the overall system for urinary acidification in those areas of the urinary tract derived from the ureteric bud is uniquely different from that in the more proximal portions of the nephron derived from the metanephric blastema (Fig. 12). In the more proximal areas of the nephron, where the bulk of filtered bicarbonate

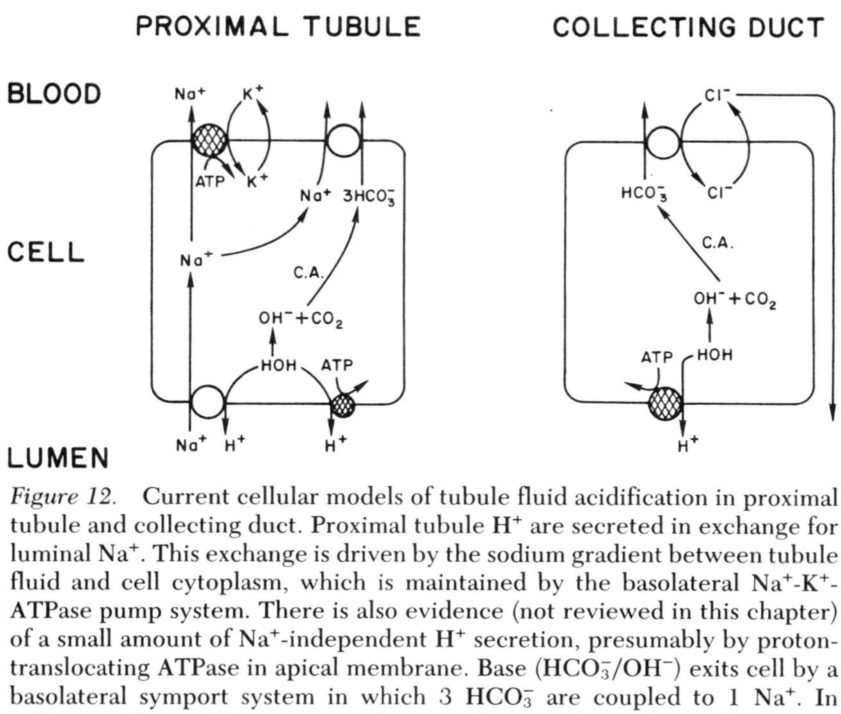

Figure 12. Current cellular models of tubule fluid acidification in proximal tubule and collecting duct. Proximal tubule H^+ are secreted in exchange for luminal Na^+. This exchange is driven by the sodium gradient between tubule fluid and cell cytoplasm, which is maintained by the basolateral Na^+-K^+-ATPase pump system. There is also evidence (not reviewed in this chapter) of a small amount of Na^+-independent H^+ secretion, presumably by proton-translocating ATPase in apical membrane. Base (HCO_3^-/OH^-) exits cell by a basolateral symport system in which 3 HCO_3^- are coupled to 1 Na^+. In collecting ducts H^+ are secreted across the apical membrane by a Na^+-independent mechanism, presumably proton-translocating ATPase. Base (HCO_3^-/OH^-) exits cell by an electroneutral exchange for Cl^-. Chloride ions recycle back across basolateral membrane by a conductive pathway. Chloride ions or luminal cations can diffuse through paracellular pathway to maintain electroneutrality.

is reabsorbed, there is a high-capacity system in which the transfer of H^+ from cell to tubule lumen is mediated primarily by a Na^+-H^+ exchanger located in the apical membrane; the transfer of bases from cell to blood is mediated by a Na^+-HCO_3^- symporter located in the basolateral cell membrane. In contrast, in the collecting ducts there is the capacity to secrete either H^+ or HCO_3^-. The hydrogen secretory system can transport H^+ from cell to tubule lumen against steep gradients and is mediated by an electrogenic sodium-independent process, probably a proton-translocating ATPase located in the apical membrane. The transfer of bases from cell to blood is mediated by the exchange of OH^- or HCO_3^- with Cl^-. The proximal system is energized by the sodium concentration gradient between the tubule fluid and cell cytoplasm, whereas the collecting duct system is energized by direct coupling to ATP.

BIBLIOGRAPHY

1. Alpern, R. J. Mechanism of basolateral membrane $H^+/OH^-/HCO_3$ transport in the rat proximal convoluted tubule: a sodium-coupled electrogenic process. *J. Gen. Physiol.* 86: 613–636, 1985.
2. Astrup, P., and J. W. Severinghaus. The history of acids and bases. In: *The History of Blood Gases, Acids and Bases*, edited by P. Astrup and J. W. Severinghaus. Copenhagen: Munksgaard, 1986, chapt. 10, p. 173–187.
3. Berliner, R. W. Renal secretion of potassium and hydrogen ions. *Federation Proc.* 11: 695–700, 1952.
4. Berliner, R. W. Some aspects of ion exchange in electrolyte transport by the renal tubules. In: *Metabolic Aspects of Transport Across Cell Membranes*, edited by Q. R. Murphy. Madison: Univ. of Wisconsin Press, 1957, p. 203–220.
5. Biagi, B. A. The effects of the anion transport inhibitor, SITS, on the proximal straight tubule of the rabbit perfused in vitro. *J. Membr. Biol.* 81: 25–32, 1985.
6. Boron, W. F., and E. L. Boulpaep. Intracellular pH regulation in the renal proximal tubule of the salamander: Na-H exchange. *J. Gen. Physiol.* 81: 29–52, 1983.
7. Boron, W. F., and E. L. Boulpaep. Intracellular pH regulation in the proximal tubule of the salamander: basolateral HCO_3 transport. *J. Gen. Physiol.* 81: 53–94, 1983.
8. Boron, W. F., and J. M. Russell. Stoichiometry and ion dependencies of intracellular pH-regulating mechanism in squid giant axons. *J. Gen. Physiol.* 81: 373–399, 1983.
9. Brodsky, W. A. Implications of urinary CO_2 tension with respect to mechanisms of urinary acidification (Abstract). *Federation Proc.* 14: 18, 1955.
10. Burg, M., J. Grantham, M. Abramow, and J. Orloff. Preparation and study of fragments of single rabbit nephrons. *Am. J. Physiol.* 210: 1293–1298, 1966.
11. Burg, M., and N. Green. Bicarbonate transport by isolated perfused rabbit proximal convoluted tubules. *Am. J. Physiol.* 233 (*Renal Fluid*

Electrolyte Physiol. 1): F307–F314, 1977.
12. CUSHNY, A. R. *The Secretion of Urine* (1st ed.). London: Longmans Green, 1917, p. 200–208.
13. DUBOSE, T. D., JR., L. R. PUCACCO, and N. W. CARTER. Determination of disequilibrium pH in the rat kidney in vivo: evidence for hydrogen secretion. *Am. J. Physiol.* 240 (*Renal Fluid Electrolyte Physiol.* 9): F138–F146, 1981.
14. FOLIN, O. The acidity of the urine. *Am. J. Physiol.* 9: 265–278, 1903.
15. FORSTNER, G. G., S. M. SABESIN, and K. J. ISSELBACHER. Rat intestinal microvillus membranes. Purification and biochemical characterization. *Biochem. J.* 106: 381–390, 1968.
16. FOSTER, M. *Lectures on the History of Physiology During the Sixteenth, Seventeenth, and Eighteenth Centuries.* Cambridge, UK: Cambridge Univ. Press, 1901, p. 120–171.
17. GALEN. *On the Natural Faculties*, translated by A. J. Brock. London: Heineman, 1916, p. 245.
18. GAMBLE, J. L. Carbonic acid and bicarbonate in urine. *J. Biol. Chem.* 51: 295–310, 1922.
19. GOOD, D. W., M. A. KNEPPER, and M. B. BURG. Ammonia and bicarbonate transport by thick ascending limb of rat kidney. *Am. J. Physiol.* 247 (*Renal Fluid Electrolyte Physiol.* 16): F35–F44, 1984.
20. GOTTSCHALK, C. W., W. E. LASSITER, and M. MYLLE. Localization of urine acidification in the mammalian kidney. *Am. J. Physiol.* 198: 581–585, 1960.
21. HENDERSON, L. J. A critical study of the process of acid excretion. *J. Biol. Chem.* 9: 403–424, 1911.
22. HOFFMAN, F. Über den Übergan von freien Säuren durch das alkalische Blut in den Harn. *Z. Biol.* VII: 338–360, 1871.
23. KINSELLA, J. L., and P. S. ARONSON. Properties of the Na^{+}-H^{+} exchanger in renal microvillus membrane vesicles. *Am. J. Physiol.* 238 (*Renal Fluid Electrolyte Physiol.* 7): F461–F469, 1980.
24. MCKINNEY, T. D., and M. B. BURG. Bicarbonate and fluid absorption by renal proximal straight tubules. *Kidney Int.* 12: 1–8, 1977.
25. MCKINNEY, T. D., and M. B. BURG. Bicarbonate transport by rabbit cortical collecting tubules. Effect of acid and alkali loads in vivo on transport in vitro. *J. Clin. Invest.* 60: 766–768, 1977.
26. MENAKER, W. Buffer equilibria and reabsorption in the production of urinary acidity. *Am. J. Physiol.* 154: 174–184, 1948.
27. MONTGOMERY, H., and J. A. PIERCE. The site of acidification of the urine within the renal tubule in amphibia. *Am. J. Physiol.* 118: 144–152, 1937.
28. MURER, H., U. HOPFER, and R. KINNE. Sodium/proton antiport in brush-border-membrane vesicles isolated from rat small intestine and kidney. *Biochem. J.* 154: 597–604, 1976.
29. NASH, T. P., and S. R. BENEDICT. The ammonia content of blood and its bearing on the mechanism of acid neutralization in the animal organism. *J. Biol. Chem.* 48: 463–488, 1921.
30. OCHWADT, B. K., and R. F. PITTS. Effects of intravenous infusion of carbonic anhydrase on carbon dioxide tension of alkaline urine. *Am. J. Physiol.* 185: 426–429, 1956.
31. PITTS, R. F. Renal excretion of acid. *Federation Proc.* 7: 418–426, 1948.
32. PITTS, R. F., and R. S. ALEXANDER. The nature of the renal tubular

mechanism for acidifying the urine. *Am. J. Physiol.* 144: 239–254, 1945.

33. Rector, F. C., Jr., N. W. Carter, and D. W. Seldin. The mechanism of bicarbonate reabsorption in the proximal and distal tubules of the kidney. *J. Clin. Invest.* 44: 278–290, 1965.
34. Schilb, T. P., and W. A. Brodsky. Acidification of mucosal fluid by transport of bicarbonate ion in turtle bladders. *Am. J. Physiol.* 210: 997–1008, 1966.
35. Sendroy, J., Jr., S. Seelig, and D. D. Van Slyke. Studies of acidosis. XXIII. The carbon dioxide tension and acid-base balance of human urine. *J. Biol. Chem.* 106: 479–500, 1934.
36. Shalhoub, R., W. Webber, S. Glabman, M. Canessa-Fischer, J. Klein, J. DeHaas, and R. F. Pitts. Extraction of amino acids from and their addition to renal blood plasma. *Am. J. Physiol.* 204: 181–186, 1963.
37. Smith, H. W. The inorganic composition of the body fluids of the chelonia. *J. Biol. Chem.* 82: 651–661, 1929.
38. Smith, H. W. *The Physiology of the Kidney.* New York: Oxford Univ. Press, 1937, p. 169–182.
39. Sorensen, S. P. S. Über die Messung und Bedeutung der Wasserstoffionenkonzentration bei biologischen Prozessen. *Ergeb. Physiol.* 12: 393–532, 1912.
40. Steinmetz, P. R. Characteristics of hydrogen ion transport in urinary bladder of water turtle. *J. Clin. Invest.* 46: 1531–1540, 1967.
41. Steinmetz, P. R. Cellular organization of urinary acidification. *Am. J. Physiol.* 251 (*Renal Fluid Electrolyte Physiol.* 20): F173–F187, 1986.
42. Steinmetz, P. R., R. S. Omachi, and H. S. Frazer. Independence of hydrogen ion secretion and transport of other electrolytes in turtle bladder. *J. Clin. Invest.* 46: 1541–1548, 1967.
43. Stone, D. K., D. W. Seldin, J. P. Kokko, and H. R. Jacobson. Anion dependence of rabbit medullary collecting duct acidification. *J. Clin. Invest.* 71: 1505–1508, 1983.
44. Van Slyke, D. D., R. A. Phillips, P. B. Hamilton, R. M. Archibald, P. H. Futcher, and A. Hiller. Glutamine as source material of urinary ammonia. *J. Biol. Chem.* 150: 481–483, 1943.
45. Vieira, F. L., and G. Malnic. Hydrogen ion secretion by rat renal cortical tubules as studied by an antimony microelectrode. *Am. J. Physiol.* 214: 710–718, 1968.
46. Vurek, G. G., D. G. Warnock, and R. Corsey. Measurement of picomole amounts of carbon dioxide by calorimetry. *Anal. Chem.* 47: 765–767, 1975.
47. Walser, M., and G. H. Mudge. Renal excretory mechanisms. In: *Mineral Metabolism: An Advanced Treatise. Principles, Processes and Systems,* edited by C. L. Comar and F. Bronner. New York: Academic. 1960, vol. I, p. 287–336.
48. Walter, F. Untersuchungen über die Wirkung der Säuren auf den tierischen Organismus. *Arch. Exp. Pathol. Pharmakol.* 7: 148–178, 1977.
49. Wearn, J. T., and A. N. Richards. Observations on the composition of glomerular urine, with particular reference to the problem of reabsorption in the renal tubules. *Am. J. Physiol.* 71: 209–227, 1924.
50. Yoshitomi, K., B.-C. Burckhardt, and E. Frömter. Rheogenic sodium-bicarbonate cotransport in the peritubular membrane of rat renal proximal tubule. *Pfluegers Arch.* 405: 360–366, 1985.

XII

Tubular Transport of Organic Anions and Cations

IRWIN M. WEINER

The disposition of an organic compound by the kidney can be quite complex. The intrarenal processes that may affect the disposition of one or another substance are glomerular filtration, active and passive reabsorption, active and passive secretion, synthesis, and metabolic destruction. In the space made available it is difficult to present a balanced view of the history of the discovery of these processes and their combined actions on various kinds of organic compounds. Rather than attempt the very difficult, I elect to give a rather idiosyncratic picture in which major emphasis is given to the controversy over the existence of tubular secretion, proof of active secretion of organic acids, the discovery of secretion of organic cations, the idea of secretion by passive mechanisms, and the idea of bidirectional transport. The central figure in this version of history is Eli K. Marshall, Jr. (1889–1966). TUBULAR TRANSPORT

Much of the material in this chapter also appears in two essays by Homer W. Smith from which I have borrowed shamelessly (60, 61). Smith, James A. Shannon, A. Newton Richards, Robert F. Pitts, Roy P. Forster, John V. Taggart, William B. Kinter, Ernest C. Foulks, and many others are given short shrift or not mentioned at all in this chapter in large part because their contributions are bound to be discussed in other chapters of this volume.

The Nineteenth Century

In 1923 Marshall and James L. Vickers (1899–1943) published a paper (39) entitled "The Mechanism of the Elimination of Phenolsulfonephthalein by the Kidney—a Proof of Secretion by the Convoluted Tubules" (Fig. 1). As is true in most "proofs" in physiology,

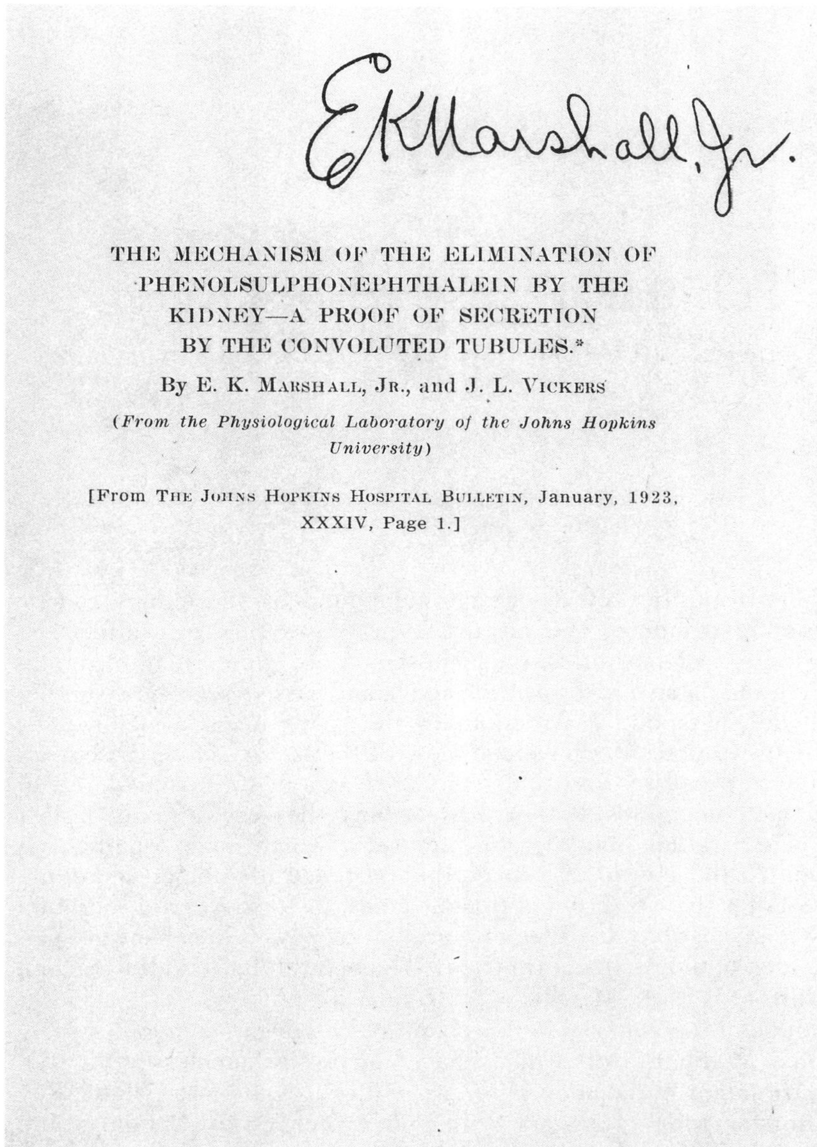

E K Marshall, Jr.

THE MECHANISM OF THE ELIMINATION OF PHENOLSULPHONEPHTHALEIN BY THE KIDNEY—A PROOF OF SECRETION BY THE CONVOLUTED TUBULES.*

By E. K. Marshall, Jr., and J. L. Vickers

(*From the Physiological Laboratory of the Johns Hopkins University*)

[From The Johns Hopkins Hospital Bulletin, January, 1923, XXXIV, Page 1.]

Figure 1. The cover of a reprint of the 1923 paper by Marshall and Vickers (39) signed by E. K. Marshall, Jr. (Courtesy of Carl W. Gottschalk.)

this one was not absolutely perfect, but it came closer to perfection than any other important proof in renal physiology up to that time. Despite its power in experiment and argument, the paper was not warmly received; indeed it took more than a decade before the idea of secretion was universally accepted in the physiological establishment. The prejudice against the idea of tubular secretion stemmed from the accidents of history that followed the disparate speculations on renal function by William Bowman (1816–1892) and Carl Ludwig (1816–1895). At almost the same time and apparently without knowledge of the existence of one another, both men observed that each glomerulus (Malpighian body) sat at the head of an individual tubule. Both were struck with the idea (9) that "*the Malpighian bodies might be an apparatus designed to separate from the blood the watery portion.*" On other matters, their ideas were quite divergent.

Ludwig's speculations were based on contemporary physics and physicochemistry. He held that fluid formation in the kidney occurred at the glomerulus by a process of ultrafiltration, more or less as we understand it today. For him the tubules were the agents of reabsorption; they acted blindly, reabsorbing the filtered fluid and its constituents by a purely physicochemical mechanism that he called endosmosis. This initial work by Ludwig was part of his thesis for the M.D. degree, the start of a long and distinguished career that put him among the premier biologists of his time (55). The breadth of Ludwig's work in physiology was enormous, but throughout the remainder of his life he maintained an interest in renal physiology. He elaborated on and modified his theory of renal function to accommodate some of the new findings from his (Fig. 2) and other laboratories. He never accepted the idea of tubular secretion despite the fact that Heidenhain made a powerful argument for its existence in 1874, some twenty-one years before death ended Ludwig's career.

Bowman was much less precise in his speculation on glomerular

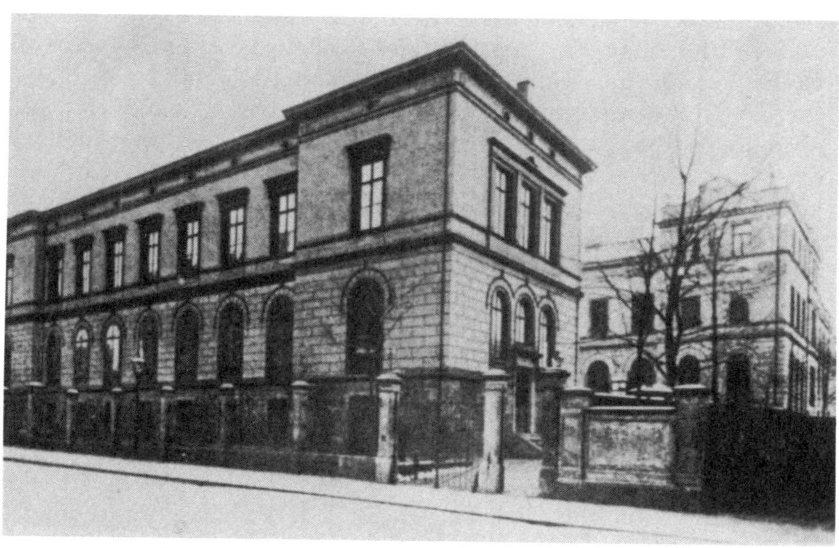

Figure 2. Ludwig's Physiological Institute at Leipzig. At the time of this photograph (ca. 1880), Ludwig was in his seventh decade. [From Rothschuh (56).]

function. He is clear on the idea that the watery part separated from blood contains salts, but the mechanism is vaguely described with the words *exude* and *transude*. Unlike Ludwig, Bowman conceived of the tubules as agents of secretion. He speculated that the waste products of the body are compacted by the tubular cells into "effete particles" that are then discharged into the luminal fluid in a manner analogous to that seen in apocrine glands. His brilliant paper on the histology of the kidney was his only contribution to the field; his later career was devoted to ophthalmology (64).

It is conceivable that had Bowman known of Ludwig's idea on filtration he would have embraced it. Bowman had seen the glomerular capillary tuft as a collection of bare capillaries. In speaking of the action of the cilia (9) he stated, "*these exquisite organs . . . tend to remove pressure from the free surface of the vessels, and so encourage the escape of their more fluid contents.*" Some fifteen years later, Charles Edward Isaacs (1811–1860) observed the epithelial layer overlying the glomerular tuft; it was he who proposed a true secretory function to the glomerulus (51), an idea later supported by Heidenhain. Thus there evolved two separate points of contention: *1*) Is the fluid elaborated by the glomerulus the product of a purely physical mechanism, or is there secretion? 2) Is transport across the tubular epithelia secretory or reabsorptive? In the context of this article, it is more fruitful to concentrate on the second question.

On the surface the question is one of pure phenomenology; but in the middle of the nineteenth century it had poignant philosophical implications that, in their extension, led to the ungracious reception accorded the Marshall and Vickers paper (39) of 1923. It was in the nineteenth century that most of the ideological contest between the vitalists and the mechanists occurred. Within each of these ideologies there was a considerable spectrum of thought. Thomas Hall (23) gives this subject a relatively succinct and very lucid treatment. In brief, the vitalists held that the behavior of living matter could not be explained by the rules of physics and chemistry that govern ordinary matter. They believed that some unique force, inherent or imposed (some believed divine), governed living systems. The mechanists believed otherwise.

Obviously Ludwig was a mechanist; he invoked nothing but physical forces in his original version of renal function. It would have been difficult for him to accept the idea of tubular secretion; there was nothing in the physical sciences of the day that could explain such a phenomenon. Ironically, the man who was to launch the most serious attack on the Ludwig hypothesis, Rudolf Peter Heinrich Heidenhain, was himself not a vitalist. Heidenhain's philosophy is exposed in this quotation from the theoretical section of his 1874 paper (25), which he believed contained proof of the secretion of the dye indigo carmine.

In the course of this presentation I have thus far avoided a question that cannot be ignored, although its solution is at present hopeless, the question being which physical and chemical processes in the epithelium mediate the secretion of indigo carmine. As long as the expression "life of the cell" is only a term describing the sum of unknown physical and chemical processes that occur in the cell, one cannot hope to better define the activity of secreting cells. The following considerations merely give leads for further investigation.

Thus, while Heidenhain was a mechanist at heart, he felt free to make observations of phenomena without attempting to reduce them to their component physical factors. In his view the latter was too formidable a task, given the complexity of the systems and the then-primitive state of knowledge. However, the lack of mechanistic explanations made his findings available for use by the vitalists in arguments for their positions, thereby tainting Heidenhain in the eyes of mechanists.

Heidenhain was born in East Prussia in 1834 and was the eldest of some twenty children (19). His father was a physician, as were five of his brothers; he manifested a childhood interest in biology as a collector of plant and animal specimens. It was quite usual at that time to attend more than one university during a course of study. He began his medical studies at Königsberg, and after two years transferred to Halle, where he came under the influence of Alfred W. Volkmann (1800–1877), an important physiologist of the time. Two years later, when he transferred to Berlin, he became a student of Emil H. du Bois-Reymond (1818–1896), a physiologist of the first rank. Heidenhain completed his studies when he was only twenty years old. His doctoral thesis dealt with the influence of the vagus nerves on the heart. It had been suggested earlier by Moritz Schiff (1823–1896) that the beat of the heart was initiated by the vagi, a suggestion disproved by Heidenhain. Heidenhain spent two additional years with du Bois-Reymond working on muscle and nerve physiology before returning to Volkmann's laboratory in Halle, where he produced his *Habilitationsschrift*, based on an improved method for estimating blood volume. In 1859 he married Volkmann's daughter Fanny, and in that same year he was called to Breslau (now Wroclaw, Poland) to be the professor of physiology. At Breslau he was greeted by a student strike; apparently the students preferred another candidate for the position. Some of the senior professors also were not enamored of Heidenhain's appointment: "*One cannot have much respect for the discipline that can be represented by a twenty-five year old teacher and master.*" Heidenhain easily overcame these difficulties and remained at Breslau for the remainder of his career. He died in 1897, two years after Ludwig; the latter was his senior by eighteen years.

Heidenhain made notable contributions to the physiology of skeletal muscle, the secretions of glands, and their control by nerves, gastric secretion, and intestinal absorption. Among the people he helped train were Ivan P. Pavlov, Ernest H. Starling, and Walter B. Cannon. One of Heidenhain's sons, Martin, became a prominent histologist (3).

It is likely that up to 1874 the Ludwig hypothesis of renal function was dominant. However, this dominance ended with the appearance of Heidenhain's paper (25) "Investigations on the Mechanism of Urine Secretion." [The subtitle indicates that the work was done in association with a medical student, Albert Neisser (1855–1916), who later discovered the causative agent of gonorrhea and became a prominent dermatologist.] Heidenhain had already made some observations that suggested the existence of tubular secretion. Moreover, his earlier work on exocrine glands and intestinal absorption prepared him to be sympathetic to the idea of epithelial transport. He set out as follows: "*If it could be proven that the epithelium of certain parts of the urinary tubules continue their secretory function while, by one method or another water filtration is suppressed, then undoubtedly safe ground could be won on which to decide between the hypotheses of Bowman* (sic) *and Ludwig.*"

Notice that at this time Heidenhain was still willing to accept the existence of filtration; by 1883 he was not (26). Thus the only question addressed in this paper (25) was the direction of tubular transport. Aided somewhat by hindsight, we can see that the premise was faulty. In one of his perceptive essays on this subject (61) Homer Smith wrote: "*Renal physiology—though perhaps no more than any other branch of science—has suffered frequently in consequence of neglect to weigh carefully and dispose of the 'alternative interpretation.'*" In this case the alternative interpretation is that while indigo carmine is secreted other substances may be reabsorbed. At later times and from different points of view, an analogous error was made by both Arthur R. Cushny and Richards (see the next section). There is another factor inherent in some of the writing of Heidenhain and others of the period that may have impeded progress, that is, the competing theories of Bowman and Ludwig were considered in their entirety: they were either entirely right or entirely wrong. Nevertheless the strong evidence for the secretion of indigo carmine was a powerful challenge to the Ludwig hypothesis. It was evidence for the activity of the tubular epithelium. The evidence, the arguments in this paper (25) and subsequent arguments (26), dominated the field for some four decades.

It is worth recounting the essence of some of Heidenhain's experiments for, in fact, half the experiments in the Marshall and Vickers paper published almost fifty years later were refinements of Heidenhain's work. Heidenhain administered saturated solutions of the sodium salt of indigo carmine, a disulfonic acid, to rabbits intravenously. Some of the rabbits had been rendered hypotensive by transection of the medulla oblongata below the atlas, on the premise that the hypotension would eliminate or virtually eliminate glomerular filtration. Some animals were killed at ten minutes after the injection of dye, others at one hour. The kidneys were removed, fixed in alcohol, transected in the sagittal plane, and subjected to gross and microscopic examination. The kidney of a hypotensive animal killed ten minutes after injection showed deep coloration of the cortex and no color in the medulla or papilla (Fig. 3). On microscopic examination the cells of convoluted tubules were stained and solid deposits of the dye were seen in the lumina. The kidney of a hypotensive animal killed an hour after injection gave a similar gross picture, but on microscopic examination the proximal epithelium was not stained; however, precipitated dye remained in the lumina. The kidney of an intact animal showed intense staining of the cortex, inner medulla, and papilla. On this basis Heidenhain envisioned a two-step process of secretion. The first step was uptake of dye from blood by the cells of the convoluted tubules. The second step was secretion of dye into the tubular lumina. In the absence of axial fluid flow, the dye would remain in the lumina near the site of secretion. There is no doubt now that Heidenhain's interpretation was entirely correct (33), but there were to be many criticisms of the experimental evidence, some of them valid (16).

It is interesting to observe that Heidenhain may well deserve credit for the concept of renal clearance. In his definitive attack on the Ludwig hypothesis (26), he made an argument based on the theoretical volume of filtrate necessary to deliver the quantity of urea excreted daily by a human. The calculated value was seventy liters, which Heidenhain considered absurd. Posterity is indebted to Cushny for correcting this misapprehension (16).

Bowman's histological tract of 1842 was in large part an exercise in comparative microanatomy of the kidney (9). He recognized that in mammals the peritubular capillary network is part of a portal circulation, that is, this network is the second of two capillary systems arranged in series, thus making the efferent arteriole analogous to the portal vein of the liver. He also recognized that in other species, for example, the boa constrictor, the peritubular network was fed also by a portal vein arising from structures in the lower parts of the body. Work by others before and after Bowman established that the existence of a renal portal vein is a common feature in amphibians, reptiles, and birds. Apparently, Moritz Nussbaum (1850–1915) was the first to recognize the possibility of utilizing this anatomical arrangement to address the problem of tubular secretion. Nussbaum was professor of anatomy at Bonn and had been at one time a student of Edward Pflüger's (1829–1910), who was a contemporary of Heidenhain in du Bois-Reymond's laboratory. In 1878 Nussbaum published two papers that gave strong support to Heidenhain's contentions (44, 45). His approach was to tie off the arterial supply to the

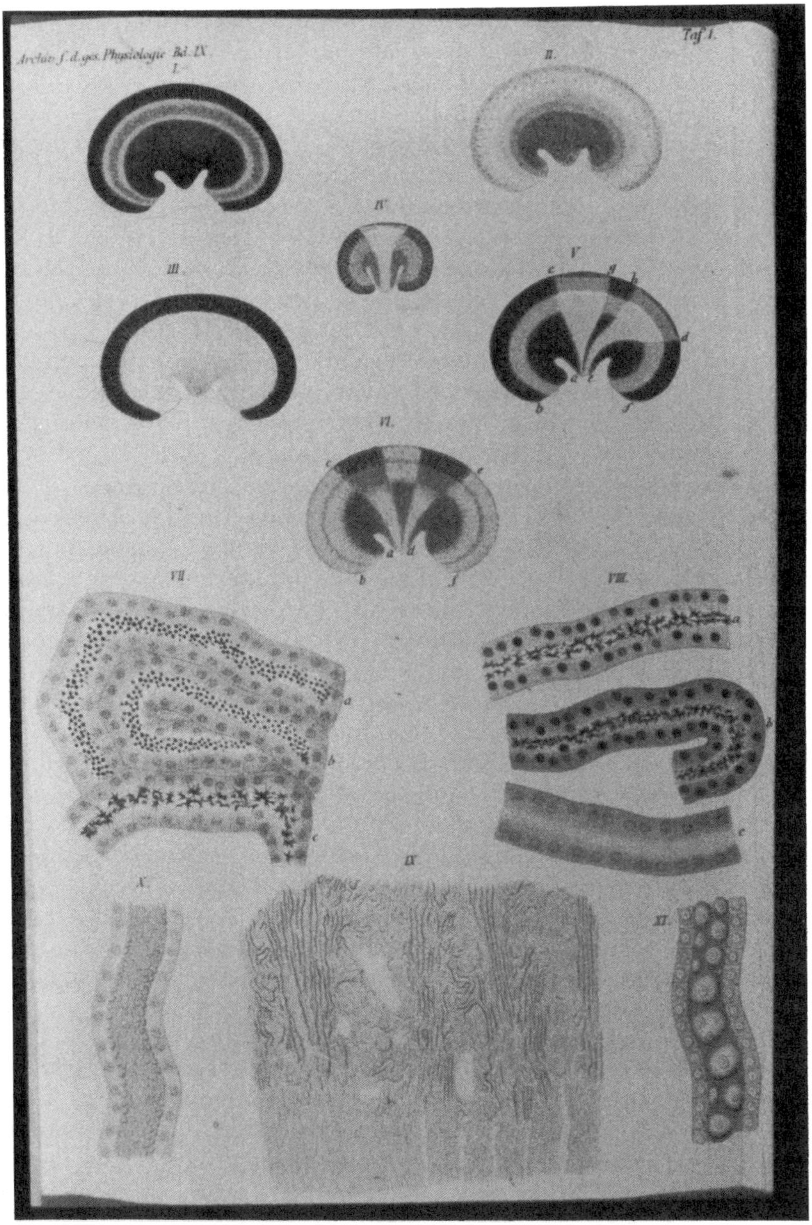

Figure 3. The plate from Heidenhain's paper of 1874. The original is in 3 colors. The figure on the upper left (I) is from a sagittal section of a kidney from a normotensive rabbit treated with indigo carmine. The figure below it (III) is from a hypotensive animal similarly treated. [From Heidenhain (25).]

kidney of the frog *Rana esculenta* and inject a test substance into the venous system, thereby giving it access to the peritubular capillaries via the renal portal vein. When indigo carmine was injected in this manner, it was seen to accumulate in renal cells and as a precipitate in the lumina. Even more remarkable, when urea was injected, the kidney (which had been anuric) reestablished the flow of urine at about a fourth of the normal rate. For control Nussbaum injected dyes into the aortas of his preparations and examined them for coloration of the glomeruli; he found none. Thus he concluded that both indigo carmine and urea are secreted and that urea carries water with it.

The elegance of Nussbaum's experiments attracted considerable attention; there were to be modifications of the technique, and a fairly extensive literature developed. Parts of this literature were summarized by Shannon (59), Smith (61), and Cushny (16). It is now appreciated that Nussbaum was correct about the secretion of indigo carmine and urea in the frog, but it is equally appreciated that his experiments were inconclusive. Despite his careful attention to detail, he did not (and probably could not at the time) recognize that his procedure did not completely dearterialize the glomeruli (31).

Felix Hoppe-Seyler (1825–1895), the famous physiological chemist and founder of the *Zeitschrift für physiologische Chemie*, is not widely remembered for his contribution to renal physiology, but in fact his was a signal contribution. In a textbook published in 1881 (29), he indicated that a passive process could not account for the difference in osmotic pressure between urine and plasma in the hydropenic animal. Thus the original Ludwig idea of the function of the tubules was disproved by the simplest of observations.

Hoppe was born in Freiburg, the tenth child of a protestant minister (56). His father died a few years after he was born and the boy was raised in the home of a brother-in-law (Seyler), who formally adopted him in 1864. He displayed an interest in experimental chemistry while still a schoolboy and continued working in the chemistry laboratory throughout his medical education in Halle. He worked subsequently at Leipzig, Greifswald, Berlin, Tübingen, and finally Strassburg, where he was appointed professor of physiological chemistry in 1872. He made important contributions to the chemistry of blood pigments and was probably the first to apply Robert Bunsen's method of spectral analysis to biological problems. Hoppe-Seyler studied the association of oxygen and hemoglobin and established that oxygen consumption occurs mainly in the tissues, not in the blood. He established the distribution of glycogen, lecithin, and cholesterol in the body; the nature of the proteins in egg white; and worked on the constitutions of bile salts and chlorophyll. His founding of the *Zeitschrift* in 1877 was one of the early steps in the fractionation of physiology, and it earned him the displeasure of

Pflüger, who had started the *Archiv für die gesamte Physiologie des Menschen und der Tiere* nine years earlier.

Thus, before the turn of the century, the physicochemical theory for tubular reabsorption had been demolished and there was substantial, if not definitive, evidence for tubular secretion. Tubular function was not a happy subject for mechanists. However, there was a plethora of other successes for them, and by the end of the century vitalism, while still alive, was no longer a powerful conceptual force. The idea of filtration was gaining strength, in large part through the efforts of Starling (1866–1927) (63), although for much of his life Starling was not convinced that filtration is as great a process as that required by the Ludwig hypothesis. It is ironic that Starling, who had worked with Heidenhain, was to develop much more along the lines of Ludwig. Starling's "law of the capillary," filtration and reabsorption by physical forces, is quite analogous to Ludwig's ideas about renal function, but it has the advantage of being correct.

Arthur Cushny

It may well be that much of the literature on renal function through the last two decades of the nineteenth and the first two decades of the twentieth century was not terribly sound. Certainly Arthur Robertson Cushny did not think much of it.

No other organ of the body has suffered so much from poor work as the kidney, and in no other region of physiology does so much base coin pass as legal tender. It was therefore necessary to sift thoroughly this mass of printed matter of over 6000 pages, and I have read it carefully, and, as far as might be, sympathetically, though I must

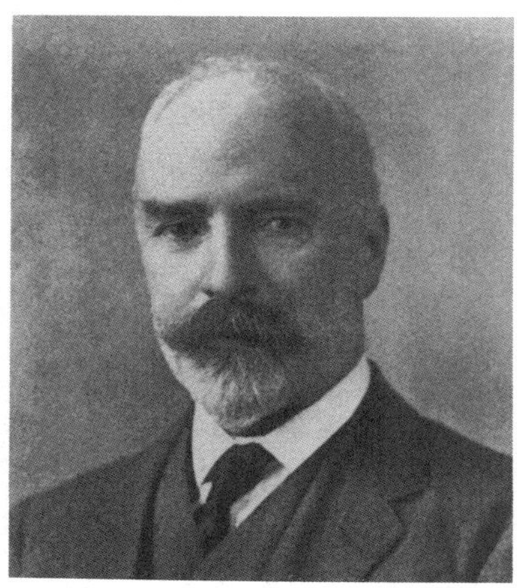

Figure 4. Arthur Robertson Cushny (1866–1926). [From Holmstedt and Liljestrand (27).]

confess that my patience has been sorely tried by some papers in which the depth bore no proportion to the length.

This quotation is from the letter of transmittal of the manuscript of the first edition of Cushny's book *The Secretion of Urine* (1917). The letter is addressed to Starling, who was the editor of a series of monographs on physiology; it is reprinted in the second edition (16), which is of greater interest in the present context because it was published in 1926 after the Marshall and Vickers paper appeared. The letter contains another notable passage.

I do not flatter myself that this treatise attains finality in regard to the secretion of the urine; that is impossible at the present time. If it serves as an advanced post from which others may issue against the remaining ramparts of vitalism, its purpose will be attained.

Cushny was the fourth son of the Reverend John Cushny of Morayshire, Scotland (1). He attended Aberdeen University, where he earned an M.A. in 1886 and a Bachelor of Medicine and Master of Surgery in 1889. The University awarded him the Thompson Fellowship, which enabled him to spend a year in Berne in the laboratory of the physiologist Hugo Kronecker (1839–1914). Kronecker had spent ten years in Leipzig with Ludwig early in his career (56). During the year in Berne, Cushny became acquainted with John Jacob Abel (1857–1938), who was studying with the biochemist Marceli von Nencki. Abel was to have a powerful influence on Cushny's career. Cushny went to Strassburg, where he worked for two years with Oswald Schmiedeberg (1838–1921), the leading exponent of the then–relatively new science of pharmacology and a former student of Ludwig. It was Schmiedeberg who recommended Abel to the University of Michigan in 1891 to chair the newly created Department of Materia Medica and Pharmacology, the first modern pharmacology department in this country. Two years later Abel was invited to chair the Department of Pharmacology at a new institution in Baltimore, The Johns Hopkins School of Medicine. He spent the summer of 1893 working in Berne, and he was commissioned by the Dean at Michigan to find his replacement. On Schmiedeberg's advice Abel persuaded Cushny to take the position, which he (Cushny) held for twelve years. In 1905 Cushny was invited to chair the Department of Materia Medica and Pharmacology at University College, London. A new institute was built for him from funds provided by Andrew Carnegie, and the department (which started from virtually nothing) prospered. In 1918 Cushny was elected to the Chair of Pharmacology at Edinburgh, where he remained until his death at age sixty from a cerebrovascular accident.

Cushny wrote the first critical textbook on pharmacology in English (14). He also wrote two important monographs, one on digitalis (15) and *The Secretion of Urine*. Of his wide-ranging research, the two most important areas were the pharmacology of the heart and the pharmacological behavior of optical isomers. He wrote only a note and a full paper on saline cathartics; he wrote six papers on renal function. His great contribution to renal physiology was the monograph (16). The book is a strange one. It is at the same time a scholarly review, an apology, and a polemic. One's opinion of it can easily change from one reading to another. For example, in his William Henry Welch lecture published in 1943 (60), Homer Smith treated the book and Cushny's ideas forgivingly; in 1959 Smith was much more critical (61).

The most cogent section of the book is the defense of the idea of filtration. Cushny successfully defused Heidenhain's idea that the magnitude of filtration required by the excretory rate of urea is absurd. Moreover, by the time of the second edition, Richard's laboratory had provided direct evidence for filtration. The weakest aspect of the book is the treatment of tubular function. As already noted, Hoppe-Seyler had destroyed the idea that all reabsorption is passive. (Remarkably, Hoppe-Seyler does not appear in the bibliography of Cushny's monograph). Cushny had to invoke the premise that reabsorption required the "vital activity" of the tubular cells. Cushny seems to want to keep this vital activity as simple as possible; he postulated that the tubules acted blindly, reabsorbing a "*perfected Locke's fluid.*" In effect he denied any regulatory function of the tubules. "*The formation of the glomerular filtrate is due to a blind physical force; the absorption in the tubules is equally independent of any discrimination, for the fluid absorbed is always the same, whatever the needs of the organism at the moment.*" With regard to tubular secretion, Cushny was far from neutral, After discussing and rejecting Marshall's work he wrote:

> *The necessity for this assumption* [secretion] *has not yet been shown, and it should be held in reserve, to be invoked only if the simpler view which I have presented proves inadequate; and perhaps not even if it fails in obscure and occasional cases, but only if it fails all along the line. There is as yet no reason to regard the two factors of filtration and reabsorption as inadequate, except such as arises from our limited knowledge of the kidney function.*

This is of course a restatement of the maxim called Occam's razor: entities are not to be multiplied without necessity. The modern biologist realizes that the necessity arises all too frequently, and in Cushny's case the necessity had already arisen.

Smith (61) chided Cushny's ghost on several other points. First, it is not clear that reabsorption of a fluid of constant composition is physiologically any less complicated a problem than reabsorption of fluids of varying composition. Second, he was displeased by Cushny's brusque treatment of Ludwig's contributions. Third, he thought that the builder of the advanced post against vitalism should have clarified the distinction between vitalism and vital activity, thereby explaining how the Cushny position was not vitalistic. Finally, Smith felt that Cushny had erected "*something of a straw man*" by attacking vitalism. By the second decade of this century, vitalism was moribund if not dead and none of the major proponents of tubular secretion had been a vitalist.

It is conceivable that Cushny became exercised about vitalism by the same event that caused Sir Lauder Brunton to speak on "*Ludwig's and other theories of the secretion of urine and the action of diuretics*" at a meeting of the Therapeutical and Pharmacological Section of the Royal Society of Medicine on 19 March, 1912 (12). Brunton (1844–1916) was a distinguished pharmacologist who supported himself by the practice of medicine, first at the Middlesex Hospital and later at St. Bartholomew's Hospital in London. He had worked with several of the important scientists on the continent, including Ludwig (27).

I should not have thought of bringing the subject before the Section to-day had it not been that in looking up a number of recent works I find that there is a good deal of uncertainty in the statement regarding the secretion of urine, and that in the Croonian Lecture of last year, given before the Royal Society, Professor Brodie makes the sweeping statement that all recent work has proved conclusively that Ludwig's explanation of the glomerular function—viz., that it is a filtering mechanism—is incorrect. A lecture given under such auspices is very likely to be accepted as possessing undoubted authority, and Ludwig's work is therefore, I fear, likely to be wrongly discredited by it.

Whatever the cause of Cushny's provocation, it is clear that his monograph was a major basis for the cool reception accorded the paper by Marshall and Vickers.

Eli K. Marshall, Jr.

The 1923 paper by Marshall (Fig. 5) and Vickers (39) describes experiments in dogs anesthetized with paraldehyde. In the first set of experiments the authors approximated Heidenhain's protocol. The dogs were made hypotensive by transection of the cord. In this case it was also necessary to destroy part of the thoracic cord to achieve anuria (arterial pressure $\leq$ 40 mmHg). Phenolsulfonphthalein (phenol red) was injected intravenously, and at various times the tissues were taken for analysis by colorimetry. The kidneys contained as much as a third of the injected dye.

As absolutely no urine flowed from the ureters in the above experiments, it is probable that phenolsulfonephthalein is either concentrated in the renal cells or transferred through the renal epithelium to the lumen of the tubules while no urine is being eliminated. As it is conceivable that filtration may be taking place in the glomeruli under

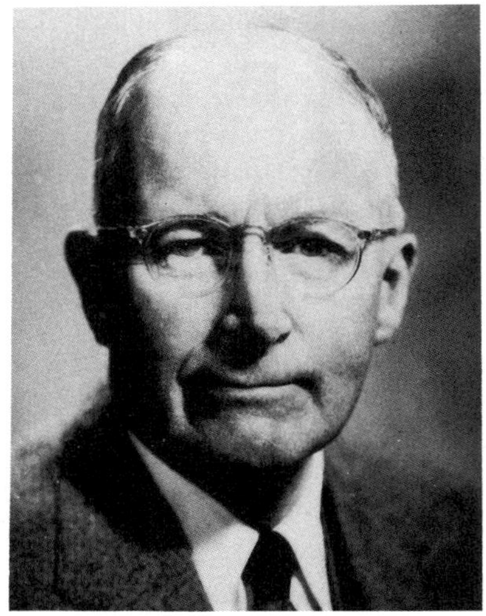

Figure 5. Eli Kennerly Marshall, Jr., (1889–1966). (Courtesy of Thomas H. Maren.)

the above conditions and all the fluid be reabsorbed in the tubules, these experiments are suggestive but not conclusive of elimination by a process other than filtration. On this hypothesis, however, filtration must cease in ten or fifteen minutes (when the phthalein content of the kidney ceases to increase) or phthalein be filtered and then reabsorbed with the water at exactly the same rate as that at which it is being filtered. Both of these assumptions would seem to be highly improbable. Evidence of another kind indicates that the phenolsulfonephthalein in the kidney is not in the lumen of the tubules or at least mainly in the cells. If one observes a kidney after longitudinal section from one of the above experiments, the contained phthalein is evident by a brilliant yellow color. It is easily noted, however, that the yellow color is confined to the cortex and that it is absent in the medullary rays of the cortex. Examination of a fresh section of such a kidney with the aid of an arc lamp and binocular microscope reveals the yellow color only in the convoluted tubules. Further examination of a teased preparation shows that the phthalein is apparently confined to the cells of the convoluted tubules and is absent from the lumen. It is, therefore, obvious that filtration cannot account for the high concentration of phthalein in the kidney, but that it is specifically taken up from the blood by the cells of the convoluted tubules.

More cogent experiments were based on the observation that phenolsulfonphthalein in plasma is to a large extent bound to circulating proteins.

Experiment 5. Dog V57, male, 10.8 kilos.

Ureters cannulated, a ten per cent solution of sodium sulphate injected intravenously (90 c.c.). At 2:52, 150 mgm of phenolsulphone-

phthalein injected. Specimens of urine and blood from the carotid obtained as follows and analyzed for phthalein. From 2:53 to 3:03, urine collected (sample I). At 2:53–3:03 blood drawn (sample I). Urine II from 3:03:40 to 3:08:50. These experiments were analyzed and gave the following results.

	RIGHT		*LEFT*	
	Volume c.c.	*Phthalein mgm*	*Volume c.c.*	*Phthalein mgm*
Urine I	*22.5*	*18.7*	*22.0*	*18.2*
Urine II	*9.8*	*7.9*	*9.0*	*8.1*

Blood I—2.86 mgm % of phthalein.
Plasma II—4.22 mgm % of phthalein.

Blood I gave 32.5 per cent corpuscles with the haematocrit. Plasma I gave by the ultrafiltration 35 per cent of the phthalein free. The kidneys together weighed 65 grams. Assuming a blood flow of 5 c.c. per gram per minute, in the five minutes during which urine sample II was collected, 1600 c.c. of blood flowed through the kidneys. Calculations from the concentration of phthalein in the blood and plasma and the hematocrit value indicate that all of the phthalein is in the plasma. Taking the value 2.86 mgm per cent which was the concentration in the blood at the commencement of the period, calculation shows that 43.8 mgm reached the kidneys. Of this, only 15 mgm were free or available for filtration. Now, since 16 mgm were eliminated by both kidneys during this time, it is obvious that filtration of all the plasma reaching the kidneys will not account for the amount eliminated.

A most remarkable graph appeared in a paper (37) published a year later (Fig. 6).

Certain scattered observations led us to believe that any direct relationship between the concentration in the blood and the rate of excretion would not be true for phenol red over any extended range of concentration. Of course, on the basis of previous work the excretion rate should depend on the amount stored in the renal cells, which should be proportional to the amount injected or the concentration in the blood. However, it is natural to suppose that at a certain concentration the renal cells would become saturated with the substance and any further increase in the rate of elimination would be brought about only by the increased amount of the free dye in the glomerular filtrate. The matter was tested as described below. Diuresis was produced in a dog. . . . The rate of excretion of urea is fairly closely proportional to the plasma concentration, while for phenol red this is true only at relatively low plasma concentrations. The kidney is much more efficient in eliminating phthalein than urea when the plasma levels are low, but exactly the reverse obtains at high plasma concentrations.

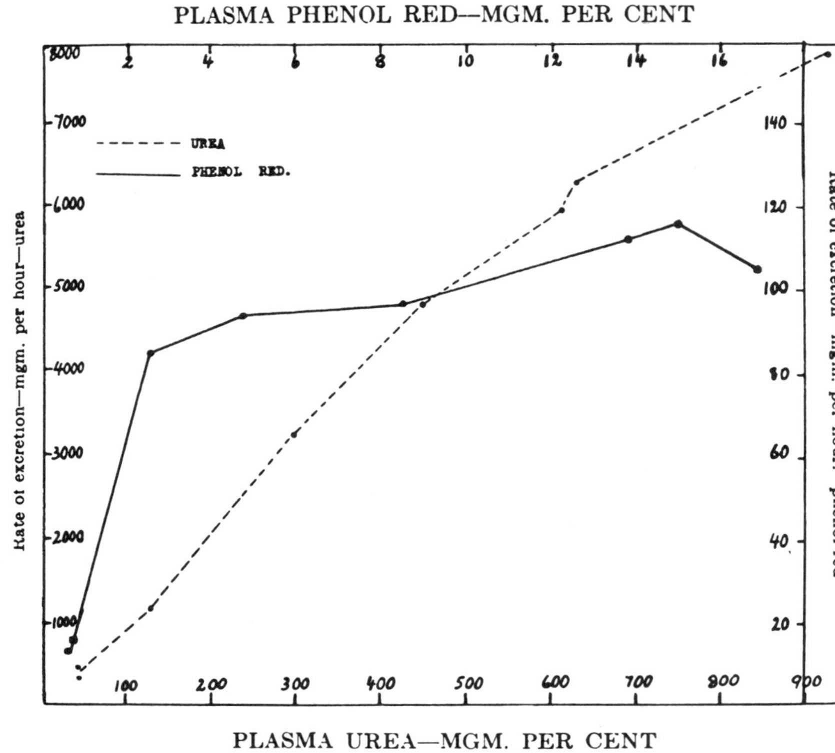

Figure 6. Figure from the 1924 paper by Marshall and Crane (37).

The gradually increased rate of elimination of the dye at the higher plasma concentrations is of course due to its increased content in the glomerular filtrate.

In this same paper (37) Marshall and Crane showed that, unlike the dog, the frog secretes urea.

Thus, over a brief span of time, Marshall and his coworkers proved the existence of tubular secretion, described saturation of the secretory mechanism, and uncovered an interesting contrast in comparative physiology. In 1928 Marshall and a medical student, Allan Lyle Grafflin (b. 1906), demonstrated the secretion of phenol red by the aglomerular kidney of the fish *Lophius piscatorius* (38). Grafflin was to chair the Department of Anatomy at Hopkins and, subsequently, became an ophthalmologist.

Cushny lived until 1926. He was aware of Marshall's papers of 1923 and 1924 and in fact met Marshall in 1923. He did not accept the existence of secretion despite the fact that E. Brice C. Mayrs in his own laboratory provided rather compelling circumstantial evidence for the secretion of urate by the avian kidney (4). After Cushny the most important holdout was A. Newton Richards (1876–1966).

It was he who, after hearing a talk of Marshall's on phenol red secretion in *Lophius*, said, "*He's found the one beast in the world that will support his theories*," or something to that effect. [The literature contains two versions of the statement and two locales for it's delivery (35, 60).] In 1937 Kempton, Bott, and Richards (33) finally demonstrated to their own satisfaction that indigo carmine is secreted in rabbits, and in 1938 Richards, Bott, and Westfall (54) demonstrated the tubular secretion of phenol red by frog kidneys. Ironically the latter study was made with doubly perfused frog kidneys, a refinement of the Nussbaum preparation.

Marshall's last major work on phenolsulfonphthalein (36) was published in 1931. He showed in dogs that the renal clearance of phenol red exceeded the clearance of creatinine and that the renal extraction of the substance can be two-thirds of that delivered by the artery. The last three pages of the paper are devoted to repudiations of the criticisms of his earlier work; it is conceivable that he enjoyed the writing.

Eli Kennerly Marshall, Jr. (1889–1966) was born in Charleston, South Carolina (35). His father's family came to this country near the beginning of the nineteenth century. His mother's family included such distinguished ancestors as a one-time governor of Connecticut and one of the founders of Yale University. The family was relatively prosperous as a result of a shoe business built up by the maternal grandfather and run by Marshall's father. Marshall was educated in private primary schools and the Charleston High School. He was a retiring youth and a good student. He attended the College of Charleston, a very small institution, where his major subject was chemistry and where he "*led a rather narrow life of the mind.*" In 1908 at the age of nineteen he matriculated at the Johns Hopkins University as a graduate student in chemistry. Here, again, he was not to be satisfied; at the conclusion of his first year at Hopkins, he arranged to transfer to the University of Chicago, but was in the end induced to return to Hopkins. Despite Marshall's dissatisfaction with the quality of the department, he enjoyed his next two years in the laboratory of Solomon F. Acree, an organic chemist. His Ph.D. thesis was a fair success; Marshall's name appears on four publications from Acree's laboratory. For reasons that are not entirely clear, he was attracted to physiological chemistry and took an assistantship in the laboratory of Walter Jones, the professor of that subject in the School of Medicine. In doing so he had moved from one weak department to another. In the summer of 1912, he traveled to Europe with a letter of introduction to the biochemist Emil Abderhalden, who was at the Physiological Institute in Halle. It was not an ideal situation for the shy American who was not adept at German and who was not favorably disposed to the Geheimrat system, but he did have an opportunity to read and become interested in enzyme action, especially the action of urease. In Baltimore later that year, he undertook chemical studies with the enzyme, eventually recognizing that it could be the basis for a highly specific assay for the estimation of urea in biological fluids. The urea method gained some visibility for Marshall and, equally important, led to his collaboration with talented clinicians interested in excretory function.

During this period Marshall attracted the attention of Abel, who arranged for his transfer to the Department of Pharmacology. It was Abel who insisted that Marshall obtain the M.D. degree, an enterprise made complex by the institutional rule forbidding members of the faculty to matriculate. He took some basic science courses at the Universities of Wisconsin and Chicago during the summers. He was never to have formal courses in physiology, pharmacology, or biochemistry, although by the time the M.D. was awarded in 1917 he had published ten papers in the *Journal of Biological Chemistry*. Fortunately for Marshall the Hopkins rule was bent; he was able to do his clinical rotations at Hopkins, and in the end he received his degree from that institution. After graduation he married his classmate, Berry Carroll, who was to become a psychiatrist. They had three children. It was wartime; Marshall was made a captain and assigned to the Chemical Warfare Service in Washington for the duration of the war to work on mustard gas. He did well by his assignment, but by happy accident he did even better by posterity. He discovered the talents and later promoted the career of Homer Smith, an enlisted man assigned to his group.

Marshall returned to Baltimore, hoping eventually to find a position in industry, but he failed. He briefly considered an offer from Peking Union Medical School, but he declined. On Abel's recommendation he was offered and accepted the Chair in Pharmacology at Washington University in St. Louis, a post he held for less than two years. The Chair in Physiology at Hopkins became available, and through Abel it was offered to Marshall, who at the time was thirty-two years old. He held the physiology position until Abel retired in 1932. The search committee for Abel's successor was chaired by Marshall, who in the end decided to accept the Hopkins pharmacology position himself. Maren (35) gives two motives for Marshall's decision: he wanted to succeed the man who had had the most influence on his career, and he felt his background in chemistry was more suited for research in pharmacology than in physiology. While still in physiology, he and his colleague Arthur Grollman did pioneering work on measurements of cardiac output using the Fick principle, work that was later extended to humans by Grollman. Most of Marshall's important work on the kidney was done in this period.

Marshall's career was characterized by a series of abrupt changes of subject (35):

In 1932 when I transferred from the Chair of Physiology to the

Chair of Pharmacology and Experimental Therapeutics [Marshall had expanded the name of the Department], *the main problem which had interested me for more than a decade in regard to renal physiology—active secretion by the convoluted tubule—was settled. It was answered in the affirmative due mainly to the investigations of myself and coworkers. A great number of problems were now apparent and waiting for solution in regard to renal excretion. These were, however, mainly a quantitative study of the qualitative framework which had been established in the past quarter of a century. I deliberately decided not to engage on them, but to seek a new field of research. Some time was spent in 1932–33 in reorganizing the laboratory course in pharmacology. This led to an interest in respiratory stimulants which lasted until the fall of 1936. One important outcome of this work was the rediscovery of the depression of respiration by oxygen and an analysis of its mechanism.*

This is not the place in which to dwell on Marshall's other and equally important contributions to science. These accomplishments are well set out by Maren (35). However, it is worth recounting an indirect contribution to renal physiologists that made many of their lives easier. Much of Marshall's monumental contribution to the pharmacology of the sulfonamides depended on a precise analytical method for the drugs. Such a method was developed and improved, culminating in the frequently cited paper by A. C. Bratton and Marshall (10) published in 1939. The work was greatly enhanced by the availability of a photoelectric colorimeter built by Morris Rosenfeld (1906–1968). Rosenfeld had worked with Abel while still a medical student and had been Marshall's collaborator in the work on respiration (8). He was well trained in physics and was a skilled instrument maker. The work on the analytical method was well known to Kenneth C. Blanchard (1900–1982), an organic chemist who was teaching biochemistry at New York University, the site of Smith's activities. Blanchard was a faithful observer of the cocktail hour, as much for the conversation as for the drinks. On one such occasion Smith was his companion and the latter bemoaned the fact that the analytical methods for the secreted substances Hippuran and Diodrast left much to be desired. Blanchard suggested that a derivative of hippuric acid bearing an aromatic amino group might have the physiological properties of Hippuran (a substituted hippurate) and be easily assayed with the Bratton-Marshall method. He synthesized a batch of *p*-aminohippuric acid for Smith. Later Blanchard joined Marshall's department, where his prodigious memory, good nature, skill at the bench, and gift as a raconteur made life easier and more entertaining for his colleagues, especially the younger of them.

Marshall was not so easily accessible. He is said to have masked his shyness by the loudness of his voice and his artful use of profanity.

He kept away from day-to-day departmental matters, leaving such things to Dorothy Wilson, the efficient and forceful secretary he had inherited from Abel. Several people have described Marshall as possessing "*absolute integrity.*" Certainly he was very direct in his speech. In scientific matters he was bold. It did not seem to worry him that a conclusion based on thoughtful analysis of carefully made observations might be wrong. For example, in 1933 Burgess, Harvey, and Marshall (11) published a paper in which they demonstrated that the characteristic response to the antidiuretic hormone could be observed only in mammals and in those birds with thin limbs of Henle's loop. They concluded that the hormone acts on the thin limb. About twenty-five years later, Robert W. Berliner gave a seminar in Baltimore on the then-emerging physiology of the countercurrent multiplier. He acknowledged the 1933 paper, and Marshall seemed pleased by the recognition of his "mistake."

Phenol Red

The use of phenol red in investigations of kidney function is one of the products of the long-standing interplay between renal and gastrointestinal physiology. Physicians and other people have been interested in cathartics since antiquity. For example, a recipe for an effective cathartic concoction is given in the Ebers papyrus (17). In the nineteenth century cathartics were the subject of investigation in the first institute for experimental pharmacology, an institute established by Rudolf Buchheim (1820–1879) at the University of Dorpat (now Tartu) in Estonia (27). Schmiedeberg, the mentor of Abel and Cushny, was Buchheim's student and successor at Dorpat before moving to Strassbourg. Both Abel and Cushny had brief encounters with the pharmacology of cathartics. Cushny did a study on saline cathartics, which (according to Smith) influenced his subsequent thinking on osmotic diuretics (60). Abel, on the other hand, studied phthalein compounds.

The cathartic action of phenolphthalein had been known since 1900, through the work of Zoltan V. Vamossy of the Pharmacology Institute of the University of Budapest. He was interested in the clinical toxicology of the compound because it had been suggested that it be used to label a certain white wine to distinguish it from illegal imitations. A sample of wine could then be alkalinized and the renal product identified by the pink color imparted by the basic form of the indicator. In his initial experiment, Vamossy ingested 1.5 grams of phenolphthalein; today the largest recommended dose is 195 mg. The efficacy of the compound was apparent shortly thereafter, the acute response lasting some ten hours and residual effects for two days. "*This observation was a warning to us to be prudent in the further choice of doses.*" (61).

Abel's goal was to discover a more soluble cathartic that could be given parenterally to patients unable to take phenolphthalein *per os*. He and his collaborator, Leonard G. Rowntree (1883–1959), studied fourteen sulfonphthaleins, among them phenol red. The compound had been synthesized in the Hopkins Chemistry Department by M. D. Sohon, who was working in the laboratory of Ira Remsen. The latter was to become president of the University. In fact, it was Remsen's leaving the chemistry department that left it in the weakened state that disappointed the graduate student Marshall. Abel and Rowntree (2) found one compound that was weakly cathartic, but it was never widely used. Of greater consequence was their observation that phenolsulfonphthalein was excreted completely by the kidneys. This finding eventually led to the development of the famous phthalein or PSP test of renal function by Rowntree and John T. Geraghty (1876–1924) in 1910 (58). The test that enjoyed widespread use in diagnosis for several decades was based on the rate of excretion of a small dose of phenol red after parenteral administration.

Rowntree was a student and collaborator of Abel for six years (61). He was born and educated in Canada, but decided to open his practice in Camden, New Jersey. After a year he felt the need for more scientific training and apprenticed himself to Abel as a volunteer. He earned his living at first by returning to Camden in the summers and working in a temporary office. By 1913 he was an Associate Professor of Pharmacology. The following year, when medicine became a full-time department, he resumed his life as a clinician. In 1916 he became Professor of Medicine at the University of Minnesota, and in 1920 he transferred to the Mayo Clinic in Rochester. In 1932 he became Director of the Philadelphia Institute for Medical Research. Shortly before World War II, he was appointed Chief of the Medical Division of the National Selective Service. Rowntree was an eminent clinical investigator. With his various colleagues, he was the first to demonstrate the nature of water intoxication; he introduced the intraveous pyelogram and the use of iodine compounds for visualization of the lungs. His book *Amid Masters of Twentieth Century Medicine* (57) gives an interesting account of his life and times.

Geraghty, a native of Minnesota, earned a Ph.D. from the St. Paul Seminary and later an M.D. from Hopkins (24). He worked his way through the ranks of the Urology Division and for the last ten years of his short life he was Professor of Clinical Urology and Assistant Director of the James Buchanan Brady Urological Institute at Hopkins. The institute is named for its benefactor "Diamond Jim" Brady. Both Geraghty and Rowntree collaborated with Marshall in his early days. Rowntree was especially influential in encouraging the work on urease.

Thus it is not surprising that Marshall had an interest in the mechanism of phenol red excretion: it was synthesized in the department where he wrote his Ph.D. thesis, he was a protege of the man who demonstrated that phenol red is excreted exclusively by the kidneys, and he was a colleague of the two men who developed the phthalein test of renal function.

The two decades after Marshall quit renal physiology were filled with remarkable discoveries by his contemporaries and juniors: the clearance of inulin was established as the measure of filtration rate, thereby allowing quantification of net secretion and reabsorption, competitive inhibition of transport was demonstrated, techniques for study of transport in vitro were developed, the micropuncture technique matured, studies of metabolic inhibitors began, and the first attempt to apply kinetic theory to renal transport was made. These matters are subjects of other chapters in this volume.

Organic Bases

This convoluted story deals next with a paper by Robert Chambers (1881–1957) and Rudolph T. Kempton (1902–1972) on the excretion of neutral red by doubly perfused frog kidneys (13). Unlike phenol red, which is a sulfonic acid, and indigo carmine, which is a disulfonic acid, neutral red is a weak organic base with a pK_a of 6.9. Chambers and Kempton observed that the dye was scarcely excreted when presented to the glomeruli via the arterial circulation, a phenomenon attributable to the extensive binding of the dye to plasma proteins. In contrast, when the dye was presented to the peritubular circulation via the renal portal system, excretion was abundant and notably greater when the urine was acid than when alkaline. These and other findings led them to postulate that the dye entered the tubular fluid by diffusion of the basic (nonionized) form, and when the urine was acid the base became protonated and thus trapped in the urine by its ionic, nonpermeant nature. This diffusion-and-capture mechanism is now commonly known as ion-trapping or nonionic diffusion. The general mechanism had been identified in other, nonrenal systems as far back as the nineteenth century. Later Kempton (32) was to show that the excretion of phenol red did not depend on the pH of urine, thus completing the contrast between a dye that is secreted by active transport and one that is apparently secreted by a passive process.

Robert Chambers was one of the most distinguished general physiologists of the first half of this century (61). He was born of Canadian parents, who at the time were Presbyterian missionaries in Turkey. He showed the inclinations of a naturalist at an early age; later he organized a Natural History Society while a student at Roberts College in Constantinople. Subsequently he earned an M.A. at Queens College in Kingston, Ontario, and a Ph.D. from the University of Munich. He held academic posts at Toronto, Cincinnati, Cornell University College of Medicine, and finally at New York

University, where he was made research professor of biology in 1928. Chambers played an important role in interesting Richards in the micromanipulator. He later developed explants of chick mesonephros and demonstrated their secretion of phenol red and the action of inhibitors thereon.

Harvey Bernhardt Haag (1900–1961) was the Professor of Pharmacology at the Medical College of Virginia from 1933 to 1947. He was a longtime student of the pharmacology of nicotine and became interested in the wide variation in urinary excretion of the toxin among smokers, despite comparable levels of intake. He and his associates were able to attribute this variation to differences in urinary pH (22), and later they extended the study to another organic base, quinine. Their interpretation was that ion trapping inhibited the reabsorption of the filtered bases somewhere in the genitourinary tract. They did not make determinations of clearances, and thus the interpretation was entirely speculative.

The renal excretion of organic bases attracted considerable attention during World War II as a result of extensive use of antimalarial drugs by troops in the Pacific theater. At the time it was difficult to estimate concentrations of drugs in plasma in the field in order to establish adequate dosage or compliance. The analytical methods were difficult, and the necessary equipment was frequently unavailable. Estimations of the rates of drug excretion were more easily obtained, but these proved to be extremely variable even when concentrations in plasma were constant. Eventually it was appreciated that the rate of drug excretion is dependent on urinary pH. The excretion of ammonia (as ammonium ion) is also pH dependent. Thus it became possible to develop formulas by which plasma levels of a drug could be roughly estimated by determining both its rate of excretion and the rate of excretion of ammonia.

Jack Orloff and Berliner (47) were the first to attempt a theoretical analysis of the excretion of bases by nonionic diffusion. They showed clearly that it is theoretically possible to achieve a high rate of renal clearance by nonionic diffusion when urine pH is acid. This treatment was extended by M. D. Milne, B. H. Scribner and M. A. Crawford (41) in a brilliant review article published in 1958. In both instances the theoretical models excluded any participation of active transport.

Quaternary Compounds

In 1947 B. R. Rennick and her colleagues (53) at the University of Michigan demonstrated the tubular secretion of the organic cation tetraethylammonium ion (TEA) in dogs, and Ivar Sperber (b. 1914) (62) of Uppsala, Sweden, demonstrated the secretion of another quaternary ion, N^1-methylnicotinamide (NMN) in chickens. The excretion of quaternary compounds was difficult to study in 1947. Such materials usually have intense pharmacological activity; for example, TEA is a powerful ganglionic blocking agent. Therefore concentrations in plasma had to be kept low and the analytical methods were too insensitive for these levels. In both instances remarkable ingenuity was required to circumvent the difficulty. The Sperber technique consisted of injecting the test compound into one thigh of a chicken and collecting urine from each kidney separately. By virtue of the renal portal circulation, the tubules on the injected side have access to the compound before it reaches the general circulation. Secretion, when it occurs, is revealed by a greater excretion of compound by the kidney on the injected side. The analogy with the Nussbaum experiment is clear. The technique has been refined and it remains quite useful.

The Michigan group used several approaches; one will serve as an example: TEA, *p*-aminohippurate, and creatinine were infused continuously into one renal artery of a dog, and urine was collected from each ureter separately. The excess of a substance appearing from the infused kidney over that from the other, divided by the rate of infusion, is a measure of its extraction by the infused kidney on the first pass of blood through it. Both *p*-aminohippurate and TEA were extracted to a greater extent than was creatinine, the latter being taken as a substance excreted by filtration only.

Barbara Ruth Rennick (Fig. 7) was a medical student at the time of this discovery. She was already proficient in laboratory work, having spent a few years as a pharmacologist in industry. At the time

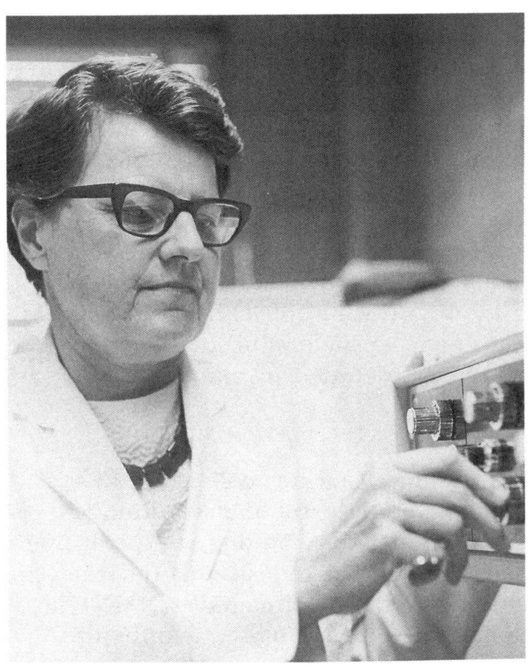

Figure 7. Barbara Ruth Rennick (b. 1919).

she earned the M.D. degree, one of her teachers and a collaborator in the 1947 study, G. K. Moe (b. 1915), moved to Syracuse to become Chairman of the Department of Physiology at the State University of New York, Upstate Medical Center. He recruited Rennick, who remained in Syracuse until 1961 when she moved to Mt. Holyoke College to direct a new physiology program. Three years later she joined the pharmacology department in Buffalo, New York, where she remained until her retirement. Rennick visited Sperber early in her career and learned his technique, which she modified and applied to great advantage in a large number of fundamental studies (52). Moe, her mentor, had only modest interest in renal function. At the time of their discovery, Moe was a major authority on the pharmacology of autonomic ganglia. He was also and remains a leading investigator of cardiac function.

Lawrence Peters (1917–1977) was among the most prolific investigators of the excretion of organic cations. His masterly review (48) clearly distinguished the separate mechanisms for the secretion of organic cations and anions. Peters, a Canadian by birth, received a Ph.D. in pharmacology at the University of Minnesota in 1942 and an M.D. from the Western Reserve University in 1950 (65). From 1942 to 1944, he worked with Beyer's group at Sharp & Dohme and was involved in the early work on the disposition of penicillin. This experience was his introduction to renal physiology. Peters served on the faculty at Western Reserve and as Chairman of the Department of Pharmacology at Tulane (1953–1955) and Kansas (1955–1964). He ended his unfortunately short career as Executive Vice President for Research at McNeil Laboratories.

Bidirectional Transport

James Augustine Shannon's (b. 1904) work and thinking in renal physiology were among the best in his time. Thus it is all the more remarkable that one of his prescient statements should have been widely ignored. In 1947, with Joseph W. Jailer (1914–1960) and Rosenfeld, he published a short, almost cryptic paper (30) on the excretion of antimalarial drugs in humans and the effects of ingesting alkalinizing and acidifying salts thereon. The work had been done in the Research Service, Third Medical Division, at the Goldwater Memorial Hospital in New York. Shannon was director of the service. Rosenfeld, the same man who worked with Marshall, was assigned to New York by the army. Jailer later became a prominent endocrinologist. The authors suggested that bases are secreted by active transport and that the extent of their reabsorption is determined by the factors that modify nonionic diffusion; that is, alkalinization of urine enhances reabsorption, whereas acidification reduces it. Certainly there was not enough evidence to establish that there is net secretion by active transport. Indeed, the Orloff and Berliner paper

(47) published nine years later provided a theoretical basis for the proposition that secretion occurs through ion trapping alone. Thus in 1956 one could argue that quaternary compounds are secreted by active transport and that amines (bases) are secreted by a passive process.

Ironically there was at the time strong, but not widely recognized, evidence against the preceding view. In 1953 Orloff, Aronow, and Berliner (46) discovered that the drug tolazoline is secreted by a saturable mechanism. Tolazoline is a base, not a quaternary, and undoubtedly Orloff et al. appreciated the importance of this observation. Indeed, they attempted to ascertain whether or not there could be competition for transport between tolazoline and the quaternary *N′*-methylnicotinamide. Unfortunately the attempt was frustrated by hemodynamic changes produced by the compounds when given together.

Mecamylamine, a ganglionic blocking agent, is another base, the renal clearance of which depends on the pH of urine. In the original publication on the subject, Baer, Paulson, Russo, and Beyer (4) demonstrated in a single animal that the renal clearance could vary from a high of over 280 ml/min to a low of 3 ml/min when urine pH was changed from 5.6 to 8.3. In this case the glomerular filtration rate of the dog was about 50 ml/min. The authors speculated that the shift in direction of transport from net secretion to net reabsorption might be a manifestation of a single active transport mechanism, the orientation of which depends on the pH of tubular fluid. This speculation was later proven wrong by Pilkington and Keyl (49), who showed that the major site of secretion is the proximal tubule and the major site of reabsorption is the distal nephron. Remarkably, however, the speculation strikes close to the mechanism by which organic cations move from cell to lumen (28).

The work on Mecamylamine is one of an enormous number of contributions that emanated from the laboratory of Karl H. Beyer, Jr. (b. 1914). Beyer's work on diuretics is discussed in the chapter by Maren, which also contains a biographical note and a portrait of him. A partial list of his other contributions to the physiology and pharmacology of the kidney would include studies on the elimination of sulfonamides, extension of the idea of competition for secretion, development of the drug carinamide, development of probenecid, studies on the transport of amino acids, studies on the excretion of synthetic organic acids and bases, and so forth (7).

John Elston Baer (b. 1917) was a longtime associate and frequent collaborator of Beyer's. Baer was trained as an organic chemist. During World War II he worked with the group at Goldwater Memorial Hospital, where he contributed largely to the development of analytical methods for antimalarials and other drugs. After joining Beyer's group at Sharp & Dohme (later the Merck Institute), he became heavily involved in the renal program. In 1971 he became Senior Director of Drug Metabolism, a position from which he is now retired.

Thus, by the latter part of the 1950s, it was fairly clear that there was bidirectional transport of organic bases, but there was no agreement with regard to mechanisms. With regard to secretion, Beyer's group, agreeing with Shannon's speculation, favored active transport; Orloff and Berliner and Milne's group favored secretion by ion trapping for at least some compounds. With regard to reabsorption, Beyer's group favored active transport; Shannon favored nonionic diffusion, as did Milne and Berliner.

The general idea of bidirectional transport was well known, the great breakthrough having come from studies of the excretion of potassium (6, 43). There were other lines of evidence as well, these stemming from studies of the excretion of sulfate and thiosulfate, creatinine, uric acid, and in the salamander *Necturus*, Diodrast and *p*-aminohippurate. In these instances the weight of evidence favored (and still favors) active transport in both directions. The literature on these subjects is summarized in a review by Berglund (5) published in 1961.

Fredrik Berglund was a major contributor to the literature on the renal excretion of sulfate and thiosulfate and many other subjects. He was born in the United States of European parents and was moved to Stockholm when he was eight. He attended the Karolinska Institutet, gaining medical licensure in 1950 and a doctorate in 1960. The years 1951 to 1957 were spent in the United States, where he had fruitful collaborations with Forster, William D. Lotspeich, Julius J. Cohen, and Rennick. He returned to the Karolinska in 1957, joined the Swedish National Institute of Public Health in 1964, and joined the Medical Research Department of KabiVitrum Pharmaceuticals in 1974.

Berglund's thinking on bidirectional active transport was influenced considerably by work on the excretion of urate and other substances in the laboratory of Alexander B. Gutman (1902–1973). Gutman was a New Yorker; he earned B.A., M.A., and Ph.D. degrees from Cornell University and the M.D. from the University of Vienna (50). From 1929 until 1947, he was on the full-time staff at the Columbia-Presbyterian Medical Center, and from 1947 to 1951 he was director of the Columbia Research Service at the Goldwater Memorial Hospital. In 1951 he was appointed Director, Department of Medicine, and Physician-in-Chief at the Mount Sinai Hospital in New York. Gutman founded the *American Journal of Medicine* in 1946 and was the editor of that journal until 1971. He was a prolific writer; much of his work dealt with gout, urate metabolism, and renal physiology. He and his longtime colleague, Ts'ai-Fan Yü (b. 1911) were the enunciators of the three-component mechanism for the excretion of uric acid (20).

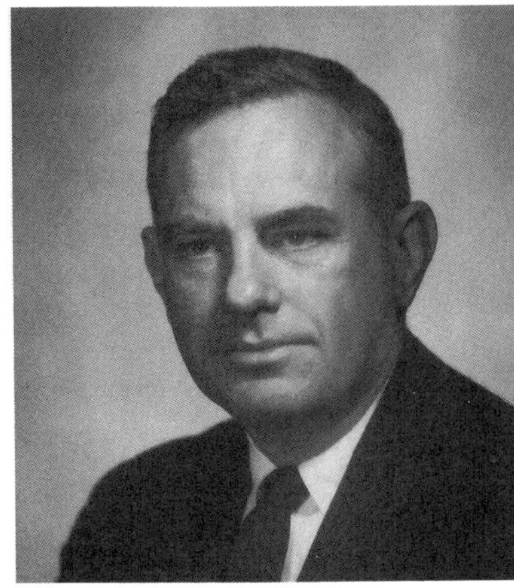

Figure 8. Gilbert Horton Mudge (b. 1915) in 1962.

An Accidental Synthesis

In 1955 Gilbert Horton Mudge (Fig. 8) was appointed successor to Marshall in the Department of Pharmacology and Experimental Therapeutics at Hopkins. Mudge, the son of an attorney, was born in Brooklyn. He attended Amherst College and later, the College of Physicians and Surgeons, Columbia University, earning the M.D. in 1941. His academic career was interrupted by service in the US Army Air Corps during World War II. At the time he was called to Hopkins, Mudge was an associate professor of medicine at Columbia and was already well established as a renal physiologist. He had worked in the laboratory of Alfred Gilman (1908–1984), the eminent pharmacologist, and was one of the discoverers of the tubular secretion of potassium. He had collaborated with John V. Taggart (b. 1916), and with Taggart he had demonstrated the inhibition in vivo of the secretion of *p*-aminohippurate by 2,4-dinitrophenol. He was a pioneer in the study of electrolyte transport by mitochondria. Mudge stayed at Hopkins for seven years. By modern standards his department was small, relaxed, and productive. He left for Dartmouth in 1962, first to be dean of the medical school, and he remained there serving in various capacities until his retirement.

One of the first projects Mudge undertook at Hopkins was an attempt to elucidate the basis for the failure of mercurial diuretics to elicit diuresis when a man or a dog is producing an alkaline urine. At one point it became desirable to learn the site in the dog nephron at which the incipient urine showed the greatest change in pH. Definitive methods were not at hand, but two factors conspired to suggest an approach to the problem. One, the stop-flow technique had recently been developed by the Michigan group (34) and was being extensively exploited by them and by Pitts and his associates.

Two, the Orloff and Berliner paper (47) on nonionic diffusion had just been published. Perhaps a stop-flow experiment would localize the site of acidification. If the pH of the voided samples didn't localize acidification, perhaps the excretory pattern of a weak electrolyte would.

Salicylic acid was chosen as the weak electrolyte. The analytical method was convenient, and Orloff and Berliner had speculated that salicylate is handled by a mechanism analogous to that of weak bases, the difference being that the effect of changes in urinary pH is opposite.

The stop-flow pattern revealed distinct evidence for active secretion in the proximal tubule and reabsorption downstream (68). Subsequent experiments revealed that the secretion could be blocked by competitive inhibitors, that reabsorption is a limitless (passive) process, that the same general pattern applies to bases, and that bases and quaternary compounds could compete for secretion (67). Marshall was amused by the findings.

Epilogue

The irony of Shannon's group suggesting the "correct" mechanisms for the excretion of many weak electrolytes with minimal evidence has already been observed. It is equally notable that Gutman et al. (21) had nearly all the evidence necessary to establish the mechanisms as early as 1955. Laudable caution and the zeitgeist prevented their making the matter explicit.

The literature after 1960 reveals many different patterns for the excretion of weak electrolytes. It also reveals a large body of information on the mechanisms underlying these phenomena. Such matters are summarized in several recent articles (17, 41, 64).

REFERENCES

1. Abel, J. J. Arthur Robertson Cushny and pharmacology. *J. Pharmacol. Exp. Ther.* 27: 265–283, 1926.
2. Abel, J. J., and L. G. Rowntree. On the pharmacological action of some phthaleins and their derivatives, with especial reference to their behavior as purgatives. I. *J. Pharmacol. Exp. Ther.* 1: 231–264, 1909–1910.
3. Alfert, M. Heidenhain, Martin. In: *Dictionary of Scientific Biography.* New York: Scribner, 1972, vol. VI, p. 223–224.
4. Baer, J. E., S. F. Paulson, H. F. Russo, and K. H. Beyer. Renal elimination of 3-methylaminoisocamphane hydrochloride (mecamylamine). *Am. J. Physiol.* 186: 180–186, 1956.
5. Berglund, F. Urinary excretion patterns for substances with simultaneous secretion and reabsorption by active transport. *Acta Physiol. Scand.* 52: 276–290, 1961.
6. Berliner, R. W., and T. J. Kennedy, Jr. Renal tubular secretion of potassium in the dog. *Proc. Soc. Exp. Biol. Med.* 67: 542–545, 1948.

7. Beyer, K. H., Jr. A career or two. *Annu. Rev. Pharmacol. Toxicol.* 17: 1–10, 1977.
8. Blanchard, K. C. Obituary—Morris Rosenfeld. *The Pharmacologist* 10: 82–83, 1968.
9. Bowman, W. On the structure and use of the malpighian bodies of the kidney, with observations on the circulation through that gland. *Philos. Trans. R. Soc. Lond.* 132: 57–80, 1842.
10. Bratton, A. C., and E. K. Marshall. New coupling component for sulfanilamide determination. *J. Biol. Chem.* 128: 537–550, 1939.
11. Brunton, L. Ludwig's and other theories of the secretion of urine and the action of diuretics. *Proc. R. Soc. Med. Ther. Pharmacol. Section* 5: 134–151, 1911–12.
12. Burgess, W. W., A. M. Harvey, and E. K. Marshall, Jr. The site of the antidiuretic action of pituitary extract. *J. Pharmacol. Exp. Ther.* 49: 237–249, 1933.
13. Chambers, R., and R. T. Kempton. The elimination of neutral red by the frog's kidney. *J. Cell. Comp. Physiol.* 10: 199–221, 1937.
14. Cushny, A. R. *A Text Book of Pharmacology and Therapeutics or the Action of Drugs in Health in Disease.* Philadelphia, PA: Lea & Febiger, 1899.
15. Cushny, A. R. *The Action and Uses in Medicine of Digitalis and Its Allies.* London: Longmans Green, 1925.
16. Cushny, A. R. *The Secretion of the Urine.* (2nd ed.). London: Longmans Green, 1926.
17. Ebbell, B. *The Ebers Papyrus, The Greatest Egyptian Medical Document.* Copenhagen: Levin & Munksgaard, 1937.
18. Grantham, J. J., and A. M. Chonko. Renal handling of organic anions and cations; metabolism and excretion of uric acid. In: *The Kidney,* edited by B. M. Brenner and F. C. Rector, Jr. Philadelphia, PA: Saunders, 1986.
19. Gruetzner, P. Zum Andenken an Rudolf Heidenhain. *Pfluegers Arch. Gesamte Physiol. Menschen Tiere* 72: 221–265, 1898.
20. Gutman, A. B., and T. F. Yü. A three-component system for regulation of renal excretion of uric acid in man. *Trans. Assoc. Am. Physicians* 74: 353–365, 1961.
21. Gutman, A. B., T. F. Yü, and J. H. Sirota. A study by simultaneous clearance techniques, of salicylate excretion in man. Effect of alkalinization of the urine by bicarbonate administration; effect of probenecid. *J. Clin. Invest.* 34: 711–721, 1955.
22. Haag, A. B., and P. S. Larson. Studies on the fate of nicotine in the body. I. The effect of pH on the urinary excretion of nicotine by tobacco smokers. *J. Pharmacol. Exp. Ther.* 76: 235–239, 1942.
23. Hall, T. S. *History of General Physiology.* Chicago, IL: Univ. of Chicago Press, 1969, vol. 2.
24. Harvey, A. M. Pharmacology's giant: John Jacob Abel. *Johns Hopkins Med. J.* 135: 245–258, 1974.
25. Heidenhain, R. Versuche über den Vorgang der Harnabsonderung. *Pfluegers Arch. Gesamte Physiol. Menschen Tiere* 9: 1–27, 1874.
26. Heidenhain, R. Die Harnabsonderung. In: *Hermann's Handbuch der Physiologie.* Leipzig, Germany: Vogel, 1883, vol. 5, p. 279ff.
27. Holmstedt, B., and G. Liljestrand. *Readings in Pharmacology.* New

York: Macmillan, 1963.
28. Holohan, P. D., and C. R. Ross. Mechanisms of organic cation transport in kidney plasma membrane vesicles. 2. ΔpH studies. *J. Pharmacol. Exp. Ther.* 216: 294–298, 1981.
29. Hoppe-Seyler, E. F. I. *Physiologische Chemie*. Berlin: Hirschwald, 1881, p. 159, 795.
30. Jailer, J. W., M. Rosenfeld, and J. A. Shannon. The influence of orally administered alkali and acid on the renal excretion of quinacrine, chloroquine and santoquine. *J. Clin. Invest.* 26: 1168–1172, 1947.
31. Kempton, R. T. Nussbaum's experiment on renal secretion. *Am. J. Physiol.* 119: 175–185, 1937.
32. Kempton, R. T. Differences in the elimination of neutral red and phenol red by the frog kidney. *J. Cell. Comp. Physiol.* 14: 73–81, 1939.
33. Kempton, R. T., P. A. Bott, and A. N. Richards. The glomerular elimination of indigo carmine in rabbits. *Am. J. Anat.* 61: 505–521, 1937.
34. Malvin, R. L., W. S. Wilde, and L. P. Sullivan. Localization of nephron transport by stop flow analysis. *Am. J. Physiol.* 194: 135–142, 1958.
35. Maren, T. H. Eli Kennerly Marshall, Jr. *Biogr. Mem. Natl. Acad. Sci.* 56: 313–352, 1987.
36. Marshall, E. K., Jr. The secretion of phenol red by the mammalian kidney. *Am. J. Physiol.* 99: 77–86, 1931.
37. Marshall, E. K., Jr., and M. M. Crane. The secretory function of the renal tubules. *Am. J. Physiol.* 70: 465–488, 1924.
38. Marshall, E. K., Jr., and A. L. Grafflin. The structure and function of the kidney of *Lophius piscatorius*. *Bull. Johns Hopkins Hosp.* 43: 205–235, 1928.
39. Marshall, E. K., Jr., and J. L. Vickers. The mechanism of the elimination of phenolsulphonephthalein by the kidney—a proof of secretion by the convoluted tubules. *Bull. Johns Hopkins Hosp.* 34: 1–6, 1923.
40. Mayrs E. B. Secretion as a factor in elimination by the bird's kidney. *J. Physiol. Lond.* 58: 276–287, 1924.
41. Milne, M. D., B. H. Scribner, and M. A. Crawford. Non-ionic diffusion and the excretion of weak acids and bases. *Am. J. Med.* 24: 709–729, 1958.
42. Møller, J. V., and I. Sheikh. The renal organic anion transport system: pharmacological, physiological, and biochemical aspects. *Pharmacol. Rev.* 34: 315–358, 1982.
43. Mudge, G. H., J. Foulks, and A. Gilman. The renal excretion of potassium. *Proc. Soc. Exp. Biol. Med.* 67: 545–547, 1948.
44. Nussbaum, M. Über die Secretion der Niere. *Pfluegers Arch. Gesamte Physiol. Menschen Tiere* 16: 139–143, 1878.
45. Nussbaum, M. Fortgesetzte Untersuchungen über die Secretion der Niere. *Pfluegers Arch. Gesamte Physiol. Menschen Tiere* 17: 580–594, 1878.
46. Orloff, J., L. Aronow, and R. W. Berliner. The transport of Priscoline by the renal tubules. *J. Pharmacol. Exp. Ther.* 109: 214–217, 1953.
47. Orloff, J., and R. W. Berliner. The mechanism of the excretion of ammonia in the dog. *J. Clin. Invest.* 35: 223–235, 1956.
48. Peters, L. Renal tubular excretion of organic bases. *Pharmacol. Rev.* 12: 1–35, 1960.

49. Pilkington, L. A., and M. J. Keyl. Stop-flow analyses of mepiperphenidol and mecamylamine in the dog. *Am. J. Physiol.* 205: 471–476, 1963.
50. Popper, H. Alexander B. Gutman, 1902-1973. *Am. J. Med.* 54: 690–693, 1973.
51. Radbill, S. X. Isaacs, Charles Edward. In: *Dictionary of Scientific Biography.* New York: Scribner, 1973, vol. VIII, p. 23–24.
52. Rennick, B. R. Proximal tubular transport and renal metabolism of organic cations and catechol. In: *Methods in Pharmacology*, edited by M. Martinez-Maldonado. New York: Plenum, 1976, vol. 4A, p. 335–356.
53. Rennick, B. R., G. K. Moe, R. H. Lyons, S. W. Hoobler, and R. Neligh. Absorption and renal excretion of the tetraethylammonium ion. *J. Pharmacol. Exp. Ther.* 91: 210–217, 1947.
54. Richards, A. N., P. A. Bott, and B. B. Westfall. Experiments concerning the possibility that inulin is secreted by the renal tubules. *Am. J. Physiol.* 123: 281–298, 1938.
55. Rosen, G. Ludwig, Carl Friedrich Wilhelm. In: *Dictionary of Scientific Biography.* New York: Scribner, 1973, vol. VIII, p. 540–542.
56. Rothschuh, K. E. *Geschichte der Physiologie.* Berlin: Springer-Verlag, 1953. History of Physiology, transl. by G. B. Riese. Huntington, N.Y.: Kreiger, 1973.
57. Rowntree, L. G. *Amid Masters of Twentieth Century Medicine.* Springfield, IL: Thomas, 1958.
58. Rowntree, L. G., and J. T. Geraghty. An experimental and clinical study of the functional activity of the kidneys by means of phenolsulphonephthalein. *J. Pharmacol. Exp. Ther.* 1: 579–661, 1909–10.
59. Shannon, J. A. Renal tubular excretion. *Physiol. Rev.* 19: 63–93, 1939.
60. Smith, H. W. Renal physiology between two wars. In: *Lectures on the Kidney.* Lawrence: Univ. of Kansas, Extension Div., 1943, p. 63–82.
61. Smith, H. W. Highlights in the history of renal physiology. *Georgetown Med. Bull.* 13: 4–48, 1959.
62. Sperber, I. The mechanism of renal excretion of some 'detoxication products' in the chicken. *Proc. Int. Congr. Physiol. Sci., 17th, Oxford, 1947*, p. 217–218.
63. Starling, E. H. Glomerular functions of the kidney. *J. Physiol. Lond.* 24: 317–330, 1899.
64. Thomas, K. B. Bowman, William. In: *Dictionary of Scientific Biography.* New York: Scribner, 1970, vol. II, p. 375–377.
65. Volle, R. L., and E. J . Walaszek. Lawrence Peters. *The Pharmacologist* 20: 27–28, 1978.
66. Weiner, I. M. Organic acids and bases. In: *The Kidney: Physiology and Pathophysiology*, edited by D. W. Seldin and G. Giebisch. New York: Raven, 1985, p. 1703–1724.
67. Weiner, I. M., and G. H. Mudge. Renal tubular mechanisms for excretion of organic acids and bases. *Am. J. Med.* 36: 743–762, 1964.
68. Weiner, I. M., J. A. Washington, and G. H. Mudge. Studies on the renal excretion of salicylate in the dog. *Bull. Johns Hopkins Hosp.* 105: 284–297, 1959.

XIII

Diuretics and Renal Drug Development

THOMAS H. MAREN

THE concept of diuresis, or the idea of a diuretic drug, is very old. Roots, plants, and minerals were known from ancient to renaissance times to increase the flow of urine, and it was thought vaguely that this was helpful in the treatment of cardiac edema, or dropsy. The word *diuretic* comes from the Greek *dia* (through) and *ouron* (urine) through Latin and Middle English.

DIURETICS

Until the end of the eighteenth century, there was no satisfactory treatment for cardiac failure, and patients suffered with enormous swellings of limbs and abdomen, as shown in Figure 1. Treatment was often mechanical, with tubes inserted into regions of edema or ascites. *Guy's Hospital Lectures in Medicine* in 1802 (Fig. 2) lists various diuretics, with remarkable attention to failures and lack of rationale for their use.

Because renal function was not given any firm base until the time of Bowman in the mid-nineteenth century, there could scarcely be a pharmacology of diuretics. In 1785 William Withering, in consultation with Erasmus Darwin, prescribed a decoction of digitalis leaf for a dropsical woman, which "*acted very powerfully upon the kidneys, for within the first twenty-four hours she made upwards of eight quarts of urine.*" But Withering (72) knew that he must dissociate the action of digitalis on the heart from that on the kidney, and that was his great triumph: "*that it has a power over the motion of the heart, to a degree yet unobserved in any other medicine, and that this power may be converted to salutary ends.*" It has taken nearly 200 years for the action of digitalis on either the heart or the kidney to receive any satisfactory physiological-chemical explanation, and there is as yet no absolute consensus.

After Bowman's extraordinary anatomy and the inspired physiol-

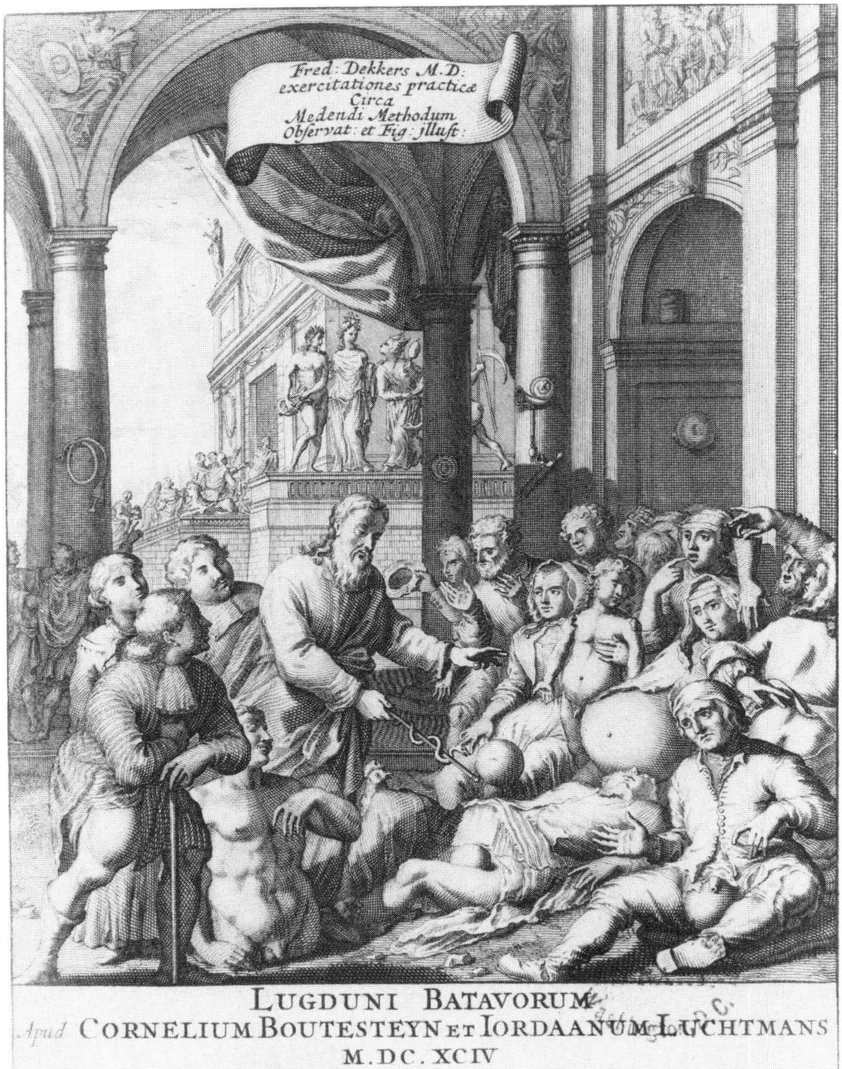

Figure 1. Frontispiece of Frederik Dekkers's *Exercitationes practical circa methodum medendi* (*Practical Exercises in Methods of Treatment*), first published in Leyden, 1673. The painting by Joseph Mueder shows the physician passing among the sick, many of whom have swollen limbs and abdomen. This book contains the first clear description of proteinuria, noting precipitation of urine with heat or acetic acid. (Courtesy of the National Library of Medicine.)

ogy of Ludwig and Heidenhain, there still was about 80 years of research, mystification, and polemics before there could be a science of renal pharmacology. It is at this point that I take up the story.

This field is two-thirds of a century old. I (the same age) have been privileged to know most of the actors on this stage and to have been

617. *Diuretics*, generally indicated, but often disappoint expectation, and of themselves rarely adequate to a cure.—Accurate comparison of their powers much wanted.—The kinds indicated under certain circumstances.—Particular articles;—Squills, and its combinations:—Colchicum; its uncertainty and frequent failure:—Lactuca Virosa,—testimony of Collin and Stoll in favour of it;—probable mode in which it operates.—Bacher's Pills.—Cuprum Ammoniatum, et vitriolatum.—Nicotiana; difficulty attending the rationale of its operation.—Digitalis; striking opposition of testimony respecting it;—attempt to explain its diuretic effect upon a new principle:—management necessary to render it safe.—Opium? occasionally operates as a diuretic.—Diluted acids, and mild saline neutrals;—Nitre,—Kali Acetatum, &c.—*Stimulant Diuretics*; Tinct. Cantharidis,—doubts and cautions respecting its employment.—Infus. Sinapeos, Raph. Rustic. et Dauci Sylv.—Decoct. Petroselini, cacuminis Genistæ, folior Cynaræ, &c.—Turpentines and Balsams,—Cerevisia Pini,—Aq. Picis;—Æthers, &c.

Figure 2. A paragraph from "General Cure of Dropsy" in *Outlines of a Course of Lectures on the Practice of Medicine*, delivered in the Medical School of Guy's Hospital by William Babington and James Curry in London (1802–1806).

one. My main themes are the interactions between industry and academics and among chemists, physiologists, pharmacologists, and clinicians. This chapter is written in hopes that it may engender to some degree the same spirited cooperation well into the next century.

The inclusion of this chapter in a physiological series indicates the inevitable and close relationship between drug research and physiological exploration. Surprisingly this has not always been the case. In the early part of this century, many of the leading contributors to renal physiology were professors of pharmacology. However, until relatively recently, these illustrious men and their successors made comparatively little use of pharmacological findings. Arthur Cushny, Professor of Pharmacology at the University of Edinburgh and at the University of Michigan, wrote the most important book (22) on renal physiology in that era; the first edition was published in 1917 and the second in 1926.

In the second edition, he stated briefly that mercury in various forms increases the secretion of urine and that this has been recognized for several centuries. He added that it is natural to suppose that diuresis arises from a direct action on the kidney, perhaps from a mild irritation, which may increase filtration at the glomerulus and at the same time dilate the vessels. A. N. Richards, Professor of Pharmacology at the University of Pennsylvania and the great pioneer in micropuncture, apparently never used a mercurial or any drug in his investigation. E. K. Marshall, Professor of Pharmacology at Johns Hopkins who proved the existence of renal secretion in 1923, appeared equally innocent of the applications of diuretics to answer the many vexing questions that arose in renal physiology in the 1920s.

A pioneering study on the action of diuretic drugs written in 1934 by the Boston clinician Herman Blumgart et al. (11) states that the nature and mechanism of their action remains obscure. Part of the reason for this was that the analysis of electrolytes was extremely difficult: Na^+ and K^+ had to be measured by cumbersome and (for Na^+) gravimetric analysis; admittedly carbon dioxide, Cl^-, and phosphate measurements were relatively simple. Importantly, there was little understanding of renal mechanisms on which to base theories of diuretic action. After Blumgart, a modest literature arose in the 1930s and 1940s on the action of mercurial diuretics. These were the only drugs of their kind, with the exception of the xanthines, which then (incorrectly) were thought to act by increasing filtration, not via a tubular mechanism.

The situation changed radically in about 1946. Homer Smith, James Shannon, and Robert Pitts had made their influence felt: there was a science of renal physiology. At the same time came the invention of the flame photometer, which meant that any laboratory could readily investigate electrolyte excretion. Some physiologists, particularly clinicians interested in cardiology and nephrology, became pharmacologists overnight. These stories are told in more detail in the sections on carbon anhydrase inhibitors (p. 436) and thiazide diuretics (p. 442). An intimate relationship arose between the men and women studying electrolyte excretion and those developing new drugs. This has lasted to the present day; the development of sophisticated methods of micropuncture and work in the isolated tubule have incorporated fully the use of these compounds, which in turn have thrown enormous light on the various reabsorptive and secretory processes in the renal tubule. This has gone so far that renal pharmacology has almost disappeared from the ranks of the Pharmacological Society, and the best and the most interesting work is done by nephrologists who are seeking mechanisms of tubular transport. However, it must be added that an important element has been lost: the chemical basis for the action of drugs on the renal tubule. The anatomical location and the effects on electrical potential and on transport are well known. But we have somewhat lost track of seeking for the chemical basis of drug action, and it fairly can be said that in the thirty years since the advent of chlorthiazide, no serious theory has evolved explaining the chemical, as distinct from the physiological, basis of any of the diuretic compounds. Perhaps an elucidation of the history of this field will provide some inspiration for studies in this neglected area.

The period about which I write begins in 1919, and the chapter is divided rather arbitrarily into seven parts: mercurials, some early organic compounds (xanthines and others), carbonic anhydrase inhibitors, thiazides or sulfonamide saluretics, high-ceiling sulfonamides, aryloxyacetic acid diuretics (ethacrynic acid), and potassium-retention and sodium-channel compounds.

Mercurials

Inorganic mercury as Hg_2Cl_2 (calomel) was known to be a diuretic by Paracelsus, who used it to treat dropsy. In the nineteenth century, along with digitalis and squill, calomel was part of the famous "Guy's Hospital Pills." Calomel was not a popular drug; it was toxic, its action was erratic, and it was a cathartic. However, it had been known since 1886 that it caused a significant loss of urinary Cl^-. At the time of World War I, the relatively nontoxic xanthine compounds were used much more.

The field of organic mercurials arose separately, entirely as antisyphilitics, beginning with their synthesis in the laboratory of the great chemist Emil Fischer. The story is well told by Alfred Vogl [Fig. 3; (70)], a major actor whom we shall meet in a moment. Several organic compounds of mercury were in use after 1909; no diuresis was reported, and in retrospect, none occurred with those compounds. In 1917 the Bayer Company introduced Novasurol (Fig. 4) after clinical trial on 900 patients; no diuresis was reported.

On 7 October 1919, a young woman with congenital syphilis came to First Medical University Clinic in Vienna. Vogl was a medical student on duty. His chief, privatdocent Paul Saxl, told the young Vogl to give salicylate of mercury parenterally, even though no one had any hope that this woman with advanced neurosyphilis would improve. Vogl could not obtain this compound that day because he had forgotten that a complicated prescription would have to be made involving its solution in oil, but he hesitated to delay treatment for fear of Dr. Saxl's wrath. Fortunately a deus ex machina appeared in the form of a retired army surgeon just demobilized from the Austro-Hungarian Army. Many such men were hanging about the clinic looking for work. One of them noticed Vogl's distress and pulled a small box from his pocket and said, "*I just got this in the mail this morning. It's a new mercurial. Why don't you use it instead of the salicylate*?" He added sadly, "*I have no patients of my own anyway.*" Institutional review boards lay fifty years in the future, so Vogl was able to inject the compound Novasurol into the young woman. Another fortunate development was at work in this clinic: a new generation of nurses was evolving; ambitious, inspired, and with

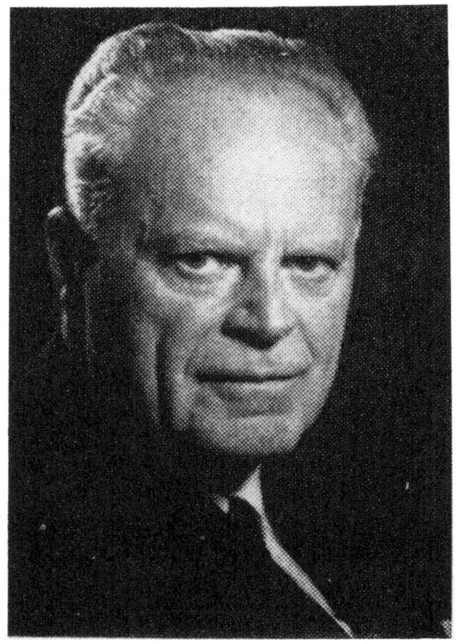

Figure 3. Alfred Vogl (1895–1973) was born in Bielitz, Austria, and received his M.D. in Vienna in 1921. He practiced medicine in Vienna until 1939, then at Guy's Hospital in London for two years, and migrated to New York in 1941. He joined the faculty of New York University and ultimately became Clinical Professor of Medicine in 1960. He was an inspired teacher and diagnostician, and exhibited much enthusiasm and energy for medical affairs, the arts, and travel. In 1969, the fiftieth anniversary of his discovery of mercurial diuretics, he received the Purquet Gold Medal at the New York Academy of Medicine.

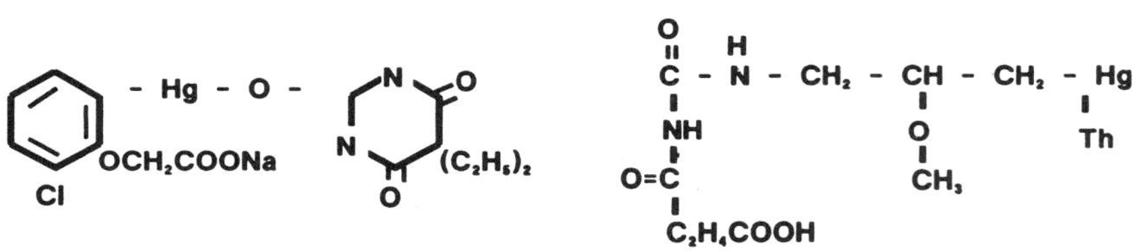

Figure 4. Chemical structures of Novasurol (*left*) and meralluride (*right*). Th, theophylline.

good educational backgrounds. They were adept particularly at making beautiful colored charts. Urine was collected and measured daily on all patients and recorded by blue vertical bars. Vogl needed only to glance at these charts to find that his young patient Joanna reached 2,000 ml by the third day. No one paid any attention to his excited comments until he discontinued the injections and promptly saw the blue lines diminish. He started again; the tall blue columns reappeared. Another syphilitic patient appeared, and he again gave 2 ml of Novasurol; he was rewarded with massive excretion of almost colorless urine, amounting in one day to over 10 liters. This man, unlike the first patient, was in congestive heart failure. Now everyone genuinely became excited. They were able to repeat these miraculous results, causing urinary deluge at will, to the mutual delight of the patients and doctors.

The action, however, remained obscure. Foremost in Vogl's mind was a connection between the action of the drug and the syphilitic process. It was recalled that other mercurials did not have this effect. The intellectual deadlock was broken when a boy with rheumatic heart disease was admitted and also responded with huge diuresis. Postmortem examination confirmed that there was no evidence of syphilis. Meanwhile, Vogl left for Berlin and docent Saxl reappeared along with Robert Heilig, Vogl's successor on the ward, and they continued the investigation. Cushny, Richards, Homer Smith, and Marshall had barely been heard from, yet Saxl and Heilig did an enormous amount of diligent labor, and their first publication appeared in 1920 (59). They left open the mechanism of action.

Surprisingly, in the decade that followed, although new diuretic mercurials were introduced and the compounds were widely used in the treatment of congestive heart failure, there was no agreement as to how they worked. It was argued by Saxl and Heilig themselves that the compounds did not work directly on the kidney. None of the renal physiologists seemed interested in this dispute or in the work. The problem of action site was attacked by Govaerts (29), who injected a dog with Novasurol and, at the height of the diuresis, transplanted the mercurialized kidney to the neck of a normal dog. The transplanted kidney continued to exhibit a diuresis, whereas the control kidney of the host excreted urine at the normal lower rate. The final proof against the extrarenal hypothesis came from Bartram (3), who obtained a unilateral diuresis by injecting small doses of a mercurial into a renal artery. Finally came the pioneering study by Blumgart et al. (11) on the effect of mercurials on electrolyte excretion in humans.

Whether the mercurials worked as part of the organic structure or whether the results were due to release of Hg^{2+} was also debated. The former seemed reasonable because many organic mercurials were not diuretics. An early study by Sollmann and Schreiber (63) demonstrated that ionized compounds are far more potent than nonionized compounds, and this led to the suggestion that it was indeed the inorganic ion that was the active agent. It was well known that mercurials were potentiated by a metabolic acidosis and that their effect was diminished by a metabolic alkalosis (27a). However, in the 1930s no one connected these findings with the molecular mechanism of the drugs. This was to come later.

By the 1940s it was clear that the excretion pattern after mercurial treatment was essentially that of Na^+ and Cl^- in the urine, but it was not clear which was the primary ion. Because mercurials increased urinary concentration of Cl^- to a greater extent than that of Na^+, it was generally accepted that they interfered primarily with the reabsorption of Cl^-. This view has been altered several times because Cl^- reabsorption was thought to be passive. In that era it had to be concluded that mercurials did act on the reabsorption of Na^+ at a distal site. Meanwhile a great argument gathered force in the middle 1950s with respect to the intact-molecule hypothesis versus the mercuric-ion hypothesis. By that time a modest number of organic mercurials were available for analysis of structure-action relations. An important drug was meralluride (Fig. 4). In a lengthy and well-documented study, Kessler, Lozano, and Pitts (36) apparently found that the intact molecule was the active moiety. They reported a relationship between the carbon length and the distance between the mercury atom and a hydrophilic group at the other end of the molecule. This hypothesis at first seemed secure, but as pointed out by Cafruny (14) in an excellent review, the experimental evidence was scanty. Fortunately the hypothesis was challenged by Mudge and Weiner (50), who reopened the question and gave evidence that it was the Hg^{2+} that was active. They showed that rupture of the carbon-mercury bond does occur, and far more rapidly in an acid medium, which explains the potentiation of mercurials in acidosis. They made the important observation that only acid-labile mercurials had diuretic actions. No acid-stable compound had any renal effect. The full study by Weiner et al. (70a) is a remarkable combination of good chemistry, pharmacology, and physiology and should probably be accepted with reservations brought to light by Burg and Green (12). They showed that mercurials inhibit the active reabsorption of Cl^- in the thick ascending limb of the loop of Henle; this may be inhibition of the Na^+-$2Cl^-$-K^+ cotransport, as described in High-Ceiling Sulfonamides, p. 447, for furosemide (32). However, in the isolated tissue the organic mercurial was not activated by lowered pH (12) as had appeared in vivo (50, 70a), and the data suggest that the intact molecule is indeed active in this segment. However, there is good evidence to show that mercurials may also play a major role distally (14), so the matter may be resolved by supposing that the intact molecule may work in the ascending limb, but in the distal segment, which produces major pH lowering, the mercurial is indeed cleaved to the ionic form (I. M. Weiner, personal communication). The specific enzymatic or chemical mechanism has not been identified.

Mercurials were never popular, but in those times they were essential for the treatment of edema and were very widely used. These drugs had to be given by injection and were potentially dangerous. Not surprisingly, then, a major goal of the pharmaceutical industry was to find an oral, nontoxic diuretic. The remainder of this chapter deals with this remarkably successful search.

After this distinguished and stormy history of some thirty years, the mercurials have disappeared from both the *Physicians' Desk*

Reference and from textbooks of pharmacology. This essay may be remarkable, if for nothing else, for being likely the last ever to be written on this fascinating subject.

Some Early Organic Compounds: Xanthines and Others

It has been known from antiquity that coffee, tea, and related beverages cause urine excretion. In the middle and end of the nineteenth century, caffeine was identified in coffee and theophylline was identified in tea; theobromine also was shown to be present in these and other beverages. After the structures were elucidated (Fig. 5), pharmaceutical chemists made hundreds of substitute pyrimidines and purines related to these compounds. Theophylline is the most effective of the three, but for many years the compound called Diuretin (theobromine with sodium salicylate) was widely used, particularly in Europe. An excellent account of the chemistry is given by deStevens (25).

It was believed for many years that caffeine and its congeners in some way stimulated the secretory activity of the renal tubule or that they had a vascular effect. This belief persisted well into the 1920s. However, the introduction of the renal clearance technique by Rehberg in 1926, when applied to the effects of theophylline, showed quite clearly that this compound, like the mercurials, had a specific effect of inhibiting the tubular reabsorption of Na^+ and Cl^- (3, 53). The problem with these compounds is simply that they are not very active and only work well in cases in which there is massive edema. Their action is not nearly as certain as that of the mercurial diuretics. As indicated by deStevens, however, this did not prevent extensive investigations into xanthines, pyrimidines, and the more distantly related triazines. In more recent years, a large number of nitrogen heterocycles have been investigated and documented by Cragoe (21).

From the historical point of view, the xanthines, and specifically theophylline, must be regarded as the first of the oral diuretics. They have low toxicity, and in the 1920s through the 1940s, some physicians preferred them to the more active but toxic mercurials, which had to be given parenterally.

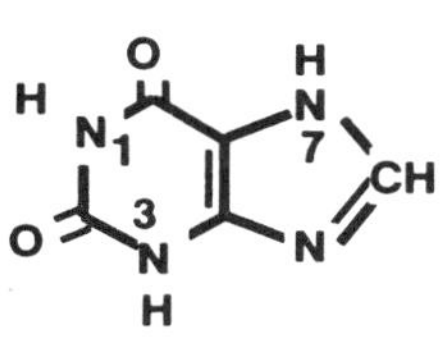

	AT N		
	1	3	7
CAFFEINE	CH_3	CH_3	CH_3
THEOBROMINE	H	CH_3	CH_3
THEOPHYLLINE	CH_3	CH_3	H

Figure 5. Chemical structures of xanthine (*left*) and related compounds (*right*).

These compounds are now relatively in disuse commercially, and investigation of their mechanism of action has been neglected. It would surely not be amiss to use them in isolated tubule preparations to determine their site of action, as has been done for other diuretic drugs.

Carbonic Anhydrase Inhibitors

When carbonic anhydrase was discovered in 1932 (48) and the specific inhibition by sulfonamides was observed in 1940 (38), there was no thought of any connection with the kidney. Some of these early compounds are shown in Figure 6. It is true that in the initial trials of sulfanilamide as an antibacterial agent, electrolyte and acid-base changes were observed. Patients studied at Johns Hopkins in 1937–1938 by Hamilton Southworth and Margaret B. Strauss developed a metabolic acidosis (64) and showed an increase in urine pH (64a). However, they could not explain the reason for these phenomena nor could Marshall and colleagues, who were doing animal experiments on sulfanilamide at the same time (46). It was Thaddeus Mann who, by a shrewd guess, made the connection between sulfanilamide and carbonic anhydrase; then in 1941, Horace Davenport found the enzyme in the kidney. This started a long series of physiological investigations that have led to the era of modern oral diuretics. The first experiment was done by the biochemist Rudolf Höber (33), who showed that sulfanilamide alkalinized frog urine. A few years later, Robert Pitts (Fig. 7) carried out his famous experiments at Cornell, showing that the normal process of urinary acidification occurred by the formation and transfer of protons from tubular cell to tubular urine. When sulfanilamide was given, both H^+ secretion and HCO_3^- reabsorption were reduced; thus both were linked to the activity of carbonic anhydrase in the tubular cells (56). The next step brought these observations into the realm of clinical medicine. William Schwartz (Fig. 8), then a fellow at the Peter Bent Brigham Hospital, saw the implication of Pitts's work with respect to Na^+ reabsorption and the treatment of congestive heart failure. He gave 10 g of sulfanilamide to a woman with rheumatic valvular heart disease (61). She was refractory to mercurial diuretics, still the sole compounds in use for the treatment of edema. As we know now,

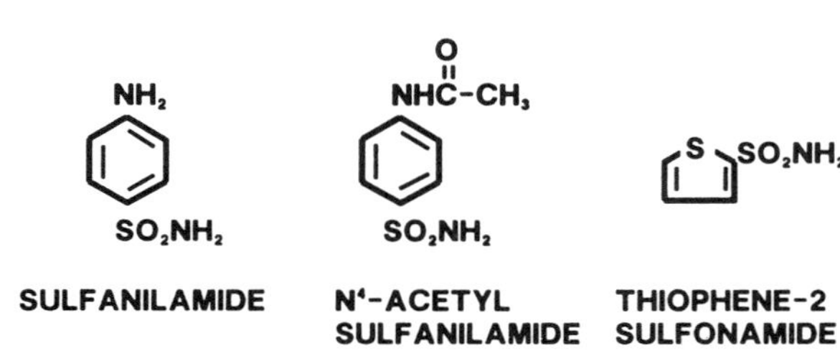

Figure 6. Some early carbonic anhydrase inhibitors.

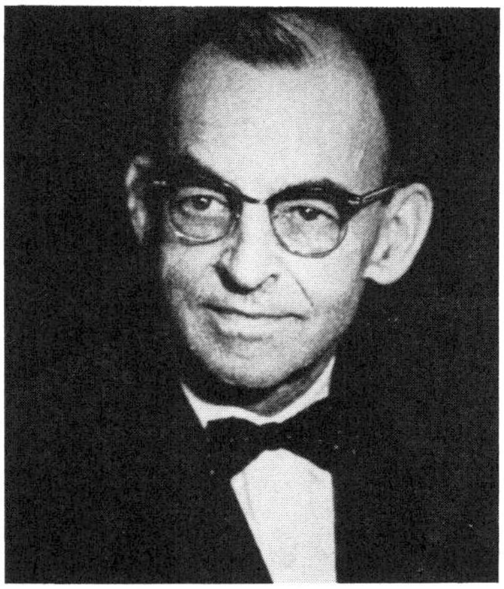

Figure 7. Robert Franklin Pitts (1908–1977) was born in Indianapolis; he received his B.S. from Butler University, his Ph.D. (physiology) from Johns Hopkins, and his M.D. from New York University. Although his early work was on the physiology of respiration, he was later influenced by Homer Smith and turned to renal physiology. After a short period as associate professor at Cornell Medical School and as Chairman of Physiology at Syracuse University, he returned to Cornell where he remained Chairman of Physiology from 1950 until retirement in 1973. He was a member of the National Academy of Sciences and a President of the American Physiological Society. His discovery of the mechanism of renal acidification had an enormous impact on physiology. He also studied the mechanism of action of diuretics and the renal handling and metabolism of ammonia. He trained many first-rate physiologists, and his impeccable standards of thought and personal laboratory skills were an inspiration to younger men and women.

this huge dose of sulfanilamide was enough to inhibit virtually all the carbonic anhydrase in the kidney. There was a very large excretion of both Na^+ and K^+. Schwartz recognized that his doses were too high to be practical and were somewhat toxic, but he understood the possibilities of developing more active drugs in the series akin to sulfanilamide (36a, 38).

Accordingly, Schwartz visited Richard O. Roblin (Fig. 9), a talented organic chemist, who was Director of the Chemotherapy Division of the American Cyanamid Company and had invented sulfadiazine ten years earlier. Roblin had already supplied Horace Davenport with thiophene-2-sulfonamide for his gastric research on carbonic anhydrase, so he was brilliantly prepared for the arrival of Schwartz and his suggestion to enter the diuretic field. From the strong base provided by Mann and Keilin (38) and by Krebs (36a), he used his great knowledge of heterocyclic sulfonamide synthesis to develop new compounds in which the benzene ring of sulfanilamide was replaced by heterocyclic rings such as thiophene, benzothiazole, and thiadiazole. In 1949 and 1950, Roblin and Clapp

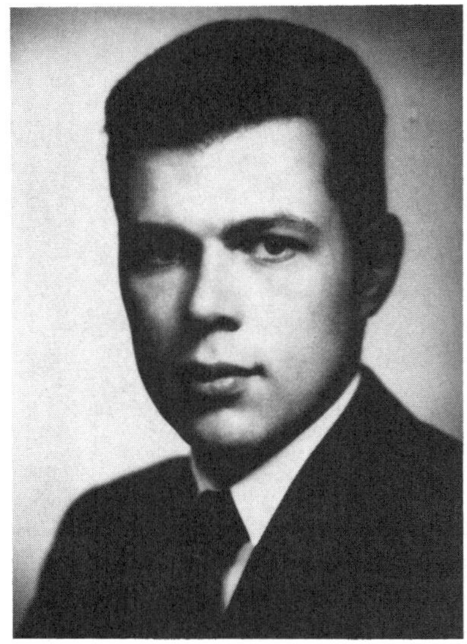

Figure 8. William Benjamin Schwartz (b. 1922) was born in Montgomery, Alabama; he received his M.D. from Duke University. He was a resident fellow at Harvard Medical School and a Markle scholar; since 1958 he has been Professor of Medicine at Tufts. He was Head of the Kidney Division, and later (1971–1976) he was Chairman of the Department of Medicine at that institution. He is currently Vannevar Bush Professor. He was a pioneer in quantitative acid-base physiology and its relation to human medicine and electrolyte disorders, and he made particular contributions to principles of whole-body buffering. Ten years ago he made a major career shift to studies of medical economics, public policy, and the application of artificial intelligence to clinical problems.

(58) synthesized dozens of these compounds. One of the first, numbered 6063, was given to Robert Berliner (Fig. 10), then at the height of his powers in renal physiology at the National Heart Institute. The structure of 6063 (Fig. 11) shows it to be a heterocyclic compound with the necessary unsubstituted sulfonamide group; Roblin knew it was a powerful carbonic anhydrase inhibitor with a dissociation constant of ~10^{-8} M, between 100 and 1,000 times more active than sulfanilamide (49). Berliner was concerned with the mechanisms of renal acidification and its relation to K^+ secretion. He and Kennedy and Orloff (5) used 6063 to show that K^+ secretion was an active process that could be inhibited by mercurials. It was this study that indicated the competition between hydrogen and potassium for a component of the distal ion-exchange mechanism. In the course of the work, however, they showed that at peak dose of 6063, 10–20 mg/kg, 30% of the filtered load of bicarbonate was excreted in the urine. Pitts and Alexander (56) had previously shown with a large dose of sulfanilamide that 12% of filtered bicarbonate was excreted; the large effect in Berliner's hands was readily ex-

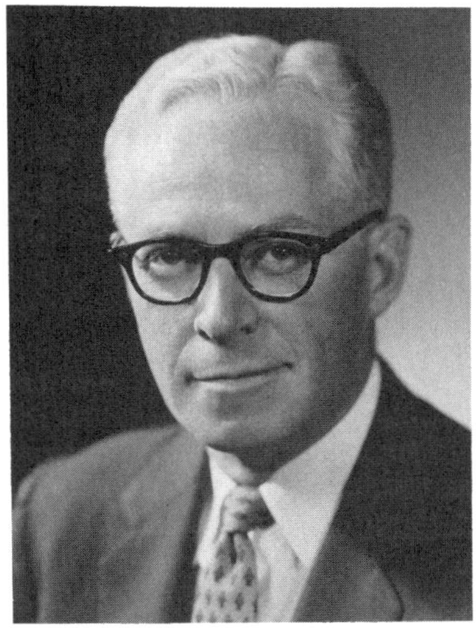

Figure 9. Richard Owen Roblin, Jr, (1907–1985) was born in Rochester, New York; he received his undergraduate degree from the University of Rochester and his Ph.D. in organic chemistry from Columbia University. He spent his entire professional life at the American Cyanamid Company; from 1938 to 1953 he was Director of its Chemotherapy Division in Stamford, Connecticut. He discovered sulfadiazine and made notable contributions to theories of action of sulfonamide drugs at a critical period in the development of the new science of chemotherapy. In addition to the carbonic anhydrase inhibitors, his unit also introduced early antibiotics, antituberculosis drugs, and anti-infectious agents for use in agriculture. In 1954 he became Vice President of Research at Cyanamid and president of their European Research Institute. His great contributions have scarcely been recognized, partly because of his personal modesty and his unwillingness to be an "organization" man.

plained by the much higher activity of 6063 against the enzyme. The new results had the important effect of switching emphasis from distal to proximal tubule to explain the effect of H^+ secretion on HCO_3^- reabsorption (4a).

Meanwhile Roblin sat in his Stamford, Connecticut, laboratory wondering which direction he should take in developing this new compound. The number of possibilities seemed remarkable. There was the problem of gastric secretion, that of the possible control of epilepsy, and questions relating to the treatment of nephrosis in childhood. Roblin had been discouraged by many of the leaders in renal physiology from developing his new drug as a diuretic because it was clear that the urine contained Na^+, K^+, and HCO_3^-—not a promising mix. However, he was able to look farther into the future and decided to gamble. At the same time, experiments by Janowitz, Colcher, and Hollander (35) showed that gastric secretion was repressed by the new drug. In December 1951 Roblin decided to go

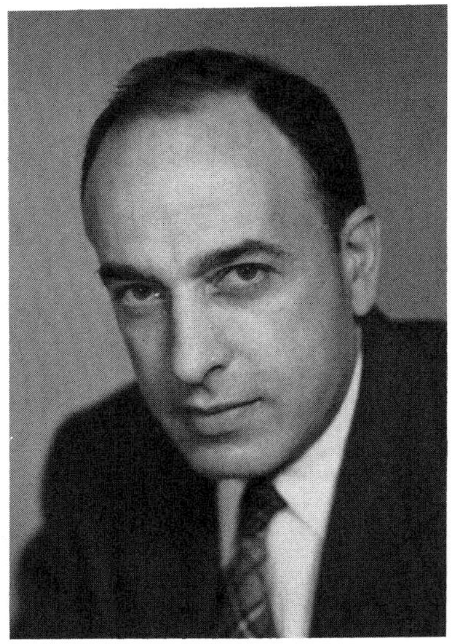

Figure 10. Robert William Berliner (b. 1915) was born in New York City; he received his B.S. from Yale University and his M.D. from Columbia University. He was a research fellow and a resident physician at Goldwater Hospital (New York) from 1942 to 1944. He was on the faculties of medicine at New York University and Columbia University until 1950 when he became the first Chief of the Laboratory of Kidney and Electrolyte Metabolism at the National Heart Institute. He developed his unit into one of the leading units of electrolyte physiology in the world. He later became Director of Research for the Heart Institute and Deputy Director of Science for the National Institutes of Health. In 1973 he became Dean of Yale Medical School from which he retired in 1985. He is a member of the National Academy of Science, received the Homer Smith Award, and was President of the American Physiological Society. He made notable personal contributions to renal physiology in the era 1945–1960, and most significantly he was an unfailing and critical guide of the careers of several generations of basic and clinical electrolyte scholars.

ahead and handed a small vial labeled 6063 to his new pharmacologist (me), who did not quite know whether it contained an inhibitor or an enzyme or indeed whether there was much difference. I had just come from Marshall's laboratory at Johns Hopkins and knew a little about handling dogs in renal and other experiments, but that was the extent of my training for the job at hand.

Of the several candidate compounds from Roblin's laboratory (all very potent inhibitors in vitro), 6063 was selected for development because of its stability in vivo and remarkable lack of toxicity. An important unsuccessful candidate drug was benzothiazole-2-sulfonamide (Fig. 11), which failed because it is very rapidly metabolized in dogs (39). As it turned out, derivatives of this compound, notably the 6-ethoxy (ethoxzolamide [Fig. 11]), were far less susceptible to

ACETAZOLAMIDE (6063)

$R = CH_3C(=O) - NH$

BENZOLAMIDE

$R = PhSO_2 - NH$

2.5 DISULFAMYL THIADIAZOLE

$R = H_2NSO_2 -$

BENZOTHIAZOLE-2-SULFONAMIDE

$R = H$

ETHOXZOLAMIDE

$R = 6- C_2H_5O$

Figure 11. Chemical structures of some carbonic anhydrase inhibitors.

such metabolic attack, and ethoxzolamide (Cardrase) became not only an important drug of this class but a very useful experimental tool (41). The metabolic pathway of benzothiazole-2-sulfonamide turned out to be novel—the first example of glutathione or cysteine attack on the C-2 atom, ultimately displacing the SO_2NH_2 group, essential for inhibitory action against carbonic anhydrase (16). These early experiments have thrown a long shadow of thirty-five years on sulfonamide development today (17).

By 1954, 6063 had a generic name (acetazolamide) and a trade name (Diamox) and was ready for the market as the "first modern oral diuretic " (43). Fortunately its toxicity was surprisingly low; the prediction that complete inhibition of carbonic anhydrase would lead to "speedy death" (24) was disproved (43), although the precise reasons remained to be discovered twenty-five years later (65).

During the development of acetazolamide, a number of physiological facts and concepts were unearthed. Perhaps the most interesting was that after the first drug day and a large diuresis of Na^+, bicarbonate, and K^+, the composition of urine reverted to normal and animals could be maintained on the drug in a sustained state of metabolic acidosis indefinitely. It was clear that in this situation bicarbonate was being reabsorbed in the absence of carbonic anhydrase. During the summer of 1953, I joined Homer Smith at the Mount Desert Island Biological Laboratory where we found that marine fish also reabsorbed all of the filtered bicarbonate without carbonic anhydrase—the enzyme was not present in these kidneys. After thirty-four years, it is now clear that this reabsorptive mechanism is simply due to a powerful acidifying system, whose chemistry is presently unknown (42a).

The work with acetazolamide on the kidney in the 1950s confirmed the basic tenets of Pitts. The kidney tubules supply a proton that is involved in the reabsorption of bicarbonate and the excretion of H^+ and NH_4^+. When carbonic anhydrase is inhibited, all of these functions decrease. A seeming paradox arose in that full carbonic anhydrase inhibition diverted only 20%–30% of filtered HCO_3^- into the urine (44), whereas ~80% reabsorption was inhibited in the proximal tubule (15). It is now clear that enzyme inhibition generates a high concentration of HCO_3^- distally, which is reabsorbed down its tubule to plasma gradient (27, 28). Thus it seems fair to say that in the normal mammalian or avian kidney, ~80% of HCO_3^- is carbonic anhydrase dependent, but when the enzyme is inhibited, a pathway independent of carbonic anhydrase is uncovered. This independent pathway is magnified in acidosis (44) and accounts for all HCO_3^- reabsorption in marine fish, as noted previously (34, 66).

Carbonic anhydrase is also present in the distal tubule and collecting duct and respectively mediates H^+ secretion for acidification and NH_4^+ formation (41); in some species it mediates HCO_3^- formation (18, 47).

Novel inhibitors with special physicochemical properties have been of great utility in unraveling the mechanism. The first was benzolamide (Fig. 11), which in low (1–3 mg/kg) doses acts only on the kidney, leaving red cell and other tissue carbonic anhydrase intact (68). The second was a dextran-bound succinyl analogue of acetazolamide, which was filtered but had access only to the enzyme at the luminal membrane (67).

Acetazolamide was used widely in the treatment of congestive heart failure in 1953–1958; results were disappointing, although by no means entirely negative. The synergism with mercurials was interesting, practically and theoretically, throwing light on both the enhanced action of mercurials in acidosis (see MERCURIALS, p. 431) and the nature of the chronic acidotic state engendered by the sulfonamides (40). As predicted, the failure to excrete Cl^- was a limiting factor in the use of acetazolamide alone (37, 57, 62). We see in the next sections that this was overcome by the development of disulfonamides (in contrast to the acetazolamide type of monosulfonamides) and their natural descendants, the thiazide and high-ceiling diuretics.

Just as acetazolamide reached the market in 1954, a new and unforeseen (by its discoverers) use was found: the treatment of glaucoma (4). This compelling story is told elsewhere, along with an account of related progress in knowledge of aqueous humor physiology generated over the past thirty years (42).

THIAZIDES OR SULFONAMIDE SALURETICS ERA

The story begins in the late 1930s when the Sharp & Dohme Company in Philadelphia hired a remarkable man, first as head of their medical group, and then as Director of Research. He was William A. Feirer, M.D., Ph.D., from Johns Hopkins, blessed with a sense of vision, an unerring capacity to judge men and science, and the bonus of equanimity and fine disposition. Within a few years he had gathered at least three men who were to leave a lasting mark on science: the pharmacologists Arnold D. Welch and Karl H. Beyer (Fig. 12) and the organic chemist James M. Sprague (Fig. 13). Their first work, not surprisingly, was on the antibacterial sulfonamides—exactly parallel to Roblin and his group at the American Cyanamid Company. Roblin had discovered sulfadiazine in 1940, and the Sharp & Dohme group developed its methylated derivatives in the same era. As we have seen, ten years later Roblin turned to the sulfonamide carbonic anhydrase inhibitors, as did Sprague at Sharp & Dohme. These two men were friends and rivals in the best tradition, alike in their chemical insights and appreciation of the quirks of biological data.

Welch left the company to become Professor of Pharmacology at Case Western Reserve and then at Yale University and became a world leader in cancer and viral chemotherapy. The others and newer associates (Fred Novello, John Baer) stayed; Sharp & Dohme was absorbed into Merck in 1953, and this inevitably increased research and marketing resources.

Beyer was fundamentally a physiologist. When he arrived at Sharp & Dohme from Wisconsin in 1943, his masters had the foresight to

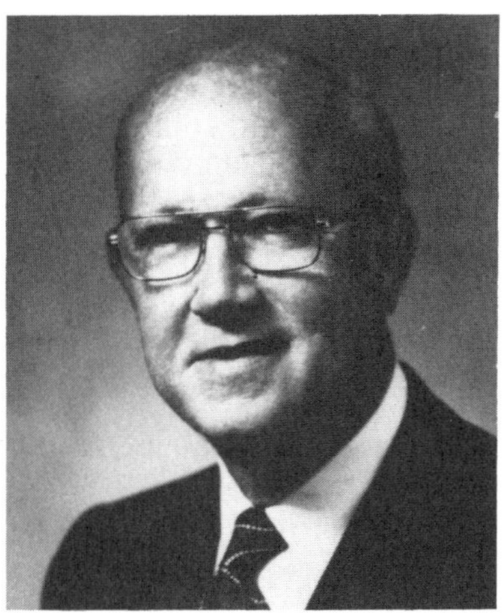

Figure 12. Karl Henry Beyer (b. 1914) was born in Henderson, Kentucky; he attended Western Kentucky State College (B.S.) and the University of Wisconsin (M.D., Ph.D.). In 1943 he joined Sharp & Dohme (which merged with Merck in 1953), rising from Assistant Director of Pharmacology to Senior Vice President. He retired in 1973 to carry out academic research at Pennsylvania State University Medical School (Hershey). In his 30 years in industry, Beyer was involved not only in diuretic development but in that of antihypertensive, anti-inflammatory, and anti-infective agents. At the same time, he made notable contributions to organized pharmacology as President of both the American Society for Pharmacology and Experimental Therapeutics and the National Academy of Science Drug Board.

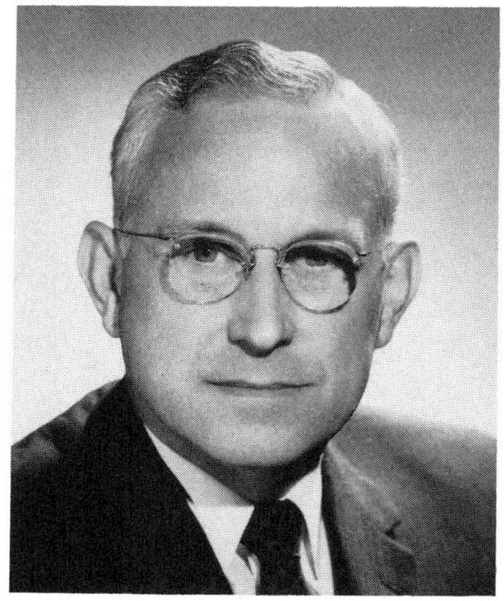

Figure 13. James Maurice Sprague (b. 1908) was born in Indiana; he received his A.B. from Franklin College and his Ph.D. from the University of Wisconsin. After three years at Yale University on a research appointment, he joined Sharp & Dohme (1937) where he soon became Director of Organic Chemistry and later became Assistant Director of Research. Following the merger of Sharp & Dohme with Merck (1953), he became Director of Medicinal Chemistry and later Vice President of Merck Sharp & Dohme research laboratories. He retired in 1972. Like so many pharmaceutical chemists of that time, his "Yale and Harvard College" was the antibacterial sulfonamides; these structures and synthetic techniques became the basis of development not only of many diuretics but of antithyroid and antidiabetic drugs. Like his doppelgänger Dick Roblin (see Fig. 9), Jim Sprague schooled himself in physiology, was modest and retiring, and left his lasting mark through the development of several classes of drugs, some of which were outside the field of diuretics. Sprague's personal and scholarly influence has now extended to the third generation of synthetic and pharmaceutical chemists at Merck and elsewhere.

send him to the laboratory of James Shannon at Goldwater Hospital. There he met the bright young men (Brodie, Axelrod, Berliner, Earle, Udenfriend) who were following Homer Smith into modern renal physiology and who later followed Shannon to create the greatness of the National Institute of Health (6).

Beyer's interest turned to compounds that would inhibit renal secretion—probenecid (Fig. 14) was the result (10). In those far-off days, it was worthwhile to repress the excretion of penicillin; probenecid also inhibited the reabsorption of uric acid and was used to treat gout. The Merck renal unit had made a scientific and commercial success (6).

Dealkylation of probenecid yields the simple unsubstituted sulfonamide *p*-carboxybenzenesulfonamide [carzenid (Fig. 14)], a carbonic anhydrase inhibitor about five times as active as sulfanilamide. In vivo carzenid modestly alkalinizes urine but also elicits a small Cl^-

excretion (7). This was the pivotal experiment; from this time onward, attention was focused on unsubstituted sulfonamides for chloruretic action.

At that time (1954) and for many years thereafter, Beyer connected the chloruresis with carbonic anhydrase inhibition (5a, 7). As will be seen, this had a significant effect on further events, although the weight of evidence is overwhelmingly against the idea (54).

Meanwhile (1950) Roblin (49, 58) had published his now-famous two papers on the new and powerful carbonic anhydrase inhibitors, including acetazolamide and other thiadiazoles (see Carbonic Anhydrase Inhibitors, p. 436). The most active inhibitor was 2,5-disulfamylthiadiazole, a compound 800 times more potent than sulfanilamide, with a dissociation constant of 10^{-8} M (see Fig. 11).

It was from this "lead," because carbonic anhydrase inhibition was the theme, that Sharp & Dohme turned to *m*-benzenedisulfonamides. It is an extraordinary but logical result that, growing out of the misconceptions that two sulfonamide groups gave superior inhibition and that such inhibition was needed for chloruresis, all future compounds of this and the high-ceiling type bear the 1,3-disulfamyl or 1-sulfamyl-3-carbonyl relation, as in compounds of Figures 14 and 15. A further irony is that the synthesis of Roblin's 2,5-disulfamylthiadiazole (see Fig. 11) cannot be (to my knowledge) reproduced, and the original details are lacking (58).

Further impetus to the Sharp & Dohme program came from the 1954 publications on the pharmacological and renal effects of Diamox (acetazolamide), as discussed in the previous section (43, 44). The decision to look for more active inhibitors was, in retrospect,

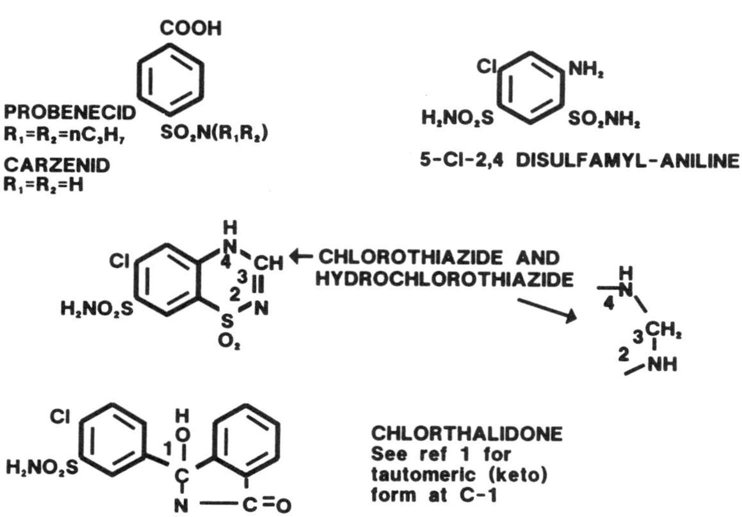

Figure 14. Chemical structures of compounds acting on renal secretion (*upper left*) and their relation to saluretics.

curious because it was clear that at small doses of acetazolamide (10 mg/kg) there was essentially complete inhibition of the enzyme, while 1,000 mg/kg appeared nontoxic. But if this was a pharmacological error, it led to stunning scientific and commercial success.

It is not known how many *m*-benzenedisulfonamides were made by Sprague and associates at Merck, by deStevens and colleagues at Ciba, and other industrial chemists. A partial list of 40 is given by deStevens (25). The crucial compound, by happy accident, was 5-Cl-2,4 disulfamylaniline (Fig. 14). This, like other disulfonamides, caused Cl^- excretion and mild HCO_3^- output, but its importance lay in its central role in the synthesis of benzothiadiazine-1,1-dioxides, referred to as "thiazides."

Novello and Sprague treated 5-Cl-2,4 disulfamylaniline with formic acid, expecting the formylamino compound. Unexpectedly cyclization occurred, yielding chlorothiazide (Fig. 14). When tested in animals and humans, the compound elicited excretion of Na^+ and Cl^-, with relatively little HCO_3^- output (7, 9). Toxicity was very low and oral absorption complete. What was thought impossible in the mercurial era had been achieved in just a few years.

The first report on chlorothiazide stated that it was 30 times as active a carbonic anhydrase inhibitor as acetazolamide (9). It was widely believed for a few years that it was this difference that led to Cl^- excretion. In fact the inhibition assay was a laboratory error, and chlorothiazide is ~1/100 as active an inhibitor as acetazolamide (7, 41). No "pure" carbonic anhydrase inhibitor (monosulfonamide) of any strength or at any dose causes chloruresis.

Structurally, then, chlorothiazide is an extension of the *m*-benzenedisulfonamides, and this regiochemical pattern leads to Cl^- excretion. It was shown that the SO_2NH_2 group could be converted to SO_2NHR or even SO_2CH_3 with complete loss of carbonic anhydrase inhibition, but activity as a chloruretic is retained (45). The basis for the crucial importance of the meta or 1,3 relationship is still not understood.

The first advance over chlorothiazide, heralding the synthesis of at least a thousand compounds of this class, was saturation of the 3-4 position to yield hydrochlorothiazide (Fig. 14). This was an important discovery by deStevens at Ciba because the new compound was 10–15 times more potent as a diuretic than chlorothiazide (on weight basis), and about 10 times less active in inhibiting carbonic anhydrase (25, 26). After nearly thirty years, this is by far the most widely used drug of the family.

The flood of compounds that followed has been described many times, notably by deStevens in 1963 (25), Peters in 1969 (54), and Allen in 1983 (1). While of great interest to the medicinal chemist, these studies have contributed little to physiology. Some compounds are 100 times more active on a weight basis than hydrochlorothiazide, making them ideal for receptor studies, which lie in the future.

It should be noted that the 1,3-disulfamyl unit can give way to a 1,3 relation between SO_2NH_2 and CONH, as in chlorthalidone (Fig. 14). Also, as indicated previously (45), SO_2NH_2 can become SO_2NHR, abolishing action against carbonic anhydrase, and chloruresis is still observed.

Studies on the renal mechanism of hydrochlorothiazide are surprisingly few. It is now thought that they work on the distal tubule, repressing a neutral NaCl cotransport reabsorptive step (69).

HIGH-CEILING SULFONAMIDES

One of many sulfonamides with modest chloruretic activities deriving from the research described in the previous section was 4-chloro-5-sulfamaylanthranilic acid (Fig. 15). It was therefore astonishing when Muschawek and Hajdu (52) reported that substitution of the NH_2 group by furfuryl leads to a large increase in activity; but further and most important, the "ceiling" or natriuretic efficiency of Na^+ or Cl^- excretion was two to three times greater than that of any known diuretic (55). This research was done in the Hoechst Laboratories in Frankfurt in 1959; the drug furosemide (Fig. 15) reached the market in 1964. Details of this discovery and development are not available in their entirety, but it is quite clear that a "high-ceiling" diuretic was not sought, but stumbled on—a classic mode of science (51).

As with the thiazides, thousands of analogues of furosemide have been made, and several clinically tested. Allen (1) has admirably documented this research. Furosemide is the largest selling diuretic in the world because it works in congestive heart failure refractory to the thiazides, and it may be more effective in hypertension than the thiazides. The ascendancy of furosemide has been challenged in the past few years by two related compounds, bumetanide and

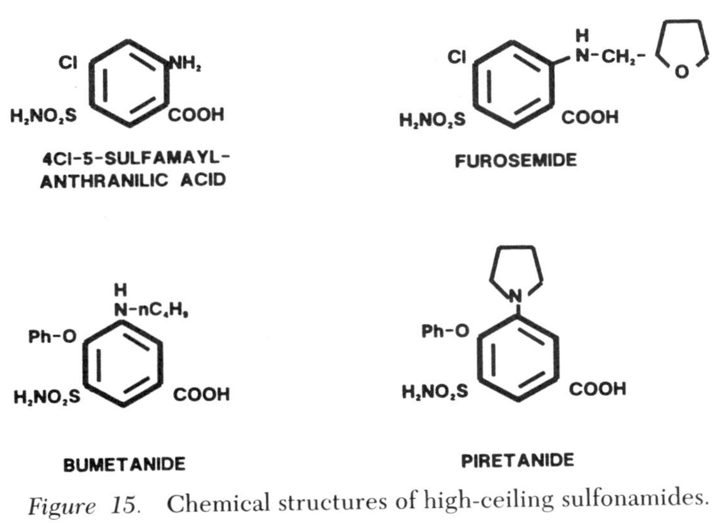

Figure 15. Chemical structures of high-ceiling sulfonamides.

piretanide, and surely there will be others. These are effective in lower doses than furosemide and have a few special features (1).

The locus of action of furosemide is the luminal border of the thick ascending limb of the loop of Henle where it diminishes Cl^- reabsorption (13). More specifically the drug appears to act on a carrier for Cl^-, which is normally pumped into the cell along with Na^+ and K^+ (30). On the blood surface, Na^+ and Cl^- are removed from the cell and exchanged for K^+ (32); this is mediated by Na^+-K^+-activated ATPase (31). Furosemide has no effect on this enzyme or on transport from the blood side. Its action is called inhibition of secondary active Cl^- transport; the changes in membrane potentials and intracellular ion activities make it clear that the luminal carrier for Cl^- (Na^+-$2Cl^-$-K^+ cotransport) is affected. Because of the very large NaCl diuresis (some 12% of filtered load), it is likely that other sites in the nephron are affected as well.

When furosemide was discovered, it was generally supposed (and taught by me, at least) that the molecular change from the thiazide type, including chlorthalidone (see Fig. 14), which (like furosemide) has SO_2NH_2 and C$=$O in meta relation, represented an augmentation of effect or an addition of an action to the fundamental chloruretic types of Figure 14.

However, this does not seem to be the case. Micropuncture data suggest that in the furosemide molecule the distal thiazide action has been abolished, and conversely the thiazide-chlorthalidone-disulfonamide (see Fig. 14) type has none of the furosemide activity in the thick ascending limb. Significantly, all furosemide-like drugs have a COOH group; the thiazides do not. Presumably a major locus of drug attachment to the luminal Cl^- carrier is the strongly anionic COO^- group. There is surely room for further research in these matters, which should stress attention to the molecular variations and the concentrations used. A remarkable paper of this type has appeared (60).

Aryloxyacetic Acid Diuretics: Ethacrynic Acid

This class of drugs, like the thiazides or sulfonamide saluretics, arose under the chemical leadership of James M. Sprague at the Merck Sharp & Dohme research laboratories. The story is well told by Edward J. Cragoe, a member of that team (19). The idea was to find compounds akin to the mercurial diuretics but lacking their toxicity. Specifically, high reactivity with SH groups was sought and found in acrylophenones, as shown here

$$X-\overset{\overset{O}{\|}}{C}-\overset{\overset{Y}{|}}{C}=CH_2 + RSH \rightleftharpoons X-\overset{\overset{O}{\|}}{C}-\underset{\underset{H}{|}}{\overset{\overset{Y}{|}}{C}}-CH_2-S-R$$

analogous to

$$Z\text{—}Hg\text{—}A + RSH \rightarrow Z\text{—}Hg\text{—}S\text{—}R$$

In the course of an imaginative and extensive synthetic program undertaken by Everett M. Schultz, attention was drawn to the acryloylphenoxyacetic acids: compounds with no further substituents on the benzene ring were weakly active against SH structures but were active enough to provide a lead and to suggest that the biochemical basis for the research might be correct. When the benzene ring was dichlorinated, both diuretic activity and reactivity against mercaptans in vitro rose at least tenfold. This compound, named ethacrynic acid (Fig. 16), was given a thorough pharmacological analysis by the Merck group, including comparison with the thiazides, the carbonic anhydrase inhibitors, and the mercurials (8).

It was at once evident that this is a high-ceiling diuretic, like furosemide. It is of particular interest in that structurally it resembles no other diuretic. In the past twenty years an enormous number of congeners have been made (19); at the same time the clinical use of ethacrynic acid has declined greatly. It provides no advantage over furosemide and is generally felt to be more toxic. Tienilic acid (ticrynafen) is related chemically but lacks the acrolyl group and is not high ceiling; this compound reached the market and had very high sales in 1979. Unlike other compounds of this (and other) classes, it was uricosuric. However, reports of liver toxicity resulted in withdrawal of the drug.

Ethacrynic acid, like furosemide, is a "loop diuretic," working chiefly on Cl^- reabsorptive mechanisms of the thick ascending limb of the loop of Henle in both cortical and medullary segments. However, pharmacological texts and reviews in nephrology inexplicably ignore the important point that their action is not the same. As noted in HIGH-CEILING SULFONAMIDES, p. 447, furosemide inhibits a carrier for "Cl^- cotransport" on the luminal surface. Ethacrynic acid acts quite differently. It does not inhibit or bind to the Cl^- carrier, yet it will block active NaCl reabsorption in this segment (60). Ethacrynic acid and its homologues affect cellular metabolism in ways yet ill defined. The cells are depolarized and cell swelling is observed (R. Greger, personal communication).

The original idea, that ethacrynic acid works by inhibiting an SH enzyme, now appears unlikely. Indeed it appears that ethacrynic

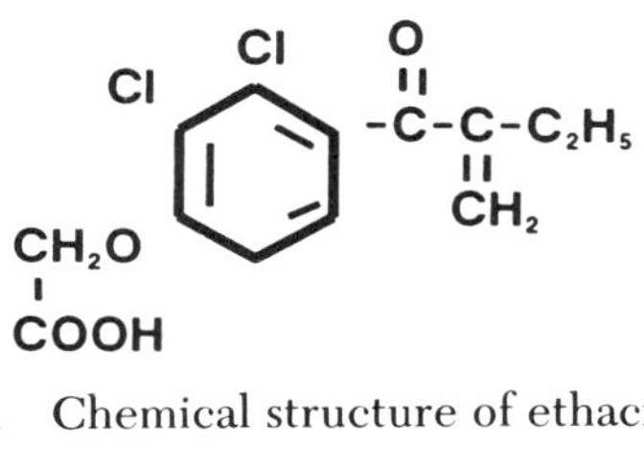

Figure 16. Chemical structure of ethacrynic acid.

acid reacts with circulatory glutathione and cysteine, and in this form it is transported to the kidney (19). Once again, however, the development of this class of drugs and the physiological insight that followed reflect creative thinking and devoted chemical and physiological research of a very high order.

Potassium-Retention and Sodium-Channel Compounds

During the early period of great synthetic activity directed toward new diuretics (1960–1970), the collaborative efforts of E. C. Taylor of Princeton and J. Weinstock of Smith Kline & French resulted in a highly active series of aminopteridines (25). Unlike the carbonic anhydrase inhibitors and thiazides (and later the high-ceiling drugs), most of the compounds elicited no K^+ loss, as shown by Wiebelhaus's pharmacological studies of triamterene (71). It was also found that activity persists in adrenalectomized rats, so it was clear that aldosterone antagonism was not involved. This separates drugs of the present section from spironolactone, which I do not consider. Cragoe has furnished a complete and scholarly account of structure-action relationships of the aminopteridines (20).

Of the many compounds tested, triamterene (Fig. 17) was selected for clinical trial and reached the market in 1964. It can be used alone as a diuretic, but its main use is in combination with hydrochlorothiazide (Dyazide) to prevent hypokalemia.

Studies of the intimate mechanism of triamterene action have lagged behind those of other diuretics, including its close pharmacological relative amiloride. It generally is agreed that triamterene acts on the cortical collection segment of the tubule, decreasing Na^+ reabsorption at a site at which this is linked to K^+ secretion. Once again a new class of drugs was discovered by accident—there is no evidence that antikaluresis was sought in the development of triamterene.

A few years later, however, Merck Sharp & Dohme directly sought a compound to elicit enhanced Na^+ and diminished K^+ output to combat K^+ loss, which followed treatment with hydrochlorothiazide. Some 25,000 compounds were screened in a rat assay. This resulted in the pyrazine compound amiloride (Fig. 17). Again Cragoe has given us a very complete account, not only of structure-action relationships but of insights into the physical chemistry of amiloride and congeners (20a).

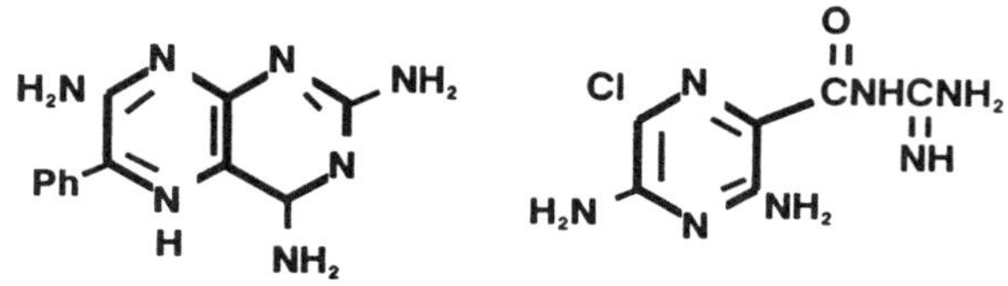

Figure 17. Chemical structures of triamterene (*left*) and amiloride (*right*).

Amiloride, like triamterene, is used in combination (Moduretic) with hydrochlorothiazide in the treatment of cardiac edema and hypertension. The Na^+ diuresis of the two drugs is additive, and K^+ loss is minimized (2).

Amiloride has been widely used in renal and electrolyte physiology (23). At 10^{-5} M it inhibits a "Na^+ channel" in cortical collecting ducts, amphibian skin, salivary ducts, and many other secretory tissues. The apical membrane in collecting tubules is depolarized (47), which appears to be the basis for marked reduction of Na^+ reabsorption and K^+ secretion (2). These are reasonably specific effects; it is interesting to see that the effect of amiloride on the Na^+-H^+ exchange on the proximal tubule is far weaker, requiring nearly a 10^{-3} M concentration.

What I have gleaned from recounting this series of tales, which are replete with scientific insight, accidents, errors, and even humor, is new respect for individual achievement and the remarkable effect that industrial effort has had on fundamental advances. The field has unusual vitality. Even in the face of the great successes in drug development, new researches ranging from organic syntheses through pharmacological development to physiological probing and clinical trial are carried on every day. The literature continues to swell; inevitably there will be a story to surpass this one by far in the twenty-first century.

BIBLIOGRAPHY

1. ALLEN, R. C. Sulfonamide diuretics. In: *Diuretics: Chemistry, Pharmacology, and Medicine*, edited by E. J. Cragoe, Jr. New York: Wiley, 1983, p. 49–200.
2. BAER, J. E., C. B. JONES, S. A. SPITZER, and H. F. RUSSO. The potassium-sparing and natriuretic activity of *N*-amidino-3,5-diamino-6-chloropyrazine carboxamide hydrochloride dihydrate (amiloride hydrochloride). *J. Pharmacol. Exp. Ther.* 157: 472–485, 1967.
3. BARTRAM, E. A. Experimental observations on the effects of various diuretics when injected directly into one renal artery of the dog. *J. Clin. Invest.* 11: 1197–1219, 1932.
4. BECKER, B. Decrease in intraocular pressure in man by a carbonic anhydrase inhibitor, Diamox. *Am. J. Ophthalmol.* 37: 13–15, 1954.

4a. BERLINER, R. W. Renal secretion of potassium and hydrogen ions. *Federation Proc.* 11: 695–700, 1952.

5. BERLINER, R. W., T. J. KENNEDY, and J. ORLOFF. Relationship between acidification of the urine and potassium metabolism. *Am. J. Med.* 11: 274–282, 1951.

5a. BEYER, K. H. The site and mode of action of some sulfonamide-derived diuretics. *Med. Clin. N. Am.* 59: 735–750, 1975.

6. BEYER, K. H. A career or two. *Annu. Rev. Pharmacol. Toxicol.* 17: 1–10, 1977.

7. Beyer, K. H., and J. E. Baer. Physiological basis for the action of newer diuretic agents. *Pharmacol. Rev.* 13: 517–562, 1961.
8. Beyer, K. H., J. E. Baer, J. K. Michaelson, and H. F. Russo. Renotropic characteristics of ethacrynic acid: a phenoxyacetic saluretic-diuretic agent. *J. Pharmacol. Exp. Ther.* 147: 1–22, 1965.
9. Beyer, K. H., J. E. Baer, H. F. Russo, and A. S. Haimbach. Chlorothiazide (6-chloro-7-sulfamyl-1,2,4-benzothiadiazine-1,1-dioxide): the enhancement of sodium chloride excretion (Abstract). *Federation Proc.* 16: 282, 1957.
10. Beyer, K. H., H. F. Russo, E. K. Tillson, A. K. Miller, W. F. Verwey, and S. R. Gass. Benemid, *p*-(di-*n*-propylsulfamyl)-benzoic acid: its renal affinity and its elimination. *Am. J. Physiol.* 166: 625–640, 1951.
11. Blumgart, H. L., D. R. Gilligan, R. C. Levy, M. G. Brown, and M. C. Volk. Action of diuretic drugs. I. Action of diuretics in normal persons. *Arch. Intern. Med.* 54: 40–81, 1934.
12. Burg, M. B., and N. Green. Effect of mersalyl on the thick ascending limb of Henley's loop. *Kidney Int.* 4: 245–251, 1973.
13. Burg, M., L. Stoner, J. Cardinal, and N. Green. Furosemide effect on isolated perfused tubules. *Am. J. Physiol.* 225: 119–124, 1973.
14. Cafruny, E. J. The site and mechanism of action of mercurial diuretics. *Pharmacol. Rev.* 20: 89–116, 1968.
15. Cogan, M. G., D. A. Maddox, D. G. Warnock, E. T. Lin, and F. C. Rector, Jr. Effect of acetazolamide on bicarbonate reabsorption in the proximal tubule of the rat. *Am. J. Physiol.* 237 (*Renal Fluid Electrolyte Physiol.* 6): F447–F454, 1979.
16. Colucci, D. F., and D. A. Buyske. The biotransformation of a sulfonamide to mercapturic acid glucuronide conjugates. *Biochem. Pharmacol.* 14: 457–466, 1965.
17. Conroy, C. W., H. Schwam, and T. H. Maren. The nonenzymatic displacement of the sulfamoyl group from different classes of aromatic compounds by glutathione and cysteine. *Drug Metab. Dispos.* 12: 614–618, 1984.
18. Coulson, R. A., and T. Hernandez. Role of carbonic anhydrase in anion excretion in the alligator. *Am. J. Physiol.* 188: 121–124, 1957.
19. Cragoe, E. J., Jr. The (aryloxy)acetic acid family of diuretics. In: *Diuretics: Chemistry, Pharmacology, and Medicine*, edited by E. J. Cragoe, Jr. New York: Wiley, 1983, p. 201–266.
20. Cragoe, E. J., Jr. Bicyclic heterocyclic diuretics. In: *Diuretics: Chemistry, Pharmacology, and Medicine*, edited by E. J. Cragoe, Jr. New York: Wiley, 1983, p. 467–482.
20a. Cragoe, E. J., Jr. Pyrazine diuretics. In: *Diuretics: Chemistry, Pharmacology, and Medicine*, edited by E. J. Cragoe, Jr. New York: Wiley, 1983.
21. Cragoe, E. J., Jr. (editor). *Diuretics: Chemistry, Pharmacology, and Medicine*. New York: Wiley, 1983.
22. Cushny, A. R. *The Secretion of Urine* (2nd ed.). London: Longmans, Green, 1926.
23. Cuthbert, A. W., G. M. Fanelli, Jr., and A. Scriabine (editors). *Amiloride and Epithelial Sodium Transport*. Baltimore, MD: Urban & Schwarzenberg, 1979, p. 180.
24. Davies, R. E. Hydrochloric acid production by isolated gastric mucosa. *Biochem. J.* 42: 609–621, 1948.

25. DeStevens, G. *Diuretics—Chemistry and Pharmacology.* New York: Academic, 1963.

26. DeStevens, G., L. H. Werner, A. Halamandaris, and S. Ricca, Jr. Dihydrobenzthiadiazine dioxides with potent diuretic effect. *Experientia* 14: 463, 1958.

27. DuBose, T. D., and M. S. Lucci. Effect of carbonic anhydrase inhibition on superficial and deep nephron bicarbonate reabsorption in the rat. *J. Clin. Invest.* 71: 55–65, 1983.

27a. Ethridge, C. B., D. B. Myers, and M. N. Fulton. The modifying effect of various inorganic salts on the diuretic action of salyrgan. *Arch. Intern. Med.* 57: 714–728, 1936.

28. Frommer, J. P., M. E. Laski, D. E. Wesson, and N. A. Kurtzman. Internephron heterogeneity for carbonic anhydrase-independent bicarbonate reabsorption in the rat. *J. Clin. Invest.* 73: 1034–1045, 1984.

29. Govaerts, P. Origine renale ou tissulaire de la diurese par un composé mercuriel organique. *C. R. Soc. Biol.* 99: 647–649, 1928.

30. Greger, R. Chloride reabsorption in the rabbit cortical thick ascending limb of the loop of Henle. A sodium dependent process. *Pfluegers Arch.* 390: 38–43, 1981.

31. Greger, R., and E. Schlatter. Properties of the basolateral membrane of the cortical thick ascending limb of Henle's loop of rabbit kidney. A model for secondary active chloride transport. *Pfluegers Arch.* 396: 325–334, 1983.

32. Greger, R., E. Schlatter, and F. Lang. Evidence for electroneutral sodium chloride co-transport in the cortical thick ascending limb of Henle's loop of rabbit kidney. *Pfluegers Arch.* 396: 308–314, 1983.

33. Höber, R. Effect of some sulfonamides on renal secretion. *Proc. Soc. Exp. Biol. Med.* 49: 87–90, 1942.

34. Hodler, J., H. O. Heinemann, A. P. Fishman, and H. W. Smith. Urine pH and carbonic anhydrase activity in the marine dogfish. *Am. J. Physiol.* 183: 155–162, 1955.

35. Janowitz, H. D., H. Colcher, and F. Hollander. Inhibition of gastric secretion of acid in dogs by the carbonic anhydrase inhibitor, 2-acetylamino-1,3,4-thiadiazole-5-sulfonamide. *Am. J. Physiol.* 171: 325–330, 1952.

36. Kessler, R. H., R. Lozano, and R. F. Pitts. Studies on structure diuretic activity relationships of organic compounds of mercury. *J. Clin. Invest.* 36: 656–668, 1957.

36a. Krebs, H. A. Inhibition of carbonic anhydrase by sulfonamides. *Biochem. J.* 43: 525–528, 1948.

37. Leaf, A., W. B. Schwartz, and A. S. Relman. Oral administration of a potent carbonic anhydrase inhibitor ("Diamox"). I. Changes in electrolyte and acid-base balance. *N. Engl. J. Med.* 250: 759–764, 1954.

38. Mann, T., and D. Keilin. Sulfanilamide as a specific inhibitor of carbonic anhydrase. *Nature Lond.* 146: 164–165, 1940.

39. Maren, T. H. (cited by Clapp, J. W.). In: A new metabolic pathway for a sulfonamide group. *J. Biol. Chem.* 233: 207–214, 1956.

40. Maren, T. H. Carbonic anhydrase inhibition. IX. Augmentation of the renal effect of meralluride by acetazolamide. *J. Pharmacol. Exp. Ther.* 123: 311–315, 1958.

41. Maren, T. H. Carbonic anhydrase: chemistry, physiology, and inhibition. *Physiol. Rev.* 47: 597–781, 1967.

42. MAREN, T. H. The development of ideas concerning the role of carbonic anhydrase in the secretion of aqueous humor: relation to the treatment of glaucoma. In: *Glaucoma: Applied Pharmacology in Medical Treatment*, edited by S. M. Drance. New York: Grune & Stratton, 1984, chapt. 15, p. 325–335.

42a. MAREN, T. H. Renal bicarbonate reabsorption in marine fish, represented by *Squalus acanthias*, is based on H^+ secretion independent of CO_2. *Bull. Mt. Desert Isl. Biol. Lab.* In press.

43. MAREN, T. H., E. MAYER, and B. C. WADSWORTH. Carbonic anhydrase inhibition. I. The pharmacology of Diamox® 2-acetylamino-1,3,4-thiadiazole-5-sulfonamide. *Bull. Johns Hopkins Hosp.* 95: 199–243, 1954.

44. MAREN, T. H., B. C. WADSWORTH, E. K. YALE, and L. G. ALONZO. Carbonic anhydrase inhibition. III. Effects of Diamox® on electrolyte metabolism. *Bull. Johns Hopkins Hosp.* 95: 277–321, 1954.

45. MAREN, T. H., and C. E. WILEY. Renal activity and pharmacology of *N*-acyl and related sulfonamides. *J. Pharmacol. Exp. Ther.* 143: 320–342, 1964.

46. MARSHALL, E. K., JR., W. C. CUTTING, and K. EMERSON, JR. The toxicity of sulfanilamide. *J. Am. Med. Assoc.* 110: 252–257, 1938.

47. MCKINNEY, T. D., and M. B. BURG. Bicarbonate absorption by rabbit cortical collecting tubules in vitro. *Am. J. Physiol.* 234 (*Renal Fluid Electrolyte Physiol.* 3): F141–F145, 1978.

48. MELDRUM, N. U., and F. J. W. ROUGHTON. Carbonic anhydrase: its preparation and properties. *J. Physiol. Lond.* 80: 113–142, 1933.

49. MILLER, W. H., A. M. DESSERT and R. O. ROBLIN, JR. Heterocyclic sulfonamides as carbonic anhydrase inhibitors. *J. Am. Chem. Soc.* 72: 4893–4896, 1950.

50. MUDGE, G. H., and I. M. WEINER. The mechanism of action of mercurial and xanthine diuretics. *Ann. NY Acad. Sci.* 71: 344–354, 1958.

51. MUSCHAWEK, R. Discovery and development of furosemides; historical remarks. In: *Diuretics: Chemistry, Pharmacology, and Clinical Applications*, edited by J. B. Puschett. New York: Elsevier, 1984, sect. 1, p. 4–11.

52. MUSCHAWEK, R., and P. HAJDU. Die salidiuretische Wirksamkeit der Chlor-N-(2-furylmethyl)-5-sulfamlanthranilsaure. *Arzneim. Forsch.* 14: 44–47, 1964.

53. NECHAY, B. R. Aminophylline and its relationship to some other diuretic agents in dogs. *J. Pharmacol. Exp. Ther.* 132: 339–344, 1961.

54. PETERS, G., and F. ROCH-RAMEL. Thiazide diuretics and related drugs. In: *Handbook of Experimental Pharmacology. Diuretica*, edited by H. Herken. Berlin: Springer-Verlag, 1969, vol. 24, p. 257–385.

55. PETERS, G., and F. ROCH-RAMEL. Furosemide. In: *Handbook of Experimental Pharmacology. Diuretica*, edited by H. Herken. Berlin: Springer-Verlag, 1969, vol. 24, p. 386–405.

56. PITTS, R. F., and R. S. ALEXANDER. The nature of the renal tubular mechanism for acidifying the urine. *Am. J. Physiol.* 144: 239–254, 1945.

57. RELMAN, A., A. LEAF, and W. B. SCHWARTZ. Oral administration of a potent carbonic anhydrase inhibitor ("Diamox"). II. Its use as a diuretic in patients with severe congestive heart failure. *N. Engl. J. Med.* 250: 800–804, 1954.

58. ROBLIN, R. O., JR., and J. W. CLAPP. The preparation of heterocyclic sulfonamides. *J. Am. Chem. Soc.* 72: 4890–4892, 1950.

59. SAXL, P., and R. HEILIG. Über die diuretische Wirkung von Novasurol- und anderen Quecksilberinjektionen. *Wien. Klin. Wochenschr.* 43: 943–944, 1920.
60. SCHLATTER, E., R. GREGOR, and C. WEIDTKE. Effect of "high ceiling" diuretics on active salt transport in the cortical thick ascending limb of Henle's loop of rabbit kidney. *Pfluegers Arch.* 396: 210–217, 1983.
61. SCHWARTZ, W. B. The effect of sulfanilamide on salt and water excretion in congestive heart failure. *N. Engl. J. Med.* 240: 173–177, 1949.
62. SCHWARTZ, W. B., A. RELMAN, and A. LEAF. Oral administration of a potent carbonic anhydrase inhibitor ("Diamox"). III. Its use as a diuretic in patients with severe congestive heart failure due to cor pulmonale. *Ann. Intern. Med.* 42: 79–89, 1955.
63. SOLLMANN, T., and N. E. SCHREIBER. Comparative diuretic response to clinical injections of various mercurials. *Arch. Intern. Med.* 58: 1067–1085, 1936.
64. SOUTHWORTH, H. Acidosis associated with the administration of para-amino-benzene-sulfonamide (Prontylin). *Proc. Soc. Exp. Biol. Med.* 36: 58–61, 1937.
64a. STRAUSS, M. B., and SOUTHWORTH, H. Urinary changes due to sulfanilamide administration. *Bull. Johns Hopkins Hosp.* 63: 41–45, 1938.
65. SWENSON, E. R., and T. H. MAREN. A quantitative analysis of CO_2 transport at rest and during maximal exercise. *Respir. Physiol.* 35: 129–159, 1978.
66. SWENSON, E. R., and T. H. MAREN. The dissociation of CO_2 hydration and renal acid secretion in the dogfish, *Squalus acanthias. Am. J. Physiol.* 250: (*Renal Fluid Electrolyte Physiol.* 19): F288–F293, 1986.
67. TINKER, J. P., R. COULSON, and I. M. WEINER. Dextran-bound inhibitors of carbonic anhydrase. *J. Pharmacol. Exp. Ther.* 218: 600–607, 1981.
68. TRAVIS, D. M., C. WILEY, B. R. NECHAY, and T. H. MAREN. Selective renal carbonic anhydrase inhibition without respiratory effect. Pharmacology of 2-benzenesulfonamido-1,3,4-thiadiazole-5-sulfonamide(CL 11,366). *J. Pharmacol. Exp. Ther.* 143: 383–394, 1964.
69. VELÁZQUEZ, H., and F. S. WRIGHT. Effects of diuretic drugs on Na, Cl, and K transport by rat renal distal tubule. *Am. J. Physiol.* 250 (*Renal Fluid Electrolyte Physiol.* 19): F1013–F1023, 1986.
70. VOGL, A. The discovery of the organic mercurial diuretics. *Am. Heart J.* 39: 881–883, 1950.
70a. WEINER, I. M., R. I. LEVY, and G. H. MUDGE. Studies on mercurial diuresis: renal excretion, acid stability and structure-activity relationships of organic mercurials. *J. Pharmacol. Exp. Ther.* 138: 96–112, 1962.
71. WIEBELHAUS, V. D., J. WEINSTOCK, A. B. MAASS, F. T. BRENNAN, G. SOSNOWSKI, and T. LARSEN. The diuretic and natruretic activity of triamterene and several related pteridines in the rat. *J. Pharmacol. Exp. Ther.* 149: 397–403, 1965.
72. WITHERING, W. An account of the foxglove, and some of its medical uses; with practical remarks on dropsy, and other diseases. Birmingham, England: M. Swinney. 1785.

XIV

Comparative Renal Physiology

WILLIAM H. DANTZLER

COMPARATIVE studies have played an important historical role in the development of the principles of renal physiology and play an even more important role today. At the same time, comparative studies in renal physiology have been among the most significant scientifically of all comparative work.

COMPARATIVE PHYSIOLOGY

There are a number of fascinating and important aspects to the study of comparative physiology. These include the possibilities of observing a particular physiological mechanism in an exaggerated form in a single species, of determining the universality of a physiological principle in a variety of species, and of using a simple preparation to study mechanisms of general physiological interest. Perhaps most people who today consider themselves comparative physiologists are intrigued by those physiological processes—and the principles reflected therein—that make it possible for diverse species to survive and indeed to thrive under widely different environmental conditions. This perhaps should be a guiding theme for all comparative research because it helps suggest those scientific studies that may reveal important general physiological principles. However, this has not always been the case. Many physiologists have initially taken the opportunity to study a single mechanism in an exaggerated form or with a simple preparation and only secondarily have become intrigued by the broader implications of their work for the organism. The results have often been no less important for both renal physiology in general and comparative physiology in particular than if the studies had been approached with a broader goal in mind.

Early Studies

The study of comparative renal physiology (and indeed the study of modern renal physiology) begins with a study in comparative anatomy, although undertaken from a functional point of view:

William Bowman's structural analysis of the renal glomerulus and renal circulation. Published in 1842, when Bowman was only twenty-six years old, "On the Structure and Use of the Malpighian Bodies of the Kidney, with Observations on the Circulation through that Gland" is certainly the classic paper in renal anatomy (6). Technically Bowman took advantage of the double-injection method (saturated solutions of potassium dichromate and lead acetate injected in succession) developed by Douere to visualize the small vessels. Conceptually, however, he considered the renal structure in many different animal species before reaching his conclusions (Fig. 1). Although even Malpighi (103) examined a number of species, Bowman appears to have taken much greater advantage of the diversity and, at the same time, the similarity of structures among the vertebrates—a true comparative analysis—to develop his ideas.

Bowman examined the kidneys of numerous mammals (including humans), birds, reptiles, amphibians, and fishes; as a result he was able to demonstrate that the Malpighian body in all species consists of "*the dilated extremity of the uriniferous tube, with a small mass of blood-vessels inserted into it*" (6). He clearly described the basement membrane of the tubules and the manner in which it was expanded to form the capsule (which we now term *Bowman's capsule*) over the glomerular tuft. Drawing especially on observations of nonmammalian vertebrates, Bowman corroborated his initial impression that in all species the glomerular capillaries hang free within the capsule and that the capsule opens directly into the lumen of the proximal tubule.

He clearly described (6) the manner in which "*all the blood of the renal artery (with the exception of a small quantity distributed to the capsule, surrounding fat, and the coats of the larger vessels) enters*" the glomerulus through the afferent arteriole, the manner in which this vessel breaks up into the glomerular capillaries, the way in which the capillaries then reunite to form the efferent arteriole, and the way in which the efferent arteriole breaks up into the peritubular capillary network that finally empties into the renal veins. Of particular interest from a comparative point of view, Bowman described the differences in the glomerular capillary bundle among numerous species: from the extreme simplicity in birds (often only a few coils of a single capillary) and reptiles to the marked complexity of a branching network in mammals (Fig. 1). These differences are better described today with modern techniques and offer a unique opportunity to understand glomerular function, but they were well demonstrated by Bowman's meticulous injection studies (Fig. 1). Bowman also described the contribution of the renal venous portal system to the peritubular capillary blood supply in most nonmammalian vertebrates, an observation exploited by later workers that permitted important comparative physiological studies of the function of renal tubules.

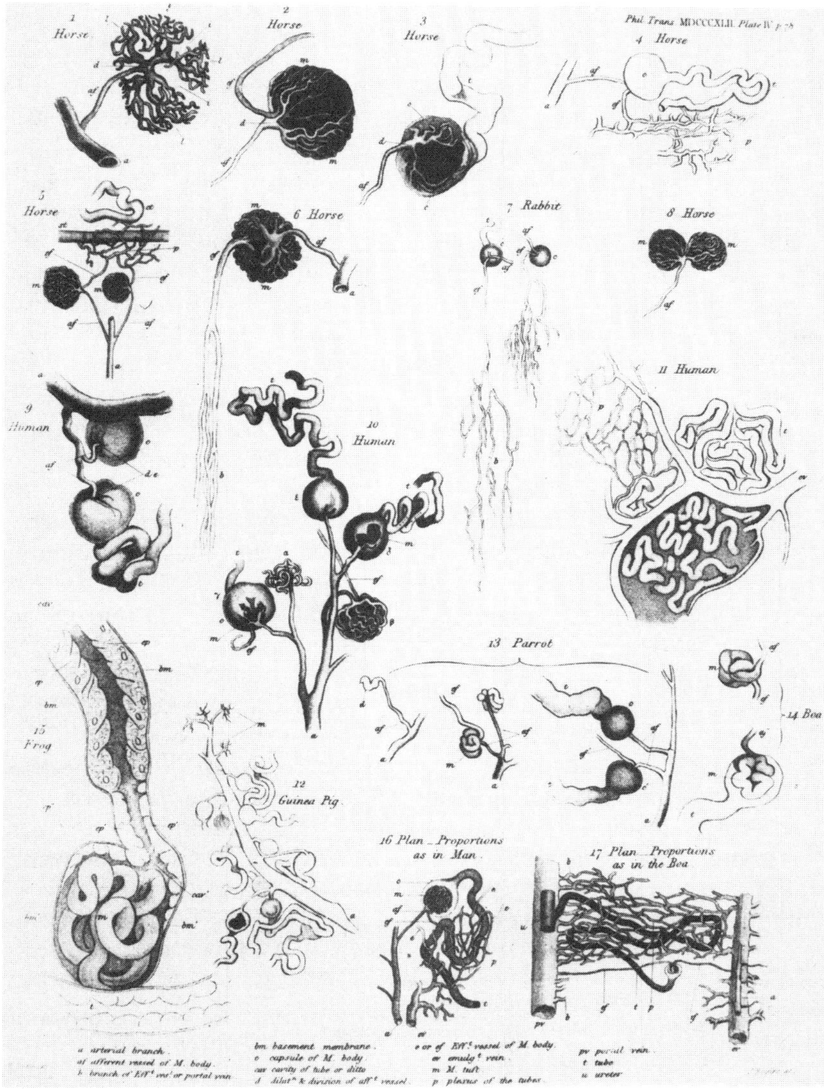

Figure 1. William Bowman's conception of the comparative anatomy of the kidney, illustrating especially comparative glomerular structure. [From Bowman (6).]

Bowman did not engage in true physiological studies but strongly suggested "*principally on anatomical grounds*" (6) that the initial process in urine formation involved the secretion of water by the glomerular capillary tuft. "*It would indeed be difficult to conceive a disposition of parts more calculated to favor the escape of water from the blood, than that of the Malpighian body*" (6). Bowman went on to suggest, although less certainly, that under normal circumstances all other constituents of urine are secreted by the renal tubules.

Although this view was supported thirty years later by the experiments of Rudolph Heidenhain (103), it was almost immediately challenged by the work of Carl Ludwig. Ludwig's theory, based on initial experiments almost certainly performed before the publication of Bowman's work and involving anatomical and chemical measurements, was first expounded in 1842 and published in 1843, probably without any knowledge of Bowman's ideas (103). Ludwig suggested that a protein-free, cell-free filtrate of the plasma, sufficient in magnitude to hold all the constitutes of urine, was produced by the hydrostatic pressure in the glomerular capillaries. He further suggested that a portion of this filtrate is reabsorbed into the peritubular capillaries by a force resulting from the concentration of the blood in these capillaries (103).

The controversy surrounding the Bowman-Heidenhain secretion hypothesis and the Ludwig filtration-reabsorption hypothesis as the major theories of renal function lasted into the second quarter of this century and is thoroughly reviewed in several chapters in this volume and elsewhere (103). However, although Ludwig studied a number of mammalian species, he did not take a true comparative approach to his work. Indeed, with the notable exception of the experiments of Maritz Nussbaum published in 1878 (82), no comparative physiological studies of renal function were done from Bowman's time through the rest of the nineteenth century.

Nussbaum took advantage of the dual blood supply of the amphibian kidney so well described by Bowman to try to determine the relative contributions of the glomeruli and tubules to the formation of urine. He attempted to eliminate any glomerular function in frogs by ligating the arterial supply to the kidney while leaving the renal venous portal system intact. When he performed this maneuver, urine flow ceased. However, when he followed the arterial ligation with an intravenous injection of urea, urine flow was restored. Nussbaum concluded that urea was secreted by the renal tubules. This experiment did not truly differentiate between secretion and filtration of fluid at the glomerulus. It only illustrated that glomerular function normally accounts for most of the urine formed and indicated that the tubules might be able to secrete urea.

Nussbaum did not enunciate any conceptual generalities with broad implications like those of Ludwig or Heidenhain. However, although his experiment did not provide the definitive information he sought, it stands out both as an attempt to take advantage of the anatomical and physiological features of a particular species to solve a problem of general physiological significance—an important use of the comparative approach—and as one of the few studies of renal function involving significant experimental physiological manipulation during the last half of the nineteenth century. The observations, later confirmed by others with a better oxygenated preparation (82), together with the original anatomical observations of Bowman apparently convinced everyone (although not until the first quarter of this century) that the glomerulus is the primary if not the sole route for removal of fluid from the blood in glomerular species.

Nussbaum's experiment was also the first to indicate the usefulness of amphibians for experimental renal studies. These animals, because of their ease of handling, adequate renal function in the pithed (or in recent years anesthetized) state, easy accessibility of the kidney and its glomeruli and tubules, large size of tubule cells, and dual renal blood supply, have played an extremely important role in the experimental determination of the principles of renal physiology. The experimental utility of the dual blood supply to the amphibian kidney was emphasized by the double-perfusion technique devised by Winifred C. Cullis (27) in 1906. By inserting one cannula into the aorta and another into the anterior abdominal vein, a collateral of the renal portal vein, she was able to present to the tubules substances not contained in the arterial fluid perfusing the glomeruli. The doubly perfused amphibian kidney preparation has been used extensively and is still used in current renal physiology, especially for studies of renal tubular transport.

The next important steps in comparative renal physiology began in the 1920s and were synonymous with major advances in renal physiology in general. They involved the work of the two leading renal physiologists of that era, Alfred Newton Richards and Eli Kennerly Marshall, Jr., and their collaborators.

Few people have contributed more to any area of experimental physiology than have Richards and his colleagues to renal physiology during the 1920s and 1930s. Because of the importance of Richards's technical developments and experiments to our present understanding of renal physiology, his accomplishments and the stories behind them have been discussed extensively previously (103) and are considered in other chapters of this volume. Only the aspects of these experiments that relate to comparative physiology are considered here.

As noted by others, Richards entered renal physiology by way of biochemistry and pharmacology (103). Apparently his interest in the pharmacological and toxicological effects of various substances (e.g., chloroform) led him and his colleagues to develop adequate systems for perfusing organs, including the kidney (103). These studies in turn led to his initial interest in the effects of perfusion pressure and epinephrine on renal function and the suggestion that filtration at the glomerulus was indeed, as Ludwig had hypothesized, the initial process in urine formation (84–86). While contemplating these findings and trying to determine how to study these problems more directly, Richards apparently read a paper by Krogh (61) describing his direct observations of the capillaries in the tongue and muscles of frogs. Krogh, who made myriad contributions to physiology during the first half of this century, had such a broad background and interest in all biological processes that he was able to find appropriate biological systems for the study of many physiological problems. In fact he enunciated what has come to be known as "the August Krogh principle," that is, for every biological problem there is a species uniquely suited for its study. Richards of course was familiar with the classic works of Nussbaum and others on renal function in frogs, and while reading Krogh's work, he conceived of directly examining the circulation in frog kidneys, perhaps even glomerular circulation, and the action of epinephrine on it (87).

Thus inspired, Richards and Carl Frederic Schmidt began in the fall of 1920 to examine glomerular circulation in living frogs (usually *R. pipiens* but sometimes *R. catesbeiana* or *R. palustris*) (87). Although this study often receives less attention than the succeeding micropuncture studies in many accounts of Richards's work, it is important not only for establishing the basic experimental approach for those later studies but particularly, in comparative renal physiology, for demonstrating aspects of glomerular regulation. Richards and Schmidt found that, under low-power magnification and with appropriately focused and cooled incident light, they could view the circulation in glomeruli on the ventral surface of the kidney. They immediately noticed that the movement of blood in glomerular capillaries varied enormously: "*in some it is of bewildering rapidity through a maze of pathways: in others, it is a slower progression of cells through fewer channels*" (87). The number and size of the capillary channels, as determined by the red cells passing through them, were seen to vary with time in individual glomeruli (Fig. 2). Richards and Schmidt also realized that the number of glomeruli through which blood circulates (i.e., the number of "active" or "functioning" glomeruli) varies markedly. This intermittent function was seen to occur spontaneously in individual glomeruli, even in apparently volume-replete animals (Fig. 3), and could be produced in such animals by the intravenous injection of epinephrine (the circulatory effects of which formed the impetus for this study) and by the stimulation of sympathetic nerves (Figs. 4 and 5). In addition the intravenous injection of pituitrin (a crude mammalian neurohypophysial extract containing both vasopressin and oxytocin) could produce cessation of glomerular function. This last observation is particularly significant in the more recent comparative studies involving glomerular intermittency and the state of hydration in non-

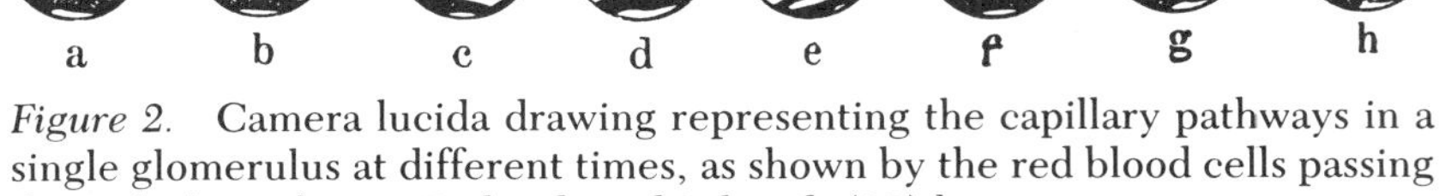

Figure 2. Camera lucida drawing representing the capillary pathways in a single glomerulus at different times, as shown by the red blood cells passing through them. [From Richards and Schmidt (87).]

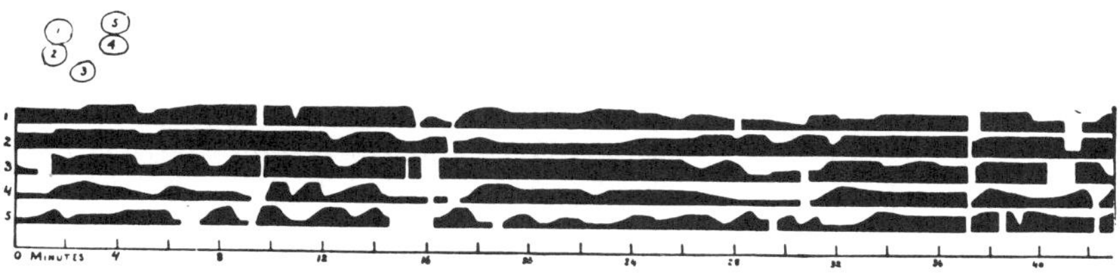

Figure 3. Chart representing spontaneous variations in blood flow through 5 adjacent frog glomeruli (positions indicated by numbered circles, *upper left*). Five telegraph keys representing the 5 chosen glomeruli were set up alongside a microscope through which the glomeruli were viewed. Each key was connected to a signal magnet arranged to write on a smoked drum. The appropriate key was pressed whenever the blood flow stopped or slowed appreciably in any glomerulus, and the meaning of the signals was recorded on the drum. *Ordinate*, glomeruli number; *abscissa*, time in minutes; broad lines, rapid flow; narrow lines, slow flow; interruptions in lines, cessation of flow. [From Richards and Schmidt (87).]

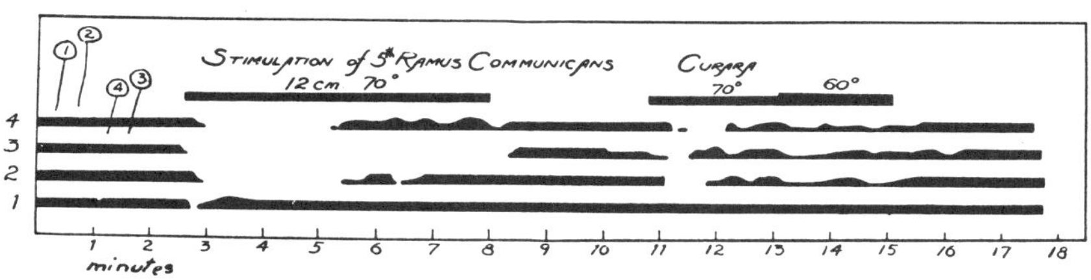

Figure 4. Chart showing variations in blood flow through 4 adjacent frog glomeruli caused by stimulation of sympathetic nerves to the kidney (5th ramus communicans). Lines and recording method, same as for Fig. 3. [From Richards and Schmidt (87).]

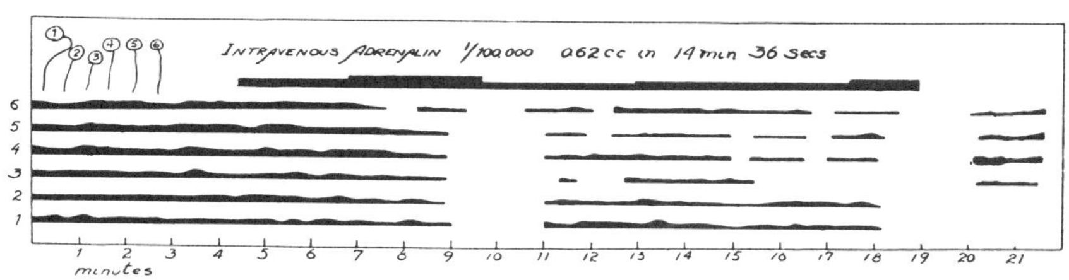

Figure 5. Chart showing variations in blood flow through 6 adjacent frog glomeruli produced by slow injection of epinephrine diluted 1/100,000. Variations in breadth of injection-signal line approximate intentional variations in injection rate. Lines and recording method, same as for Fig. 3. [From Richards and Schmidt (87).]

mammalian vertebrates (see Regulation of Glomerular Filtration, p. 467). The authors saw no evidence that the capillaries contracted; they interpreted their data, without direct observation, as indicating that contraction and relaxation occur at the level of the arterioles—a view generally supported by many later studies.

Because of the changes observed in the number of capillaries through which blood flows, Richards and Schmidt suggested that variation in the functioning glomerular surface area must be considered a major factor in glomerular urine formation. This concept emerged before Richards and his colleagues had provided strong evidence that ultrafiltration actually occurs at the glomerulus, although Richards clearly believed that Ludwig was correct in this regard. The idea that surface area (now expressed as the area available for filtration) is important for renal function continues to be a significant concept in current studies on glomerular regulation in all vertebrates.

Richards and Schmidt stressed the idea of "*glomerular intermittence*" (Fig. 3) and concluded that not all glomeruli are functioning at any one time in the normal kidney. Glomerular intermittence, like variations in the number of capillaries through which blood is flowing in a given glomerulus, is important in determining the total surface area available for filtration. This concept of intermittent glomerular function, derived as it was from studies on accessible glomeruli in the amphibian kidney, may not apply to normal mammals, but it continues to play an important role in all thinking on comparative renal function in nonmammalian vertebrates (35).

The development of this amphibian preparation for direct observation of glomeruli led to the original micropuncture experiments for which Richards and his colleagues are so well known. The story of the initiation of these experiments, of the technical developments, and of the major findings has been told so often by Richards (83, 110) and by others (103) that it does not need repeating here. However, a few observations are particularly important with regard to comparative renal physiology. The definitive demonstration of glomerular ultrafiltration in amphibians [both anurans (frogs) and urodeles (*Necturi*) (82, 88)] and its later confirmation in mammals (108) not only established the universality of this process and the utility of nonmammalian vertebrates for its study but also permitted and made scientifically legitimate future comparative studies of the regulation of the filtration process, especially in nonmammalian vertebrates. Similarly the micropuncture studies of segmental function along the nephrons of amphibians, particularly *Necturi*, not only demonstrated the major tubular sites for certain processes (e.g., glucose absorption in proximal tubules and acidification in distal tubules) but also illustrated the usefulness of amphibian nephrons for more detailed studies of tubular transport in the future (82).

Simultaneously with Richards's studies in the 1920s, Marshall was deliberately taking advantage of the comparative approach to demonstrate that renal tubules secrete as well as reabsorb substances. His studies are often cited as an outstanding example of the importance of comparative physiology and as an application of the August Krogh principle (the deliberate selection of a species in which a particular function is so exaggerated that it can be studied readily). As with Richards's micropuncture experiments, the story of Marshall's studies on tubular secretion has been told so often and so well, particularly by Homer Smith (103) and Bodil Schmidt-Nielsen (93), that it scarcely needs repeating here. However, some points related to the development of comparative renal physiology deserve to be stressed.

Although Richards's initial studies in the 1920s confirmed the existence of glomerular ultrafiltration and with it the occurrence of tubular reabsorption (many filtered substances disappeared from the filtrate as it flowed along the tubules), they provided no evidence on the process of tubular secretion. No adequate filtered-volume marker was available to indicate the extent of fluid absorption or whether the increased concentration of a substance along the tubules was a result of such fluid reabsorption or net secretion.

Even at the beginning of the 1920s, Marshall believed that the possibility of tubular secretion should not be summarily dismissed, as Arthur R. Cushny had done in his influential volume *The Secretion of Urine* (28) in 1917. In 1923 Marshall's work with Vickers on phenol red excretion in dogs (71), which indicated that the amount excreted probably could not be explained by any reasonable estimate of filtration and that the dye accumulated in the renal cortex even when blood pressure was reduced to the point that urine flow ceased, provided the first convincing, if indirect, evidence for tubular secretion in mammals. Of more importance from a comparative viewpoint, however, was Marshall's study with Crane (69) indicating that as plasma levels of urea and phenol red were increased, phenol red excretion but not urea excretion leveled off in dogs and both urea excretion and phenol red excretion leveled off in frogs (*R. catesbeiana*). They reasoned that this leveling off of excretion indicated "saturation" of a secretory process in the renal tubules and concluded that whereas urea was excreted solely by filtration in dogs (and other mammals), phenol red in dogs and both urea and phenol red in frogs were excreted by filtration and tubular secretion. Although this was the first really conclusive evidence of tubular secretion, at the time of its publication most people, including Richards, were not convinced.

At this same time, E. Brice C. Mayrs (72) developed similar evidence that uric acid excretion in chickens exceeded that level that could be filtered. These studies, performed in Cushny's laboratory in Edinburgh, failed to convince Cushny or anyone else, except those already convinced, of the presence of tubular secretion.

Marshall knew that he needed more direct evidence of tubular secretion. However, this initial comparative study apparently convinced him that there were distinct differences in the development of renal function in the different classes of vertebrates that could and indeed must be exploited to fully understand renal function.

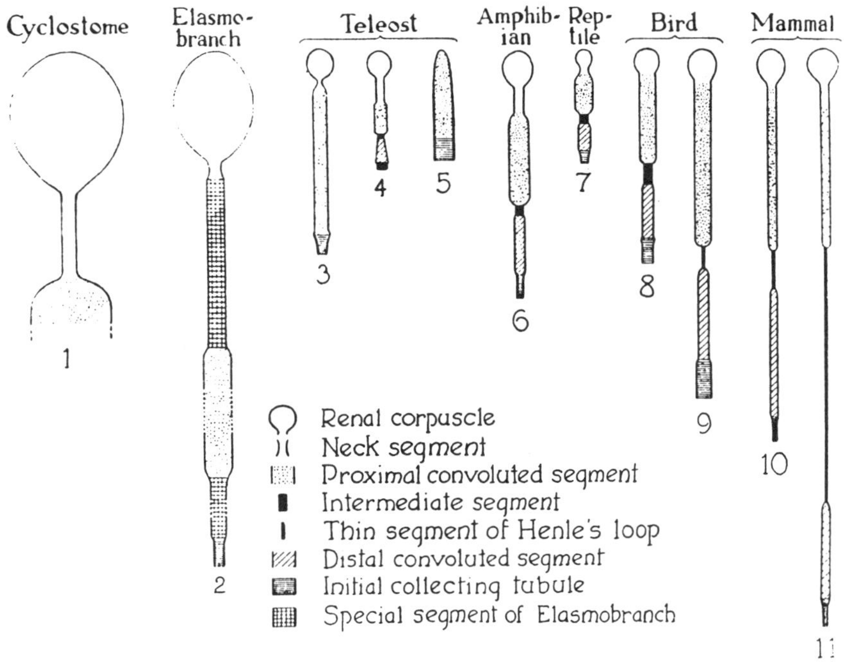

Figure 6. Schematic representation of vertebrate nephron segments. [From Marshall (68).]

Therefore he began to search the literature for information on the comparative physiology of the kidney.

This search of course led to his becoming aware that certain fish, most notably the goosefish (*Lophius piscatorius*), have kidneys with nephrons that apparently lack both glomeruli and an arterial blood supply (only the renal portal blood supply remains). On finding that *Lophius* could be obtained in the coastal waters of Maine, he went to Mount Desert Island Biological Laboratory in the summer of 1926. With Grafflin he began the well-known anatomical and physiological studies that led to the confirmation of the aglomerular nature of these kidneys and the definitive demonstration of tubular secretion and its involvement in urine formation (70). With these studies the three major general processes involved in renal function—glomerular filtration, tubular reabsorption, and tubular secretion—were well documented and generally accepted.

Marshall's appearance at Mount Desert Island Biological Laboratory in the summer of 1926 was very important for the development of comparative renal physiology. Not only did it apparently convince Smith to concentrate on renal research, leading to many fruitful studies in comparative renal physiology and in renal physiology in general, it also led to the emphasis on the comparative approach to studying the steps in tubular transport of organic molecules as well as fluid and electrolytes that has extended to the present (see Tubular Transport, p. 476). Marshall continued his comparative studies of tubular structure and function for the next six years, concentrating on teleost fishes, reptiles, and amphibians, and culminating in his well-known comparison of the tubular segments in vertebrate kidneys [Fig. 6; (68)]. Although Marshall left renal physiology at this point, saying (as he has often been quoted) that he had answered the questions that interested him and that he was not interested in the second decimal, he left behind the legacy of the comparative approach to the solution of problems in renal physiology.

Expanding Studies in Comparative Renal Physiology

As Smith turned his full attention to renal physiology and associated problems from the middle 1920s on and, by the force of his personality and the example of his work, attracted many young workers to the field, studies in comparative renal physiology (as well as in renal physiology in general) expanded greatly. As Smith noted in his own comments on Marshall's work, "*Comparative study of renal function in all classes of vertebrates was essential to the proper understanding of this complicated problem*" (103). Except for the hiatus during World War II, the number and type of such studies have increased even more dramatically to the present day.

Smith's major contributions to renal physiology and their place in the historical development of the field are well covered elsewhere in this volume. The important comparative studies by Smith and others can be considered within three broad areas in the development of comparative renal physiology from the 1920s to the present: *1*) glomerular filtration regulation, *2*) tubular transport, and *3*) urine dilution and concentration. Even within these general directions of development, only a few workers and studies can be considered.

Regulation of Glomerular Filtration

As noted above, Richards and Schmidt (87) described apparent intermittent blood flow (and by inference intermittent filtration) in the glomeruli of living frogs. Hayman (52), working in Richards's group, indirectly but elegantly estimated the afferent arteriolar and glomerular capillary pressures in living frogs by controlling the pressure on Bowman's capsule and watching the blood flow in the glomerular capillaries while blocking flow down the proximal tubule. He demonstrated that glomerular capillary pressure must be adequate for filtration. From that time until the 1970s, comparative studies of the regulation of glomerular filtration were generally more indirect.

The search for an adequate marker for the measurement of glomerular filtration and for fluid movements along the renal tubules—an inert substance that was freely filtered but neither secreted nor reabsorbed—proceeded during the 1920s and into the 1930s. The search involved many of the leading workers of that time, including Marshall, Richards, and Smith as well as Poul Brandt Rehberg in Copenhagen. Smith and Richards apparently independently and simultaneously began using inulin in 1933 (82). The story of this development, although aided by comparative studies, is really the subject of other discussions (see the chapter by Bradley in this volume). However, no one championed the clearance approach for the study of glomerular filtration and tubular transport as much as Smith and his colleagues, and this approach dominated the comparative studies of the regulation of glomerular filtration until the 1970s.

In the late 1930s, Smith and his colleagues (79) suggested that the question of glomerular intermittency could be approached indirectly in the intact kidney by studying the maximum rate of tubular reabsorption of filtered glucose. They reasoned that if changes in glomerular filtration rate were the result of changes in the amount filtered by each nephron, but all nephrons continued to function, the maximum reabsorptive rate for glucose would not change. However, if changes in glomerular filtration rate were the result of changes in the number of functioning glomeruli, the tubular maximum would vary with the glomerular filtration rate because tubule cells distal to nonfiltering glomeruli would not receive glucose to reabsorb. The studies by Smith and his co-workers on mammals, including humans, indicated that under normal conditions nephrons did not function intermittently (79, 99).

However, Roy P. Forster, who in 1938 began spending his summers at Mount Desert Island Biological Laboratory, decided to apply this approach to studies on frogs (apparently the bullfrog *R. catesbeiana*), the animals in which Richards and Schmidt (87) had directly observed apparent intermittent glomerular blood flow. Forster (46) had previously found that the glomerular filtration rate in these animals was proportional to urine flow and had concluded on the basis of this observation and the observations of Richards and Schmidt (87) that variations in the whole-kidney glomerular filtration rate were associated with corresponding variations in the number of functioning nephrons. When he found that the tubular maximum for glucose reabsorption varied directly with glomerular filtration rate (Fig. 7) as predicted, he took this evidence as confirmation of glomerular intermittence in the intact unanesthetized animal (47). In view of Richards and Schmidt's earlier observations (87), this study by Forster also appeared to validate this indirect approach to determining glomerular intermittence. In a later study on frogs (*R. clamitans*), Forster and B. Schmidt-Nielsen (95) found that it made no difference whether the maximum rate of tubular transport was measured for a substance reabsorbed by the renal tubules (such as glucose) or for a substance secreted by the renal tubules [such as *p*-aminohippurate (PAH)] because in both cases the tubular maximum

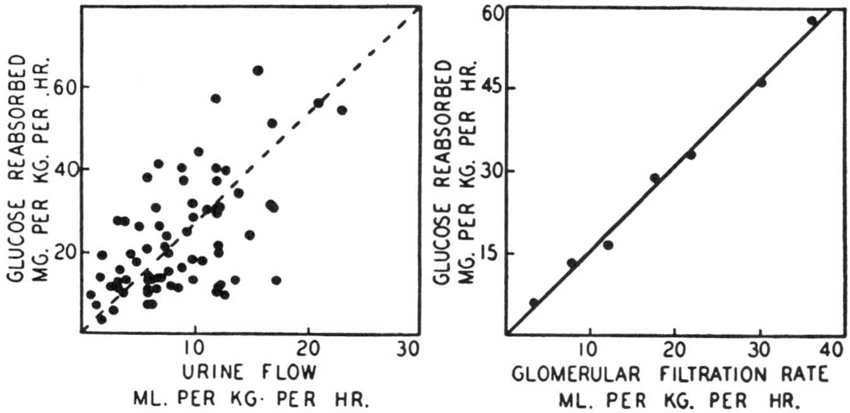

Figure 7. Relationship between maximum rate of glucose reabsorption and simultaneous rates of urine flow and glomerular filtration in frogs. [From Forster (47).]

varied directly with the glomerular filtration rate. This approach became widely used for the determination of possible intermittent glomerular function in nonmammalian vertebrates.

In between these studies by Forster and Schmidt-Nielsen, W. H. Sawyer (then at Harvard) examined the effect of neurohypophysial extracts on renal function in frogs (*R. pipiens*) by combining clearance measurements of glomerular filtration with the direct visualization of glomerular circulation in a manner similar to that employed earlier by Richards and Schmidt (87). Published in 1951, this study (90) indicated that injections of mammalian pituitary extract produce decreased urine flow and whole-kidney glomerular filtration rate (creatinine clearance) and a cessation of blood flow through the glomerular capillaries. (In regard to very recent studies, note that Sawyer has commented to me that, although it was easy to see the red cells stop moving in a single capillary, it was not possible to be certain that all plasma flow also ceased at that time.) This study thoroughly documented the decrease in whole-kidney glomerular filtration rate, apparently as a result of a decrease in the number of filtering nephrons, in response to neurohypophysial extracts. Sawyer's work also indicates that Pitocin (mammalian oxytocin) is apparently more potent than Pitressin (mammalian arginine and lysine vasopressin) in producing this glomerular effect, presaging the later demonstration by Sawyer, Munsick, and van Dyke (91) at Columbia University that arginine vasotocin is the naturally occurring neurohypophysial antidiuretic hormone in amphibians and all other nonmammalian tetrapods.

In their 1954 study on *R. clamitans*, Schmidt-Nielsen and Forster interpreted the decrease in whole-kidney glomerular filtration rate and apparent number of filtering glomeruli during dehydration as an effect of neurohypophysial antidiuretic hormone. By this time the concept of glomerular intermittence in amphibians, controlled at least in part by neurohypophysial antidiuretic hormone, was widely accepted. However, the situation for other nonmammalian vertebrates was much less clear. Although Marshall and his colleagues (18) had shown that the injection of mammalian neurohypophysial extracts into an alligator (probably *Alligator mississippiensis*) apparently produced a decrease in urine flow and glomerular filtration rate (measured as xylose clearance), nothing was really known about possible glomerular intermittence in reptiles or its regulation. During the early 1960s, while working with Schmidt-Nielsen at Duke University (40), I found that in freshwater turtles (*Pseudemys scripta*) and desert tortoises (*Gopherus agassizii*) the maximum rate for tubular secretion of PAH varies directly with the glomerular filtration rate, indicating that nephrons filter intermittently. In freshwater turtles the glomerular filtration rate decreases with dehydration and increases with hydration. From this and preliminary observations that a crude neurohypophysial extract produces a decrease in whole-kidney glomerular filtration rate, we concluded that in chelonian reptiles the number of filtering nephrons is regulated in part by the neurohypophysial antidiuretic hormone arginine vasotocin. The role of arginine vasotocin in regulating the number of filtering nephrons in chelonian reptiles was confirmed some years later by Butler (19) at the University of Toronto.

Shortly after the initial studies on chelonian reptiles, I used a similar approach to examine glomerular intermittence and the regulatory role of arginine vasotocin in ophidian reptiles (the water snake *Natrix sipedon*) (30). Again the correlation between the tubular maximum for PAH and whole-kidney glomerular filtration rate supported the concept of glomerular intermittence, and at physiological levels arginine vasotocin appeared to play an important role in regulating the number of filtering nephrons.

Although the general concept of glomerular intermittence and a probable regulatory role for antidiuretic hormone in this process were accepted for reptiles and amphibians by the middle 1960s, the situation for birds was much less clear. Birds, like mammals, are homeotherms with relatively high, well-controlled arterial blood pressure, making glomerular intermittence seemingly less likely. However, unlike mammals and like reptiles and amphibians, birds have a renal portal system that can supply the tubule cells with oxygen and nutrients in the absence of a postglomerular arterial blood supply, making glomerular intermittence at least a possibility.

The study of this possibility in birds was complicated by the structure of the avian kidney. As depicted by Braun and me (11) in 1972, the avian kidney contains nephrons resembling both those in reptilian kidneys and those in mammalian kidneys (Fig. 8). Most nephrons (~70%–90%, depending on the species) are of the reptilian

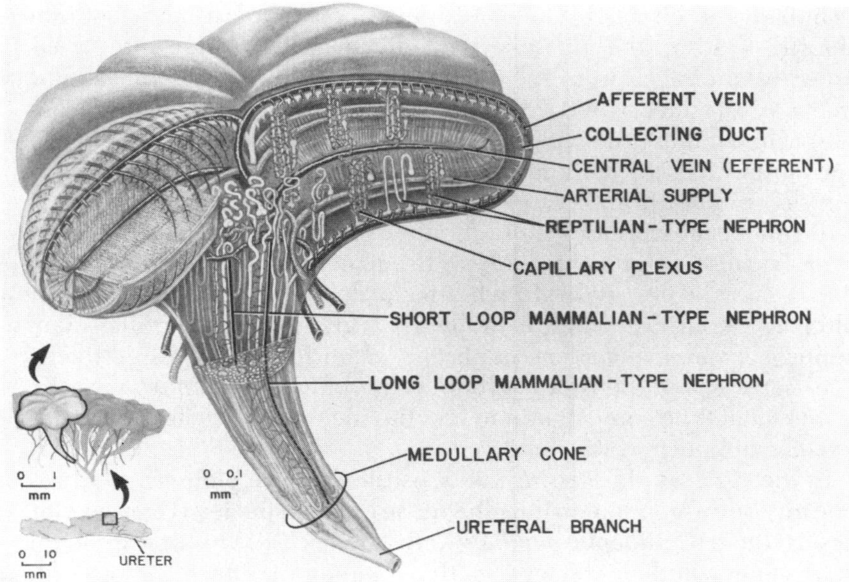

Figure 8. Three-dimensional drawing of a section of avian kidney (Gambel's quail *Callipepla gambelii*) showing types of nephrons present, their relative positions in the kidney, and their relationships to each other and to other renal structures. [From Braun and Dantzler (11).]

type. These nephrons, which lack loops of Henle, are located superficially in the kidney and empty at right angles into collecting ducts. They are not arranged in a manner that would be expected to permit them to contribute directly to a mechanism for production of a urine hyperosmotic to the plasma. However, some nephrons (~10%–30%, depending on the species) are of the mammalian type. These nephrons, which have loops of Henle, are situated deep to the reptilian type. The loops of Henle, the vasa recta (which arise from the efferent arterioles of glomeruli of mammalian-type nephrons), and the collecting ducts (which drain both the reptilian-type and the mammalian-type nephrons) are bound together in parallel by a connective tissue sheath into a tapering medullary cone (Fig. 8). This arrangement, as in mammalian kidneys, would be expected to permit the avian kidney to produce a urine hyperosmotic to the plasma.

With the ability, however modest, to produce a urine hyperosmotic to the plasma, it was not clear that any reduction in glomerular filtration rate in response to dehydration or the need to excrete an osmotic load would be advantageous under normal circumstances. Nevertheless I decided to examine this possibility and to try to determine whether a change in glomerular filtration rate, if it occurred, reflected a change in the number of filtering nephrons. I examined the effects of an acute intravenous hyperosmotic sodium chloride load on the whole-kidney glomerular filtration rate (measured as inulin clearance) and on the maximum rates of tubular transport of glucose and PAH in domestic fowl (*Gallus domesticus*) (29). The whole-kidney glomerular filtration rate decreased and the maximum rates for glucose and PAH transport varied directly with the glomerular filtration rate, indicating that the decrease in filtration rate reflects a decrease in the number of filtering glomeruli. However, because of the complexity of the structure of the avian kidney, these data did not indicate whether a decrease in the number of filtering nephrons, if it did indeed occur, involves reptilian-type nephrons, mammalian-type nephrons, or both. We suggested that if only nephrons of the reptilian type ceased filtering, nephrons of the mammalian type could continue functioning together, allowing maintenance of concentrating ability.

In the process of assessing the sensitivity of the glomerular filtration rate of a nondomestic gallinaceous avian species (Gambel's or desert quail *Callipepla gambelii*), Braun and I (11) attempted to determine whether changes in the number of filtering glomeruli involved only one type of nephron or both types. Initially we observed that, as in the case of domestic fowl, the whole-kidney glomerular filtration rate decreased with the hyperosmotic sodium chloride load and the tubular maximum for PAH transport decreased with it. We also obtained histological evidence that the number of open proximal tubule lumina in the superficial areas of the kidney (the area of the reptilian-type nephrons) decreases as the whole-kidney glomerular filtration rate decreases. Because the lumen of a proximal tubule tends to collapse when filtration ceases and the fluid in the lumen is reabsorbed, these data support the concept of a decrease in the number of filtering reptilian-type nephrons. However, we could not differentiate histologically between the proximal tubules of the deeper reptilian-type nephrons and mammalian-type nephrons.

At this point in our studies of the avian kidney, de Rouffignac et al. (43), in Saclay, France, published their constant-infusion version of the sodium ferrocyanide–precipitation technique for measurement of the filtration rates of individual nephrons. This technique, a substantial modification of one introduced some years earlier by Hanssen (51) in Oslo, Norway, makes possible the determination of filtration rates in nephrons inaccessible to direct micropuncture (see the chapter by Windhager in this volume for details of the technique). On reading de Rouffignac's paper, I was struck by the possibility of applying this technique, which had first been used on rats, to birds in an attempt to assess the filtration rates of nephrons in the two populations and to determine whether both types undergo intermittent function. Braun agreed with this approach and immediately set about validating the technique for the avian kidney. The results clearly demonstrate that under control conditions all mammalian-type nephrons filter at about twice the rate per nephron as reptilian-type nephrons (11). Moreover, even under these control conditions, only ~70% of reptilian-type nephrons filter. During a hyperosmotic sodium chloride load that produces a marked decrease in whole-kidney glomerular filtration rate, all reptilian-type nephrons cease filtering while all mammalian-type nephrons continue filtering at the control rate. Braun (8) went on to demonstrate with vascular-injection studies that this reduction in the number of filtering reptilian-type nephrons apparently results from vasoconstriction at the level of the afferent glomerular arterioles. Later studies indicate that physiological doses of arginine vasotocin can reduce the whole-kidney glomerular filtration rate by reducing the number of filtering reptilian-type nephrons without affecting the filtration rates of functioning nephrons of either type (12). Acute hydration, however, produces a doubling of the single-nephron filtration rates and causes all reptilian-type as well as all mammalian-type nephrons to filter (13). This effect of hydration probably results in part from suppression of arginine vasotocin release, although increased renal blood flow from acute volume expansion may also be important.

By the middle 1970s, the concept of intermittent function of reptilian-type nephrons in the avian kidney and at least partial control of this process by arginine vasotocin was well supported by these studies. However, the constant-infusion sodium ferrocyanide–precipitation technique, although permitting the measurement of filtration rates in nephrons throughout the kidney, only permits such measurements at one point in time. It is not possible to determine filtration rates in the same animal under two different sets of circumstances. Realizing this problem, Laverty and I (64) adapted the micropuncture techniques originally pioneered by Richards to the study of the superficial reptilian-type nephrons of the avian kidney. This approach, although limited to only a portion of one population of nephrons, should permit further analysis of the control of intermittence in these nephrons. Indeed direct observations confirm such intermittent function.

Although the fishes, beginning with Marshall's work in the 1920s, had become important experimental subjects for renal research (attracting both those interested only in the general concepts of renal function and those interested in the adaptations of renal function to an aqueous environment), most attention had focused on tubular transport (see Tubular Transport, p. 476). Glomerular regulation in these animals attracted little attention. In the middle 1960s, however, Hickman (54) at the University of Alberta in Canada suggested that one species of freshwater teleost (the northern pike *Esox lucius*) that had a rudimentary renal portal system (55) might exhibit glomerular intermittence. This assumption was based primarily on the correlation between urine flow and glomerular filtration rate and on the absence of any correlation between tubular water reabsorption and glomerular filtration rate. Shortly thereafter, Mackay, then a graduate student at the University of Alberta, and Beatty (66) demonstrated in another freshwater teleost (the white sucker *Catostomus commersonii*) that the maximum rate of glucose reabsorption varies directly with glomerular filtration rate, suggesting intermittent glomerular function. The glomerular filtration rate in this species shows large natural variations with time (55). It is not clear, however, whether these animals have even a rudimentary renal portal system. At approximately this same time, Lahlou (62), working at the Station Zoologique in Villefranche-sur-Mer, France, found that when the glomerular filtration rate of a euryhaline teleost (the flounder *Platichthys flesus*) varied with changes in salinity the tubular maximum for glucose reabsorption varied directly with it. He also interpreted these findings as indicating intermittent glomerular function. Like all euryhaline teleosts studied (55), these animals have a true renal portal system.

There was little further information on the possibility of glomerular intermittence in fishes until the late 1970s. At this time Henderson and his colleagues at the University of Sheffield and Rankin and his students at the University College of North Wales (both in Great Britain) began exploring this question and others related to glomerular filtration in fishes. Henderson worked with a species of euryhaline teleost (the rainbow trout *Salmo gairdneri*), whereas Rankin worked with a species of primitive lamprey (*Lampetra fluviatilis*). As noted previously, euryhaline teleosts have a true renal portal system, which can supply the tubule cells with blood in the absence of postglomerular blood flow, whereas the primitive lampreys do not (55).

Henderson and his colleagues (14, 15) applied the constant-infusion sodium ferrocyanide–precipitation technique to the problem of measuring single-nephron glomerular filtration rates and determining glomerular intermittence. The adaptation of this technique for use with these fish formed part of the dissertation research of Brown (14, 15). These studies showed that in rainbow trout, ~45% of the nephrons filter in animals adapted to freshwater, whereas only ~5% filter in animals adapted to seawater. This difference in the number of nephrons filtering in freshwater-adapted and seawater-adapted animals corresponds to the difference in whole-kidney glomerular filtration rate under the same set of circumstances. In addition the remaining nephrons filtering during adaptation to seawater do so at an average rate greater than that of nephrons filtering during adaptation to freshwater. These studies also indicate that during changes in the whole-kidney filtration rate, the filtration rates of individual functioning nephrons can change. The physiological effects of arginine vasotocin in fishes are by no means clear, but studies by Rankin (2) and Henderson (53) and their colleagues suggest that this hormone may play a role in the described glomerular adjustments of euryhaline teleosts to seawater.

Rankin and his co-workers (74) applied micropuncture techniques to the measurement of single-nephron glomerular filtration rates in lampreys. Their recent work suggests that when the whole-kidney glomerular filtration rate in these animals decreases with adaptation to brackish water, the filtration rates of all individual nephrons decrease, but none cease filtering (80). Again it must be stressed that these animals have no renal portal system to supply the tubules in the absence of postglomerular arterial blood flow.

Although the concept of changes in the number of filtering glomeruli as the primary process by which the whole-kidney glomerular filtration rate is regulated in nonmammalian vertebrates has developed and generally been supported by experimental work over the sixty years since the observations of Richards and Schmidt (87), it has always been apparent that variations in filtration rate of filtering nephrons occur and must play some role in the observed changes in whole-kidney glomerular filtration rate. In the first observations of glomerular blood flow in frogs (before the process of glomerular ultrafiltration was proven), Richards and Schmidt (87) noted that within a given glomerulus flow could cease in a portion of the capillaries and continue in the rest. Richards and Bordley (5) made similar observations on blood flow in the glomeruli of a few snakes. My colleagues and I suggested that some variation in the filtration rate of filtering nephrons should occur in reptiles and birds (32, 37), and Braun and I (11, 13) documented such changes in birds with the sodium ferrocyanide–infusion technique. Similarly both Hickman (54) and Henderson and his co-workers (14) suggested that in teleosts gradations in filtration by functioning glomeruli could be superimposed on the process of glomerular intermittence, and Henderson and his co-workers demonstrated such changes with the sodium ferrocyanide–infusion technique. However, this technique gives measurements at only one point in time, and in most species few if any glomeruli are directly accessible to micropuncture or direct observation. Therefore very little quantitative information is available on the relative importance of changing blood flow or filtration among functioning glomeruli in nonmammalian vertebrates.

However, in a direct continuation of the historical tradition of the micropuncture work begun by Richards and the microcirculatory studies begun by Krogh, Yokota, working first in my laboratory and then in his own laboratory at the University of West Virginia, is applying the most recent advances in these techniques to glomerular function in ophidian reptiles. Yokota recognized that in these animals (the garter snake *Thamnophis sirtalis*) not only the tubular elements but also the glomerulus and the entire lengths of the afferent and efferent glomerular arterioles are exposed on the dorsomedial surface of the kidney. As noted nearly a century and a half ago by

Bowman (see Early Studies, p. 457) the glomerular capillaries form only a few loops.

Because the kidney cannot be transilluminated, Yokota is using epifluorescent intravital video microscopy to observe and record blood flow to and within the glomeruli. Fluorescein isothiocyanate–labeled albumin is injected intravenously, and with appropriate illumination and filters the red cells can be visualized through a microscope against the fluorescent background. The images are recorded with an appropriate video camera for later off-line analysis of red blood cell velocity with the video dual-slit method (56). These studies are already quantitatively documenting intermittent blood flow and indicating (as expected) that the number of nephrons exhibiting cessation of blood flow increases with the plasma osmolality and that cessation of blood flow can be produced by arginine vasotocin. At the same time, these studies are providing quantitative measurements of blood flow rates in functioning glomeruli. Yokota is beginning to combine these methods with simultaneous direct measurements of pressures in the glomerular arterioles and capillaries with a modern servo-null pressure-measuring system (112) and of glomerular filtration with micropuncture techniques. These studies are taking advantage of the anatomical arrangement of the ophidian kidney—as so often in comparative studies—and of the modern versions of the approaches pioneered by others to analyze glomerular function continuously in real time. Such quantitative methods should offer the possibility of analyzing glomerular regulation far more effectively than previous static determinations.

Tubular Transport

Tubular Secretion

Organic Substances

Studies of tubular secretion, particularly the tubular secretion of organic substances, have formed one of the major research trends in comparative renal physiology for more than half a century. The initial impetus for such studies apparently arose directly from the pioneering work of Marshall that demonstrated tubular secretion (see Early Studies, p. 457). Many comparative studies also represent important steps in the development of renal physiology in general and are discussed in detail in the chapters by Kleinzeller and Weiner in this volume. Only those studies of particular importance for the development of comparative renal physiology are considered here.

As noted previously, during the 1920s and early 1930s, Marshall and his co-workers demonstrated that a number of organic substances, including creatinine, were secreted by the renal tubules of aglomerular fish. Glucose and other sugars were found to be not secreted by these aglomerular tubules, although a much later study indicated that a tiny net secretory flux of glucose could occur (67). During the 1930s, studies by Smith and his colleagues, most notably James A. Shannon, demonstrated tubular secretion of organic substances (both organic acids and bases) by glomerular as well as aglomerular fish (98). These studies at the Mount Desert Island Biological Laboratory took advantage of easily obtainable and readily studied elasmobranchs (the dogfish *Squalus acanthias*) and teleosts (the flounder *Pseudopleuronectes americanus*). These comparative studies of tubular secretion permitted Shannon (98) to analyze the transport process in 1939, at least as a first approximation, in terms of the type of chemical kinetics used in so many studies since then.

Of particular interest in terms of the comparative physiology of tubular transport and of later work on the mechanism of tubular transport is a series of in vivo and in vitro studies in the early 1930s on the secretion of phenol red (or chlorphenol red) by the proximal tubule cells of chick embryos. These studies by Robert Chambers, the same Robert Chambers whose work with micromanipulators inspired Richards a decade earlier, and his colleagues in the Department of Biology at New York University were somewhat out of the developing mainstream of renal physiology. Although the work was surely noted at the time, the potential of studies of this type for the understanding of the transport process was largely ignored for the next fifteen years.

In the late 1920s, Chambers, a true cell physiologist, became interested in the determination of the pH of cell cytoplasm and nuclei by microinjection of indicator dyes. By the beginning of the 1930s, Chambers and Cameron (21) had begun working with cells in tissue culture and noted that the cultured cells of chick mesonephros took up phenol red. Therefore they did not have to inject the sulfonphthalein indicators into these cells to determine pH. Although others had noted that renal tubule cells could become colored by such dyes, Chambers and Cameron (21) took advantage of this property to estimate the intracellular pH of the cultured cells and arrived at a value of ~6.8. Of greater importance for renal physiology, Chambers and Kempton (22) systematically evaluated the transport of phenol red by these mesonephric and (in a few cases) metanephric cells.

Phenol red injected into the amniotic cavity, yolk sac, or extraembryonic vein of a 9-day-old chick embryo rapidly appeared in the allantoic fluid. The proximal tubule cells, but not the other kidney cells or the cells of other organs, were rapidly colored by the dye. This color faded within a few minutes as the dye entered the tubule lumina and moved distally.

The primary in vitro studies involved fragments of teased mesonephric tubules from an 8- to 10-day-old chick embryo incubated at 39°C in an undefined culture medium consisting of equal parts chicken plasma and embryo extract diluted 9:1 with Tyrode solution.

These explants functioned for at least 4 days (usually longer), and Chambers and Kempton found that they could easily differentiate the proximal from the distal tubules (Fig. 9). Within the first 1–2 h of incubation, the broken ends of the tubules became filled with a plug of cells that gradually formed into a single cell layer continuous with the wall of the tubule. In this way the healthy but broken incubated tubules were converted into closed cylinders of various lengths. The lumina of the proximal convoluted, but not the distal, tubule cylinders became distended with fluid within 24 h and after 3–4 days were so distended that the cuboidal epithelium of the walls was flattened. The shorter tubule segments actually became converted into globular cysts (Fig. 9). If these tubules or cysts were punctured with a micropipette and the fluid drained from them, the volume of the lumen was reduced and the cells rapidly returned to

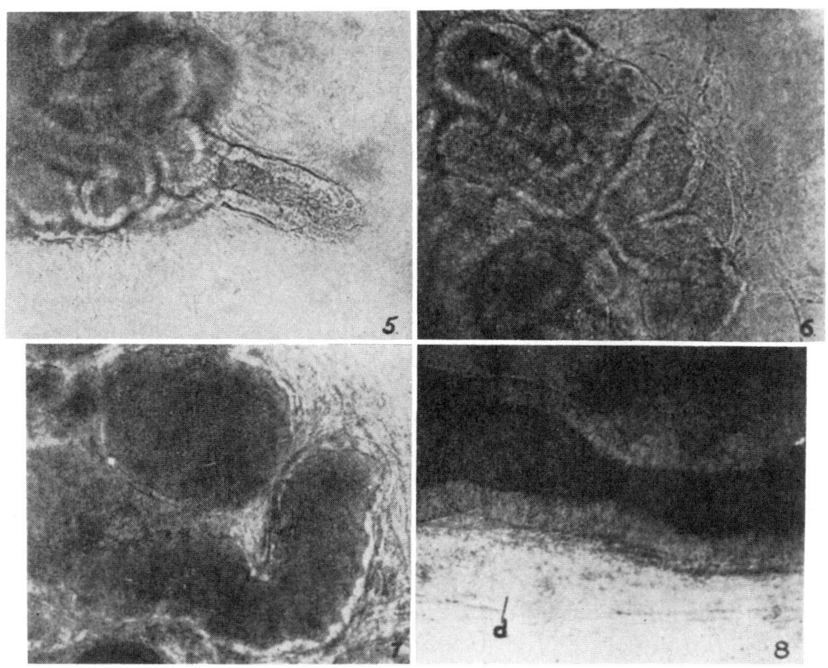

Figure 9. Tissue culture explants of mesonephros from 9-day-old chick embryo. *Panel* 5: 24-hour culture. Broken end of proximal tubule projecting from margin of explant with a plug of cells from which a sheet of epithelium is beginning to grow. *Panel* 6: 24-hour culture. Several closed segments of proximal tubule beginning to distend. *Panel* 7: 72-hour culture. Two closed proximal segments with continued secretion of phenol red that has greatly distended their lumina (*dark areas*). *Panel* 8: proximal and distal segments lying side by side. Proximal segment only (*black area*) is distended with phenol red. Proximal tubule wall (*dark area*) is yellow. Wall of distal tubule (d) is colorless and glassy. [From Chambers and Kempton (22).]

their normal cuboidal form. When the pipette was removed, the hole closed and the tubule became distended again within a few hours. These observations indicate some form of fluid secretion in these tubule segments, but Chambers and Kempton did not explore the process further. However, these remain important initial observations relative to current comparative studies on this process.

With the addition of small amounts of phenol red (or chlorphenol red) to the culture medium at 39°C, the cells of the proximal tubule cylinders or cysts, but not other cells, became faintly to moderately colored. Although Chambers and Kempton suggested that this color was considerably more intense than the medium, indicating concentration of the dye within the cells, they did not attempt to quantitate it. As long as the temperature was maintained at 39°C, the dye was rapidly discharged into the distended lumina, apparently reaching a concentration (estimated from the intensity of the color) of 20–30 times that of the medium (Figs. 9 and 10). When the temperature was lowered to room temperature (probably between 20°C and 25°C), the color remained in the cells but did not enter the lumina. When the temperature was again raised to 39°C, the dye rapidly entered the lumina. At very low temperatures (5°C), dye did not enter the cells or the lumina from the medium and there was apparently no fluid secretion into the lumina. Again this situation was rapidly reversed by warming to 39°C. When the preparation was acidified by incubation in a carbon dioxide and air mixture, secretion was not affected and the color of the cells did not change;

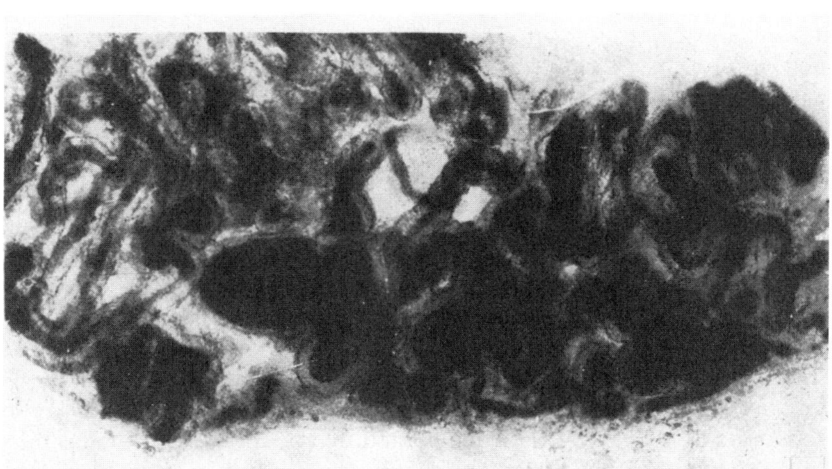

Figure 10. Twenty-four-hour culture of chick mesonephros incubated with phenol red. Lumina (*black areas*) of convoluted proximal tubules are distended with phenol red. Walls of tubules (*dark areas*) are yellow. [From Chambers and Kempton (22).]

however, the luminal fluid appeared to be acidic, as judged by the color of the dye. Phenol red injected into the lumina of distended tubule segments appeared to enter the cells very slowly, indicating that the primary mode of entrance was via the peritubular side. Additional studies demonstrated that transport of phenol red from the incubation medium into the cells and lumina was inhibited by cyanide and iodoacetate (3, 20).

Occasionally distal tubule segments in the explants were found attached to proximal tubule segments. Although the distal tubule cells never took up phenol red from the medium, dye secreted into a proximal tubule lumen could occasionally move distally into an attached distal segment. When this happened, the color changed from red to yellow, indicating acidification.

Although rarely explicitly noted by later workers, Chambers and Kempton showed similar uptake and secretion by cultured metanephric proximal tubules in a few experiments with 18- to 19-day-old chicks and even with explants of 1-wk-old mouse kidneys; however, only a few of the mouse tubules functioned well after 2 h of incubation.

These studies were the first to really begin to indicate the steps in organic anion secretion by the renal tubules. Moreover they suggested an approach to renal studies that was only taken up and developed further fifteen or more years later. Like other important comparative studies, these not only indicated how a particular tissue could be used for the study of a given phenomenon but also indicated how the techniques might be applied to other tissues. It is not clear why analogous approaches were not followed for so many years. Perhaps it was because most of the studies involved the mesonephric kidney; most people appear to have ignored the portion involving the metanephric kidney. More likely, the time simply was not ripe for more quantitative studies involving this approach to tubular transport, and Chambers's own interests lay in other directions. In any case this approach was not really followed again until Forster (48) began studies in this area in the late 1940s.

At that time Forster (48), working at Mount Desert Island Biological Laboratory, began using thin kidney slices and isolated renal tubules from poikilothermic nonmammalian vertebrates to attempt a quantitative assessment of the tubule secretory processes. The most significant aspect of this development involved the use of isolated fish tubules, particularly those of the winter flounder *Pseudopleuronectes americanus.* Forster found that when freshly cut fragments of kidney tissue were placed in a properly balanced saline solution the tubules could be separated readily by agitation and gentle teasing. This permitted each tubule to be exposed to the bathing medium. As with the chick mesonephric tubules studied by Chambers, the cut ends of the flounder tubules rapidly contracted and closed so that substances only entered the lumen across a wall of cells. In the proper medium at a temperature of 24°C–30°C, the tubules concentrated phenol red in their lumina for several hours.

This preparation was a continuation of the experimental development begun fifteen years earlier by Chambers, but it had the distinct advantages of being easier to prepare and maintain and of involving a chemically defined incubation medium. Moreover Forster and Taggart (50, 106) used this preparation to make a semiquantitative assessment of the transport of phenol red. The use of this preparation (as it developed) not only supplied insight into secretory transport in nonmammalian vertebrates but also provided an approach to the understanding of the mechanisms involved in such transport in vertebrates in general. Taggart, as noted elsewhere (see the chapter by Kleinzeller in this volume), went on to develop the kidney-slice approach for renal transport studies in mammalian vertebrates.

With this flounder tubule preparation, Forster and Taggart (50, 106) established a semiquantitative scale for visual assessment of phenol red accumulation in the lumina. They found that the dye concentration in the lumina reached a steady state within 30–60 min. The uptake and maintenance of the steady state depended on the presence of oxygen and were reversibly inhibited by cold. They were also inhibited by agents that interfered with aerobic processes, such as cyanide, aresenite, and azide; by agents known to interrupt aerobic phosphorylation, such as 2,4-dinitrophenol and related compounds; by agents known to inhibit anaerobic glycolysis, such as iodoacetate; by sulfhydryl-binding heavy metals such as mercury; and by other organic anions known to be secreted by the renal tubules of fish, such as PAH and penicillin, but not by organic cations known to be secreted by the renal tubules of fish, such as creatinine. At no time did these investigators observe phenol red accumulation in the tubule cells.

These first studies, although only semiquantitative, employed most of the evaluative steps (at least in terms of metabolic or competitive inhibition) used in later comparative studies of organic anion secretion. However, shortly thereafter another group of investigators—Theodore Puck, Karlman Wasserman, and Alfred Fishman—also working at the Mount Desert Island Biological Laboratory with the advice of Forster and Smith developed a more quantitative assessment of phenol red transport by these flounder tubules and took advantage of the chemically defined medium to assess the ionic requirements for such transport (78). These investigators devised a system for direct visual comparison of the color of the dye in the tubules with standards of known concentration. Although the technique was so crude that it permitted errors as great as 50%–100% in a single reading, the concentrations attained in the tubule lumina were so great that the results were still reasonably reliable. They were certainly the most rigorous measurements of single-tubule transport of organic substances up to that time.

This study indicated that under control conditions the transepithelial secretory process became saturated, but no dye was observed in the cells. When potassium was removed from the medium, no dye appeared in the lumina or cells. When calcium was removed from the medium, no dye appeared in the lumina but a small amount seemed to be present in the cells. In the absence of calcium, an increase in the potassium concentration produced an apparent marked increase of dye in the cells. Both PAH and iodopyracet, another organic acid secreted by the renal tubules, inhibited transport into the lumina in the standard medium and transport into the cells in calcium-free, high-potassium medium. These investigators proposed that net secretion involved two active transport steps, one from the medium into the cells that requires potassium and another from the cells into the lumina that requires calcium.

In an attempt to make these types of secretory studies more quantitative, Kinter (60), working at the Mount Desert Island Biological Laboratory during the summers of 1963–1965, devised a spectrophotometric method to measure chlorphenol red uptake during the course of the experiments. This study showed the time course of saturable transport into the lumina of flounder tubules, permitted an approximate determination of the Michaelis constant (K_m) and the maximum velocity (V_{max}), and indicated directly that other organic anions such as PAH and probenecid were competitive inhibitors of such transport. However, Kinter obtained no evidence of cellular accumulation of the dye during transport. Of course one of the problems of determining the intracellular concentrations of these dyes from the intensity of the color is that the color changes with pH. This was an advantage for Chambers, who was really interested in determining the intracellular pH, but it was a disadvantage for those interested in determining transepithelial transport.

The problem of the intracellular concentration of these exogenous anions during transepithelial transport was resolved with the next development in these studies of tubular transport: the application of the isolated perfused-tubule technique devised by Maurice Burg and his colleagues (16) at the National Institutes of Health (see the chapter by Windhager in this volume). Perfusion of flounder and rabbit tubules by Burg and his colleagues (17, 107) and of snake (*Thamnophis* spp.) and frog (*Rana catesbeiana*) tubules by my colleagues and me (e.g., 34) revealed that transport occurred from bath to lumen against a concentration gradient but that during this transport process the concentration in the cells was always greater than that in the bath or lumen. Therefore the primary energy-requiring transport step is at the peritubular side. These recent studies, which are in the main historical line of determining the details of organic anion secretion that Marshall first demonstrated so clearly (although in much more detail than Marshall thought interesting), have permitted further analysis of the membrane permeabilities and the factors influencing transport at both the peritubular and luminal sides. The most detailed studies, on snake renal tubules, have indicated that the step from cells to lumen is carrier mediated, probably involves anion exchange, and is influenced by calcium (34, 38). However, the calcium effect probably involves calcium entry into the cells (38, 39). The anion exchange process at the luminal membrane is supported (at least for flounder tubules among the nonmammalian vertebrates) by studies involving current membrane vesicle techniques (45) (see the chapter by Kleinzeller in this volume). As indicated in earlier studies, the peritubular transport step (at least in snake tubules) depends on potassium (34). However, it also depends on sodium and apparently on the entry of calcium into the cells (34, 38, 39). The details of these relationships are not yet well understood, but coupled cation and anion countertransport processes may be involved. Clearly work will continue on the comparative aspects of this process in the tradition begun by Marshall.

Studies of tubular transport (particularly tubular secretion) of the end products of nitrogen metabolism have also played a prominent historical role in comparative renal physiology. Urate is the major excretory end product of nitrogen metabolism in birds, in reptiles (except some of the Testudinidae); and even in some of the anuran amphibians (33). Net tubular secretion of urate was first suggested for birds by the work of Mayrs in 1924 (see EARLY STUDIES, p. 457) even before the process of net tubular secretion had been definitively demonstrated by Marshall. This was confirmed by Shannon (97) in 1938, after the acceptance of inulin as a marker for glomerular filtration, when he clearly demonstrated that urate clearance exceeded the simultaneous inulin clearance. Since that time net tubular secretion of urate has been demonstrated by a number of investigators using clearance methods in all uricotelic vertebrates studied (33). Additional advances in understanding these secretory transport processes have only come with the application of in vitro microperfusion and in vivo micropuncture methods (see the chapter by Windhager in this volume).

Following the tradition of the micropuncture experiments begun by Richards and his colleagues but employing current analytical techniques (electron microprobe and high-performance liquid chromatography), Laverty and I (64) have shown in birds that net urate secretion occurs early in the proximal tubule of the superficial reptilian-type nephrons. Whether additional urate secretion or reabsorption occurs beyond this portion of the reptilian-type nephrons in birds has not yet been determined with certainty, but the data suggest that such reabsorption or secretion would be small. More importantly, it has not yet been possible to determine whether any significant urate secretion occurs in the mammalian-type nephrons in which precipitation of urates could interfere with flow through the loops of Henle. The answer to this question may have to await the application of in vitro microperfusion to the proximal tubules of the mammalian-type nephrons, which are inaccessible to micropuncture, a step that has not yet proven possible.

During the past fifteen years, my colleagues and I have examined net urate secretion by reptilian renal tubules (snake *Thamnophis* spp.) isolated and perfused in vitro. In fact we began attempting to perfuse these tubules in the late 1960s specifically to study the steps in the urate secretory process. The attempt grew out of a question I was asked at the Fall Meeting of the American Physiological Society at Howard University, Washington, DC, in 1967. At that time, Jared J. Grantham (then of the National Institutes of Health and now of the University of Kansas Medical Center), after listening to my presentation on urate and PAH secretion by snake kidneys and viewing a diagram of a snake nephron, asked whether these nephrons could be teased from the renal tissue without enzymatic digestion. It appeared unlikely, but we were so interested in understanding the striking urate secretory process in reptiles that late in 1968 we tried. Much to our surprise we found that we could tease out nephron segments in vitro and that with practice this process became progressively easier. Thus began our attempts to perfuse these tubules (34).

As for the other organic anions, these perfusion studies showed that the primary energy-requiring transport step for urate is located at the peritubular membrane (34). We found that the transport of urate occurs throughout the length of the proximal tubule, whereas the transport of other organic anions occurs only in the distal portion of the proximal tubule, thereby confirming the partial spatial separation of transport sites for urate and other organic anions indicated in earlier studies involving alterations in the portal blood flow (31). Moreover there is no competition between urate and PAH for this transport step into the cells on the peritubular membrane. The transport step for urate, like that for other organic anions, may involve an anion-exchange process. However, in contrast to that for other anions, it depends on the presence of potassium but not sodium or calcium. Also, in contrast to PAH and other anions, the movement of urate from the cells into the tubule lumen cannot be shown to be a carrier-mediated process. These studies on nonmammalian renal tubules that only show mediated secretory transport for urate—again the selection of a particular species in which one particular process dominates—have been fruitful in determining the steps in such transport.

Urea is another excretory end product of nitrogen metabolism whose transport by renal tubules has been important in the development of comparative renal physiology as well as of renal physiology in general. The major features of urea excretion are covered elsewhere (see the chapter by Schmidt-Nielsen in this volume), but a few aspects related to urea secretion by the renal tubules are of particular importance in the development of comparative renal physiology. Net tubular secretion has been well documented for a number of primarily aquatic anuran amphibians of the genus *Rana* (*R. catesbeiana*, *R. pipiens*, and *R. clamitans*) (35). A tubular secretory process appears advantageous for these semiaquatic animals that have low filtration rates during dehydration or adaptation to cold (see REGULATION OF GLOMERULAR FILTRATION, p. 467). Net tubular secretion of urea apparently can occur under some circumstances in a few other nonmammalian vertebrates (Atlantic hagfish *Myxine glutinosa*, lizards *Lacerta viridis* and *Sceloporus cyanogenous*, rhyncocephalian reptile *Sphenodon punctatum*, and ducks *Anas platyrhynchos*) (35).

Almost all studies of the urea secretory process have involved freshwater frogs (primarily *R. catesbeiana*). Before tubular secretion had been clearly demonstrated and before an adequate glomerular filtration marker was known, Marshall and Crane (69) suggested that the saturability of urea excretion in *R. catesbeiana* indicated a tubular secretory transport system. The idea of a carrier-mediated, energy-requiring transepithelial transport process for a small, neutral polar molecule to which membranes are highly permeable has always been intriguing, and beginning in the 1950s, attempts were made to learn more about such a process by taking advantage of the apparent secretory transport in frogs.

Initial in vivo studies by Forster, Schmidt-Nielsen, and their colleagues clearly indicated that the secretory system saturates and that the urea concentration in the kidney tissue is greater than that in the plasma, suggesting that an active transport step into the tubule cells exists at the peritubular membrane (35). This possibility is supported by observations that thiourea, probenecid, and PAH inhibit net tubular secretion of urea, probably in a competitive fashion, and that both net tubular secretion and the tissue accumulation of urea and thiourea are eliminated by 2,4-dinitrophenol (35). At the time of this inhibition, passive net absorption of filtered urea is revealed (35). In addition William Scott Long, working in the early 1970s as a graduate student in B. Schmidt-Nielsen's laboratory, showed by micropuncture methods that net urea secretion occurred in the proximal and distal tubules but not in the collecting ducts (35).

However, in vitro studies have led to no further understanding of this transport process. Schmidt-Nielsen found no evidence of active uptake into kidney slices, and James M. Irish III, working in my laboratory in the early 1970s, found no evidence of either primary or secondary active transport in isolated, perfused proximal tubules (35). Although other transport systems (e.g., PAH and sodium) appeared to be intact in these tubules, some specific factor necessary for urea transport may have been missing in vitro. In any case, as intriguing as this apparent tubular secretory process is, it has not yet been possible to take advantage of its presence in these renal tubules to gain a more detailed understanding of active urea transport—a puzzling, but still intriguing, failure in the comparative approach.

Inorganic Ions

Tubular secretion of inorganic ions—particularly potassium, calcium, phosphate, magnesium, and sulfate—has been of considerable interest in comparative renal physiology. However, with the exception of potassium and, to a much lesser extent, phosphate, studies on these processes were very limited prior to the last few years. Although net potassium secretion has been demonstrated in representatives of all classes of nonmammalian tetrapods, freshwater teleosts, marine elasmobranchs, and euryhaline teleosts adapted to freshwater, detailed studies of the secretory process have only been performed in recent years, and then only on urodele and anuran amphibians (*Rana catesbeiana*, *Necturus maculosus*, and *Amphiuma means*) (35). However, these studies have formed part of the main line of research involved in the understanding of renal tubular transport of potassium in general and are discussed in the chapter by Giebisch in this volume.

Phosphate secretion by the tubules of nonmammalian vertebrates has attracted somewhat more attention over the years than calcium, magnesium, and sulfate secretion, probably because it is so clearly regulated by parathyroid hormone in birds and reptiles. In 1957 Levinsky and Davidson (65), then at the National Institutes of Health, first showed that chickens were capable of net tubular secretion of phosphate when given a phosphate load. This property of avian renal tubules was confirmed twenty years later in clearance studies on European starlings (*Sturnus vulgaris*) by Clark, Braun, and Wideman (23), working at the University of Connecticut. They demonstrated that phosphate secretion could be produced by the administration of parathyroid hormone. Shortly thereafter they showed that in starlings net secretion is converted to net reabsorption by parathyroidectomy and that net secretion in parathyroidectomized animals cannot be restored by phosphate loading alone but can be restored by the administration of parathyroid hormone with or without phosphate loading (25, 111). Even more recently Laverty and I (63, 64) demonstrated in micropuncture studies on starlings that net reabsorption or net secretion of phosphate can occur along the proximal tubule of the reptilian-type nephrons and that net secretion can be produced or enhanced by parathyroid hormone.

In a similar fashion, Clark and I (24) found in the early 1970s that net phosphate secretion dependent on parathyroid hormone occurs in water snakes of the genus *Nerodia*. The degree of phosphate secretion in response to parathyroid hormone in some of these clearance studies suggests that the hormone stimulates a secretory step for phosphate transport rather than inhibits a reabsorptive step, as in mammals (24). This intriguing possibility, if pursued in detail, could lead to increased understanding of the interaction of a hormone with an epithelial transport process. However, initial in vitro studies with isolated reptilian renal tubules have yet to show any stimulation of secretory transport.

Fluid

Fluid secretion by aglomerular nephrons has been noted by investigators since its initial demonstration by Marshall and others over half a century ago. However, the mechanism involved in such secretion has until recently attracted little attention. The lack of detailed study possibly reflected the assumption that fluid secretion was a unique occurrence in a few fishes and that water movement was simply coupled to the secretion of divalent ions such as calcium, magnesium, or sulfate. Beginning in the middle 1970s, however, clearance studies of Schmidt-Nielsen and Renfro (81, 96) provided evidence that fluid secretion is a significant component of urine volume even in some glomerular teleosts. Similarly Yokota, Benyajati, and I (114) even found evidence for some fluid secretion during clearance studies on sea snakes. It should also be recalled that in 1933 Chambers and Kempton (22) obtained evidence of fluid secretion in cultured chick mesonephric tubules although no such evidence was reported for the few metanephric tubules studied. In any case the observations in fishes led Beyenbach (4), working at Cornell University and at Mount Desert Island Biological Laboratory, to use a modification of the isolated, perfused-tubule technique to demonstrate fluid secretion directly in nephrons from glomerular marine teleosts (flounder *Pseudopleuronectes americanus*) and marine elasmobranchs (dogfish *Squalus acanthias*). Interestingly, such secretion apparently depends on the secretion of sodium and chloride, and not on the secretion of divalent ions (4). Beyenbach, in conjunction with Eberhardt Frömter of Frankfurt, is continuing to explore the mechanism involved in this fluid secretion. The secretory process may be a very primitive one that is present to some degree in all vertebrates, including mammals. Its ready observance in aglomerular fish as part of Marshall's initial demonstration of the general process of tubular secretion now appears to be leading to intriguing new studies on the coupling of solute and water movement.

Tubular Reabsorption

Organic Substances

Although the reabsorption of amino acids by the renal tubules of nonmammalian vertebrates has been recognized for a number of years, only a few attempts have been made to examine comparative differences in the amounts reabsorbed among the various vertebrates (35). Even fewer attempts have been made to localize the transport sites or to examine the transport mechanisms. Part of the problem of course has stemmed from the lack of adequate techniques to measure the transport of individual amino acids. Only in 1978 did Oken and Weise (77), working at the Medical College of Virginia, publish micropuncture data on urodele amphibians (*Necturus maculosus*) showing proximal tubular reabsorption of amino acids but indicating that absorption may occur beyond the end of the proximal tubule. This is of considerable interest, but thus far little is known about the mechanism of absorption, even in the proximal tubules of nonmammalian vertebrates.

The excretion of urea has long been of interest in comparative studies. Because it plays a special role in the renal concentrating mechanism in mammals (see the chapter by Berliner in this volume), its reabsorption by the renal tubules of different mammalian species has been of particular interest for renal physiology in general. [Studies of this process in mammals are discussed in detail elsewhere (see the chapter by Schmidt-Nielsen in this volume).] However, tubular reabsorption of urea in marine elasmobranchs (in which high extracellular urea concentrations offset the high osmolarity of the seawater environment), like the tubular secretion of urea in frogs, has been particularly intriguing because it may involve an active transport process. Starting in the late 1950s, studies by Forster (49) that later involved Schmidt-Nielsen, Leon Goldstein, and their colleagues at Mount Desert Island Biological Laboratory indicated that transport in vivo occurs against a concentration gradient but is not saturable and is not inhibited by the usual metabolic inhibitors. Preliminary micropuncture studies by Schmidt-Nielsen (92) and others in the 1960s suggested that the reabsorptive process must occur between the end of the proximal tubule and the beginning of the collecting duct, apparently in the distal tubule, which is inaccessible to micropuncture. The lack of conclusive evidence for an active transport process and the observation that, in those elasmobranchs studied, the terminal segment of the nephron (the portion in which urea reabsorption apparently takes place) is intimately surrounded by loops of proximal tubule led Boylan (7), while working at Mount Desert Island Biological Laboratory, to propose a complex countercurrent model to account for the reabsorption by passive means. However, later studies at Mount Desert Island Biological Laboratory in the 1970s indicated that the reabsorptive process for urea is shared by amide-containing compounds (e.g., acetamide) but not thiourea, is sodium linked, and is suppressed by inhibitors of sodium reabsorption and phloretin (35). Although these data suggest that the reabsorption of urea may involve some form of active transport process, there is insufficient information to decide whether an active (either primary or secondary) or a passive process or both play a role in urea reabsorption. As with the apparently active secretion of urea by frog proximal renal tubules, this process remains an intriguing and potentially very important observation in comparative renal physiology.

Inorganic Ions

Although clearance studies over many years have shown net tubular reabsorption of the major filtered inorganic ions (sodium, chloride, and usually potassium) in all the vertebrate classes, until very recently the only detailed studies of tubular transport processes in nonmammalian vertebrates have involved urodele amphibians (primarily *Necturus maculosus* and *Amphiuma means*). These studies, beginning with the micropuncture experiments of Richards and his colleagues and continuing with studies of isolated perfused renal tubules in recent years, have formed a major portion of the work involved in understanding these tubular transport processes in general.

However, there is one similarity in distal tubule reabsorption among the vertebrates that has become apparent in recent years and is important in understanding both past studies and future trends in comparative research. Studies with isolated perfused renal tubules, first in amphibians by Larry C. Stoner at the National Institutes of Health in the early 1970s and more recently in freshwater fish and birds by Hiroko Nishimura and her colleagues at the University of Tennessee Center for Health Sciences, have demonstrated that in those species capable of producing a dilute urine (see DILUTION AND CONCENTRATION OF URINE, p. 491) there is apparently a common diluting area in the distal tubule (75, 76, 104). In birds this area appears to involve at least the thick ascending limb of the loop of Henle of the mammalian-type nephrons and the early distal tubule of the reptilian-type nephrons. In amphibians this area also appears to involve the early distal tubule. In all cases there is a lumen positive voltage and avid sodium and chloride reabsorption, both of which are inhibited by furosemide. This pattern appears to be very similar to that observed in the thick ascending limb of the loop of Henle and the early distal tubule of mammalian nephrons. Indeed the very large cells of the early distal tubule of *Amphiuma* permit a detailed analysis of the transport process that suggests that it is the same as that in the mammalian thick ascending limb but easier to study (104) (see the chapter by Giebisch in this volume). Therefore it appears that a similar mechanism for diluting the urine has evolved in all vertebrates in which such dilution occurs and that it can be approached most directly in some nonmammalian vertebrates.

Fluid

Over the years numerous clearance studies have indicated that the bulk of the filtered fluid is reabsorbed by the renal tubules of all nonmammalian tetrapod vertebrates (35). However, a number of micropuncture studies have shown that although 60%–80% of the filtrate is reabsorbed along the proximal tubules of mammalian nephrons, only 30%–50% is reabsorbed along the proximal tubules of amphibian, reptilian, and reptilian-type avian nephrons (35). Apparently a much larger fraction is reabsorbed in the distal portions of these nephrons or collecting ducts than in mammals. Moreover in birds, reptiles, and amphibians further reabsorption of fluid, depending on the requirements of the animal, can take place in regions distal to the kidney (e.g., colon, cloaca, or bladder). In addition some primitive marine cyclostomes (e.g., the Atlantic hagfish *Myxine glutinosa*) conform to their environment and no fluid at all is reabsorbed along their primitive archinephric ducts (35).

A number of micropuncture or microperfusion studies extending from Richards's day to the present have indicated that fluid absorption in the proximal tubules of amphibians, reptiles, birds, and freshwater lampreys is always an isosmotic process (35). Of particular importance in the development of the understanding of the proximal tubule reabsorptive process in vertebrates in general is the micropuncture and microperfusion study performed on *Necturus maculosus* at the end of the 1950s by Windhager, Whittembury, Oken, Schatzmann, and Solomon (113), working in Solomon's laboratory at Harvard Medical School. This study indicates that apparently isosmotic fluid absorption depends on the absorption of sodium. Thus, in a continuation of the type of comparative study involving an accessible tubule preparation pioneered by Richards, the first basic information on the coupling of solute and water movement in the vertebrate proximal renal tubule was obtained on a urodele amphibian. Since that time many additional studies on this problem have involved mammals as well as amphibians and, although adding to the complexity of the problem, have not really contradicted the basic finding of this initial study.

However, although the dependence of fluid reabsorption in the proximal tubule on sodium reabsorption normally may hold for all mammalian as well as nonmammalian vertebrates, studies on isolated perfused snake proximal renal tubules (*Thamnophis* spp.) in my laboratory in the late 1970s suggest that this does not always have to be the case (36). While examining the effects of sodium substitutions on organic anion transport, we were astounded to discover that isosmotic fluid reabsorption in these tubules apparently can proceed at control rates when lithium is substituted for sodium or when some other substitution is made for sodium or chloride or both in the perfusate and bathing medium simultaneously. The nature of this process, which apparently requires metabolic energy, is not understood. However, recent preliminary structural studies by Larry W. Welling and Daniel J. Welling of the University of Kansas Medical Center performed in collaboration with me indicate that the area of the luminal and basolateral cell membranes doubles within a few minutes after the replacement of sodium with choline in the perfusate and bathing medium. This increase in cell membrane area may permit a small driving force to become highly effective in producing fluid reabsorption. In any case these additional comparative studies suggest new possibilities in the coupling of solute and water fluxes.

Dilution and Concentration of Urine

Dilution

During the past half century, clearance studies and even studies involving simple urine collections have shown that representatives of all the tetrapod vertebrate classes as well as many fishes are capable of producing urine that is hyposmotic to their plasma (35). As noted previously this ability is associated with the possession of distal tubule or loop of Henle segments that avidly reabsorb sodium and chloride without water. The possession of such a distal diluting segment by the urodele amphibians in particular permits fundamental physiological studies of this process (see Tubular Transport, p. 476, and the chapter by Giebisch in this volume). Of additional importance in this area of comparative physiological research are the studies by Schmidt-Nielsen and some of her colleagues and students (41, 89, 94) at Duke and Case Western Reserve Universities in the early 1960s. They observed that some saurian and crocodilian reptiles with distal tubules are apparently unable to dilute their ureteral urine at all. Electron-microscope studies at that time suggested that these reptiles lack the early distal cell type that might be responsible for dilution (41, 89). Although this could be important in understanding the comparative physiology of dilution, no detailed physiological studies have yet explored this question. Any reabsorption of solutes without water in these species, if necessary, apparently occurs in structures distal to the actual kidneys.

Concentration

As early as 1927, Crane (26) clearly stated that only birds and mammals produce a urine hyperosmotic to the plasma and even related this to the possession of loops of Henle by birds as well as mammals. Comparative anatomical studies of mammalian nephrons, their structure and their relationship to each other and to the medullary vascular supply, played an important role in the development of our current understanding of the mammalian concentrating mechanism. In fact, more refined comparative anatomical studies are today contributing to an even more detailed understanding of the function of the countercurrent multiplier system and especially of the role of urea in the mammalian concentrating process. The development of these ideas and a discussion of the individuals involved are covered in the chapter by Berliner in this volume.

The function of the avian concentrating mechanism, although very important from a comparative point of view and offering some possible insights into the function of the mammalian system, has been far less well studied than the mammalian system. Birds evolved from reptiles earlier than mammals and quite independent of them. As previously noted (see Fig. 8), most avian nephrons resemble reptilian nephrons; only a small fraction of the nephrons resemble mammalian nephrons and are arranged with loops of Henle parallel to the vasa recta and the collecting ducts that drain both types of nephrons. Because birds, like reptiles, excrete uric acid and almost no urea, this system did not need to evolve to permit the excretion of urea while water was being conserved. However, it does permit the concentration of electrolytes and some additional conservation of water. Nevertheless such additional concentration of electrolytes in solution is modest. Measurements of avian urine osmolality, dating from the early years of this century, indicate that only one of the species studied (the salt marsh savannah sparrow *Passerculus sandwichensis beldingi*) is capable of concentrating its urine to more than 2–3 times the plasma osmolality (35).

However, several other observations are important in assessing the significance of this relatively modest concentrating ability in the conservation of water and the elimination of electrolytes. First, Braun and I (37) observed that during water deprivation the plasma osmolality of birds increases much more than that of mammals with no ill effects. The reason for this lability of the plasma osmolality is unknown, but clearly the osmolar urine-to-plasma ratio in birds cannot be compared directly with that in mammals in determining its significance. Second, beginning in the early 1970s, several investigators, most notably McNabb, McNabb, and Hinton (73) at Virginia Polytechnical Institute and State University and Braun (9), found significant quantities of sodium and potassium combined with urate precipitates in the ureteral urine of birds. The actual quantities of inorganic cations combined with urate precipitates, the chemical structure of these precipitates, and the manner in which the cations combine with them are not yet clearly defined (35). However, these organic cations in the urate precipitates can be excreted without contributing to the osmotic pressure of the ureteral urine. Therefore the limited concentrating ability of the avian kidney does not reflect its true capacity for excreting inorganic cations. Finally, Skadhauge (101) in Copenhagen and Braun (10) demonstrated that after the urine of birds enters the cloaca, it can move retrograde into the colon where significant solute-linked water reabsorption can occur against a modest osmotic gradient. Braun (10) has suggested that the lack of a highly concentrated urine permits this process to function efficiently.

Because of the general anatomical relationship of the loops of Henle to the vasa recta and collecting ducts in the medullary cones and the resemblance of this arrangement to that in the mammalian medulla, it has been assumed that the concentrating mechanism functions in the same manner as that of mammals. However, the physiological studies of this process in birds are by no means as complete as in mammals, and there are a number of structural, biochemical, and physiological differences between birds and mammals that point to differences in the function of this process.

In the middle 1960s, Skadhauge and Schmidt-Nielsen (102), then working in Cleveland, were able to show an osmotic gradient in the medullary cones of domestic fowl that was analogous to that in the mammalian renal medulla. A few years later, William B. Kinter and Nona Emery, then at the State University of New York–Upstate Medical Center in Syracuse, and Thomas L. Poulson, then at the University of Notre Dame, demonstrated a similar osmotic gradient in the medullary cones of two small passerine species (budgerigars *Melopsittacus undulatus*, and savannah sparrows *Passerculus sandwichensis rostratus*) (44). Moreover, during the 1960s and 1970s, Oscar W. Johnson, at Moorhead State College in Minnesota, and a number of colleagues (including Skadhauge) showed that the relative length of the medullary cones correlates with concentrating ability (57, 59). These studies and others certainly pointed to the function of the loops of Henle as a countercurrent multiplier system and the general function of the concentrating mechanism in a manner analogous to that in the mammalian kidney.

Birds, however, excrete almost no urea, and the study by Skadhauge and Schmidt-Nielsen (102) indicated that the osmotic gradient in the medullary cones is formed by sodium, chloride, and to a lesser extent, potassium, with virtually no urea. This absence of urea in the medullary tissue contrasts strikingly with the situation in the mammalian medulla. Moreover Johnson's histological studies (58) during the late 1960s and the microdissection studies of Braun (10) over the past fifteen years have shown that the descending limb of the loop of Henle thickens before the bend in all species studied. Thus, like the short-looped nephrons in the mammalian kidney, the mammalian-type nephrons in the avian kidney have no thin ascending limbs. These observations suggest that the thin limb is not necessary in the absence of urea and that, by analogy with the thick ascending limb of mammalian nephrons, the countercurrent multiplier system in the avian kidney depends solely on the transport of sodium and chloride out of the entire length of the thick ascending limb. Although these structures are inaccessible to micropuncture, initial studies on isolated perfused fragments of the thick ascending limb of young Japanese quail (*Coturnix coturnix japonica*) by Nishimura et al. (75) suggest that this segment does indeed function very much like the thick ascending limb of mammalian nephrons. Also, as previously noted, dilution appears to occur in the early distal tubules of the reptilian-type nephron. Thus recent work is beginning to clarify the countercurrent multiplication process in the avian kidney.

However, the exact manner in which antidiuretic hormone (arginine vasotocin) functions with the countercurrent multiplier system in birds to produce a concentrated urine is not yet clear. Skadhauge and his colleagues (1, 100) demonstrated in the early 1960s and 1970s that the increase in urine osmolality observed with dehydration could be mimicked by the administration of apparently physiological doses of arginine vasotocin. Because of these observations, it has generally been assumed that the antidiuretic effect results primarily from an increase in the permeability of the collecting ducts to water, permitting the fluid in them to equilibrate with the surrounding hyperosmotic interstitium of the medullary cones. However, an effect of arginine vasotocin on the permeability of the collecting ducts to water has not been demonstrated directly, and the effects of changes in volume flow rate through the collecting ducts on equilibration have not been evaluated. Arginine vasotocin does reduce the number of filtering reptilian-type nephrons in a manner analogous to that observed with dehydration or a salt load. This is practical for nephrons of this type that do not function in concert to produce the osmotic gradient in the medullary cones. Such a mechanism can conserve water at the expense of excreting some ions and uric acid. More importantly, perhaps, it reduces the volume flow rate through the collecting ducts. Because all reptilian-type nephrons contribute to the fluid flowing through the collecting ducts in the medullary cones [see Regulation of Glomerular Filtration, p. 467; (see Fig. 8)], a reduction in the number of nephrons filtering reduces the volume flow rate through the collecting ducts and may do more than any increase in tubular permeability to water to enhance the concentrating ability of the avian kidney (12). However, a definite description of the actions of arginine vasotocin awaits direct measurements of its effects on the permeability of the collecting ducts and of the effects of volume flow rate through these structures on the equilibration process.

Conclusion

The comparative approach to renal physiology began with the anatomical studies of Bowman and was reinforced by the success of Marshall's and Richards's work in the 1920s and 1930s and by the leadership of Smith and his colleagues during the 1930s and 1940s. In the last forty years, comparative studies have expanded dramatically to involve many investigators, to lead to new insights into renal adaptations and basic physiological mechanisms, and to suggest possible future avenues for research into fundamental physiological problems.

The preparation of this chapter and the personal research mentioned herein were supported by National Science Foundation Research Grant DCB-8501260 and preceding grants and National Institutes of Health Grant RO1AM16294.

BIBLIOGRAPHY

1. AMES, E., K. STEVEN, and E. SKADHAUGE. Effects of arginine vasotocin on renal excretion of Na^+, K^+, Cl^-, and urea in the hydrated chicken. *Am. J. Physiol.* 221: 1223–1228, 1971.
2. BABIKIR, M. M., and J. C. RANKIN. Neurohypophysial hormone control of kidney function in the European eel (*Anguilla anguilla* L.) adapted to sea-water or fresh water. *J. Endocrinol.* 76: 347–358, 1978.
3. BECK, L. V., and R. CHAMBERS. Secretion in tissue cultures. II. Effect of Na iodoacetate on the chick kidney. *J. Cell. Comp. Physiol.* 6: 441–455, 1935.
4. BEYENBACH, K. W. Direct demonstration of fluid secretion by glomerular renal tubules in a marine teleost. *Nature Lond.* 299: 54–56, 1982.
5. BORDLEY, J., III, and A. N. RICHARDS. Quantitative studies of the composition of glomerular urine. VIII. The concentration of uric acid in glomerular urine of snakes and frogs, determined by an ultramicroadaptation of Folin's method. *J. Biol. Chem.* 101: 193–221, 1933.
6. BOWMAN, W. On the structure and use of the Malpighian bodies of the kidney, with observations on the circulation through that gland. *Philos. Trans. R. Soc. Lond. B Biol. Sci.* 132: 57–80, 1842.
7. BOYLAN, J. W. A model for passive urea reabsorption in the elasmobranch kidney. *Comp. Biochem. Physiol.* 42: 27–30, 1972.
8. BRAUN, E. J. Intrarenal blood flow distribution in the desert quail following salt loading. *Am. J. Physiol.* 231: 1111–1118, 1976.
9. BRAUN, E. J. Renal response of the starling (*Sturnus vulgaris*) to an intravenous salt load. *Am. J. Physiol.* 234 (*Renal Fluid Electrolyte Physiol.* 3): F270–F278, 1978.
10. BRAUN, E. J. Comparative aspects of the urinary concentrating process. *Renal Physiol.* 8: 249–260, 1985.
11. BRAUN, E. J., and W. H. DANTZLER. Function of mammalian-type and reptilian-type nephrons in kidney of desert quail. *Am. J. Physiol.* 222: 617–629, 1972.
12. BRAUN, E. J., and W. H. DANTZLER. Effects of ADH on single-nephron glomerular filtration rates in the avian kidney. *Am. J. Physiol.* 226: 1–8, 1974.
13. BRAUN, E. J., and W. H. DANTZLER. Effect of water load on renal glomerular and tubular function in desert quail. *Am. J. Physiol.* 229: 222–228, 1975.
14. BROWN, J. A., B. A. JACKSON, J. A. OLIVER, and I. W. HENDERSON. Single nephron filtration rates (SNGFR) in the trout, *Salmo gairdneri*. *Pfluegers Arch.* 377: 101–108, 1978.
15. BROWN, J. A., J. A. OLIVER, I. W. HENDERSON, and B. A. JACKSON. Angiotensin and single nephron glomerular function in the trout *Salmo gairdneri*. *Am. J. Physiol.* 239 (*Regulatory Integrative Comp. Physiol.* 8): R509–R514, 1980.
16. BURG, M., J. GRANTHAM, M. ABRAMOW, and J. ORLOFF. Preparation and study of fragments of single rabbit nephrons. *Am. J. Physiol.* 210: 1293–1298, 1966.
17. BURG, M. B., and P. F. WELLER. Iodopyracet transport by isolated perfused flounder proximal renal tubules. *Am. J. Physiol.* 217: 1053–1056, 1969.

18. BURGESS, W. W., A. M. HARVEY, and E. K. MARSHALL, JR. The site of the antidiuretic action of pituitary extract. *J. Pharmacol. Exp. Ther.* 49: 237–249, 1933.
19. BUTLER, D. G. Antidiuretic effect of arginine vasotocin in the western painted turtle (*Chrysemys picta belli*). *Gen. Comp. Endocrinol.* 18: 121–125, 1972.
20. CHAMBERS, R., L. V. BECK, and M. BELKIN. Secretion in tissue cultures. I. Inhibition of phenol red accumulation in the chick kidney. *J. Cell. Comp. Physiol.* 6: 425–439, 1935.
21. CHAMBERS, R., and G. CAMERON. Intracellular hydrion concentrations studies. VII. The secreting cells of the mesonephros in the chick. *J. Cell. Comp. Physiol.* 2: 99–103, 1932.
22. CHAMBERS, R., and R. T. KEMPTON. Indications of function of the chick mesonephros in tissue culture with phenol red. *J. Cell. Comp. Physiol.* 3: 131–166, 1933.
23. CLARK, N. B., E. J. BRAUN, and R. F. WIDEMAN, JR. Parathyroid hormone and renal excretion of phosphate and calcium in normal starlings. *Am. J. Physiol.* 231: 1152–1158, 1976.
24. CLARK, N. B., and W. H. DANTZLER. Renal tubular transport of calcium and phosphate in snakes: role of parathyroid hormone. *Am. J. Physiol.* 223: 1455–1464, 1972.
25. CLARK, N. B., and R. F. WIDEMAN, JR. Renal excretion of phosphate and calcium in parathyroidectomized starlings. *Am. J. Physiol.* 233 (*Renal Fluid Electrolyte Physiol.* 2): F138–F144, 1977.
26. CRANE, M. M. Observations on the function of the frog's kidney. *Am. J. Physiol.* 81: 232–243, 1927.
27. CULLIS, W. C. On secretion in the frog's kidney. *J. Physiol. Lond.* 34: 250–266, 1906.
28. CUSHNY, A. R. *The Secretion of Urine.* London: Longmans Green, 1917.
29. DANTZLER, W. H. Renal response of chickens to infusion of hyperosmotic sodium chloride solution. *Am. J. Physiol.* 210: 640–646, 1966.
30. DANTZLER, W. H. Glomerular and tubular effects of arginine vasotocin in water snakes (*Natrix sipedon*). *Am. J. Physiol.* 212: 83–91, 1967.
31. DANTZLER, W. H. Comparison of renal tubular transport of urate and PAH in water snakes: evidence for differences in mechanisms and sites of transport. *Comp. Biochem. Physiol.* 34: 609–623, 1970.
32. DANTZLER, W. H. Renal function (with special emphasis on nitrogen excretion). In: *Biology of the Reptilia. Physiology A*, edited by C. G. Gans and W. R. Dawson. San Francisco, CA: Academic, 1976, vol. 5, p. 447–503.
33. DANTZLER, W. H. Urate excretion in nonmammalian vertebrates. In: *Handbook of Experimental Pharmacology. Uric Acid*, edited by W. N. Kelley and I. M. Weiner. Berlin: Springer-Verlag, 1978, vol. 51, p. 185–210.
34. DANTZLER, W. H. Studies on nonmammalian nephrons. *Kidney Int.* 22: 560–570, 1982.
35. DANTZLER, W. H. Comparative aspects of renal function. In: *The Kidney. Physiology and Pathophysiology*, edited by D. W. Seldin and G. Giebisch. New York: Raven, 1985, p. 333–364.
36. DANTZLER, W. H., and S. K. BENTLEY. Fluid absorption with and without sodium in isolated perfused snake proximal tubules. *Am. J Physiol.* 234 (*Renal Fluid Electrolyte Physiol.* 3): F68–F79, 1978.

37. DANTZLER, W. H., and E. J. BRAUN. Comparative nephron function in reptiles, birds, and mammals. *Am. J. Physiol.* 239 (*Regulatory Integrative Comp. Physiol.* 8): R197–R213, 1980.
38. DANTZLER, W. H., and O. H. BROKL. Effects of low [Ca^{2+}] and La^{3+} on PAH transport by isolated perfused renal tubules. *Am. J. Physiol.* 246 (*Renal Fluid Electrolyte Physiol.* 15): F175–F187, 1984.
39. DANTZLER, W. H., and O. H. BROKL. Verapamil and quinidine effects on PAH transport by isolated perfused renal tubules. *Am. J. Physiol.* 246 (*Renal Fluid Electrolyte Physiol.* 15): F188–F200, 1984.
40. DANTZLER, W. H., and B. SCHMIDT-NIELSEN. Excretion in fresh-water turtle (*Pseudemys scripta*) and desert tortoise (*Gopherus agassizii*). *Am. J. Physiol.* 210: 198–210, 1966.
41. DAVIS, L. E., and B. SCHMIDT-NIELSEN. Ultrastructure of the crocodile kidney (*Crocodylus acutus*) with special reference to electrolyte and fluid transport. *J. Morphol.* 121: 255–276, 1967.
42. DAVIS, L. E., B. SCHMIDT-NIELSEN, and H. STOLTE. Anatomy and ultrastructure of the excretory system of the lizard, *Sceloporus cyanogenys*. *J. Morphol.* 149: 279–326, 1976.
43. DE ROUFFIGNAC, C., S. DIESS, and J. P. BONVALET. Détermination du taux individuel de filtration glomérulaire des néphrons accessibles et inaccessibles á la microponction. *Pfluegers Arch.* 315: 273–290, 1970.
44. EMERY, N., T. L. POULSON, and W. B. KINTER. Production of concentrated urine by avian kidneys. *Am. J. Physiol.* 223: 180–187, 1972.
45. EVELOFF, J., R. KINNE, and W. B. KINTER. *p*-Aminohippuric acid transport into brush border vesicles isolated from flounder kidney. *Am. J. Physiol.* 237 (*Renal Fluid Electrolyte Physiol.* 6): F291–F298, 1979.
46. FORSTER, R. P. The use of inulin and creatinine as glomerular filtrate measuring substances in the frog. *J. Cell. Comp. Physiol.* 12: 213–222, 1938.
47. FORSTER, R. P. The nature of the glucose reabsorptive process in the frog renal tubule. Evidence for intermittency of glomerular function in the intact animal. *J. Cell. Comp. Physiol.* 20: 55–69, 1942.
48. FORSTER, R. P. Use of thin kidney slices and isolated renal tubules for direct study of cellular transport kinetics. *Science Wash. DC* 108: 65–67, 1948.
49. FORSTER, R. P. Active tubular transport of urea and its role in environmental physiology. In: *Urea and the Kidney*, edited by B. Schmidt-Nielsen and D. W. S. Kerr. Amsterdam: Excerpta Med., 1970, p. 229–237.
50. FORSTER, R. P., and J. V. TAGGART. Use of isolated renal tubules for the examination of metabolic processes associated with active cellular transport. *J. Cell. Comp. Physiol.* 36: 251–270, 1950.
51. HANSSEN, O. E. Method for comparison of glomerular filtration in individual rat nephrons. In: *2nd Int. Congr. Nephrol., Prague, 1963*, edited by J. Vostal and G. Richet. Amsterdam: Excerpta Med. Found., 1964, p. 527–529. (Int. Congr. Ser. vol. 76.)
52. HAYMAN, J. M., JR. Estimations of afferent arteriole and glomerular capillary pressures in the frog kidney. *Am. J. Physiol.* 79: 389–409, 1927.
53. HENDERSON, I. W., and N. A. M. WALES. Renal diuresis and antidiuresis after injections of arginine vasotocin in the freshwater eel (*Anguilla anguilla* L.). *J. Endocrinol.* 61: 487–500, 1974.

54. Hickman, C. P., Jr. Studies on renal function in freshwater teleost fish. *Tran. R. Soc. Can.* 3: 213–236, 1965.
55. Hickman, C. P., Jr., and B. F. Tramp. The kidney. In: *Fish Physiology. Excretion, Ionic Regulation, and Metabolism*, edited by W. S. Hoar and D. J. Randall. New York: Academic, 1969, vol. 1, p. 91–239.
56. Intaglietta, M., N. R. Silverman, and W. R. Tompkins. Capillary flow velocity measurement in vivo and in situ by television methods. *Microvasc. Res.* 10: 165–179, 1975.
57. Johnson, O. W. Relative thickness of the renal medulla in birds. *J. Morphol.* 142: 277–284, 1974.
58. Johnson, O. W., and J. N. Magaas. Quantitative and organizational features of the avian renal medulla. *Condor* 3: 288–292, 1970.
59. Johnson, O. W., and E. Skadhauge. Structural-functional correlations in the kidneys and observations of colon and cloacal morphology in certain Australian birds. *J. Anat.* 120: 495–505, 1975.
60. Kinter, W. B. Chlorphenol red influx and efflux: microspectrophotometry of flounder kidney tubules. *Am. J. Physiol.* 211: 1152–1164, 1966.
61. Krogh, A. The supply of oxygen to the tissues and the regulation of the capillary circulation. *J. Physiol. Lond.* 52: 457–474, 1919.
62. Lahlou, B. Mise en évidence d'un "recrutement glomérulaire" dans le rein des Téléostéens d'après la mesure du Tm glucose. *C. R. Acad. Sci. Paris Ser. D* 262: 1356–1358, 1966.
63. Laverty, G., and W. H. Dantzler. Micropuncture of superficial nephrons in avian (*Sturnus vulgaris*) kidney. *Am. J. Physiol.* 243 (*Renal Fluid Electrolyte Physiol.* 12): F561–F569, 1982.
64. Laverty, G., and W. H. Dantzler. Micropuncture study of urate transport by superficial nephrons in avian (*Sturnus vulgaris*) kidney. *Pfluegers Arch.* 397: 232–236, 1983.
65. Levinsky, N. G., and D. G. Davidson. Renal action of parathyroid extract in the chicken. *Am. J. Physiol.* 191: 530–536, 1957.
66. MacKay, W. C., and D. D. Beatty. The effect of temperature on renal function in the white sucker fish, *Catostomus caommersonii*. *Comp. Biochem. Physiol.* 26: 235–245, 1968.
67. Malvin, R. L., and I. B. Fritz. Renal transport of urea and some carbohydrates in *Lophius piscatorius*. *J. Cell. Comp. Physiol.* 59: 111–115, 1962.
68. Marshall, E. K., Jr. The comparative physiology of the kidney in relation to theories of renal secretion. *Physiol. Rev.* 14: 133–159, 1934.
69. Marshall, E. K., Jr., and M. M. Crane. The secretory function of the renal tubules. *Am. J. Physiol.* 70: 465–488, 1924.
70. Marshall, E. K., Jr., and A. L. Grafflin. The structure and function of the kidney of *Lophius piscatorius*. *Bull. Johns Hopkins Hosp.* 43: 205–230, 1928.
71. Marshall, E. K., Jr., and J. L. Vickers. The mechanism of the elimination of phenolsulphonephthalein by the kidney—a proof of secretion by the convoluted tubules. *Bull. Johns Hopkins Hosp.* 34: 1–7, 1923.
72. Mayrs, E. B. Secretion as a factor in elimination by the bird kidney. *J. Physiol. Lond.* 58: 276–287, 1924.
73. McNabb, R. A., F. M. A. McNabb, and A. P. Hinton. The excretion of

urate and cationic electrolytes by the kidney of the male domestic fowl. (*Gallus domesticus*). *J. Comp. Physiol.* 82: 47–57, 1973.
74. Moriarty, R. J., A. G. Logan, and J. C. Rankin. Measurement of single nephron filtration rate in the kidney of the river lamprey, *Lampetra fluviatilis* L. *J. Exp. Biol.* 77: 57–69, 1978.
75. Nishimura, H., M. Imai, and M. Ogawa. Sodium chloride and water transport in the renal distal tubule of the rainbow trout. *Am. J. Physiol.* 244 (*Renal Fluid Electrolyte Physiol.* 13): F247–F254, 1983.

76. Nishimura, H., M. Imai, and M. Ogawa. Transepithelial voltage in the reptilian- and mammalian-type nephrons from Japanese quail (Abstract). *Federation Proc.* 42: 304, 1983.
77. Oken, D. E., and M. Weise. Micropuncture studies of the transport of individual amino acids by the Necturus proximal tubule. *Kidney Int.* 13: 445–451, 1978.
78. Puck, T. T., K. Wasserman, and A. P. Fishman. Some effects of inorganic ions on the active transport of phenol red by the isolated tubules of the flounder. *J. Cell. Comp. Physiol.* 40: 73–88, 1952.
79. Ranges, H. A., H. Chasis, W. Goldring, and H. W. Smith. The functional measurement of the number of active glomeruli and tubules in kidneys of normal and hypertensive subjects. *Am. J. Physiol.* 126: 603P, 1939.
80. Rankin, J. C., V. Griffiths, and A. J. McVicar. Control of kidney function in the river lamprey, *Lampetra fluviatilis* L. *Abstracts of Papers, Ninth International Symposium on Comparative Endocrinology*, 1981, p. 190.
81. Renfro, J. L. Relationship between renal fluid and Mg secretion in a glomerular marine teleost. *Am. J. Physiol.* 238 (*Renal Fluid Electrolyte Physiol.* 7): F92–F98, 1980.
82. Richards, A. N. Urine formation in the amphibian kidney. *Harvey Lect.* 30: 93–118, 1934–1935.
83. Richards, A. N. Physiology of the kidney. *Bull. NY Acad. Med.* 14: 5–20, 1938.
84. Richards, A. N., and O. H. Plant. Urine formation by the perfused kidney: preliminary experiments on the action of caffeine. *J. Pharmacol.* 7: 485–509, 1915.
85. Richards, A. N., and O. H. Plant. Urine formation in the perfused kidney. The influence of alterations in renal blood pressure on the amount and composition of the urine. *Am. J. Physiol.* 59: 144–183, 1922.
86. Richards, A. N., and O. H. Plant. Urine formation in the perfused kidney. The influence of adrenalin on the volume of the perfused kidney. *Am. J. Physiol.* 59: 184–190, 1922.
87. Richards, A. N., and C. F. Schmidt. A description of the glomerular circulation in the frog's kidney and observations concerning the action of adrenalin and various other substances upon it. *Am. J. Physiol.* 71: 178–208, 1924.
88. Richards, A. N., and A. M. Walker. Methods of collecting fluid from known regions of the renal tubules of amphibia and of perfusing the lumen of a single tubule. *Am. J. Physiol.* 118: 111–120, 1937.
89. Roberts, J. S., and B. Schmidt-Nielsen. Renal ultrastructure and excretion of salt and water by three terrestrial lizards. *Am. J. Physiol.* 211: 476–486, 1966.

90. Sawyer, W. H. Effect of posterior pituitary extracts on urine formation and glomerular circulation in the frog. *Am. J. Physiol.* 164: 457–464, 1951.

91. Sawyer, W. H., R. A. Munsick, and H. B. van Dyke. Pharmacological evidence for the presence of arginine vasotocin and oxytocin in neurohypophysial extracts from cold-blooded vertebrates. *Nature Lond.* 184: 1464, 1959.

92. Schmidt-Nielsen, B. Renal transport of urea in elasmobranchs. In: *Transport Mechanisms in Epithelia*, edited by H. H. Ussing and N. A. Thorn. Copenhagen: Munksgaard, 1972, p. 608–621, (Alfred Benzon Symp. V).

93. Schmidt-Nielsen, B. A history of renal physiology at the Mount Desert Island Biological Laboratory. *Physiologist* 26: 261–266, 1983.

94. Schmidt-Nielsen, B., and L. E. Davis. Fluid transport and tubular intercellular spaces in reptilian kidneys. *Science Wash, DC* 159: 1105–1108, 1968.

95. Schmidt-Nielsen, B., and R. P. Forster. The effect of dehydration and low temperature on renal function in the bullfrog. *J. Cell. Comp. Physiol.* 44: 233–246, 1954.

96. Schmidt-Nielsen, B., and J. L. Renfro. Kidney function of the American eel *Anguilla rostrata*. *Am. J. Physiol.* 228: 420–431, 1975.

97. Shannon, J. A. The excretion of uric acid by the chicken. *J. Cell. Comp. Physiol.* 11: 135–148, 1938.

98. Shannon, J. A. Renal tubular excretion. *Physiol. Rev.* 19: 63–93, 1939.

99. Shannon, J. A., S. Farber, and L. Troast. The measurement of glucose T_m in the normal dog. *Am. J. Physiol.* 133: 752–761, 1941.

100. Skadhauge, E. Effects of unilateral infusion of arginine vasotocin into the portal circulation of the avian kidney. *Acta Endocrinol.* 47: 321–330, 1964.

101. Skadhauge, E. Renal and cloacal salt and water transport in the fowl (*Gallus domesticus*). *Dan. Med. Bull.* 20, Suppl. I: 1–82, 1973.

102. Skadhauge, E., and B. Schmidt-Nielsen. Renal medullary electrolyte and urea gradient in chickens and turkeys. *Am. J. Physiol.* 212: 1313–1318, 1967.

103. Smith, H. W. Renal Physiology. In: *Circulation of the Blood. Men and Ideas*, edited by A. P. Fishman and D. W. Richards. New York: Oxford, 1964, p. 545–606.

104. Stoner, L. C. Isolated, perfused amphibian renal tubules: the diluting segment. *Am. J. Physiol.* 233 (*Renal Fluid Electrolyte Physiol.* 2): F438–F444, 1977.

105. Stoner, L. C. The movement of solutes and water across the vertebrate distal nephron. *Renal Physiol.* 8: 237–248, 1985.

106. Taggart, J. V., and R. P. Forster. Renal tubular transport: effect of 2,4-dinitrophenol and related compounds on phenol red transport in the isolated tubules of the flounder. *Am. J. Physiol.* 161: 167–172, 1950.

107. Tune, B. M., M. B. Burg, and C. S. Patlak. Characteristics of *p*-aminohippurate transport in proximal renal tubules. *Am. J. Physiol.* 217: 1057–1063, 1969.

108. Walker, A. M., P. A. Bott, J. Oliver, and M. C. MacDowell. The collection and analysis of fluid from single nephrons of the mammalian kidney. *Am. J. Physiol.* 134: 580–595, 1941.

109. Wayland, H., and P. C. Johnson. Erythrocyte velocity measurement in microvessels by a two-slit photometric method. *J. Appl. Physiol.* 22: 333–337, 1967.
110. Wearn, J. T., and A. N. Richards. Observations on the composition of glomerular urine, with particular reference to the problem of reabsorption in the renal tubules. *Am. J. Physiol.* 71: 209–227, 1924.
111. Wideman, R. F., Jr., N. B. Clark, and E. J. Braun. Effects of phosphate loading and parathyroid hormone on starling renal phosphate excretion. *Am. J. Physiol.* 239 (*Renal Fluid Electrolyte Physiol.* 8): F233–F243, 1980.
112. Wiederhelm, C. A., J. W. Woodbury, S. Kirk, and R. F. Rushmer. Pulsatile pressures in the microcirculation of frog's mesentery. *Am. J. Physiol.* 207: 173–176, 1964.
113. Windhager, E. E., G. Whittembury, D. E. Oken, H. J. Schatzman, and A. K. Solomon. Single proximal tubules of *Necturus* kidney. III. Dependence of H_2O movement on NaCl concentration. *Am. J. Physiol.* 197: 313–318, 1959.
114. Yokota, S. D., S. Benyajati, and W. H. Dantzler. Renal function in sea snakes. I. Glomerular filtration rate and water handling. *Am. J. Physiol.* 249 (*Regulatory Integrative Comp. Physiol.* 18): R228–R236, 1985.

Contributors

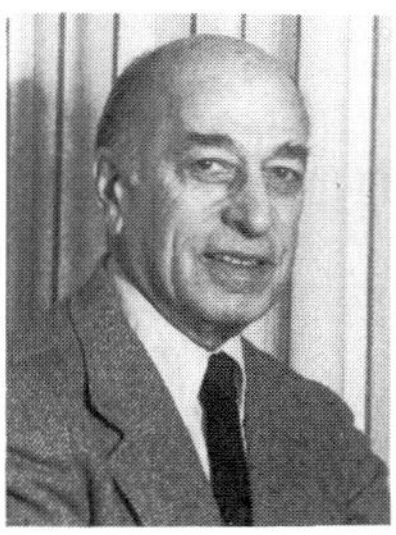

ROBERT W. BERLINER, *Professor Emeritus of Physiology and Medicine, Yale University School of Medicine, New Haven, Connecticut*

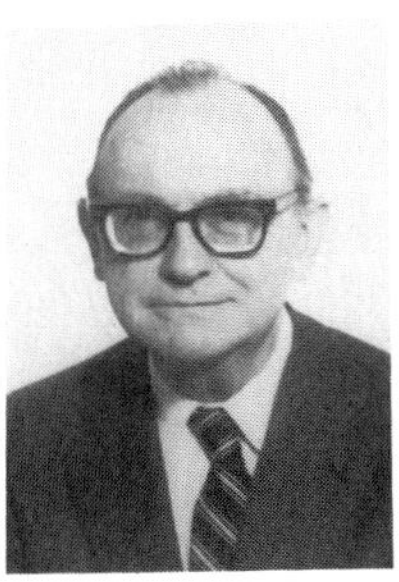

STANLEY E. BRADLEY, *Samuel Bard Professor Emeritus of Medicine, Department of Medicine, Columbia University College of Physicians and Surgeons, New York, New York*

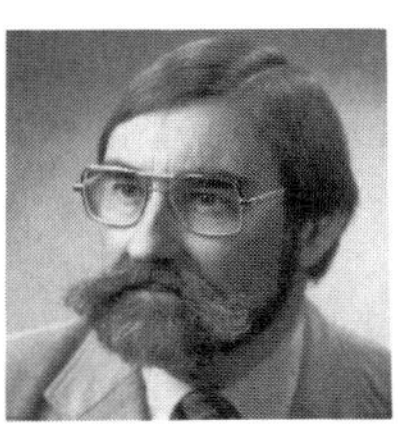

WILLIAM H. DANTZLER, *Professor of Physiology, Department of Physiology, University of Arizona College of Medicine, Tucson, Arizona*

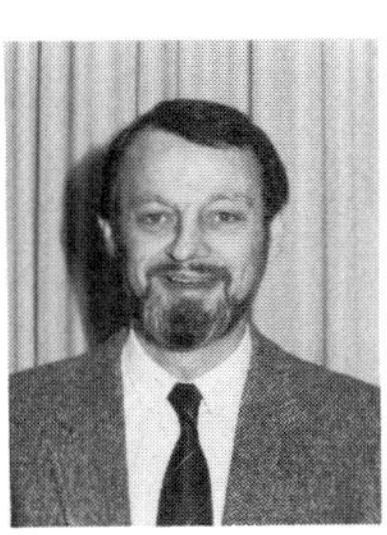

JOHN DAVIS, *Scientific Assistant, Institute of Physiology, University of Munich, Munich, Federal Republic of Germany*

RENAL PHYSIOLOGY

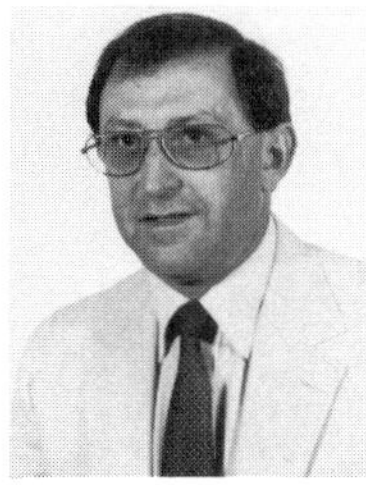

LEON G. FINE, *Professor of Medicine and Chief, Division of Nephrology, Department of Medicine, University of California School of Medicine, Los Angeles, California*

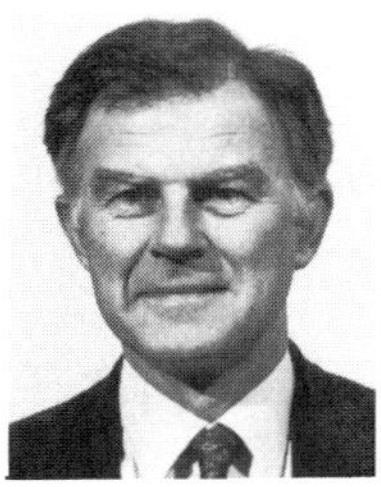

JAMES T. FITZSIMONS, *Reader in Physiology, University of Cambridge; Fellow of Gonville and Caius College, Cambridge, England*

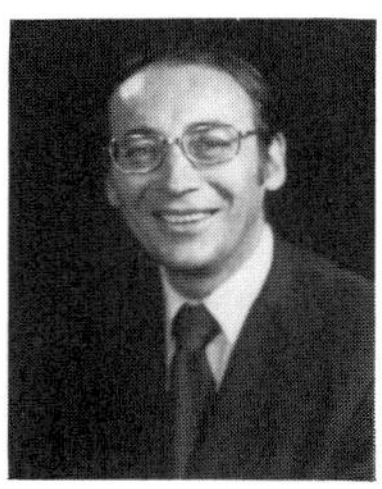

GERHARD GIEBISCH, *Sterling Professor of Physiology, Department of Cellular and Molecular Physiology, Yale University School of Medicine, New Haven, Connecticut*

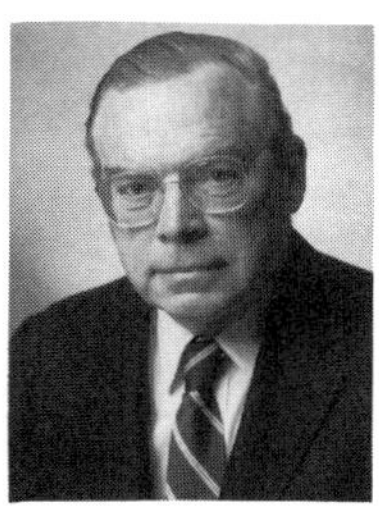

CARL W. GOTTSCHALK, *Career Investigator, American Heart Association; Kenan Professor of Medicine and Physiology, Department of Medicine, University of North Carolina School of Medicine, Chapel Hill, North Carolina*

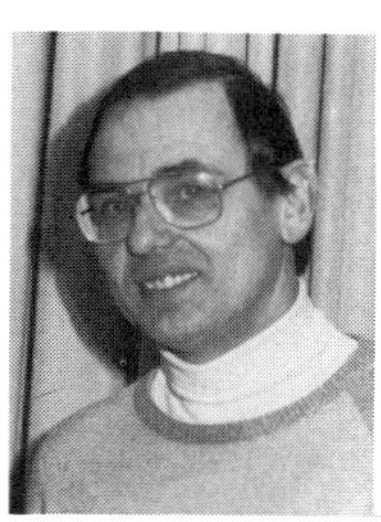

DIETER HÄBERLE, *Professor of Physiology, Institute of Physiology, University of Munich, Munich, Federal Republic of Germany*

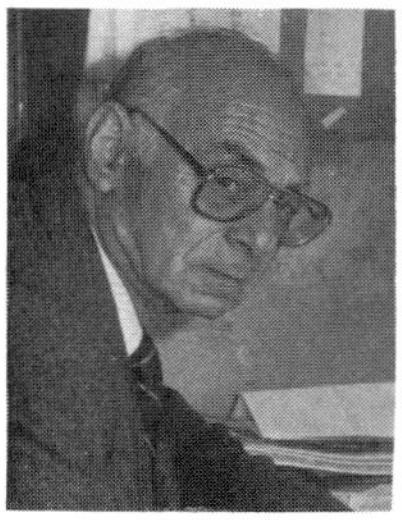

ARNOST KLEINZELLER, *Professor Emeritus, Department of Physiology, University of Pennsylvania School of Medicine, Philadelphia, Pennsylvania*

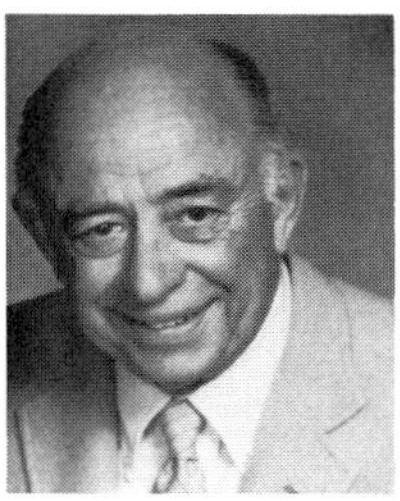

THOMAS H. MAREN, *Graduate Research Professor, Department of Pharmacology and Therapeutics, University of Florida College of Medicine, Gainesville, Florida*

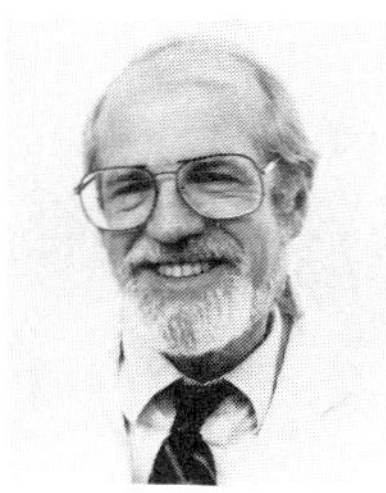

FLOYD C. RECTOR, JR., *Professor of Medicine and Physiology, Division of Nephrology; Senior Scientist, Cardiovascular Research Institute, University of California School of Medicine, San Francisco, California*

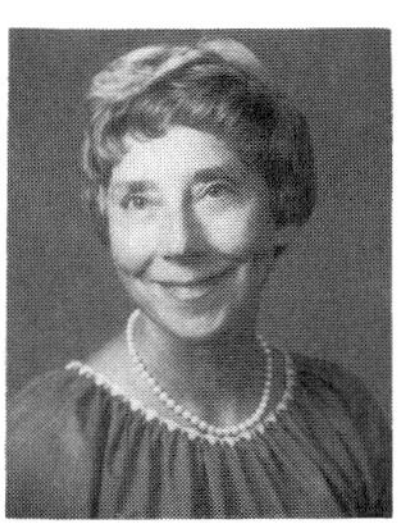

BODIL SCHMIDT-NIELSEN, *Retired Research Scientist, Mount Desert Island Biological Laboratory, Salisbury Cove, Maine; Adjunct Professor, Department of Physiology, University of Florida, Gainesville, Florida*

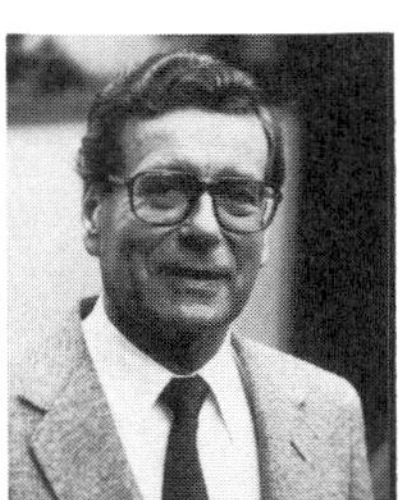

KLAUS THURAU, *Professor of Physiology and Chairman, Institute of Physiology, University of Munich, Munich, Federal Republic of Germany*

RENAL PHYSIOLOGY

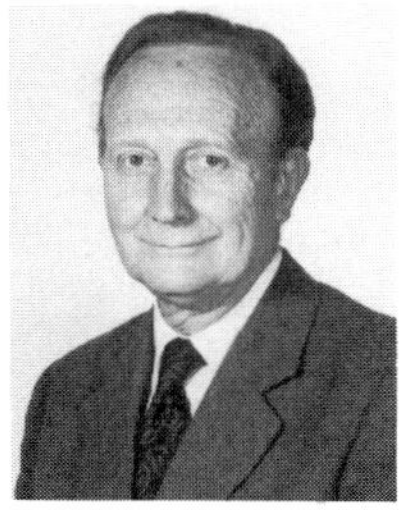

HUGH E. DE WARDENER, *Emeritus Professor of Medicine, University of London; Research Laboratories, Charing Cross and Westminster Medical School, London, England*

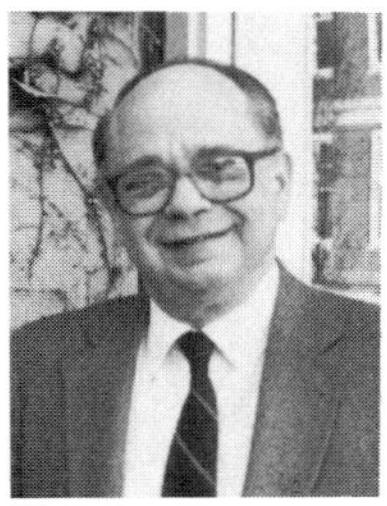

IRWIN M. WEINER, *Dean, College of Medicine, State University of New York Health Science Center, Syracuse, New York*

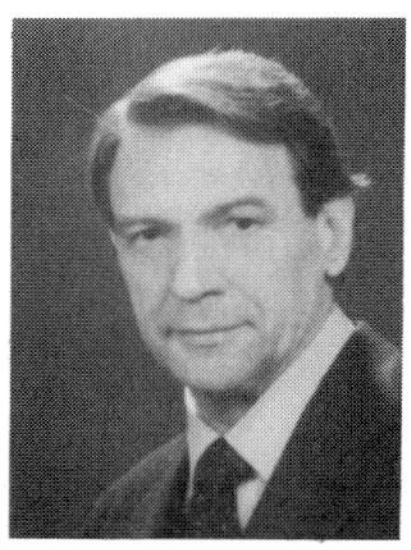

ERICH E. WINDHAGER, *Professor and Chairman, Department of Physiology, Cornell University Medical College, New York, New York*

Index